Essentials of Diagnostic Gynecological Pathology

Laurence Brown
Editor

Pathology of the Vulva and Vagina

Springer

Editor
Laurence Brown, B.Sc., MBBS, FRCPath
Department of Histopathology
Leicester Royal Infirmary
Leicester
UK

W. Glenn McCluggage, FRCPath
Department of Pathology
Royal Group of Hospitals
Belfast
Northern Ireland

Series Editors
Naveena Singh, MBBS, M.D., FRCPath
Department of Cellular Pathology
Barts and the London NHS Trust
London
UK

ISBN 978-0-85729-756-3 ISBN 978-0-85729-757-0 (eBook)
DOI 10.1007/978-0-85729-757-0
Springer Dordrecht Heidelberg New York London

Library of Congress Control Number: 2012946615

Printed on acid-free paper

Springer is part of Springer Science+Business Media (www.springer.com)

This series is dedicated to the respected memory of Professor Harold Fox (1931–2012), one of the foremost gynecological pathologists of all time, in recognition of the ageless legacy of his teaching and written word which will continue to inspire many generations of gynecological pathologists.

Preface to the Series

Gynecological pathology forms a large proportion of the diagnostic workload of most histopathology laboratories. There are frequent changes in diagnostic criteria, ancillary techniques, and staging systems, as well as descriptions of new entities that the diagnostic pathologist needs to keep up to date with, particularly in view of the ever increasing pressure from government, the public, and clinicians for accurate and timely diagnosis. This updating needs to be an individual and continuous exercise of professional development, through reading papers and attending conferences and courses as well as through self-study using published texts.

The female genital tract is a complex system with several different organs. In-depth knowledge of all areas is not necessarily the requirement of all pathologists. Many pathologists have more limited needs; for example, the bulk of the diagnostic work in a United Kingdom district general hospital is formed by cervical screening program-related biopsies, endometrial biopsies, benign uterine pathologies, and miscarriage-related as well as placental pathology, while due to current cancer treatment guidelines, most complex surgical specimens, particularly ovarian, cervical, and vulval cancers, are dealt with in cancer centers. Dermatopathologists may have an interest in vulval pathology but not in other areas of gynecological pathology. Pathology texts are also of interest to researchers and clinicians in particular specialties, for example, dermatologists and oncologists, and their interest will often be restricted to one particular area.

The British Association of Gynecological Pathologists (BAGP) aims to support the development and maintenance of the highest standards of clinical diagnostic practice in gynecological pathology. This aim is achieved through various educational activities, including courses, meetings, and cases of interest on its website, www.thebagp.org. The idea for a series of textbooks, each covering a specific area in gynecological pathology, was conceived while serving within the council of the BAGP. The series is intended for consultant pathologists and trainees who may have a requirement or interest in one or more areas of gynecological pathology due to their particular work situation. These books are intended to provide clear updated information on currently accepted classifications, nomenclature, diagnostic criteria, management implications, staging, and the role of ancillary techniques for neoplastic and nonneoplastic gynecological pathologies. For those interested in all areas of gynecological pathology, this series of smaller individual books holds greater potential for timely responsiveness to major changes in the field in subsequent editions, by virtue of having multiple contributors and a more limited scope in comparison to larger available texts. Dividing up the field also makes individual volumes more affordable for those in need of access to detailed information in a specific area in gynecological pathology.

We hope that the successive volumes in this series will present the essentials of current diagnostic gynecological pathology comprehensively and in a compact format for practicing and trainee pathologists as well as others.

March 2012

W. Glenn McCluggage
Naveena Singh

Preface to This Volume

The vulva has featured in ritual and Palaeolithic art since the dawn of humanity. Starting with simple line drawings scratched on rock, then evolving into three-dimensional carvings, the vulva is prominent in that apotheosis of the fertility symbol, the Venus of Willendorf [1, 2].

In later history, Sheela-na-gig stylized vulvas, disembodied or not, were a common sight in medieval Europe, placed above the lintels of simple country churches [3]. However, women growing up in most modern societies rarely uncover their vulvas in public, and perhaps because of this, vulval disease tends to be neglected. Groups such as the International Society for the Study of Vulvovaginal Disease (http://www.issvd.org) and the affiliated British Society for the Study of Vulval Disease (http://www.bssvd.org) have been raising awareness of the medical and psychosocial aspects of conditions affecting these sites and are now increasing their attention to the pathological understanding of those diseases.

Yet, of the many gynecological histology specimens received in a routine laboratory, those derived from the vulva or vagina constitute only a small fraction. Vulval diseases are relatively rare and vaginal lesions almost vanishingly so. Though this is possibly one of the factors that make their histological diagnosis problematic—even for specialist gynecological pathologists—this is by no means the only factor. While women readily seek medical advice for symptoms related to vaginal bleeding, discharge, or pelvic symptoms, for psychosocial reasons, they may be more hesitant with a visible lesion or symptoms related to the vulva. Consequently, secondary changes in long-standing lesions, compounded by occlusion, moisture, scratching, and possibly self-medication, are common. Secondly, while many rare, site-specific lesions occurring in the vulva are known to gynecological pathologists, they may be less familiar with dermatological conditions involving vulval skin. Furthermore, recent years have seen the description of many new lesions and refinement in the diagnostic criteria of existing entities.

This book illustrates with stylish artist-drawn graphics the basic anatomy and embryology necessary to understand the range of lesions and symptoms occurring here. The misery of vulval itch, swelling, soreness, or pain is explained by detailed descriptions of the extensive range of tropical and non-tropical infections to affect the site with clear descriptions of the noninfectious dermatological and mucosal dermatoses that may also be seen. The chapter on benign and malignant glandular lesions includes our increasing awareness of prostatic-like tissues in the lower female genital tract. Recent advances in the understanding of human papilloma virus in the causation of vulval squamous carcinoma, nonviral causes of carcinoma, and the underlying conditions of differentiated VIN, lichen sclerosus, and lichen simplex chronicus are explained at length. Other chapters cover the diagnosis of the earliest stages in the development of squamous carcinoma, the concept of sentinel node biopsy, the mimics of squamous neoplasia, and the wide and often difficult differential diagnoses of soft tissue and melanocytic lesions. A final chapter covers extramammary Paget's disease, outlines the difference to Paget's disease of the breast, and reviews the concept of anogenital mammary type glands and their role in glandular neoplasia in this site.

All these factors and others make the study of vulvovaginal disease interesting but also difficult. Clinically, these conditions may fall within the remit of general practice, gynecology, or dermatology teams. In the approach to the morphological diagnosis of vulvovaginal diseases, the most cogent advice that can be offered is to be aware of these factors and to promote close working between gynecological and dermatological pathologists. The chapters that follow are authored by experts in the pathology of gynecology, dermatology, and genitourinary medicine with exactly these points in mind.

March 2012

Naveena Singh
Laurence Brown

References

1. Wendt H. From Ape man to Adam. 2 edn. Omega; 1972, London.
2. Nelson B. Goddess worship in ancient Europe. At: http://espanol.reocities.com/Area51/Keep/3779/oldeuropegoddess.doc. Accessed on 10 Jan. 2012
3. Jerman JA. The 'Sheela-na-Gig' carvings of the British Isles: suggestions for a re-classification, and other notes. J County Louth Archaeol Hist Soc. 1981;20:10–24.

Contents

Contributor

Laurence Brown, B.Sc., MBBS, FRCPath Department of Histopathology, Leicester Royal Infirmary, Leicester, UK

Thomas Brenn, M.D., Ph.D., FRCPath Department of Pathology, Western General Hospital and The University of Edinburgh, Edinburgh, UK

Eduardo Calonje, M.D., DipRCPath Department of Dermatopathology, St. John's Institute of Dermatology, St. Thomas' Hospital, London, UK

Asma Zaman Faruqi, MBBS, LMCK, FRCPath Department of Cellular Pathology, The Royal London and St. Bartholomew's Hospitals, London, UK

C. Simon Herrington, M.A., MBBS, D.Phil., FRCP, FRCPath Department of Pathology, Ninewells Hospital and Division of Cancer Research, Jacqui Wood Cancer Centre, University of Dundee, Dundee, UK

Denisa Kacerovska, M.D., Ph.D. Sikl's Department of Pathology, Medical Faculty Hospital, Charles University, Pilsen, Czech Republic

Dmitry V. Kazakov, M.D., Ph.D. Sikl's Department of Pathology, Medical Faculty Hospital, Charles University, Pilsen, Czech Republic

Boštjan Luzar, M.D., Ph.D. Medical Faculty, Institute of Pathology, University of Ljubljana, Ljubljana, Slovenia

W. Glenn McCluggage, FRCPath Department of Pathology, Royal Group of Hospitals, Belfast, Northern Ireland

Michal Michal, M.D. Sikl's Department of Pathology, Medical Faculty Hospital, Charles University, Pilsen, Czech Republic

Richard Oparka, BMSc, MBChB Department of Pathology, Ninewells Hospital, Dundee, UK

Pratistadevi K. Ramdial, FCPath (SA) Anat Department of Anatomical Pathology, University of Kwazulu-Natal, Durban, South Africa

Naveena Singh, MBBS, M.D., FRCPath Department of Cellular Pathology, Barts and the London NHS Trust, London, UK

1 Development and Anatomy: Disorders of Development

Naveena Singh

Abstract

An overview of the complex embryological development of the lower female genital tract, some of which remains incompletely understood, is useful for the understanding of many neoplastic and nonneoplastic vulvovaginal lesions. The Fallopian tubes, uterus, and cervix develop from the paramesonephric (Mullerian) ducts. The vagina has a dual origin with the upper portion, including the vaginal fornices, arising from the paramesonephric ducts and the lower portion from the urogenital sinus. The development of the mesoderm surrounding the female genital tract in humans is incompletely understood. Experimental studies demonstrate that complex stromal epithelial interactions are crucial for site-specific epithelial differentiation, especially for development of glandular epithelia. Development of external genitalia occurs under the influence of sex hormones through proliferation of the mesoderm and ectoderm lateral and ventral to the cloaca. The area bounded by the vaginal orifice and the urogenital sinus enlarges to form the vestibule and is of endodermal origin. This is morphologically and functionally distinct from the rest of vulval tissues which are mesodermally and ectodermally derived. This difference in origin is reflected in differences in responses to sex hormones and other stimuli. A variety of abnormalities in development can therefore occur as a result of structural and hormonal disturbances, including external influences such as in utero exposure to diethylstilbestrol.

Development of the Vulva and Vagina

An overview of the embryological development of the lower female genital tract is useful for the understanding of many neoplastic and nonneoplastic lesions that occur at this site. Although there have been many advances in the study of the development of the human embryo, the development of parts of urogenital system remains incompletely understood [1].

N. Singh, MBBS, M.D., FRCPath
Department of Cellular Pathology,
Barts Health NHS Trust,
2nd Floor, 80 Newark Street, London E1 2ES, UK
e-mail: n.singh@bartshealth.nhs.uk

L. Brown (ed.), *Pathology of the Vulva and Vagina*, Essentials of Diagnostic Gynecological Pathology,
DOI 10.1007/978-0-85729-757-0_1, © Springer-Verlag London 2013

The Fallopian tubes, uterus, and cervix develop from the paramesonephric (Mullerian) ducts. The vagina develops by contributions from the Mullerian ducts as well as the urogenital sinus. The paired Mullerian ducts originate in the fifth week as longitudinal grooves in the urogenital ridge, lying lateral to the mesonephric (Wolffian) ducts. The ducts grow caudally by cellular proliferation as solid tubes which canalize as they elongate. Caudally, these cross to the midline in front of (ventral to) the mesonephric ducts. The Mullerian ducts approach, fuse with each other, forming the uterovaginal canal, and join with the urogenital sinus in the seventh week (Fig. 1.1a) [2]. The proximal vertical portions of the ducts develop into the Fallopian tubes, retaining their funnel-shaped opening into the coelomic cavity at their origin as their fimbrial ends. The caudal fused portion gives rise to the uterine corpus and isthmus. The junction of the Mullerian duct with the urogenital sinus is the site of a solid mass of cells known as the Mullerian tubercle. The growth and canalization of this structure produces the cervix, upper vagina, and vaginal fornices (Fig. 1.1b) [3, 4].

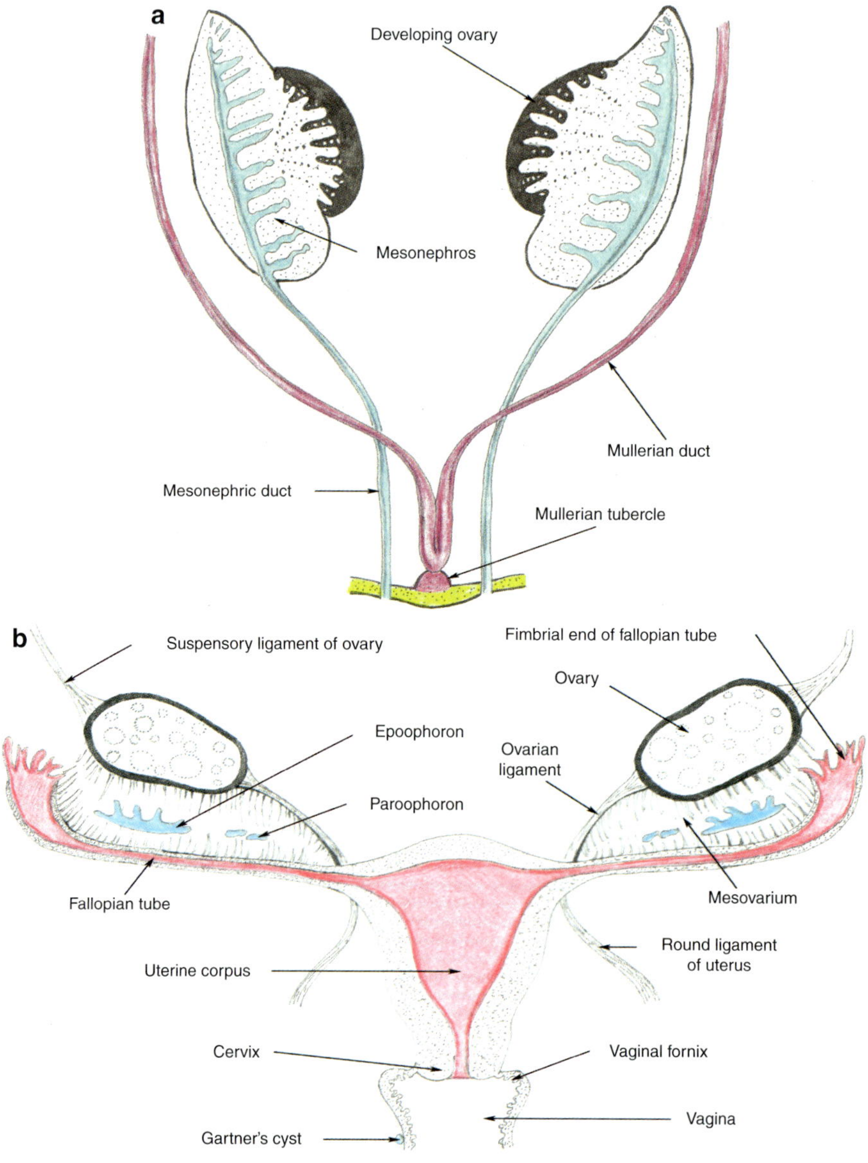

Fig. 1.1 (**a**) Mullerian and paramesonephric duct development. (**b**) The female genital tract fully developed with remnants of the mesonephric ducts in *blue*

Around day 66, there is an upward migration of squamous epithelial cells from the urogenital sinus. This structure, initially a solid cylinder of cells which later canalizes, is known as the vaginal plate and is unique to the human embryo [5]. Proliferation at the cranial end of the vaginal plate results in elongation of this outgrowth which becomes fully canalized by the fifth month. The caudal end of this plate is the site of the hymen. The vagina therefore has a dual origin with the upper portion, including the vaginal fornices, arising from the paramesonephric ducts and the lower portion from the urogenital sinus (Figs. 1.2, 1.3, 1.4).

More proximally endocervical mucinous glands appear between the 13th and 15th weeks together with differentiation of endometrial and serous epithelia in the upper genital tract. The development of the mesoderm surrounding the female genital tract in humans is incompletely understood, but experimental studies demonstrate that complex stromal epithelial interactions are crucial for site-specific epithelial differentiation [6]. The mesoderm consists of two layers. The inner layer forms the endometrium and endocervical stroma, tapering distally and possibly extending into the vagina and vulva. It is this inner layer of mesenchyme that is believed to induce tubal,

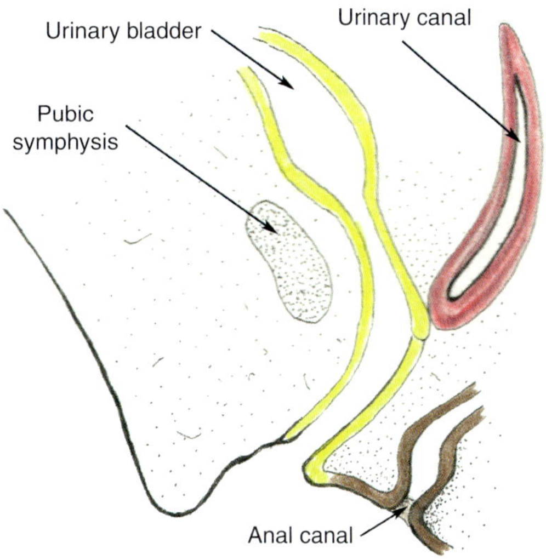

Fig. 1.2 Sagittal section through the developing uterovaginal canal at 9 weeks showing the Mullerian tubercle of paramesonephric and vaginal plate of urogenital sinus origin

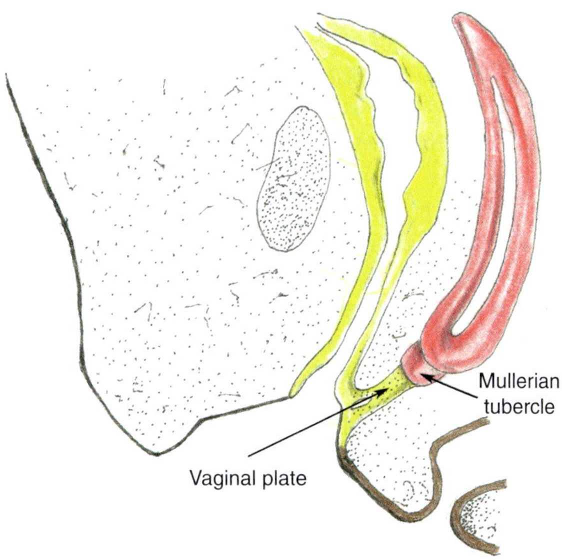

Fig. 1.3 The vagina at the end of the third month

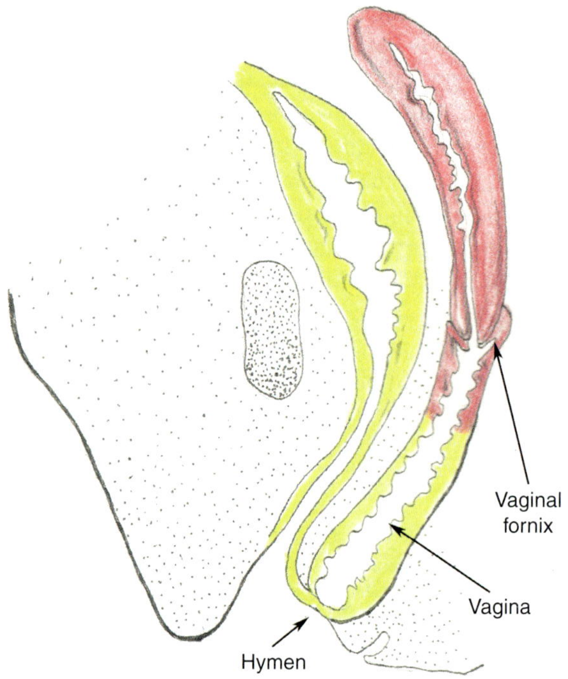

Fig. 1.4 The fully canalized vagina in the newborn female

endometrial, and endocervical types of glandular epithelial development [7]. The outer layer forms the muscle wall of the Fallopian tube, the myometrium, the outer cervical stroma, and the muscle wall of the vagina.

Development of external genitalia occurs under the influence of sex hormones [8]. In the fourth week, the cloaca begins to divide into the rectum dorsally and the urogenital sinus ventrally. By the sixth week, the urorectal membrane, a layer of mesoderm dividing the cloaca in a coronal plane, fuses with the cloacal membrane demarcating the urogenital sinus anteriorly and the anal canal posteriorly (Fig. 1.5a). Proliferation of the mesoderm and ectoderm lateral and ventral to the cloaca results in the formation of a pair of ectodermal elevations which are fused ventrally forming the genital tubercle and form two pairs of parallel ridges laterally. The medial pair is termed the urogenital folds, while the lateral pair are the labioscrotal folds (Fig. 1.5b). The genital tubercle, urogenital folds and labioscrotal folds give rise to the clitoris, labia minora and labia majora, respectively (Fig. 1.5c). The ventral portions of the labioscrotal folds fuse medially to produce the mons pubis. The labioscrotal folds fuse posteriorly within the urogenital membrane anterior to the anus.

The area bounded by the vaginal orifice and the urogenital sinus enlarges to form the vestibule (see below), which is therefore largely of endodermal origin apart from a variable area anterior to the urethra. This is morphologically and functionally distinct from the rest of vulval tissues which are mesodermally and ectodermally derived, reflected in differences in responses to sex hormones and other stimuli. Typically, irritation in endodermally derived areas is perceived as burning in contrast to the itching felt in ectodermal epithelia.

Anatomy and Histology of the Vagina

The vagina is an anteroposteriorly collapsed hollow fibromuscular tube about 9 cm in length in the adult female. This opens into the vulva inferiorly. Superiorly, the vagina communicates with the cervix. The axis of the vagina lies in an oblique line with the top of the vagina lying superior and posterior to the introitus. The axis of the

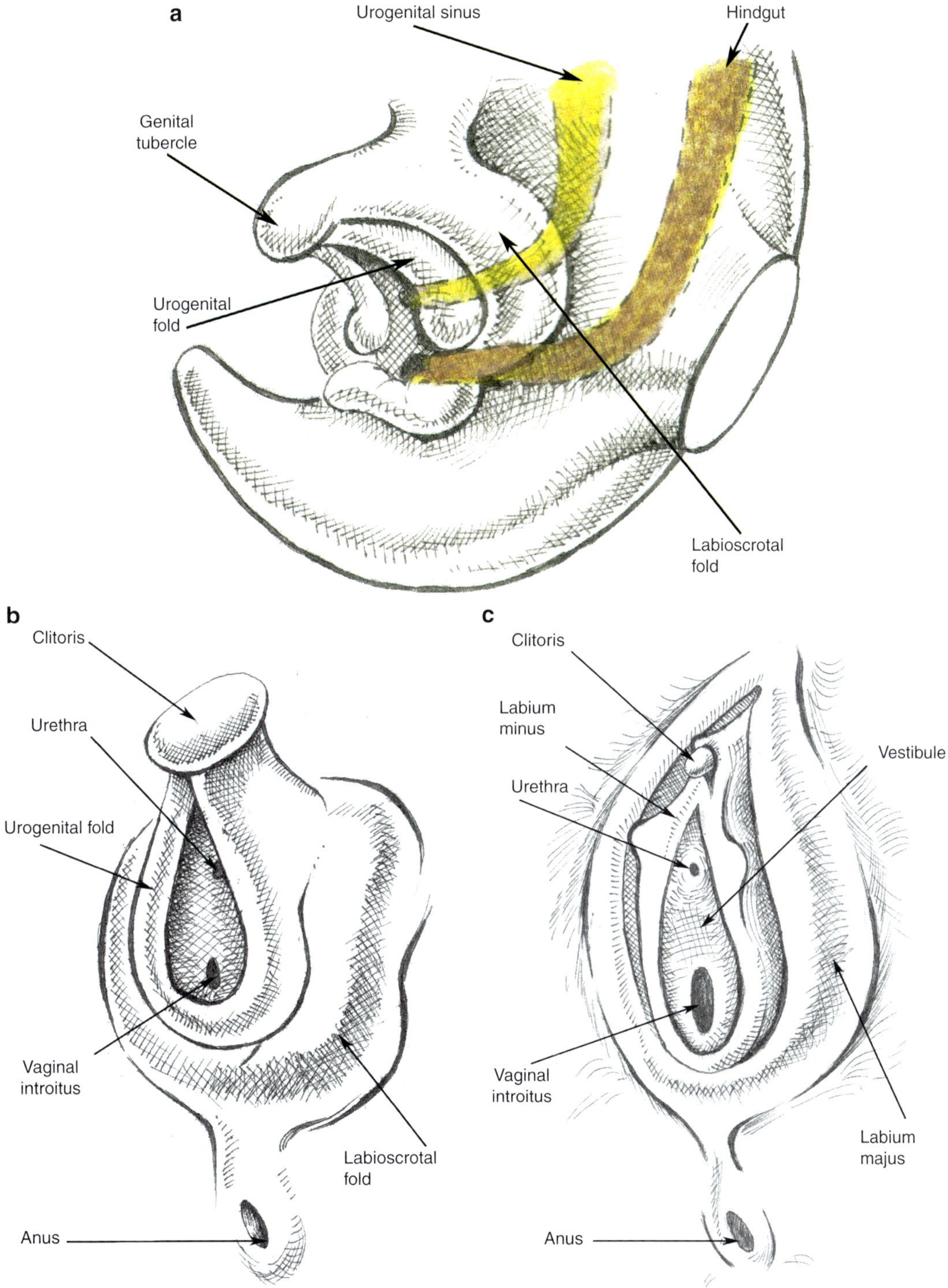

Fig. 1.5 (**a**) Development of the external genitalia begins with the appearance of the genital tubercle, labioscrotal fold, and urogenital fold; the cloaca has divided into the urogenital sinus and the hindgut. (**b**) The labioscrotal and urogenital folds remain separate in the female, enclosing the vestibule which receives the openings of the urethra and vagina (in the male, these pairs of folds fuse to form the scrotum). (**c**) The genital tubercle, urogenital folds, and labioscrotal folds give rise to the clitoris, labia minora, and labia majora, respectively

normally anteverted uterus and cervix forms an obtuse angle with that of the vagina, such that the external os of the cervix faces the posterior vaginal wall. The cervix bulges into the upper vagina and the blind folds of vaginal mucosa that surround the cervix are known as the fornices, being deepest posteriorly.

The inner surface of vagina is covered by a dull lining that bears many horizontal folds or rugae to enable stretching. There are normally no glands in the vagina and the secretions that are seen as part of the arousal response appear to be derived from transudate resulting from increased blood flow in mural vessels, with contributions from Bartholin's, sebaceous, sweat, Skene's, and endocervical glands [9, 10]. The vaginal fluid has a slightly acidic pH which varies with the phase of the menstrual cycle and during the arousal response when it has a higher pH and is rich in enzymes and immunoglobulins. The vaginal wall becomes more soft and relaxed during pregnancy and parturition.

The structures anterior to the vagina are the base of the urinary bladder and the urethra. The distal 2/3rds of the urethra is closely apposed to the anterior vaginal wall, separated only by a dense fused fascial layer. Posteriorly, the upper 1/4th of the vagina wall, including the posterior fornix, forms the anterior boundary of the cul-de-sac in the pelvic peritoneal cavity known as the pouch of Douglas which represents the deepest part of the peritoneal cavity. The distal part of the posterior wall of the vagina is separated from the rectum by the rectovaginal septum. The distal part of the posterior wall lies in relation to the perineal body and anorectal sphincters, separating the vagina from the anal canal. The most significant lateral relations are the ureters, which pass forward to enter the urinary bladder crossing beneath the uterine arteries just above the lateral fornices. The remaining lateral relations are the muscles that support the pelvic structures and form the pelvic floor, with the caudal most being the bulbocavernosus, which forms a sphincter around the distal vagina.

The vagina receives a richly anastomotic blood supply from the uterine, vaginal, middle rectal, and internal pudendal branches of the internal iliac arteries. Venous drainage is into a vascular plexus following the arterial supply and draining ultimately via the internal iliac vein.

Lymphatic drainage of the vagina is complex. Broadly, the superior and anterior portion follows the uterine artery and drains into the external iliac lymph nodes. The posterior vagina drains into inferior gluteal, sacral, and anorectal lymph nodes. The distal vagina, like the vulva, drains into inguinofemoral lymph nodes. Rich anastomosis, however, means that any part of the vagina may drain into any of these three nodal sites: pelvic, anorectal, or inguinofemoral [10].

Four layers are seen on histological examination of the vaginal wall [9]. The surface epithelium is of nonkeratinizing stratified squamous type. This consists of basal, parabasal, intermediate, and superficial squamous cells, identical to the layers of the ectocervix and similarly responsive to hormonal stimuli. Thus, the thickness and maturation of the epithelium varies with age and menstrual phase. Basal cells are cuboidal with uniformly hyperchromatic nuclei and high nuclear to cytoplasmic ratio. Parabasal cells form a layer that is 2–5 cells thick. These cells are polygonal with round dark nuclei and show mitotic activity. As maturation proceeds, the cells become larger and flatter and the nuclei progressively smaller. Loss of maturation occurs after the menopause and in other low estrogen states. The intermediate and superficial epithelial cells are glycogenated. Breakdown of glycogen by lactobacilli normally resident in the adult vagina contributes to the protective acidic pH through production of lactic acid. Glycogenation imparts a perinuclear clear zone resulting in a resemblance to koilocytosis which should only be diagnosed in the presence of abnormal nuclear features.

The epithelium rests on a variably distinct lamina propria composed of a loose fibrovascular stroma with collagen and elastic tissue. There may be occasional stellate and multinucleated cells present in this layer (see Chap. 8). The major portion of the thickness of the vaginal wall is formed by the dense fibromuscular layer. The smooth muscle is poorly demarcated into inner circular and outer longitudinal layers which

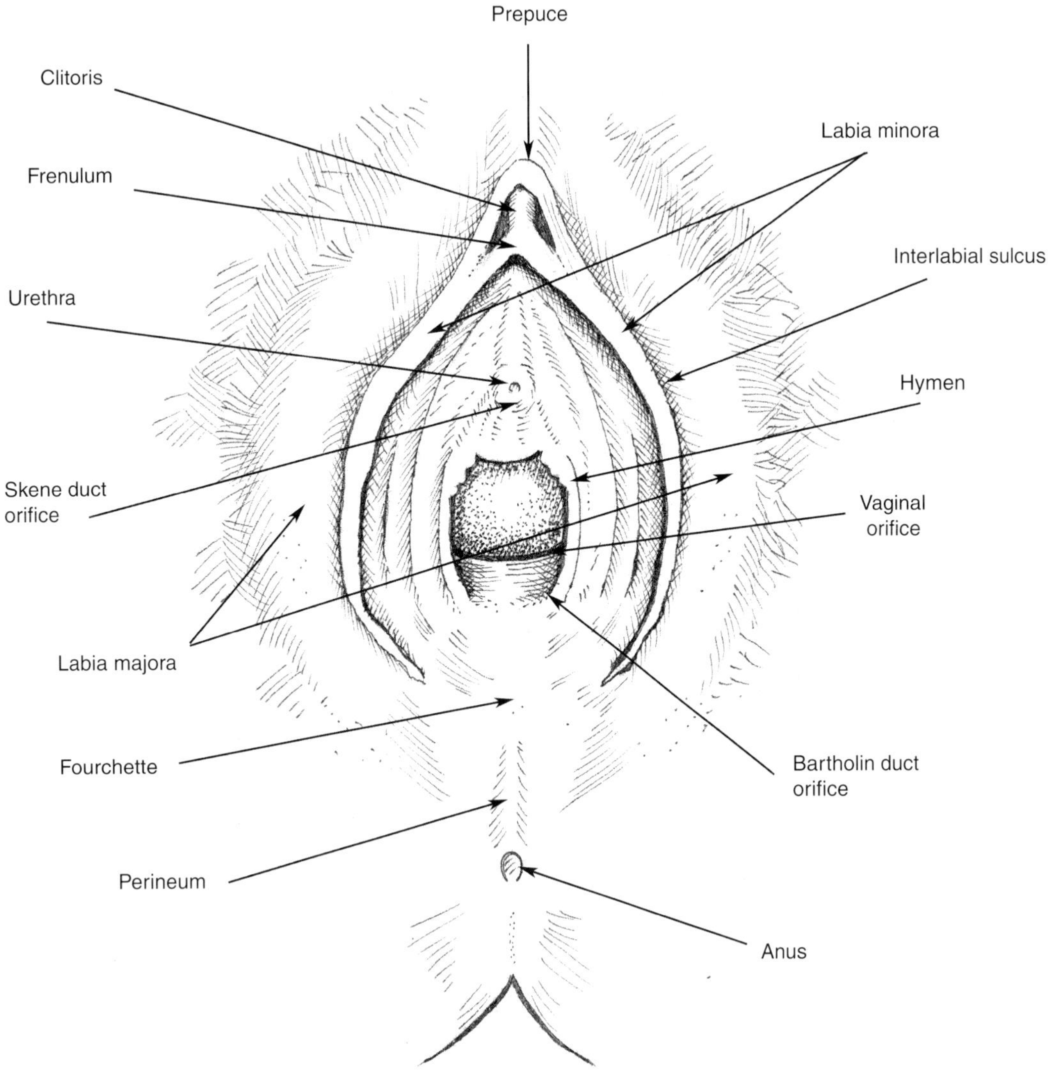

Fig. 1.6 The external adult genitalia showing the clitoris with prepuce and frenulum, paired outer lips—the labia majora, paired inner lips—the labia minora, medial urethra, vaginal introitus, and fourchette. A pair of Skene's glands opens in to the anterior vestibule and paired Bartholin's glands into the posterior vestibule. The perineum and anus lie posteriorly

merge with adjacent pelvic muscles. An adventitial fibroadipose layer lies outermost.

Remnants of the mesonephric ducts or Gartner's duct may be seen in the vaginal wall usually in a lateral position though rarely elsewhere (Fig. 1.1b) [11]. These consist of a ductal structure surrounded by smooth muscle and variable numbers of glands. The glands are lined by non-ciliated and non-mucinous cells with a high nuclear to cytoplasmic ratio, scanty pale or clear cytoplasm, and bland nuclei. The luminal spaces characteristically contain eosinophilic material.

Anatomy and Histology of the Vulva

The vulva constitutes the external genitalia of the human female (Fig. 1.6). Anteriorly, including and bounded by the mons pubis, the vulva lies between the inguinogluteal folds laterally and the anus posteriorly. Structures included in the vulva are the mons pubis and labia majora, labia minora, clitoris, and vestibule, the last containing the vaginal introitus and urethra as well as openings of the major vestibular (Bartholin's), periurethral (Skene's), and minor vestibular glands. The proximal boundary at the vaginal introitus is the hymen, the inferior surface of which forms the roof of the vestibule. An imaginary line, the vestibular line of Hart, demarcates the vestibule, of endodermal (urogenital sinus) origin from the rest of the vulva which is ectodermal in origin [9]. Functionally and histologically, this line demarcates sebaceous gland-bearing skin of the medial labia majora from the hormone sensitive and glycogenated nonkeratinized stratified squamous epithelium of the labia minora and vestibular structures. The line is formed by the prepuce anteriorly, the labia minora laterally, and posteriorly by the perineal body, a poorly defined fibromuscular node midway between the two ischial tuberosities where the muscles of the pelvic floor converge [12].

The mons pubis and labia majora consist of skin, subcutaneous fat, and some smooth muscle. The labia majora are bounded medially by the interlabial sulcus and posteriorly by the perineal body. At the onset of puberty, coarse, short, and curly pubic hair appears over the mons pubis and lateral surface of the labia majora. The medial surface of the labia majora is devoid of hair, and sebaceous and apocrine glands open directly onto the skin surface. These may be visible to the naked eye as small, white Fordyce spots. The histology of the skin covering these structures is identical to that elsewhere over the body [9, 13].

The labia minora are folds of nonkeratinizing stratified squamous epithelium and subepithelial connective tissue that includes richly vascular erectile tissue and elastic fibers. These folds are devoid of adipose tissue, hair, and sebaceous glands except close to the interlabial sulcus and on their posterolateral aspects. Anteriorly, each labium minus forks to contribute to the prepuce anterior and the frenulum posterior to the clitoris.

The clitoris is an erectile structure formed, like the penile shaft, of two columns of incompletely demarcated erectile tissue, the corpora cavernosa. These have richly innervated fibrous sheaths. The surface is covered by keratinized stratified squamous epithelium. There are no glands. The prepuce forms a fold over the clitoris and consists of keratinized stratified squamous epithelium and fibrovascular stroma. Posteriorly, the clitoris is bounded by the frenulum, the junction of the labia minora. The corpus spongiosum is divided in the female into bilateral vestibular bodies composed of erectile connective tissue, lying deep within the vestibule, lateral to the vaginal orifice [2].

The vestibule is covered by glycogenated nonkeratinized stratified squamous epithelium resting on loose connective tissue with variable amounts of erectile tissue included. This epithelium merges with transitional lining of the urethra and ductal epithelia of the major (Bartholin's) and minor vestibular glands as well as the periurethral (Skene's) glands. The vestibule of the vulva corresponds to the male urethra where this area is absorbed within the penile shaft.

The urethral meatus is a 0.1–1 mm opening with slightly rolled edge, directly anterior to the vaginal orifice and about 2.5 cm posterior to the clitoris. This is covered by nonkeratinizing stratified squamous epithelium, which merges with transitional mucosa at a variable distance within the urethra, an anteroposteriorly collapsed tubular structure measuring about 4 cm in length and 6 mm in diameter in adult females [2].

The vaginal introitus is the inferior opening of the vagina, marked by the hymen. The apposed anterior and posterior walls of the vagina make this a closed structure requiring insertion of a speculum to separate the walls during examination. The hymen is an incomplete membrane present at the introitus. This may range from being an indistinct rim to being annular, cribriform, or imperforate. The hymen may be torn by coitus, instrumentation, or use of tampons. Following parturition, the remnants of the hymen may appear as tags—the carunculae myrtiformes. The hymen consists of glycogenated nonkeratinizing stratified squamous epithelium with scant fibrovascular stroma.

The periurethral Skene's glands are paired structures about 1.5-cm maximum dimension that are analogous to the male prostate. These mucinous glands have openings directly into the vestibule posterior and lateral to the urethra as well as within the distal posterolateral urethra. The glands are lined by pseudostratified mucin-secreting columnar epithelium and the ducts by transitional epithelium, merging with vestibular squamous epithelium close to their orifices [13].

The major vestibular or Bartholin's glands are paired branching tubuloalveolar mucinous glands that lie in the posterolateral aspect of the vulva deep to the labia majora, labia minora, and posterior part of the hymen. These correspond to the bulbourethral or Cowper's glands in the male. The glands are composed of acini lined by simple mucin-secreting columnar epithelium. Each gland opens through a single Bartholin's duct which measures about 2.5 cm in length. The ducts are lined by mucinous epithelium close to the acini, changing to transitional epithelium and distally merging with squamous epithelium. The gland openings are situated in the posterolateral part of the vestibule, inferior to the hymen. Additional minor vestibular glands are simpler superficial tubular mucinous glands within the subepithelial stroma that open directly onto the vestibular surface. These are analogous to the urethral Littre glands in the male. These glands and their ducts show a variable degree of squamous metaplasia and occasionally become completely replaced by squamous epithelium.

Additional anogenital glands are present within the interlabial sulcus. These are similar morphologically and immunohistochemically to mammary glands and may consist of simple or more complex lobular units opening into a duct [14]. The structures are surrounded by a variably fibrotic stroma and lined by a dual layer of luminal cuboidal to columnar layer resting on a myoepithelial layer. The luminal cells are of apocrine type, but a milk line of vestigial mammary glands does not exist in humans (see Chap. 9) [15].

The fourchette is the posterior portion of the vestibule marked by the junction of the labia minora. The union of the labia majora is indistinct posteriorly and the 2.5–3 cm area between this and the anus forms the gynecological perineum. Deep to this lies the perineal body composed of the junction of the anal sphincter, bulbocavernosus, and superficial perineal muscles of the pelvic floor [2, 12].

Blood supply to the vulva is derived from the femoral artery, via superficial and deep external pudendals, and internal iliac artery, via the internal pudendal [9, 13]. These give rise to the anterior and posterior labial vessels. The clitoris, including its erectile apparatus, is supplied through a separate anterior clitoral artery. The vestibule derives its supply from the anterior vaginal artery. Venous drainage follows the arterial supply.

The lymphatic drainage of the vulva is to the superficial inguinal and femoral lymph nodes [9, 13]. Drainage is ipsilateral though the clitoris and midline perineal structures drain bilaterally. The lymphatics course anteriorly and superiorly from the more medial structures and proceed laterally with channels from the labia majora to enter the femoral and inguinal lymph nodes. The superficial inguinal lymph nodes are divided into two groups by the ligament of Poupart. The superior group is situated above the ligament and the inferior between the ligament and the junction of saphenous vein and fascia lata.

Disorders of Development

Developmental Abnormalities of the Vagina

Imperforate Hymen and Transverse Vaginal Septum

Imperforate hymen is a rare abnormality in which the vaginal orifice is covered completely by a membrane composed of fibrovascular stroma covered by stratified squamous epithelium. The condition, estimated to occur in about 1/1,000 females [16], may be diagnosed at birth as a result of a bulge due to collected mucus. Usually, the diagnosis is made at puberty, when hematocolpos results from collected menstrual blood. If long-standing, this can be complicated by retrograde passage of menstrual products into the pelvic cavity leading to adhesion formation, endometriosis, and infertility [11].

A more severe abnormality is the presence of a transverse vaginal septum [11]. This may be complete or incomplete and seen at any level of the vagina. The inferior portion of the canal may be fully developed and lined by normal nonkeratinizing stratified squamous epithelium. The upper surface is lined by glandular epithelium, reflecting the dual origin of the vagina and the need for communication between the Mullerian and urogenital sinus-derived portions for its normal development. Complete septa may result in complications due to retrograde menstruation.

Septate Vagina

Septate vagina is rare and usually associated with severely abnormal uterine development in the form of a duplicated uterus and cervix [16].

Other Vaginal Developmental Disorders

Vaginal adenosis refers to persistence of glandular epithelium in the vagina. This is seen frequently, but not invariably, in women exposed to diethylstilbestrol (DES) in utero [16]. The glandular epithelium is usually mucinous but can also be tuboendometrial, especially in cases following exposure to DES in the vagina. The underlying defect in such cases is hypothesized to be a failure of normal segregation of the inner layer of mesenchyme, which induces the development of mucinous and tuboendometrial epithelium and failure of normal upgrowth of the urogenital sinus that appears to be necessary for limiting this differentiation to the upper female genital tract [4]. Vaginal adenosis is probably the developmental disorder of greatest importance to the gynecological pathologist, and its diagnosis is dealt with in the chapter on glandular abnormalities (see Chap. 4).

Congenital opening of the urethra or the anus into the vagina occurs due to abnormal cloacal development. In its most severe form, there may be retention of a common cloacal opening communicating with the rectum, uterus, and urinary bladder [16].

Developmental Abnormalities of the Vulva

Ambiguous genital development is rare and may occur with virilizing syndromes or various forms of hermaphroditism [13]. This manifests as clitoral hypertrophy and a variable degree of labial fusion. Congenital asymmetry of the vulva due to hypogenesis or hypertrophy is also rarely reported.

References

1. Robboy SJ, Prade M, Cunha G. Vagina. In: Sternberg SS, editor. Histology for pathologists. New York: Raven Press; 1992.
2. Gray H, Williams PL, Warwick R, editors. Splanchnology, in Gray's anatomy. Edinburgh/London/Melbourne/New York: Churchill Livingstone; 1980. p. 1432–4.
3. Sadler TW. Urogenital system, in Langman's medical embryology. Baltimore: Lippincott Williams & Wilkins; 2006.
4. Robboy SJ. A hypothetic mechanism of diethylstilbestrol(DES)-induced anomalies in exposed progeny. Hum Pathol. 1983;14(10):831–3.
5. Kurman RJ, Sherman ME, Wilkinson EJ. Embryology of the lower female genital tract. In: AFIP atlas of tumor pathology, Tumors of the cervix, vagina and vulva, vol. 4. Silver Springs: Armed Forces Institute of Pathology; 2010.
6. Cunha GR. Epithelial-stromal interactions in development of the urogenital tract. Int Rev Cytol. 1976;47:137–94.
7. Cunha GR, Shannon JM, Taguchi O. Epithelial-mesenchymal interactions in hormone induced morphogenesis. In: Sawyer FJ, Fallon JF, editors. Epithelial-mesenchymal interactions in development. New York: Praeger; 1983.
8. Jaubert F, Robboy SJ, Mutter GL, Fellous M. Embryology. In: Robboy SJ, Mutter GL, Prat J, Bentley RC, Russell P, Anderson MC, editors. Robboy's pathology of the female reproductive system. London: Churchill Elsevier; 2009.
9. Kurman RJ, Ronnett BM, Sherman ME, Wilkinson EJ. Anatomy of the lower female genital tract. In: AFIP atlas of tumor pathology, Tumors of the cervix, vagina and vulva, vol. 4. Silver Springs: Armed Forces Institute of Pathology; 2010.
10. Zaino RJ, Robboy SJ, Kurman RJ. Diseases of the vagina. In: Kurman RJ, editor. Blaustein's pathology of the female genital tract. New York: Springer; 2002.
11. Robboy SJ, Russell P. Vagina. In: Robboy SJ, Mutter GL, Prat J, Bentley RC, Russell P, Anderson MC, editors. Robboy's pathology of the female reproductive tract. London: Churchill Livingstone Elsevier; 2009.

12. Drake RL, Vogl AW, Mitchell AW, editors. Pelvis and perineum, in Gray's anatomy for students. Churchill Livinstone: Elsevier; 2004.
13. Wilkinson EJ, Xie DL. Benign diseases of the vulva. In: Kurman RJ, editor. Blaustein's pathology of the female genital tract. New York: Springer; 2002.
14. Kazakov DV, Spagnolo DV, Kacerovska D, Michal M. Lesions of anogenital mammary-like glands: an update. Adv Anat Pathol. 2011;18(1):1–28.
15. van der Putte SC. Mammary-like glands of the vulva and their disorders. Int J Gynecol Pathol. 1994;13(2): 150–60.
16. Boyd TK, Elvin J, Crum CP. Female genital tract development and disorders of childhood. In: Crum CP, Lee KR, editors. Diagnostic gynecologic and obstetric pathology. Philadelphia: Elsevier Saunders; 2006.

Vulvovaginal Infections

2

Pratistadevi K. Ramdial and Eduardo Calonje

Abstract

Vulvovaginal infective diseases encompass a spectrum of primary and secondary bacterial, viral, fungal, and parasitic, including protozoal, infections that variably affect females of different age groups and in varying global, geographic locations. In addition, the disease spectrum is also influenced by the underlying immune status of the patients. The primary vulvovaginal infections are dominated by the sexually transmitted diseases that are grouped under the rubric "genital ulcer disease" and encompass syphilis, chancroid, donovanosis, lymphogranuloma venereum, and herpes simplex virus infection. Syndromic medical management of genital ulcer disease has not only decreased the need for diagnostic biopsies but has also limited the exposure of pathologists to the wide range of histopathological features, mimicry, and pitfalls of these ulcerative entities and the associated diagnostic challenges. Hence, familiarity with the spectrum of features that characterize the disease is critical to avoid misdiagnosis of other inflammatory disease mimickers. The histopathological diagnosis of vulvovaginal involvement by systemic infections is plagued by clinical underrecognition of vulvovaginal involvement by systemic infections and the attendant-altered clinicopathological morphology because of exposure of the vulvovaginal area to friction, moisture, and pruritus. The biopsy therefore plays a pivotal diagnostic role in the confirmation of an increasing range of infections, including those that are unsuspected clinically.

P.K. Ramdial, FCPath (SA) Anat
Department of Anatomical Pathology,
University of Kwazulu-Natal,
Durban, South Africa

E. Calonje, M.D., DipRCPath (✉)
Department of Dermatopathology,
St. John's Institute of Dermatology,
St. Thomas' Hospital, Westminster Bridge Road,
London SE1 7EH, UK
e-mail: jaime.calonje@kcl.ac.uk

Introduction

A spectrum of primary and secondary infective processes may involve the vulvovaginal area. While some of these infections represent primary genital tract infections, other vulvovaginal infections are acquired, either by contiguous spread from adjacent organs or as part of system dissemination. The primary vulval infections are

L. Brown (ed.), *Pathology of the Vulva and Vagina*, Essentials of Diagnostic Gynecological Pathology,
DOI 10.1007/978-0-85729-757-0_2,

dominated by sexually transmitted diseases that are grouped under the rubric "genital ulcer disease." While the vulvovaginal manifestations of systemic infections may share phenotypic features of the diseases in extravulvovaginal locations, the exposure of the vulvovaginal area to friction, moisture, and pruritus may alter the morphological diagnostic features. The clinical phenotype of vulval infections overlaps with those of noninfective vulval dermatoses, posing clinical diagnostic challenges. Vulvovaginal infections may be assessed, for the first time, by a spectrum of health-care professionals including family practitioners, venereologists, dermatologists, gynecologists, or infectious disease specialists. Hence, clinical suspicion of vulvovaginal infections varies as no single practitioner oversees the spectrum of diseases. The biopsy may therefore be pivotal in the diagnostic confirmation of many vulvovaginal infections, including those that are not suspected clinically.

Predominantly Primary Vulvovaginal Infections

Genital Ulcer Disease

Syphilis

Syphilis, caused by *Treponema pallidum*, is a predominant sexually transmitted infectious disease of worldwide distribution [1]. Congenital and acquired forms of syphilis are characterized by cutaneous involvement, including vulval manifestations [2]. Acquired syphilis is divided into primary, secondary, latent, and tertiary stages [3]. *Clinical features*: The manifestations of primary syphilis occur 10–90 days postinfection as a painless "chancre" at the site of inoculation in association with local lymphadenopathy [3]. Rarely, more than one chancre may be present. Although resolution of the chancre occurs, vascular invasion facilitates the secondary stage, 2–6 months later [3]. In addition to mucocutaneous lesions, visceral and constitutional symptoms occur. The cutaneous clinical phenotype of secondary syphilis is heterogeneous and includes maculopapular, annular, psoriasiform, lichenoid, pustular, and ulcerative lesions [4]. In flexural and anogenital skin, fleshy verrucous papules referred to as "condylomata lata" may be present. Tertiary syphilis occurs many years after disease onset but this may be accelerated in the setting of HIV infection [5, 6]. Cutaneous lesions, described in 70% of patients, include nodular tertiary and benign gummatous syphilis. Classical serologic testing for syphilis encompasses nontreponemal (rapid plasma reagin or Venereal Disease Research Laboratory) and treponemal tests (*T. pallidum* hemagglutination assay or *T. pallidum* particle agglutination) [7]. These tests may be negative in primary syphilis, and the serological tests are limited by low sensitivity and specificity [8].

Interactions between HIV and *T. pallidum* cause an accelerated disease course of both infections, altered clinical and laboratory profiles, increased risk for complications, and a decreased response to antisyphilitic treatment [9–11]. Serological confirmation of syphilis in HIV-infected patients may be hampered by an increased rate of negative serological tests in primary and secondary syphilis, increased false-negative nontreponemal antibody tests due to the prozone phenomenon [12], failure to clear nontreponemal antibody after treatment, and seroreversion of specific treponemal antibody tests to a negative state after treatment [13]. The accelerated cutaneous syphilitic lesions manifest as lues maligna with severe cutaneous ulceration and pseudolymphomatous mycoses-fungoides like lesions [14, 15]. The curative treatment schedule should include higher doses of penicillin [16, 17].

Microscopic features: *Primary syphilis* (*chancre*): The initial microscopic features of primary syphilitic encompass endothelial swelling and proliferation and an associated superficial and deep perivascular mononuclear inflammatory cell infiltrate. There is subsequent luminal occlusion as a result of endothelial hyperplasia and endarteritis obliterans and increased density of the mononuclear inflammatory cell in infiltrate, variable ulceration, and associated pseudoepitheliomatous hyperplasia. *Secondary syphilis*: Two main reactional patterns characterize secondary syphilis: psoriasiform (Fig. 2.1a, b) and lichenoid (Fig. 2.2a) [9]. The psoriasiform pattern (Fig. 2.1a,

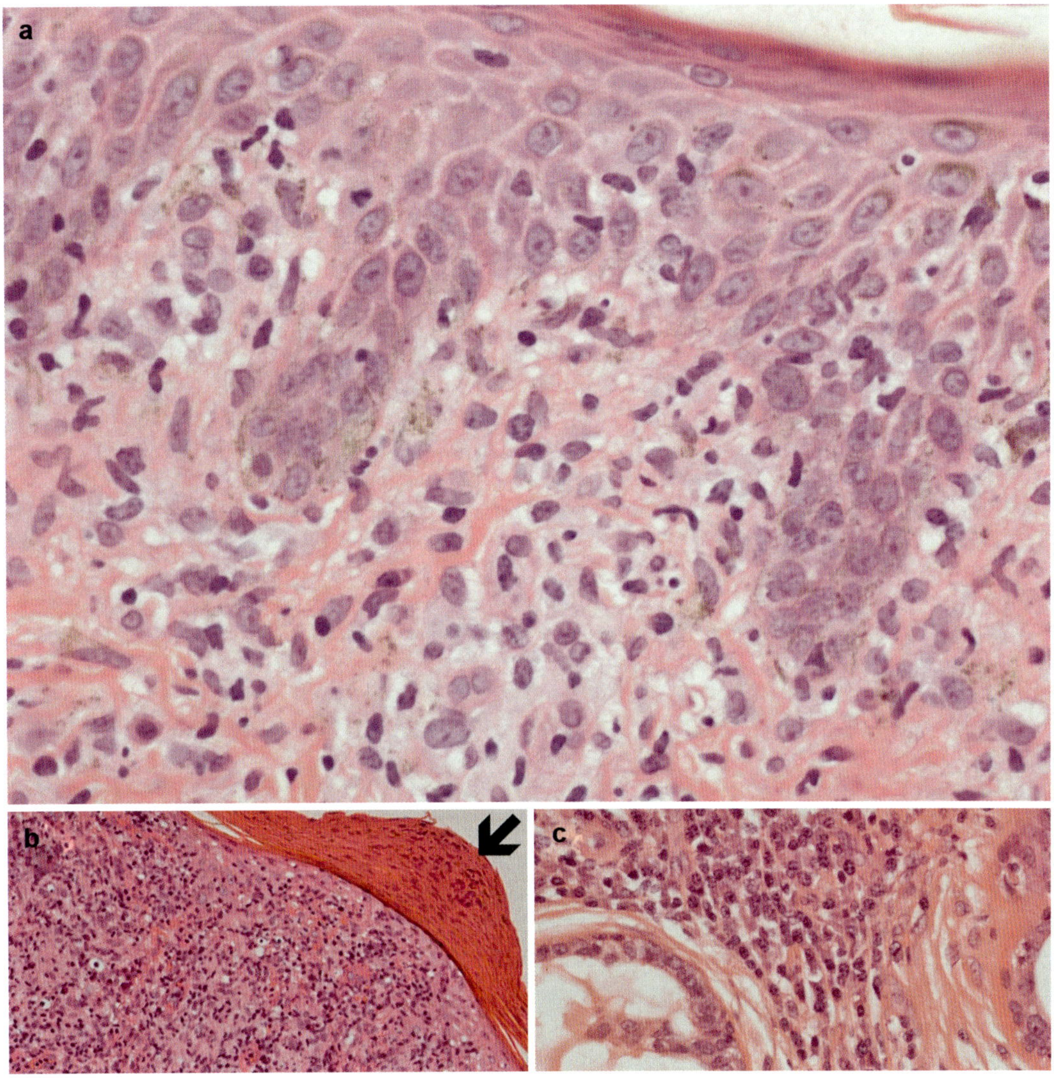

Fig. 2.1 Secondary syphilis: psoriasiform epidermal hyperplasia (**a**) with confluent parakeratotic crust (**b**, *arrow*) and plasma cells within eccrine secretory coil (**c**)

b) demonstrates epidermal acanthosis and club-shaped elongation of the rete ridges while the lichenoid pattern is typified by a band-like interface inflammatory infiltrate (Fig. 2.2a). The epidermis also demonstrates variable parakeratosis, apoptosis, erythrocyte extravasation, and transepidermal neutrophils and eosinophils (Figs. 2.1a, b and 2.2a, b). The dermal inflammatory cell infiltrate, composed mainly of CD8+ T lymphocytes, plasma cells, and macrophages, may extend deep into the dermis in perivascular and periappendageal locations (Fig. 2.1c) [18]. Other variable findings include the presence of nonnecrotizing granulomas (more common in older lesions) and neutrophilic eccrine hidradenitis and the absence of plasma cells. Condylomata lata demonstrate more pronounced epidermal hyperplasia and intraepidermal microabscesses [19]. Lues maligna is characterized by thrombotic endarteritis obliterans (Fig. 2.2c), most pronounced at the dermal-subcutaneous junction, cutaneous infarction, ischemic ulceration, and a dense plasmacytic and histiocytic infiltrate. Pustular syphilis is characterized by folliculocentric

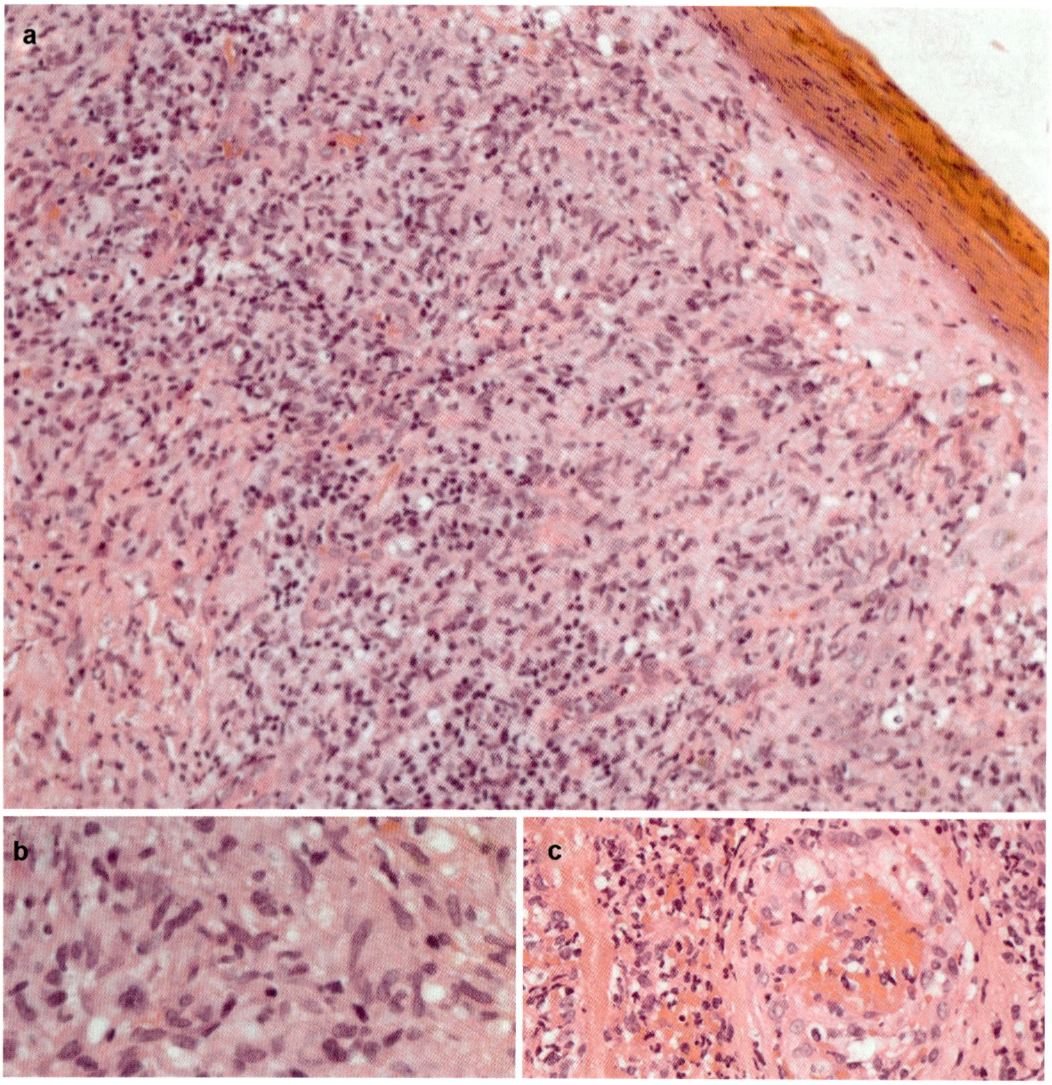

Fig. 2.2 Secondary syphilis: lichenoid inflammatory reaction pattern (**a**) with granulomatous inflammation (**b**). Thrombotic vasculitis in lues maligna (**c**)

suppurative inflammation and a surrounding perivascular lymphoplasmacytic infiltrate. Spirochetes are easily identified on silver stains. *Tertiary syphilis*: nodular tertiary syphilis is characterized by a dermal and subcutaneous perivascular plasmacytic infiltrate, variable granulomatous inflammation, and endarteritis obliterans (Fig. 2.3a). Benign gummatous syphilis is characterized by necrotizing granulomatous inflammation in which broad, irregular, acellular debris is surrounded by epithelioid histiocytes, multinucleate giant cells of Langhans type, lymphocytes, plasma cells, and fibroblasts (Fig. 2.3b).

Traditionally, *T. pallidum* has been identified using silver-impregnation staining, including Warthin Starry, Steiner, and Levaditi stains (Fig. 2.3c) [20]. The introduction of direct and indirect immunofluorescence and immunohistochemical spirochetal detection methods on fresh or archival wax block tissue has decreased the diagnostic challenges associated with nonspecific artefactual arygyrophilia of cutaneous elements, including melanin pigment and connective tissue elements [20–22]. While spirochetes are demonstrated in primary and secondary, and to a lesser extent, tertiary, syphilis, significantly different

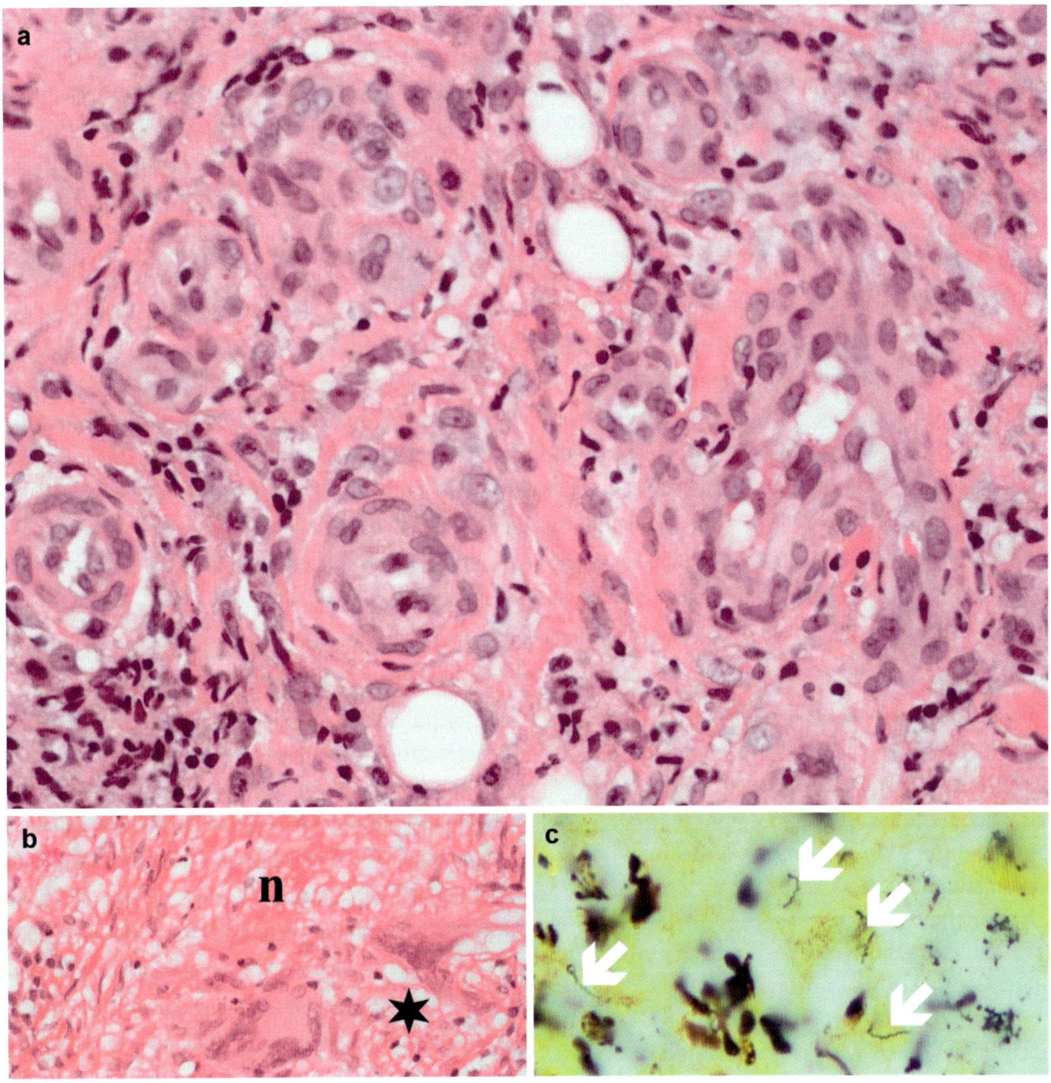

Fig. 2.3 Endarteritis obliterans (**a**) in nodular tertiary syphilis and necrotizing (*n*) granulomatous inflammation (*asterisk*) in syphilitic gumma (**b**). Warthin Starry silver stain demonstrating spirochetes (**c**, *arrows*)

distribution patterns have been documented in immunohistochemical and ultrastructural studies [20]. An epitheliotropic pattern typified by abundant spirochetes in an intercellular location in the lower epidermis has been described in secondary syphilis. Primary syphilis displays a mixed epitheliotropic and vasculotropic pattern with spirochetes being identified in and around blood vessels. The immunohistochemical detection of *T. pallidum* is hampered by false positivity for other spirochetal infections and borreliosis [7]. Molecular detection of *T. pallidum* using the polymerase chain reaction technique appears more specific [23–25]. Amplification products specific to the *tp47* gene have been confirmed by the *tp47* hybridization probe; *tp47* lacks homology with other bacteria [7].

Differential diagnosis: While the lichenoid infiltrate of secondary syphilis mimics lichen planus, lichenoid drug eruptions, and pityriasis lichenoides chronica, the psoriasiform epidermal pattern mimics psoriasis and psoriasiform drug reaction. The inflammatory infiltrate extends deeper into the dermis in a predominant perivascular location in secondary syphilis. Marked spongiosis and dyskeratosis are not associated with lichen planus or psoriasis vulgaris. While granulomatous foci may mimic sarcoidosis, granuloma annulare, and leprosy [26], a dense inflammatory component may mimic cutaneous lymphoma. Perifollicular pustular syphilis may resemble folliculitis. Gummatous syphilis may mimic gummatous tuberculosis, but the central necrotic zone of the former has an acellular appearance in which ghost outlines of cells are seen without the characteristic caseative nature of tuberculosis [27]. In addition, the large numbers of plasma cells are not a typical feature of tuberculosis. The syphilitic gumma differs from sarcoidosis by the presence of necrosis and the plasma cell-rich inflammatory background.

Chancroid

Chancroid, caused by *Haemophilus ducreyi*, a Gram-negative, facultative, anaerobic coccobacillus and strict human pathogen, is associated with suppurative lymphadenitis (buboes) [28, 29]. It is endemic in developing countries where a high HIV infection and AIDS prevalence coexist [28–30]. Chancroid causes a 25-fold increased HIV acquisition and transmission rate [30]. After entering the skin through microabrasions, the organism incites a local reaction. After 3–5 days, an erythematous papule develops at the entry site. This subsequently evolves into a pustule that undergoes necrosis to form a tender ulcer.

Clinical features: The ulcer has a necrotic, dirty appearance with an undermined edge and perilesional erythema. The ipsilateral lymph nodes form fluctuant masses that may rupture and result in draining inguinal sinuses. Clinical variants include dwarf, giant, follicular, transient, serpiginous, and phagedenic chancroid [31, 32]. While early studies documented atypical manifestations of chancroid in HIV-infected patients, subsequent studies have reported little difference in the clinical course, histomorphology, and response to therapy between HIV-naïve and HIV-seropositive patients [30]. *Diagnosis*: Apart from the histopathological diagnosis, *H. ducreyi* infection may be confirmed by culture, immunofluorescence tests, and PCR. *H. ducreyi* is a fastidious organism and is difficult to isolate from culture because it requires immediate inoculation on enriched medium, such as chocolate horse blood agar [31, 33]. 16S rDNA sequencing techniques may allow definitive diagnosis [23, 29]. The potential virulence factors of *H. ducreyi* include pili, lipopolysaccharide, iron-regulated proteins, cytotoxins and hemolysins, heat shock proteins, and outer membrane proteins [29]. Antiphagocytic mechanisms, critical to the survival of *H. ducreyi* because it is an extracellular pathogen, are mediated by two homologous, large supernatant proteins, LspA1 and LspA2 [34], and fibrinogen binder A. *H. ducreyi* resistance to serum-mediated bactericidal activity occurs through the outer membrane protein, ducreyi serum resistance protein A.

Pathological features: Biopsy of the ulcer bed demonstrates a typical triple zonation phenomenon characterized by a superficial, necrotic zone that contains fibrin, neutrophils, erythrocyte, and necrotic debris (Fig. 2.4a); an edematous granulation tissue zone dominated by proliferating capillaries, display with thromboses or fibrinoid necrosis; and a third deep layer containing lymphocytes and plasma cells [35]. Pus aspirates or biopsies of the ulcer edge demonstrate coccobacilli on Giemsa (Fig. 2.4b), silver, or Gram stains. The arrangement of the organisms in clusters, and in parallel rows, is referred to as "school of fish," "railroad," or "chaining." [35, 36] Ultrastructurally, *H. ducreyi* is largely extracellular and contains a trilaminar cell wall, typical of Gram-negative bacteria. B and T lymphocytes are preferentially located perivascularly in the middle and third zones, respectively [36]. Biopsies of the ulcer edge lack a zonation phenomenon but demonstrate a cell-mediated response dominated by CD4 and CD8 T lymphocytes, NK cells, macrophages, and plasmacytoid dendritic cells [34].

Donovanosis

Granuloma inguinale is caused by *Calymmatobacterium granulomatis*, a Gram-negative facultative, obligate intracellular pleomorphic bacterium [37, 38]. The natural history, treatment, disease classification, and nomenclature are controversial [37]. While originally labeled "serpiginous ulcer" in 1882, "granuloma inguinale" was introduced

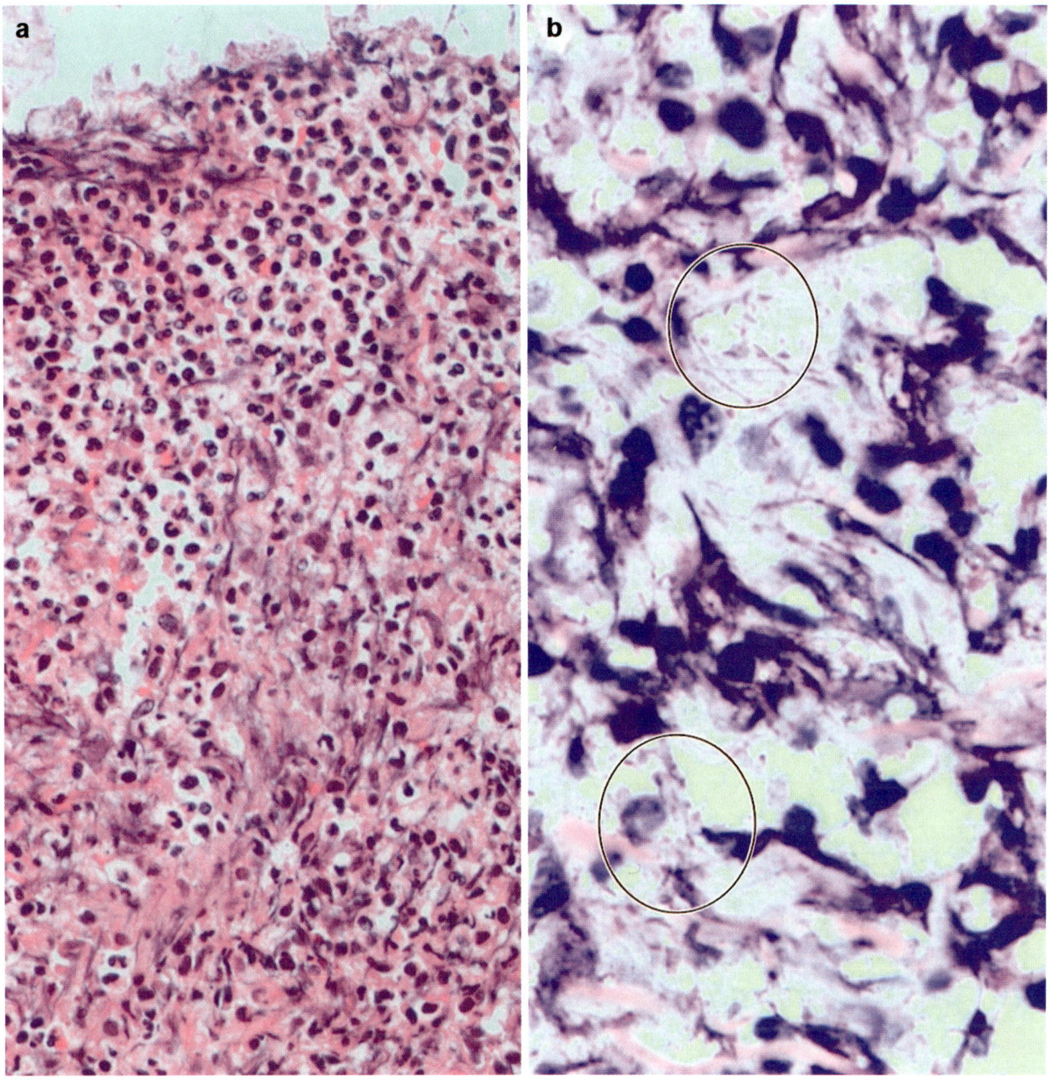

Fig. 2.4 Chancroid: ulcer with superficial necrotic debris and acute and chronic inflammatory cells (**a**) and "school of fish" appearance of coccobacilli (**b**, *encircled*)

thereafter to incorporate granulation tissue and the frequent localization of granuloma inguinale to the inguinal area [39]. The rubric "donovanosis" was coined in 1950 in honor of Donovan, who, in 1905, pioneered the discovery of the causative infective agent [39]. The name of the organism mirrors its pseudoencapsulated appearance in tissue sections ("Kalymma": Greek for "hood" or "veil"). It has been proposed that the organism be reclassified as *Klebsiella granulomatis* because of the approximate 99% phylogenetic similarity with *K. pneumoniae* and *K. rhinoscleromatis* [37]. Granuloma inguinale occurs in New Guinea, the Caribbean, South Africa, Southeast Asia, Australia, Brazil, and parts of India [40]. Granuloma inguinale is generally regarded as a sexually transmitted infection with an incubation period of 2 weeks to 6 months [41, 42].

Clinical features: Cutaneous and subcutaneous papules and nodules form at the site of inoculation. They may then evolve into large ulcers that bleed easily to touch [37, 39]. Hypertrophic, verrucous, or foul-smelling destructive, deep

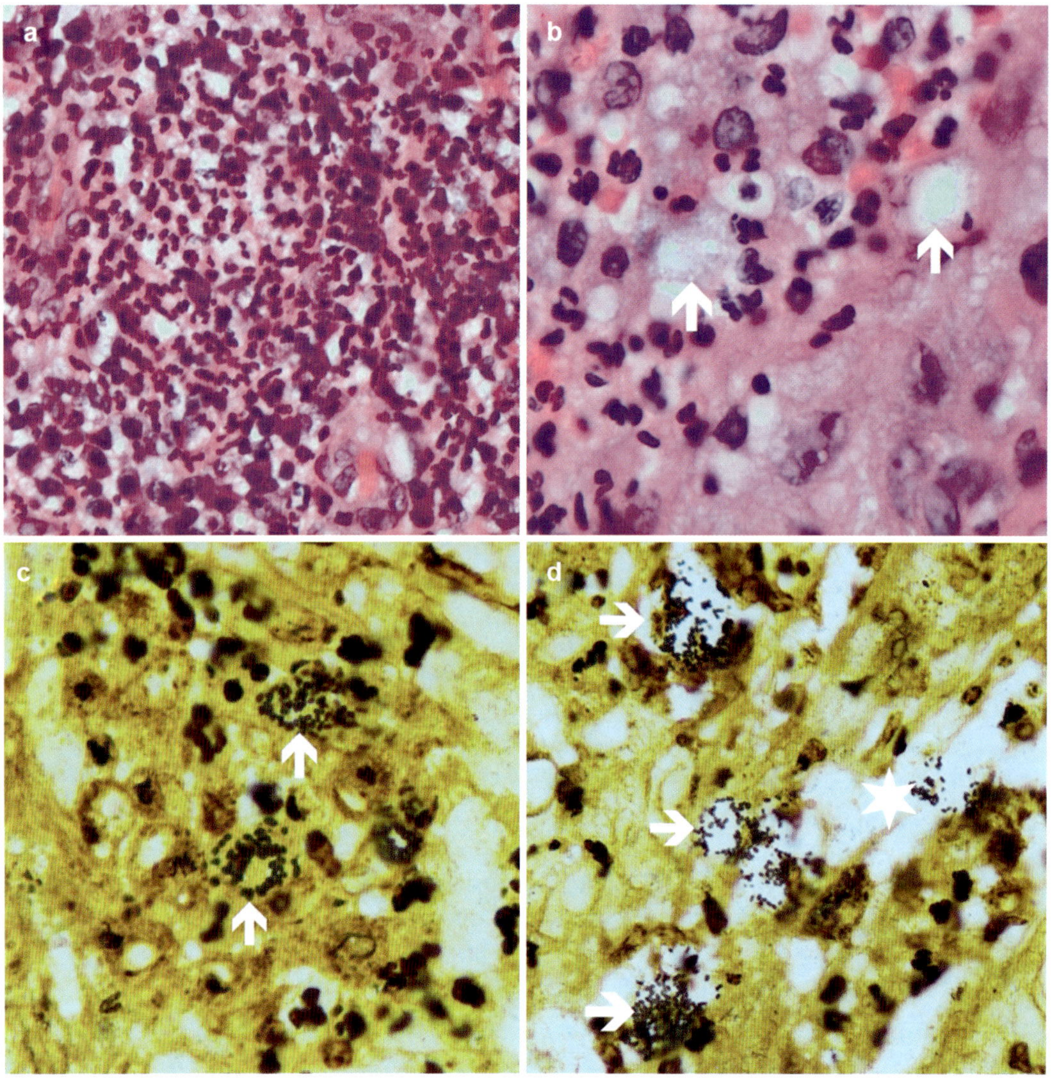

Fig. 2.5 Dense inflammatory infiltrate composed of neutrophils and plasma cells (**a**), Donovan bodies (**b**, *arrows*), highlighted with Warthin Starry silver stain (**c**, *arrows*). Transepidermal (*asterisk*) elimination of Donovan bodies (**d**, *arrows*)

ulcers; deformative, fibrosing, cicatrizing lesions; abscesses; or fistulae are documented [37, 39, 41]. *Treatment and outcome*: Granuloma inguinale resolves if appropriate treatment is instituted promptly. Doxycycline, azithromycin, cotrimoxazole, erythromycin, and aminoglycosides are effective. Treatment delays may result in significant morbidity [38]. HIV coinfection may result in persistent ulcers with greater tissue destruction that may require more aggressive and prolonged therapy [38]. Smears and histopathological assessment of lesional tissue will demonstrate the presence of Donovan bodies. However, in partially treated lesions, Donovan bodies may be elusive. In such settings, PCR studies are helpful in confirming the diagnosis [42].

Histopathology: The diagnostic features of granuloma inguinale include a granulation tissue response with a dense inflammatory component composed of plasma cells, macrophages, aggregates of neutrophils, and few, if any, lymphocytes (Fig. 2.5a). The macrophages are large with voluminous, vacuolated cytoplasm in which 1–2-μm bacilli, the Donovan bodies, are seen on routine stains (Fig. 2.5b). The organisms are demonstrated to better effect on Warthin Starry-(Fig. 2.5c) or Giemsa-stained sections where they have the typical bipolar appearance of safety pins because of the bipolar condensation of the stain. Transepidermal elimination of the organisms is described (Fig. 2.5d). The edge of the ulcer may demonstrate pseudoepitheliomatous hyperplasia. *Differential diagnosis*: The extent of neutrophilic infiltration in a background of granulation tissue and chronic inflammation mimics the chronic suppurative prototypical inflammatory response of an abscess. This may be particularly important in deep subcutaneous nodules. More superficial biopsies with pseudoepitheliomatous hyperplasia may mimic squamous cell carcinoma. Squamous cell carcinoma coexists with granuloma inguinale rarely [40]; strict criteria for malignancy must be adhered to, to avoid misdiagnosis. In patients who have received symptomatic treatment, Donovan bodies may be elusive. In such instances, when the inflammatory background is compelling for granuloma inguinale, PCR testing and nucleotide sequencing investigations will confirm the histopathological suspicion. Fungal (histoplasmosis, cryptococcosis, and pneumocystosis) [43] and protozoal (toxoplasmosis, leishmaniasis) [44] infections also contain intracytoplasmic organisms within histiocytes, but these infections are typified by a granulomatous response, the histiocytes may have a foamy appearance, and the infecting agents are larger and have a round to oval rather than elongated bacillary shape.

Lymphogranuloma Venereum

Although lymphogranuloma venereum (LGV) was described as early as 1786 [45], it was only established as a distinct clinicopathological entity in 1913. Reported uncommonly, LGV accounts for 2–10% of genital ulcers in India and Africa [46]. It is caused mainly by one of three invasive LGV biovar stains of *C. trachomatis* serotypes L1, L2, and L3. *C. trachomatis* is an obligate intracellular parasite. The L1, L2, and L3 serotypes parasitize histiocytes [47, 48]. Three stages typify the life cycle of *C. trachomatis*. In stage 1, elementary particles, referred to as the infective particles, penetrate the host cell. In stage 2, the elementary particle evolves into a reticulate body. The reticulate body exists exclusively intracellularly, is metabolically active, and divides by binary fission. Eventually, in stage 3, reticulate bodies transform into elementary bodies that leave the host cell by exocytosis [45].

Clinical features: LGV also occurs in three clinicopathological stages. Following an incubation period of 3–30 days, a small papule, ulcer, or herpetiform lesion develops at the site of inoculation [38, 45, 48]. The secondary or inguinal stage evolves over an average of 10–30 days after the primary stage [45, 49]. Inguinal, femoral, and deep pelvic lymphadenopathy occurs and is followed by necrosis and subsequent chronic edema, ulcers, and sclerosing fibrosis. The tertiary stage, referred to as the genitoanorectal syndrome, encompasses proctocolitis, perirectal abscesses, fistulae, stenosis, and strictures of the rectum [38]. Lymph stasis results in severe vulval edema, known as esthiomene [50]. *Diagnosis*: Is based on the isolation of *C. trachomatis* by culture and cell typing of the isolate [38]. Isolation is undertaken in a coculture system or in the yolk sac of eggs. LGV also induces a strong immune response. In the presence of clinical clues of LGV, a complement fixation antibody titre of >1:64 or a fourfold increase in titer is diagnostic of chlamydial infection. Molecular confirmation of LGV using PCR techniques and DNA sequencing of the variable segments of the *OMP1* gene is used to determine the serovars/serotype [51].

Microscopic features: The ulcer of the first stage is characterized by superficial fibrin and neutrophils and deep mixed inflammation, including neutrophils, mononuclear cells, and giant cells [45, 50, 52]. The features at this stage are nonspecific [35]. The lymph nodes demonstrate follicular hyperplasia and foci of necrosis that evolve into stellate abscesses with a zone of palisaded epithelioid cells, giant cells, and lymphocytes (Fig. 2.6a, b). The foci of central necrosis become eosinophilic, acellular, and homogeneous. Fibrosis supervenes. *Differential diagnosis*: The

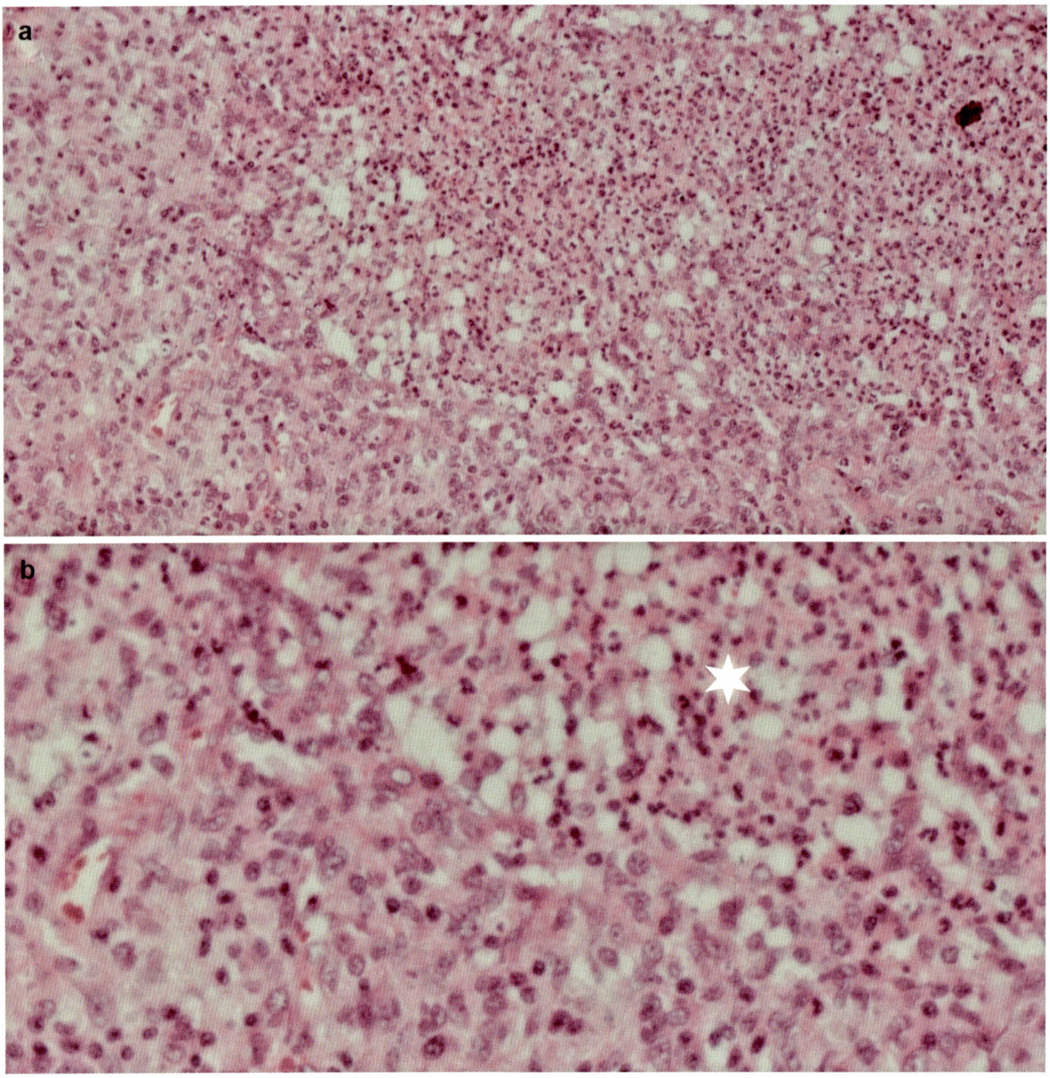

Fig. 2.6 Lymphogranuloma venereum: part of a stellate abscess in an inguinal lymph node (**a**, low power) and high power (**b**) demonstration of central suppuration (*asterisk*) and adjacent histiocytic response

microscopic features of the genital ulcer mimic an abscess, early cat scratch disease, syphilis, and herpetic and aphthous ulcers.

Herpes Simplex Virus Infection

Derived from the ancient Greek word meaning to crawl or creep, "*herpes*" refers to the family of viruses of which the ubiquitous, immunologically distinct *herpes simplex virus-1* (HSV-1) and *herpes simplex virus-2* (HSV-2) are the most aggressive human pathogens [53]. Genital herpes is the most common cause of genital ulceration worldwide [38]. While HSV-2 is the more common cause of genital herpes, an increasing prevalence of HSV-1-induced genital ulcers is being recognized [54]. The virus spreads during asymptomatic and symptomatic viral shedding. Viral replication at the site of inoculation is followed by neural transmission to the dorsal root ganglia, where the virus remains in a latent state, until reactivation occurs. The latter may be a consequence of fever, stress, immunosuppression, or immunocompromise [55–57]. HSV-1 infections are less likely to recur than HSV-2 infections [58].

Clinical features: Primary genital herpes ulcers and vesicles are typically asymptomatic, occurring within 3 days to 2 weeks, with an average of 5 days, after HSV exposure. However, a systemic prodrome, inclusive of fever, myalgia, and headache, occurs. Secondarily infected or recurrent herpetic lesions are very painful. The recurrent lesions manifest as vesicles on an erythematous base with variable crusting, pustulation, and erosions. These lesions heal with scarring. Recurrent disease is typified by systemic spread, prominent regional lymphadenopathy, and adjacent skin and soft tissue involvement of the buttock, perineum, and cervix. Unusual clinical appearances include nodular vulvitis and a Well's syndrome (eosinophilic cellulitis), presentation with vulvar edema [59, 60], and exophytic masses. Genital herpes in HIV-infected patients may have severe and atypical clinical presentations, including an increased number and size of lesions, increased pain, slower healing, and a verrucous clinical appearance [54]. *Diagnosis*: HSV infection can be confirmed by their direct identification in cultures, direct immunofluorescence, immunohistochemistry, in situ hybridization, and PCR techniques. Viral culture involves the inoculation of lesional tissue into HeLa cells, amnion, or fibroblasts with resultant demonstration of viral cytopathic effects. Appropriate primers or pyrosequencing can be employed to subtype the herpesvirus [61]. *Outcome*: Topical, oral, or intravenous antiviral agents (acyclovir, valaciclovir, famciclovir) are effective in primary or recurrent disease. Intravenous use may be effective in immunocompromised hosts. HSV may develop acyclovir resistance because of mutations in the viral *thymidine kinase* gene [53]. HSV may thus be either deficient in thymidine kinase or may contain thymidine kinase that is incapable of phosphorylating acyclovir.

Pathologic features: The epithelium undergoes ballooning and reticular degeneration to form an intraepithelial vesicle. Ballooning degeneration is characterized by intense eosinophilia of the cytoplasm with loss of intracellular cohesion and attachment, resulting in secondary acantholysis [62]. Molding of these cells may be prominent. Reticular degeneration is characterized by hydropic swelling and rupture of the epidermal cells and ulceration (Fig. 2.7a). Eosinophilic intranuclear inclusions are an important diagnostic feature. They measure 3–8 μm in diameter, are surrounded by a halo, and may be identified in epidermal cells, endothelium, sebaceous and eccrine, epithelium, fibroblasts, macrophages, and endoneurial cells [62, 63]. Multinucleation may be present (Fig. 2.7a). Neutrophils, sebaceous gland involvement, folliculitis, and neuritis may be variably noted. The neural alterations include neuronal atrophy and Schwann cell hypertrophy [62, 63]. Herpetic syringitis, associated with eccrine epithelial necrosis and syringosquamous metaplasia, is documented rarely, mainly in immunocompromised patients [64, 65]. HSV-2-associated eosinophilic cellulitis (Well's syndrome) has been documented in biopsies of acute, edematous blistering vulval dermatitis [60]. In this setting, epidermal spongiosis, massive eosinophil infiltration of the dermis, and eosinophilic flame figures partially surrounded by histiocytes are observed [60]. Biopsies of exophytic or nodular masses demonstrate variable ulceration and pseudoepitheliomatous hyperplasia of the epidermis and a dense inflammatory dermal response [66, 67]. Pseudolymphomatous features that are observed include a dense lymphoid infiltrate with atypical lymphocytes, angiotropism and a variable eosinophilic component (Fig. 2.7b, c) [68, 69]. The immunophenotype of the lymphoid infiltrate is predominantly $CD3^+$, with variable of CD4, CD8, CD30, CD56, and T1A1 immunopositive cells. A wedge-shaped infiltrate with atypical lymphocytes, some CD30 positive, may resemble lymphomatoid papulosis. The infiltrate may demonstrate polyclonality or monoclonality on molecular investigation of the TCR-γ gene [69]. Ultrastructural examination demonstrates virus particles, 90–130 μm in diameter, in the nuclei of basal epidermal cells [62].

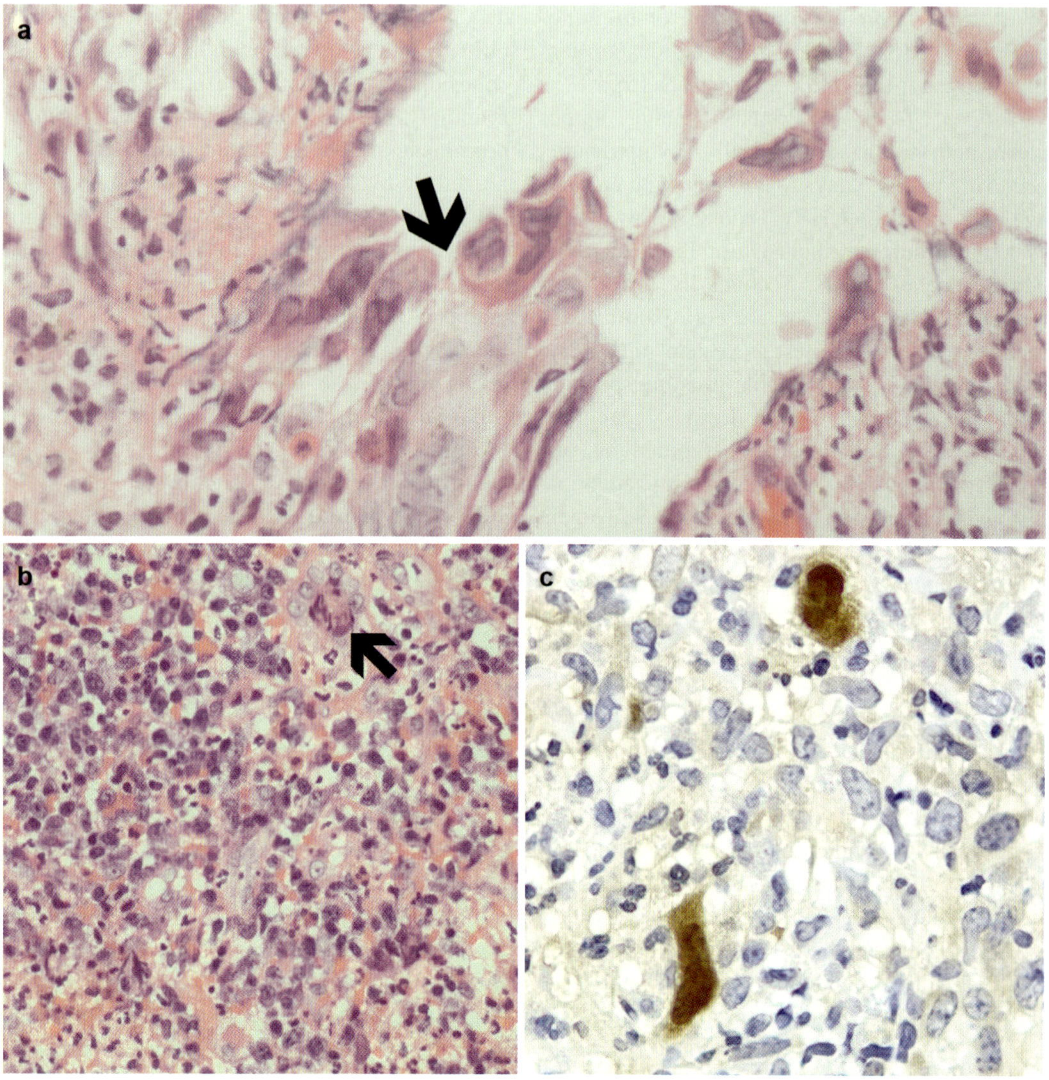

Fig. 2.7 *Herpes simplex virus* infection: Epithelial ulceration with intranuclear inclusions (**a**, *arrows*) and giant cell transformation. Pseudolymphomatous response around *herpes simplex virus*-infected cell (**b**, *arrow*), highlighted by *herpes simplex virus* immunostain (**c**)

Other Predominantly Primary Genital Infections

Other Bacterial Infections and Malakoplakia

Bacterial vaginosis is typified by a decrease in the quantity and prevalence of hydrogen peroxide-producing lactobacilli; the microecologic imbalanced replacement by *Gardnerella vaginalis*, anaerobes, and *Mycoplasma hominis*; and the consequent production of malodorous vaginal discharge, vulvovaginal pruritus, and irritation [70, 71]. The diagnosis is usually made by the presence of clue cells on vaginal smear (Fig. 2.8a) and a positive whiff test. The latter refers to the production of a fishy odor when the vaginal discharge is exposed to potassium hydroxide [72].

Superficial and deep staphylococcal folliculitis and abscess formation, occurring secondary to physical trauma or chemical injury, are characterized by perifollicular erythema and variable follicular suppuration, destruction, and granulomatous

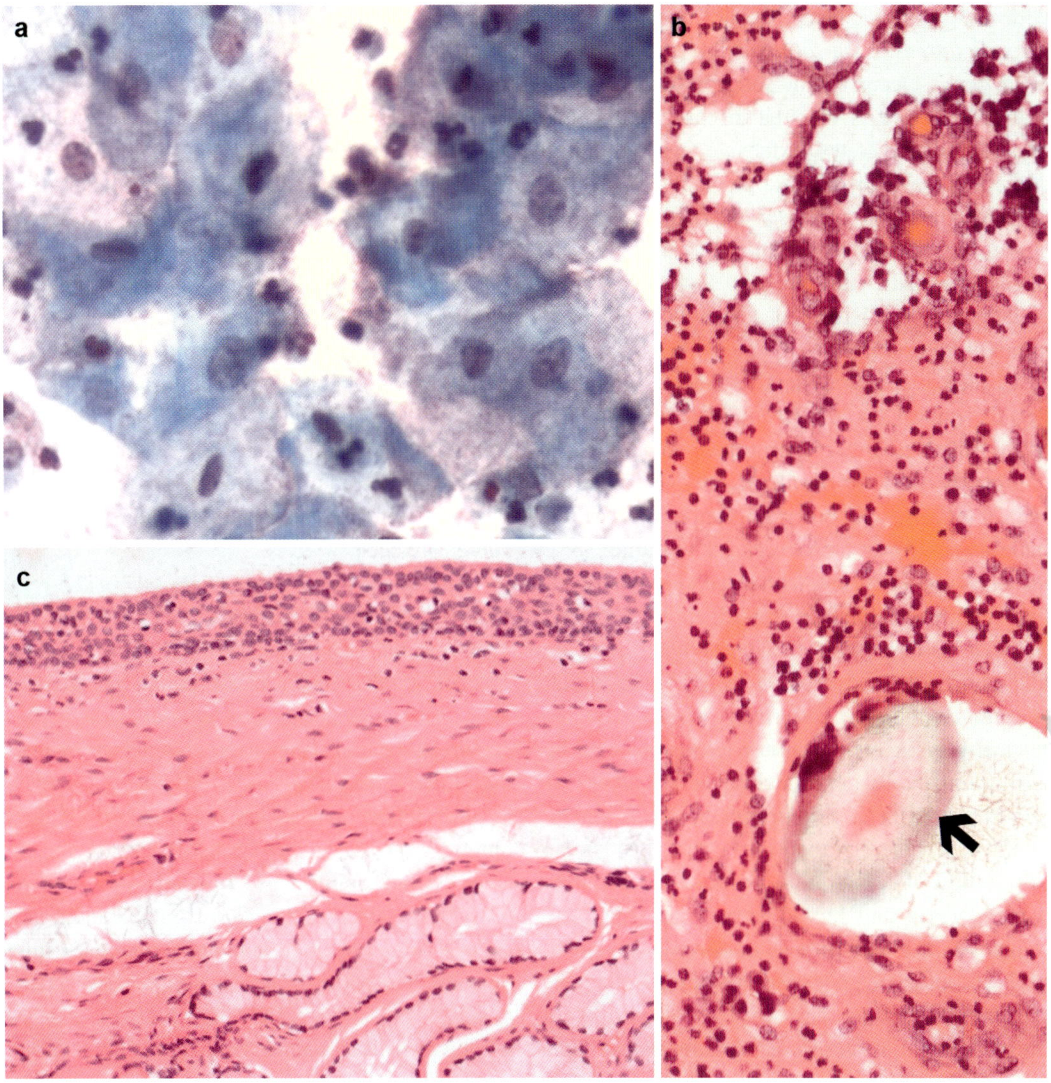

Fig. 2.8 Bacterial vaginosis (**a**) characterized by squamous epithelial cells covered by coccobacilli (clue cells). Bartholin duct cyst (**b**) with superficial epithelium and mucous glands in wall. Pilonidal sinus (**c**) with a granulation tissue-lined tract with suppuration and hair shafts (*arrow*)

inflammation, similar to that in other anatomic sites. Bullous impetigo and staphylococcal scalded skin syndrome are typified by flaccid bullae. Rupture of the bullae in staphylococcal scalded skin syndrome results in exfoliation of confluent areas of the epidermis. In patients with recurrent vulvovaginal abscesses, infection caused by methicillin-resistant *S. aureus* should be considered as an etiological agent [73–75]. Abscesses in the vulvovaginal area may arise in dilated and inflamed Bartholin (Fig. 2.8b), Gartner, or Skene ducts, hidradenitis suppurativa, pilonidal sinuses (Fig. 2.8c), and urethral diverticula. *S. aureus* is implicated in most of these settings but *Bacteroides*, *E. coli*, *N. gonorrhoea*, *K. pneumoniae*, and *Chlamydia* have been implicated in Bartholin abscess [76–79].

Streptococcal infections of the vulvovaginal area are heterogeneous. Superficial streptococcal disease encompasses a perianal dermatitis with vulvovaginal spread. Necrotizing gangrene, a fulminant life-threatening condition, is caused by a wide range of organisms, including *C. perfringens, S. aureus, P. mirabilis, P. aeruginosa*, and *S. viridans*. Occurring in patients with diabetes mellitus, peripheral vascular disease, and immunocompromised states, extensive surgical debridement is the gold standard of management [80, 81]. Microscopic appraisal of debrided tissue demonstrates extensive tissue necrosis including fascial necrosis, thrombosis, and obliterative endarteritis of subcutaneous vessels and leukocytic infiltration [80].

Erythrasma, a superficial cutaneous infection that is caused by *Corynebacterium minutissimum*, involves the intertriginous spaces most commonly [82]. It occurs mainly in diabetic, obese, elderly, and other immunocompromised patients and those with excessive sweating [83]. Patients usually present with large, slowly spreading, confluent, slightly raised, reddish-brown macular patches with variable central clearing and poorly defined borders [82]. A superficial scale maceration is present in dry and moist areas, respectively. While the cutaneous lesions may be asymptomatic, moderate itching or discomfort is recorded [82]. *C. minutissimum* is a Gram-positive, aerobic diphtheroid rod that invades the upper third of the stratum corneum and proliferates in warm and humid conditions [83]. The diagnosis of erythrasma is confirmed by coral-pink fluorescence under Wood's lamp and by the presence of Gram-positive rods on smears or in the superficial stratum corneum in biopsy sections [82–84]. Methylene blue-stained smears demonstrate the presence of dark blue granules. Erythrasma may be confused with seborrheic dermatitis and may coexist with *Malassezia* species [82–85]. However, the latter is characterized by spores and thick hyphal forms that demonstrate green autofluorescence under Wood's lamp.

Malakoplakia, initially described by Michaelis and Gutmann in 1902, is a chronic inflammatory disease that is associated with a range of bacterial infections [86]. While malakoplakia involves the mucosa of the urinary tract most commonly and a wide range of extraurinary sites may be involved, vulvovaginal involvement is documented rarely [86, 87]. However, of the genital organs, vaginal involvement is most common [87]. The pathogenesis of malakoplakia is controversial, but an infective basis, altered histiocytic activity, altered immune response, and abnormal gut flora have been implicated [88–90]. *E. coli* is implicated in more than two-thirds of cases, but other known infective associations include *Klebsiella, Mycobacterium tuberculosis, Staphylococcus aureus, Proteus* species, and *Rhodococcus equi* [88–90]. Malakoplakia is characterized by the presence of solitary or widespread soft plaques and nodules [90]. Microscopically, sheets of swollen histiocytes with eosinophilic granular or vacuolated cytoplasm, referred to as von Hansemann cells, containing periodic acid Schiff-positive and diastase-resistant inclusions and Michaelis-Gutmann bodies are seen.

Vulvovaginal Candidiasis

Vulvovaginal candidiasis affects approximately 75% of women in the reproductive age at least once in their lifetime, with approximately 50% experiencing ≥1 recurrence and 5–8% experiencing multiple annual episodes [91, 92]. Occurring in association with a normal vaginal pH (pH range = 4.0–4.5), vulvovaginal candidiasis is caused most commonly by *Candida albicans* [91, 93]. Risk factors for vulvovaginal candidiasis include diabetes mellitus, antibiotic use, high reproductive hormone levels, and genetic predisposition [94, 95]. Clinically, patients have a white, curd-like vaginal discharge, vulvovaginal erythema, edema, and fissures. Microscopically, there is epidermal hyperkeratosis, parakeratosis, and hyperplasia with subcorneal or spongiotic pustules (Fig. 2.9a) and periodic acid Schiff-positive budding yeasts, 3–6 μm diameter, round to oval in shape, and pseudohyphae, 2–4 μm in length (Fig. 2.9b). In biopsies, the epidermal alterations may resemble that of psoriasis vulgaris, lichen simplex chronicus, and eczematous dermatitis. Periodic acid Schiff identification of the fungal forms is pivotal to the diagnosis.

Trichomoniasis

Trichomoniasis, caused by the flagellate protozoan *T. vaginalis*, is believed to be the most frequent sexually transmitted infection and is a risk

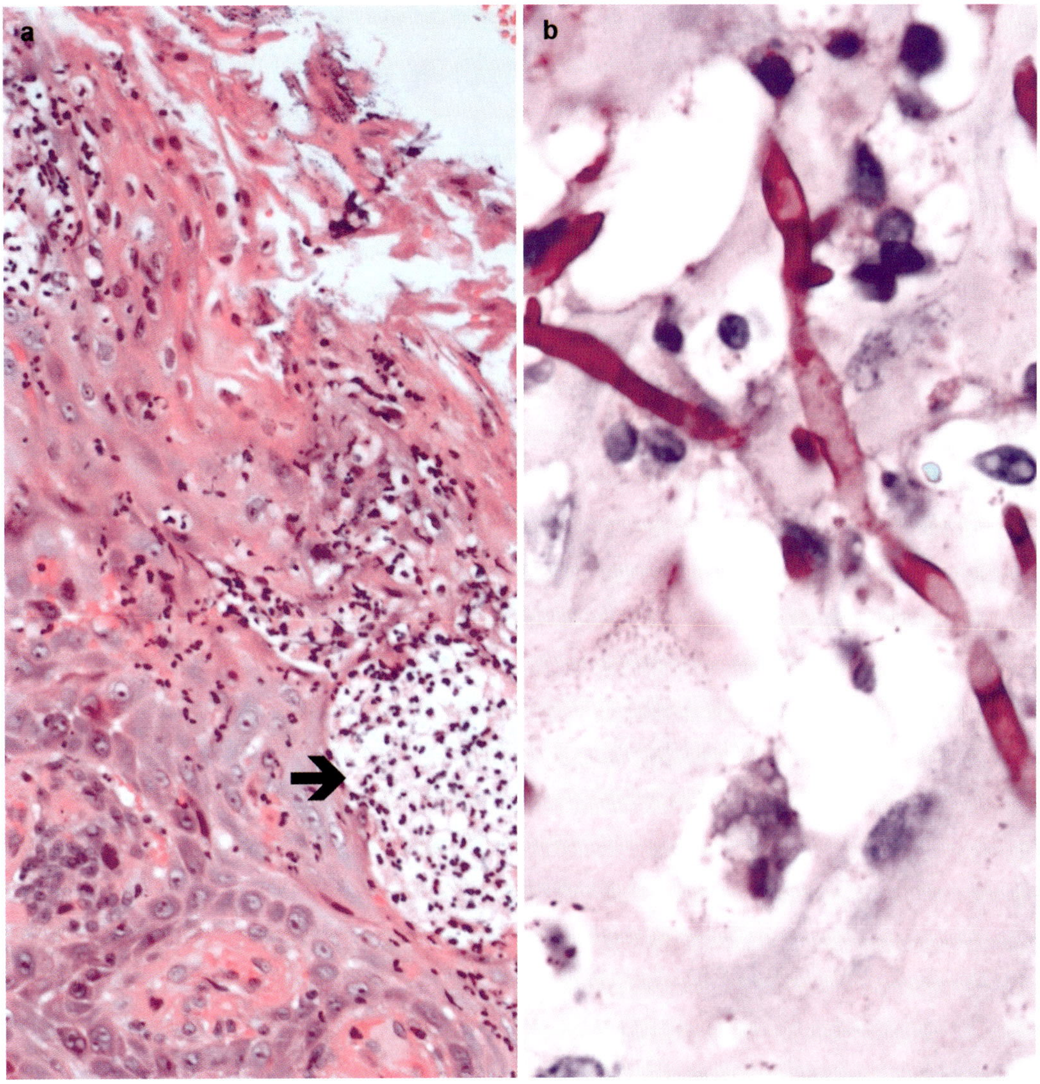

Fig. 2.9 Vulvovaginal candidiasis: Hyperparakeratotic, acanthotic epithelium (**a**) with pustules (*arrow*) and superficial debris. Periodic acid Schiff-positive pseudohyphae (**b**)

factor for HIV transmission [96, 97]. It usually parasitizes the vagina, prostate gland, and urethra [98]. *T. vaginalis* trophozoites are 23–39 μm in length and 5–8 μm wide. They contain four anterior flagella and a fifth flagellum that is present within the undulating membrane [98, 99], spanning approximately two-thirds of the distance to the posterior end of the body [98, 99]. Patients present with a foul-smelling, yellow-green vaginal discharge, acute vaginitis, and vulvovaginal tenderness [100]. The vulvovaginal mucosa demonstrates intense erythema and edema [98, 101]. Diagnosis is made on direct wet mount examinations of vaginal secretions (Fig. 2.10a), culture, Papanicolaou smears, and serologic and PCR investigation; the latter has been found to be 100% specific and sensitive [102]. Oral metronidazole is the current drug of choice.

Pediculosis Pubis

Pubic lice (pediculosis pubis, crab lice) infest over 10% of human populations worldwide [103]. Caused by *Phthirus pubis*, crab louse disease is usually transmitted sexually in association with

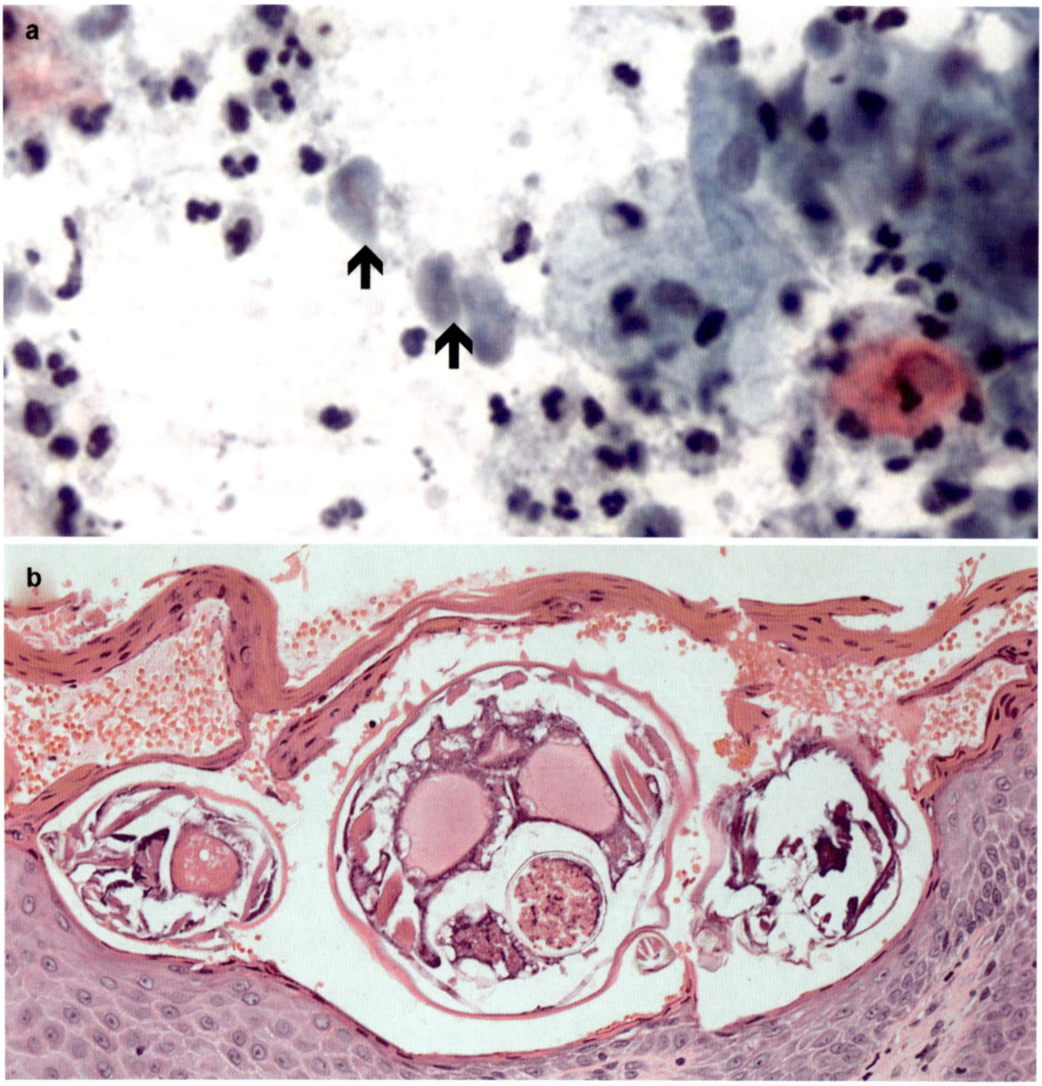

Fig. 2.10 Trichomoniasis: pear-shaped organisms (**a**, *arrows*) on a Papanicolaou-stained smear. Hyperparakeratotic, acanthotic epidermis with *S. scabiei* mites (**b**)

another concomitant sexually transmitted disease in 30% of patients [104]. Crab louse infestation is typified by their attachment to pubic hairs. Established infestation is accompanied by bluish-gray macules on the thighs and lower abdomen that are a consequence of hemorrhage and hemosiderin deposition. Excoriations may be present as a consequence of pruritus. Diagnosis depends on the identification of the 0.8- to 1.2-mm long adult organisms and viable eggs (nits) on hair shafts [103].

Scabies

Scabies is caused by the female mite of the genus *Sarcoptes scabiei* var *hominis*. It is spread by close human contact. The female mite lives in epidermal burrows. Norwegian or crusted scabies is associated with immunosuppression. Microscopically, scabies is associated with intraepidermal mites or scabietic fecal material or ova, epidermal spongiosis, intraepidermal eosinophils, and a lymphoeosinophilic infiltrate around the superficial and deep vascular plexuses.

Norwegian scabies is characterized by a psoriasiform epidermal reaction pattern with epidermal hyperkeratosis, parakeratosis, and large numbers of organisms (Fig. 2.10b) [54, 105].

Secondary Vulvovaginal Infection

Contiguous Spread from Adjacent Organs

Amoebiasis

Cutaneous amoebiasis is a rare disease [106, 107]. Caused by *Entamoeba histolytica*, it may be the exclusive expression of amoebiasis, or it may represent contiguous spread from a local site. *E. histolytica* has phagocytic, proteolytic, and cytolytic capabilities [108, 109]. Cytolysis is induced by amoebapores, small peptide that form pores in lipid bilayers [110]. Cytokines and chemokines released by disrupted epithelial cells attract neutrophils and macrophages to the site of disease [111, 112]. Neutrophil lysis and cysteine proteinases released by *E. histolytica* exacerbate the tissue damage [113]. Despite the proximity of the vulva to the gastrointestinal tract, vulval amoebiasis is reported rarely [114]. The cutaneous manifestations include painful ulcers with necrotic bases and variably raised edges, fistulae, abscesses, sinuses, and polypoid and warty outgrowths. Cutaneous amoebiasis occurs by direct or indirect routes. The former comprises contiguous spread from an adjacent visceral amoebic focus in the colon, rectum, or liver. Indirect cutaneous involvement occurs by vascular invasion and hematogenous and lymphatic spread. *Outcome*: If diagnosed and treated in a timely manner, healing of cutaneous lesions occur. Intravenous or oral metronidazole is the drug of choice.

Pathologic features: While the biopsy findings may differ based on the pathogenesis of the disease, the hallmark of the disease is liquefactive necrosis and trophozoites with ingested erythrocytes, hematophagous trophozoites (Fig. 2.11a). Pseudoepitheliomatous hyperplasia, atrophy, sinuses, and fistulae are variable findings. Vascular invasion and intraluminal amoebae may be identified, especially in lesions with deep involvement. Neutrophils with leukocytoclasis may be prominent. The periodic acid Schiff stain highlights hematophagous amoebic trophozoites (Fig. 2.11b) but degenerate trophozoites do not stain, and amoebae may be missed in densely neutrophilic foci. *Differential diagnosis*: The clinical differential diagnosis includes tuberculosis, syphilis, herpetic ulceration, Crohn's disease, and carcinoma, all of which are microscopically distinctive.

Schistosomiasis

Blood flukes of the genus *Schistosoma* are the infective agents of schistosomiasis that afflicts >200 million people worldwide [115]. The three major pathogenic species include *S. mansoni*, *S. japonicum*, and *S. haematobium*. *S. haematobium* is most commonly associated with female genital tract schistosomasiasis [116]. Schistosomiasis is endemic in Egypt, Middle East, and Africa and is transmitted by freshwater snails [44]. Cercariae swim through fresh water and penetrate human skin with the aid of proteolytic enzymes [117]. Schistosomes form, shed off a surface glycocalyx and become schistosomules. These migrate to the lung and then settle in the pelvic or hepatic venous plexuses [117]. Cutaneous disease, in general, assumes four forms: cercarial dermatitis, urticarial lesions, papular granulomatous or warty lesions, and extragenital cutaneous lesions. Vulvar schistosomiasis is typified by papules, nodules, ulcers, polyps, warty outgrowths, exophytic tumor masses, and vulval edema. The lesions may be pruritic and painful [118, 119]. It has been suggested that genital schistosomiasis may be a risk factor for HIV transmission [116]. Sequestration of ova in the mucocutaneous epithelium of the genitalia causes friable contact bleeding foci. At these points, genital schistosomiasis is hypothesized to expose the deeper mucocutaneous tissue to HIV. *Diagnosis*: If patients have hematuria, microscopic examination of a midday or filtered terminal urine specimen may demonstrate ova. *S. haematobium* has a characteristic terminal spine, in contrast to *S. mansoni* ova that have lateral spines. *S. japonicum* does not possess a spine. While the entire wall of *S. mansoni* and

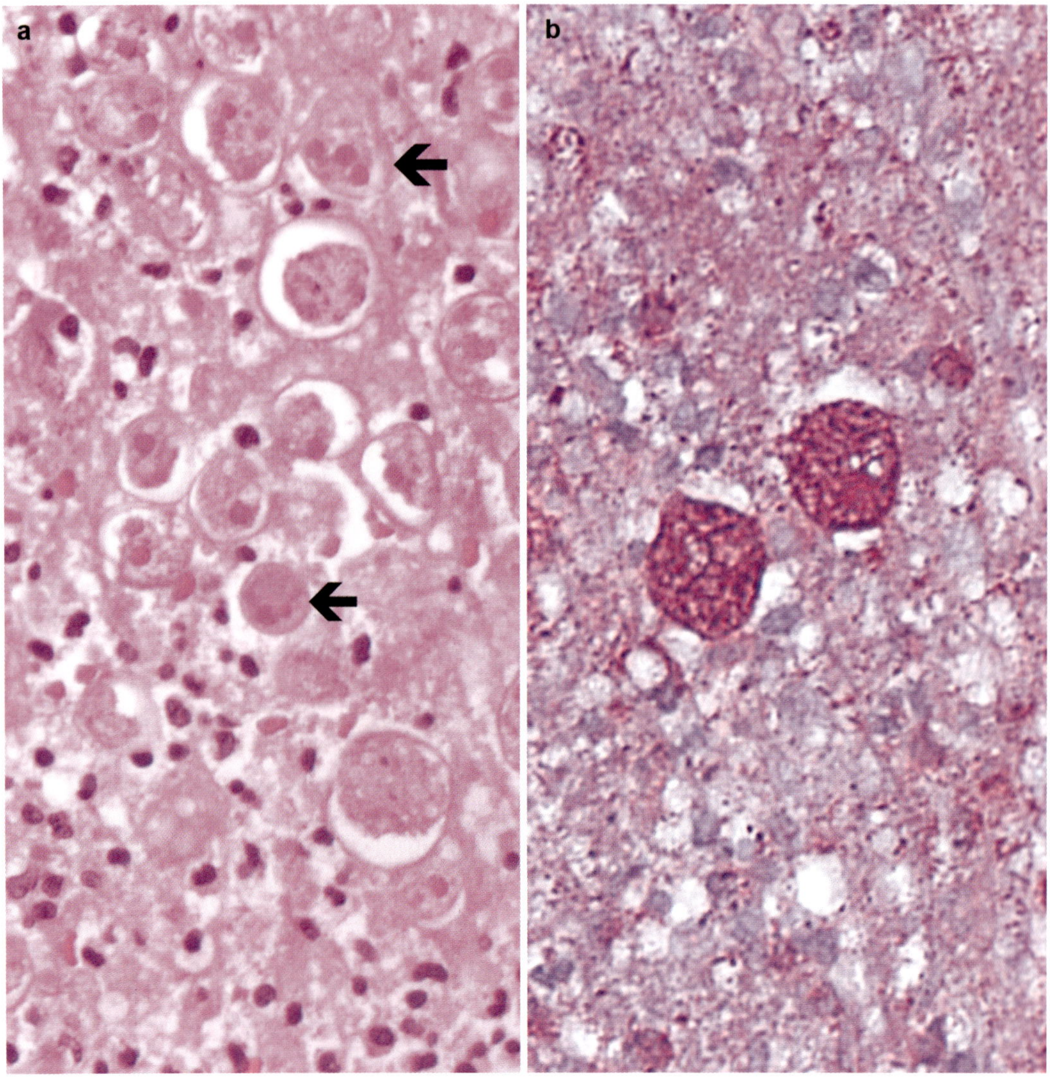

Fig. 2.11 Amoebiasis: hematophagous amoebic trophozoites (**a**, *arrows*) highlighted by periodic acid Schiff stain (**b**)

S. japonicum ova is acid fast by Ziehl Neelsen staining, only the terminal spine of *S. haematobium* is acid fast [117]. ELISA methods have been developed to confirm schistosomal infection. *Outcome/treatment*: Praziquantel is the current drug of choice for schistosomiasis with a cure rate of 60–90% in individuals from endemic areas and 100% for those in nonendemic areas [120, 121]. High pretreatment schistosomal load, high rate of reinfection, drug resistance, the circulation of immature parasitic organisms unaffected by drugs, and noncompliance are causes for a suboptimal response to praziquantel [120, 121]. Current molecular investigational tools include the Taq Man real-time PCR assay for early detection of *Schistosoma* species, the role of increased CD23^{+} B lymphocytes in drug-resistant schistosomiasis, genotypic analyses for the monitoring of mass drug administration campaigns, and the role of the phosphotyrosine signaling network in the development of novel antischistosomal therapy [115, 122, 123].

Pathology: Genital or perineal biopsies demonstrate ulceration, sinuses, and pseudoepitheliomatous hyperplasia. Free-lying, variably calcified ova may be accompanied by a florid granulomatous

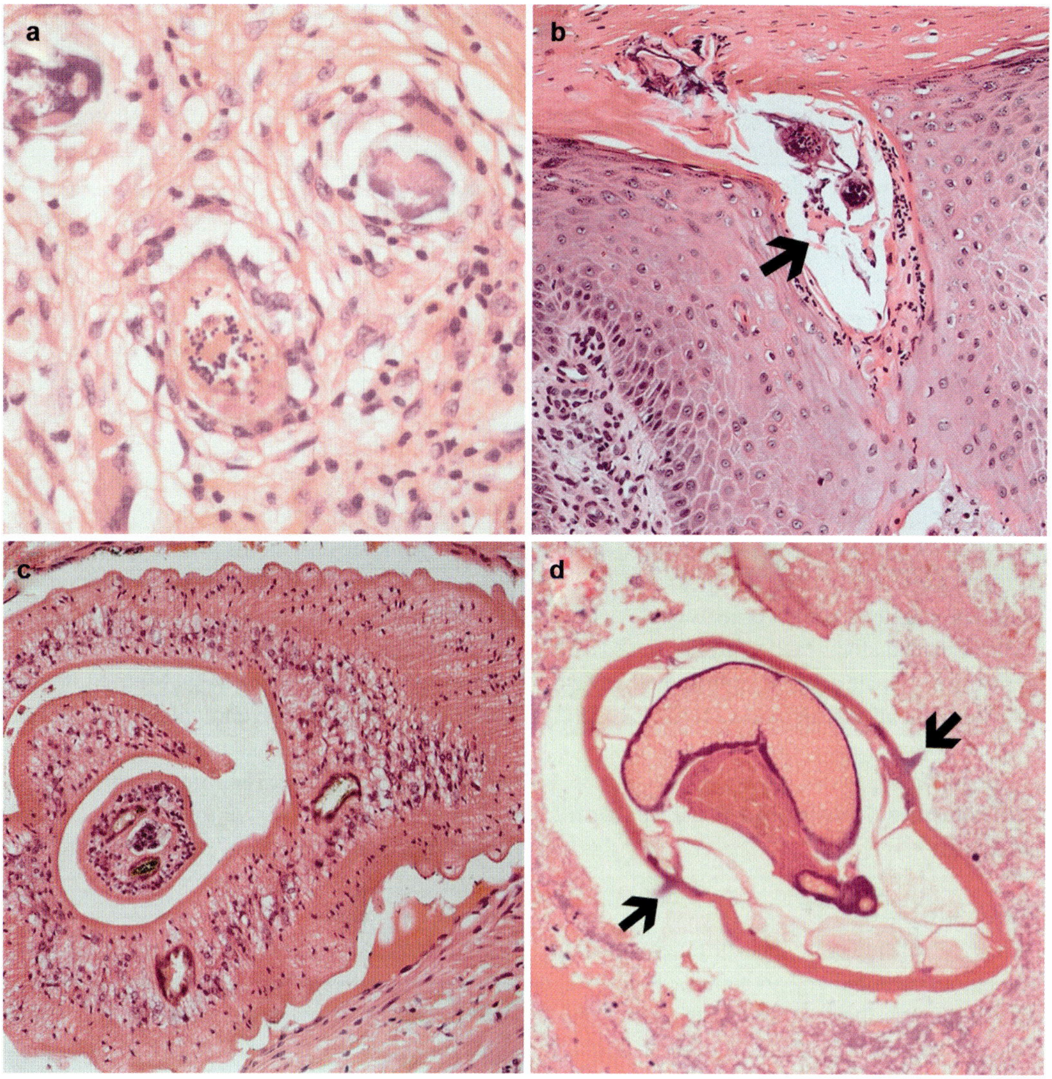

Fig. 2.12 *S. haematobium* ova within a dermal granuloma (**a**). Transepidermal elimination of viable ova (**b**, *arrow*) and intravenous schistosomal worms (**c**). *E. vermicularis* with lateral alae (**d**, *arrows*)

reaction (Fig. 2.12a) with eosinophils, eosinophil flame figures, and the Splendore-Hoeppli phenomenon [44, 118]. The ova may be degenerate or viable with identifiable miracidia. Transepidermal elimination of schistosomal ova may be present (Fig. 2.12b), especially in biopsies demonstrating pseudoepitheliomatous hyperplasia [123]. Fibrosis and intravenous worms (Fig. 2.12c) are a variable finding.

Enterobiasis

Enterobiasis, a worldwide infection, caused by *Enterobius vermicularis*, is spread by overcrowding and the sharing of clothing. *E. vermicularis* is an intestinal parasite, residing mainly in the ileocecal area, colon, rectum and vermiform appendix [124]. Following copulation in the colonic lumen, the adult male worm dies. The gravid female migrates to the anal region where ova are deposited, causing intense pruritus ani and serving as a nidus for ano-oral transmission of the organism. The ingested ova that contain first-stage larvae hatch in the duodenum and are carried to the colon where they develop into adult worms [124, 125]. Retrograde infection may occur when ova hatch on the skin of the buttocks and larvae migrate through the anus to the colon [124]. Because of the proximity of the vulva to the anus, adult worms migrate to the vulva, vagina, cervix, endometrium, ovaries, and peritoneal cavity, with resultant deposition of ova. Vulval involvement by *E. vermicularis* is rare, with patients presenting with vulvovaginitis or a vulval mass [125–127].

Microscopic features: There is pseudoepitheliomatous epidermal hyperplasia that mimics squamous cell carcinoma. An inflammatory response to subepithelial ova or worms is present. This may be granulomatous in nature with a variable eosinophilic component. The inflammatory component can assume a lichenoid pattern [124]. The ova are approximately 50–60 μm by 20–30 μm in dimension and contain a thick two-layered shell. The cuticle of adult worms is expanded into alae that extend along each side (Fig. 2.12d). The uterus of the female adult worm fills the body cavity and is distended with ova [124, 125].

Vulvovaginal Involvement by Systemic Infection

Tuberculosis

Although tuberculosis has afflicted mankind throughout recorded and archeological history, it remains among the leading causes of morbidity and mortality worldwide [128, 129]. Caused by *M. tuberculosis*, a member of the *M. tuberculosis* complex that includes six other closely related species, cutaneous tuberculosis accounts for 1.5% of extrapulmonary disease [130]. Less than 2% of genital tuberculosis occurs in the vulva and vagina, with the vulva being the least common site for genital tuberculosis [131, 132]. Primary vulval inoculation tuberculosis, first described in 1888 [132], is rare. Vulval tuberculosis is usually associated with systemic disease, especially pulmonary tuberculosis or tuberculosis higher in the genital tract, including the fallopian tubes, uterus, and ovaries [130].

Clinical features: Vulval tuberculosis presents as ulcers with variable sinus formation, hypertrophic lesions, id reactions, or rarely, esthiomene [133–137]. Lupus vulgaris and scrofuloderma have been described, the former more commonly [130, 138, 139]. Vulval tuberculids are documented rarely. While lichen scrofulosorum and papulonecrotid tuberculid may involve the vulva, the latter is the only documented vulval tuberculid, described as part of localized or more widespread disease [140, 141]. Lichen scrofulosorum, a widely disseminated rash composed of 2-mm-diameter, variably scaly, folliculocentric papules, may involve the vulva as part of a generalized process [142]. *Differential diagnosis*: Ulcerative manifestations may resemble sexually transmitted diseases including LGV, chancroid and syphilis, schistosomiasis, Crohn's disease, and amoebiasis. Hypertrophic lesions may resemble carcinoma while the papular tuberculids may resemble sarcoidosis. *Diagnosis*: Apart from the histomorphological confirmation of tuberculosis, mycobacterial PCR can be employed for diagnosis [143]. Microbiological culture not only allows genotypic analysis of the culture isolates but also facilitates drug sensitivity testing. *Treatment*: The first-line drug schedule includes isoniazid, rifampicin, ethambutol, and pyrazinamide. Patients with multidrug- and extreme-drug-resistance tuberculosis require alternate schedules.

Microscopic features: Necrotizing granulomatous inflammation with caseative necrosis and a surrounding histiocytic, palisaded, or granulomatous inflammatory response with Langhans giant cells is the prototypical reaction pattern. Ziehl Neelsen staining demonstrates acid fast bacilli. In scrofuloderma, tuberculous lymphadenitis ruptures more commonly to the skin and to the surface with resultant sinus formation. The center of the lesion demonstrates suppurative or abscess-like morphology. The deep aspect of the lesion is composed of the prototypical necrotizing granulomatous histomorphology with identifiable acid fast bacilli. Papulonecrotic tuberculid is characterized by a wedge-shaped zoned inflammatory reaction pattern. Superficial crust, acute inflammatory exudate, coagulative necrosis, granulomatous inflammation, and vasculitis are stratified from the superficial to deepest location (Fig. 2.13a). Acid fast bacilli are not identified on special

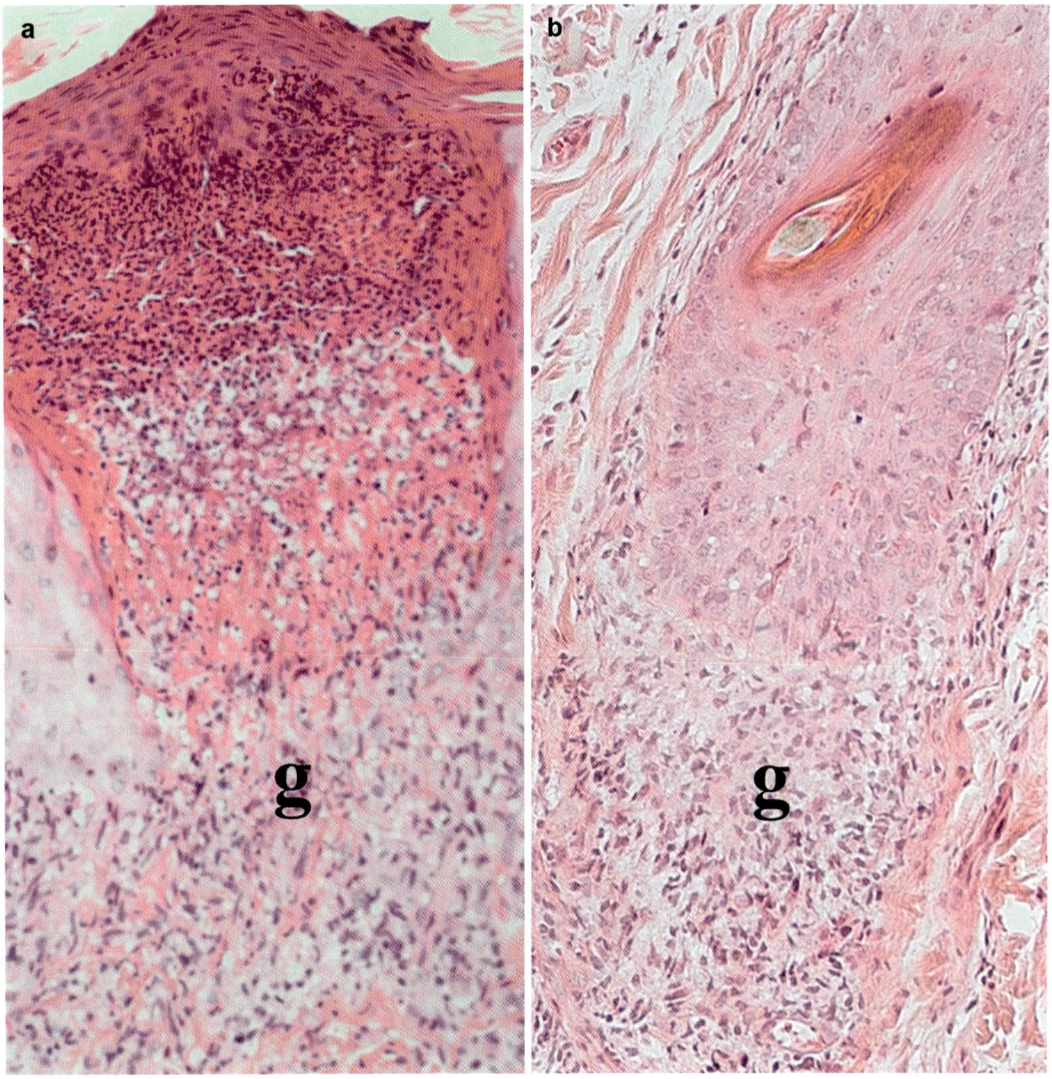

Fig. 2.13 Papulonecrotid tuberculid (**a**) with a "zoned" inflammatory, including deep granulomatous (*g*), response. Nonnecrotizing perifollicular granulomatous inflammation (*g*) in lichen scrofulosorum (**b**)

mycobacteria stains. Biopsy of lichen scrofulosorum demonstrates subepidermal, periappendageal, and interstitial microgranulomas (Fig. 2.13b).

Bacillary Angiomatosis

Bacillary angiomatosis is caused by members of the *Bartonella* spp., *B. quintana*, and *B. henselae* [144–146]. Although known for more than 100 years, *Bartonella* spp. are still considered emerging infectious agents [147, 148]. *B. henselae* that also causes cat scratch disease and peliosis hepatitis is transmitted mainly by cat fleas. *B. quintana*, residing in humans, also causes trench fever and is transmitted by body lice, cat fleas, and ticks. It is associated with poor living conditions and homelessness. Bacillary angiomatosis is associated with clinical heterogeneity, presenting as solitary or multiple lesions. Ulcers, papules, nodules, and pyogenic granuloma-like and warty lesions are documented in the skin. Vulval bacillary angiomatosis is documented rarely [149–151].

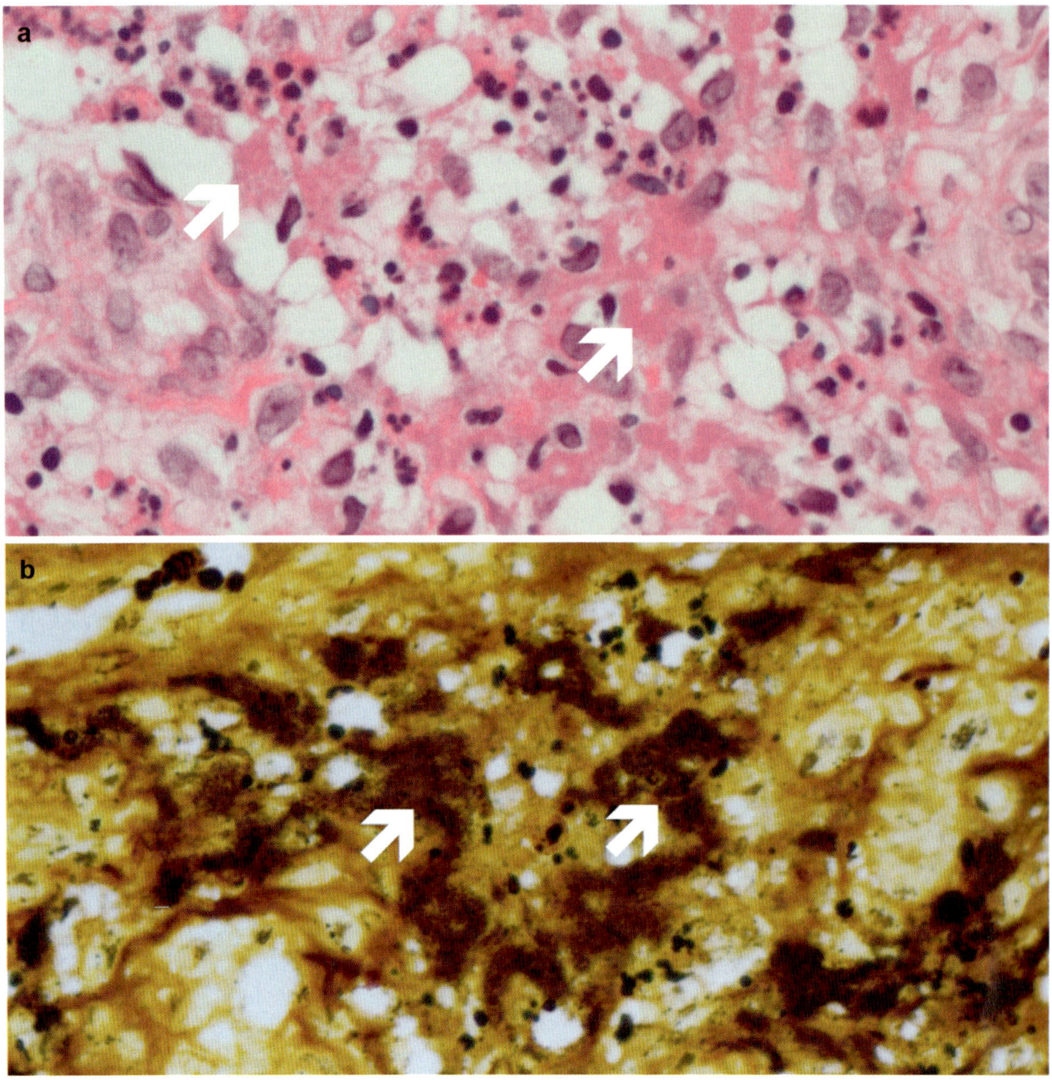

Fig. 2.14 Bacillary angiomatosis: vasculature lined by plump endothelial cells (**a**), intervascular neutrophils, karyorrhectic debris, and paravascular eosinophilic material (*arrows*), confirmed to be argyrophilic organisms on Warthin Starry stain (**b**, *arrows*)

Microscopic features: Bacillary angiomatosis is characterized by lobular vascular proliferation, interstitial neutrophils, and karyorrhectic debris (Fig. 2.14a). The vascular channels are lined by epithelioid endothelial cells. Paravascular clumps of argyrophilic organisms are present (Fig. 2.14b). Ulceration, pseudoepitheliomatous hyperplasia, and a confluent neutrophilic infiltrate are less common microscopic findings. *Differential diagnosis*: Deep lesions may mimic abscess because of confluent suppuration or they may have a solid appearance with minimal debris, resembling tumors with an epithelioid endothelial phenotype, including angiosarcoma, epithelioid hemangioendothelioma, and cutaneous epithelioid angiomatous nodule. Bacillary angiomatosis with spindle cells mimic Kaposi sarcoma. The diagnosis may be confirmed on a biopsy, with exact bacillary confirmation being obtained by molecular investigation. Serological and microbiological studies, the latter typified by specialized techniques, may also aid the diagnosis.

Cytomegalovirus Infection

Cytomegalovirus (CMV) is a member of the Herpesviridae family of DNA viruses [152]. A major cause of mortality and morbidity in immunocompromised individuals, it is one of the most common fatal systemic infections in patients with AIDS [153].

Clinical features: Cutaneous manifestations, documented rarely, include a generalized maculopapular rash, ulcers, indurated hyperpigmented nodules, vesicles, petechiae, plaques, and pseudoangiomatous lesions that mimic a range of dermatoses [153]. Nonpathognomonic ulcers involve the genital, perineal, and perianal areas [152, 154]. They may be single or multiple and vary in size [155]. The significance of CMV in the cutaneous lesions is controversial [156, 157]. While CMV may be pathogenic, it may also be an epiphenomenon and colonizer of endothelial cells during CMV viraemia [157]. It has been questioned why localized CMV ulceration has a propensity for genital or perineal involvement [155]. It has also been suggested that these anatomic locations serve as latency sites for CMV. The intraneural location of CMV inclusions in genital and perineal skin, similar to shingles, has supported such a view. *Diagnosis*: According to some workers, light microscopy of routine hematoxylin-and-eosin-stained sections is the most sensitive diagnostic tool [157]. Immunohistochemistry, in situ hybridization, and molecular investigations may be employed for diagnostic confirmation. *Outcome*: Localized infection has a better outcome than disseminated disease. Ganciclovir, foscarnet, and valganciclovir are used for treatment.

Microscopic features: There is capillary dilatation with endothelial localization of large, eosinophilic intranuclear inclusions, approximately 10 μm in size (Fig. 2.15a) [62, 158]. These inclusions may be present within the granulation tissue in the ulcer base, with resultant leukocytoclastic vasculitis and thrombosis [62, 155, 157]. Inclusions are also present in keratinocytes, eccrine epithelium, macrophages, and fibroblasts [157].

Epstein-Barr Virus Infection

While Epstein-Barr virus (EBV)-associated genital ulcers were first documented in 1977, in 1913 Lipschütz described an acute disease with fever, genital ulcers, and lymphadenopathy in young women that was labeled "Lipschütz syndrome" [159]. It is possible that some patients with Lipschütz syndrome have primary EBV infection. EBV-associated genital ulcers occur in patients with a mean age of 14.5 years (range = 2–51 years) [159].

Clinical features: The ulcer may be single and >1 cm in diameter or multiple and small [160]. The ulcers are deep and necrotic with irregular edges and a yellow adherent membrane. Pain is the main presenting symptom, but a prodrome of fatigue, headache, and fever precedes the ulcer symptoms. Signs of infectious mononucleosis may also be present, including lymphadenopathy and tonsillitis [159, 160]. The ulcers respond to systemic corticosteroid therapy or may resolve spontaneously within approximately 2 weeks [160]. *Diagnosis*: Clinical suspicion is pivotal to diagnostic confirmation. The initial presence of IgM in the absence of antibody to EBV nuclear, and a subsequent identifiable IgG antibody response to viral capsid, confirms a primary EBV infection. The genital ulcers may therefore be a manifestation of a viremia [159]. PCR testing of the ulcer may be helpful to confirm the diagnosis. *Differential diagnosis*: The differential diagnosis includes primary syphilis, which is painless in comparison to the EBV ulcer. Aphthous ulcers can be excluded by the results of clinical serological tests. Other infective ulcers, including those due to herpes simplex virus infection and candidiasis, demonstrate identifiable organisms.

Microscopic features: Biopsies demonstrate nonspecific features including granulation tissue with mixed acute and chronic cells and debris, similar to that seen in aphthous ulcers. Thrombosis and lymphocytic vasculitis may be present.

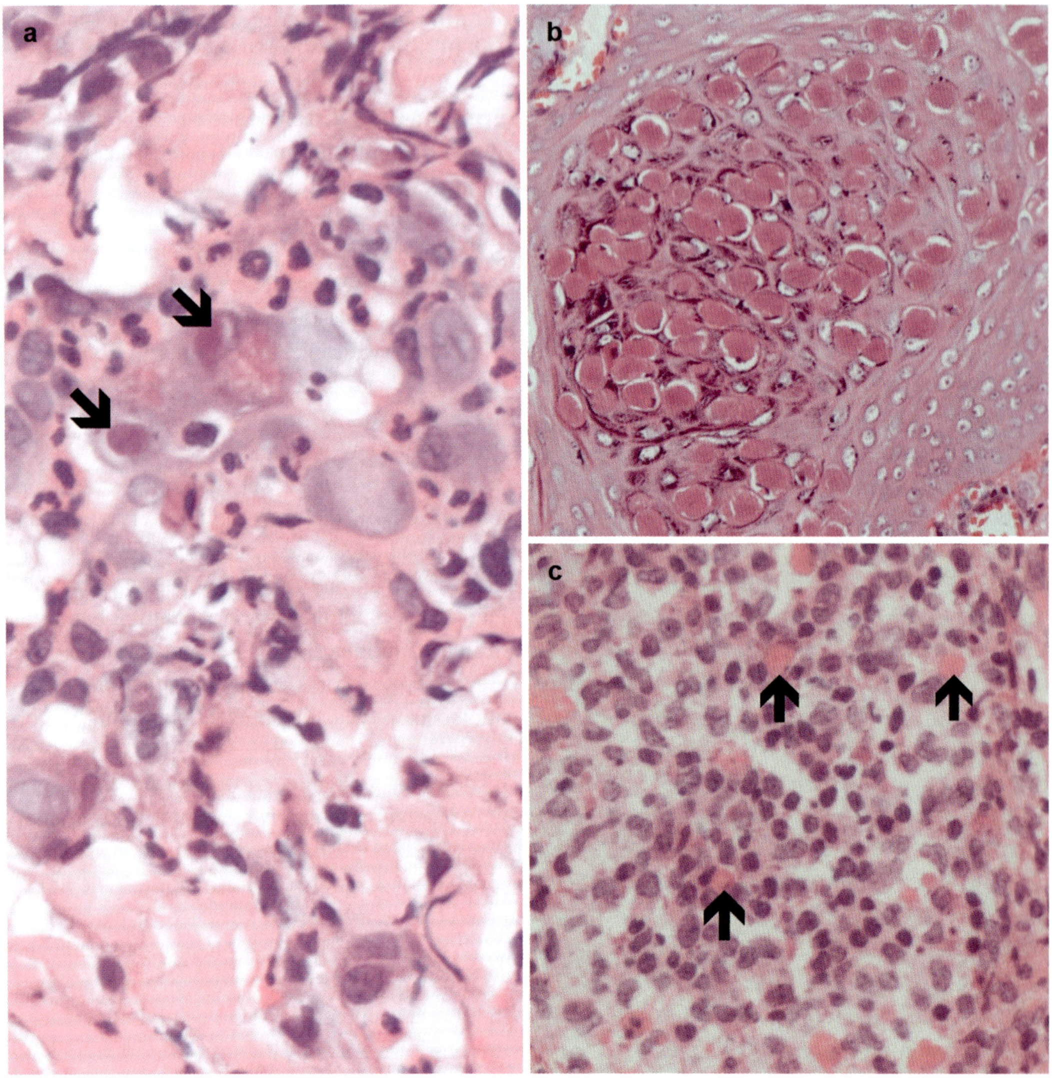

Fig. 2.15 *Cytomegalovirus* infection: vasculitis and "owl's eye" inclusions in endothelial cells (**a**, *arrows*). Inclusions of *Molluscum contagiosum virus* within epithelial crater (**b**). Pseudolymphomatous inflammatory reaction to degenerate dermal molluscum bodies (**c**, *arrows*)

Molluscum Contagiosum

Molluscum contagiosum, a worldwide infection, is caused by *Molluscum contagiosum virus*, the most common poxvirus that infects humans [161]. It occurs in individuals of all ages, but it commonly affects children, sexually active adolescents, and immunocompromised persons [162]. Molluscum contagiosum in women is usually a sexually transmitted disease, but spread through fomites, direct bodily contact, or minor abrasions also occurs. It manifests as waxy, skin-colored papules, 2–5 mm in dimension, in multiple anatomical locations on the labia majora, labia minora, and mons pubis as a sexually transmitted disease [163, 164]. In patients with AIDS, giant molluscum contagiosum often measuring more than 1 cm occurs. In children, vulval involvement usually occurs as part of disseminated disease. Exclusive vulval molluscum contagiosum in children is unusual [165]. In adult women, exclusive vulval molluscum contagiosum occurs as a sexually transmitted infection

[164]. While molluscum contagiosum is a self-limited disease, curettage or cryosurgery may be used as physical treatment modalities. Topical application of 5% imiquimod cream may also be effective.

Microscopic features: A cup-shaped lesion composed of acantholytic epidermis with viral inclusion bodies is seen. In the lower epidermis, ovoid, eosinophilic inclusion bodies, the molluscum, or Henderson-Patterson bodies are seen in a peripheral location. At the granular layer level, the molluscum bodies appear basophilic. Central disintegration of the stratum corneum results in crater formation and the release of molluscum bodies therein. While the dermis is usually uninvolved, rupture of the crater discharges molluscum bodies and keratinous debris into the dermis (Fig. 2.15b). In this setting and when the molluscum contagiosum undergoes spontaneous involution, intense dermal inflammation, including a pseudolymphomatous response (Fig. 2.15c), is seen.

Superficial Dermatophytic Infection and Pityriasis Versicolor

The superficial dermatophytes include organisms of three genera: *Microsporum*, *Trichophyton*, and *Epidermophyton*. Tinea cruris, a dermatophytic infection of the groin, perineum, and perianal area, is caused by organisms of all three genera, but *T. rubrum* is the most common. Erythematous patches, plaques, pustules, and vesicles may be present. Biopsies demonstrate variable epidermal acanthosis, parakeratosis, spongiosis, and fungal yeasts and hyphae [43]. Majocchi granuloma, caused most commonly by *T. rubrum*, presents with perifollicular disease in immunocompetent and deep plaque/nodular lesions in immunocompromised patients [166]. It has been reported rarely in the vulva [166]. *Microscopically*, there is granulomatous perifolliculitis and an infiltrate of neutrophils, lymphocytes, and histiocytes. Vulval diseases caused by *Malassezia furfur* include pityriasis versicolor and folliculitis, both of which may occur in the vulva [167]. Pityriasis versicolor is characterized by reddish-brown to white scaly macules on the labia majora. *Microscopically*, fungal yeasts and hyphae are noted in the stratum corneum.

Histoplasmosis

Histoplasmosis is caused by *Histoplasmosis capsulatum*, a dimorphic fungus that exists worldwide but is endemic in the central United States, Latin American, and Caribbean countries [168–170]. Found in moist, acid soil with a high organic content, histoplasmosis is acquired by the inhalation of spores from soil contaminated by bird and bat guano [170, 171]. Ninety percent to ninety-five percent of new *H. capsulatum* infections are asymptomatic [172]. The rest present with symptomatic acute, disseminated, and chronic pulmonary forms of the disease [172]. Cutaneous histoplasmosis usually occurs in the setting of disseminated histoplasmosis, secondary to progression of primary pulmonary disease, in approximately 6% of patients with disseminated histoplasmosis [43, 168]. The patients who are afflicted are mainly patients with hematological malignancies, inborn errors of immunity, or AIDS. Mucocutaneous histoplasmosis of the female genital tract is rare, being reported twice to date, once as part of chronic disseminated histoplasmosis [173] and once as primary conjugal histoplasmosis [174].

Clinical appearance: The cutaneous spectrum of histoplasmosis includes ulcers, papules, nodules, plaques, molluscum-like lesions, purpura, erythroderma, and panniculitis [170, 175]. *Diagnosis*: Serological testing, fungal culture, histopathological appraisal, and PCR testing are useful diagnostic measures. Fungal morphologic in cultures at temperatures <35°C are those of a mycelial phase while at 37°C, the organism assumes a yeast-like form [168, 172]. *Differential diagnosis*: Organisms that reside in an intracellular location include those that cause donovanosis, leishmaniasis, toxoplasmosis, and leprosy. *H. capsulatum* is the only microorganism that parasitizes histiocytes and stains with the usual fungal stains. *Treatment*: Oral itraconazole is effective for less severe forms of the disease and for maintenance therapy. Amphotericin-B is used in patients with severe disease and AIDS.

Microscopic features: Necrotizing or nonnecrotizing granulomatous (Fig. 2.16a) or diffuse histiocytic reaction patterns occur. The former

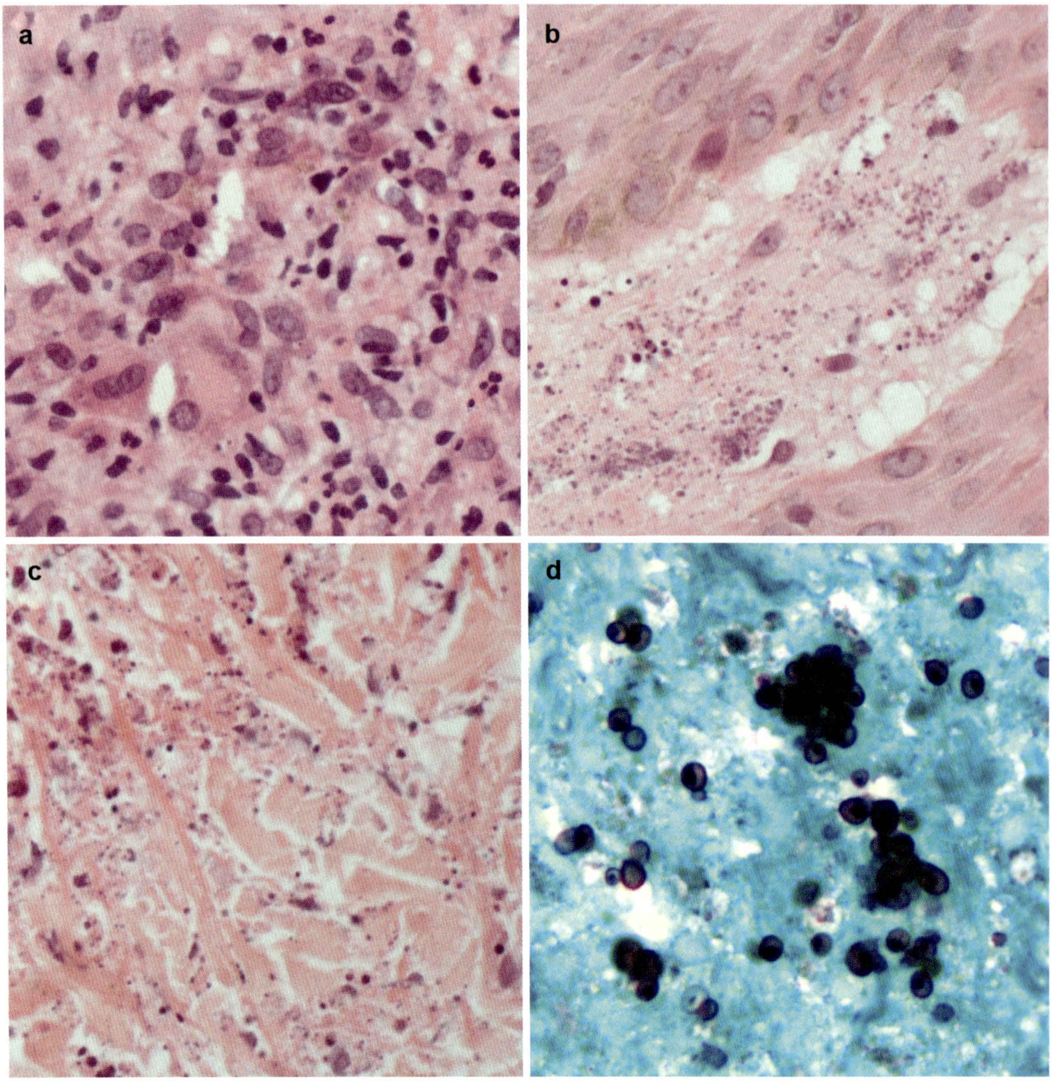

Fig. 2.16 Histoplasmosis: granulomatous response (**a**). Diffuse histiocytic infiltrate with intracytoplasmic microorganisms (**b**) and abundant dermal karyorrhexis (**c**). Gomori-Grocott methenamine silver-stained *H. capsulatum* yeast forms (**d**)

is unusual in skin locations. The histiocytic reaction pattern is typified by sheets and nodular aggregates of dermal histiocytes in which abundant intracytoplasmic organisms are seen (Fig. 2.16b) [168, 170]. Karyorrhexis is variably present (Fig. 2.16c) [170, 176]. The individual organisms are round to oval 2–4-μm spores that are surrounded by a halo. The spores demonstrate variable narrow-necked budding and stain with periodic acid Schiff and silver stains (Fig. 2.16d).

Cryptococcosis

Cryptococcosis, caused by *C. neoformans*, is a fungal infection of worldwide occurrence [177]. It is a ubiquitous saprophyte of soil, being most abundant in environments contaminated by bird excreta [177]. Although usually acquired by inhalation of yeasts, primary cutaneous cryptococcosis occurs rarely [43]. Cryptococcosis occurs mainly in patients with malignancies, patients on immunosuppressive or corticosteroid therapy, and in transplant recipients [178]. Pulmonary

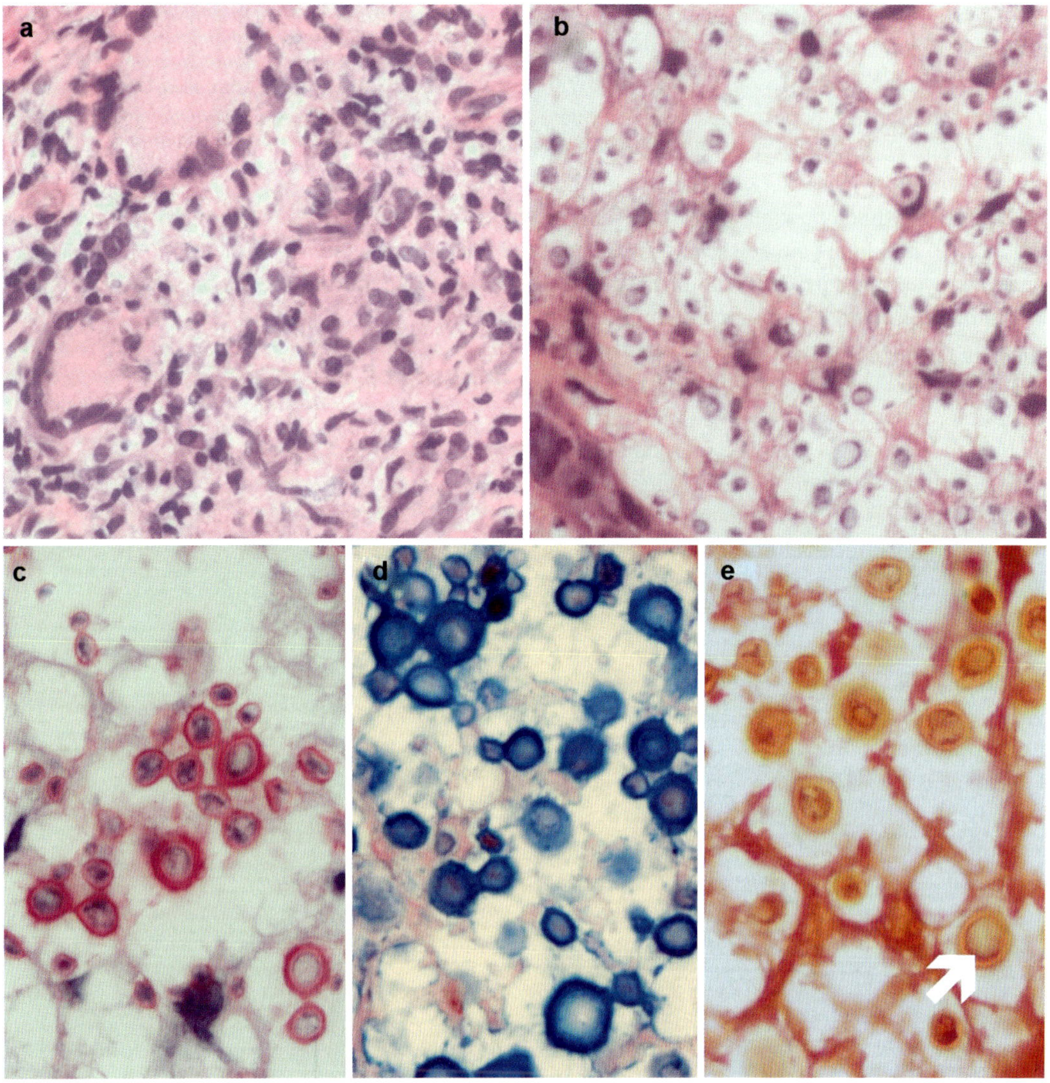

Fig. 2.17 Cryptococcosis: granulomatous (**a**) and paucicellular, "gelatinous" (**b**) patterns. Carminophilous organisms (**c**, Southgate mucicarmine), alcian *blue*-positive capsules (**d**), and Fontana-Masson-positive cell walls (**e**, *arrow*)

disease may be symptomatic or asymptomatic. The most important clinical manifestation is meningitis that is fatal if untreated [179]. Disseminated cryptococcosis occurs in 10–15% of immunocompromised patients [180]. Cutaneous disease, involving mainly the face, scalp, and neck, occurs in approximately 10% of patients with disseminated cryptococcosis [180]. Genital tract involvement by *C. neoformans* is rare [181, 182]. Cutaneous disease is heterogeneous with papules, ulcers, nodules, plaques, molluscum-like lesions, tumor-like swellings, and ecchymoses being documented most commonly [43, 178]. They may be solitary or multiple. Vulvovaginal cryptococcus has been documented in less than five patients to date [181, 183, 184]. *Treatment*: Antifungal agents, including amphotericin B, fluconazole, and itraconazole form the backbone of therapeutic schedules, with fluconazole emerging as the drug of choice for maintenance therapy [178].

Microscopic features: The microscopic appearances include granulomatous (Fig. 2.17a) and paucicellular infiltrates (Fig. 2.17b–e). Paucicellular reactions are typified by aggregates of histiocytes, parasitisized by yeast forms, many in a narrow-necked budding state (Fig. 2.17b). The organism is a 4- to 12-μm diameter round to oval yeast with a carminophilous, mucoid, capsule. Southgate mucicarmine (Fig. 2.17c), periodic acid Schiff, and alcian blue (Fig. 2.17d) stains highlight the capsule while Fontana Masson staining (Fig. 2.17e) highlights the cell wall. The latter is important when capsule-deficient forms are present. In biopsies with a necrotizing granulomatous appearance, the organisms are fewer and less readily visible than in those with a paucicellular, gelatinous appearance. Unusual appearances include those with abscess-like morphology and a pseudotumoral spindle cell-reaction pattern [182]. In biopsies from patients on antiretroviral therapy, immune reconstitution may result in an intense, including neutrophilic, inflammatory response with dense granulation tissue. In such biopsies, cryptococci may be elusive and require the full panel of infective stains for diagnosis.

Leishmaniasis

Leishmaniasis, caused by protozoa of the gender *Leishmania*, is one of the most common protozoan diseases worldwide [44]. Sandflies are the arthropod vectors of *Leishmania* species [185]. Sandflies belong to the genus Phlebotomus in the Old World and to Lutzomyia and Psychodopygus in the New World [44]. Mucocutaneous genital tract ulcers are documented in men more than in women [185–189]. Following a sting by the infected sandflies, promastigotes transform into amastigotes within macrophages. Leishmaniasis is classified into acute and chronic forms of the disease. The acute forms that may be localized or diffuse last approximately 3 months and are composed of a diffuse infiltrate of histiocytes with intracytoplasmic, 2–4-μm-diameter, Leishman-Donovan bodies. Representing amastigotes, these Leishman-Donovan bodies are typified by a round, basophilic nucleus and a rod-shaped, paranuclear kinetoplast that is optimally demonstrated by the Giemsa stain [44]. Chronic cutaneous leishmaniasis refers to disease that remains unresolved after 1–2 years of symptomatic cutaneous disease. It is characterized by diffuse or nodular, tuberculoid-type granulomatous inflammation with intracytoplasmic Leishman-Donovan bodies. *Differential diagnosis*: Includes diseases with intracytoplasmic organisms. The Donovan bodies of granuloma inguinale are smaller than Leishman-Donovan bodies and stain positively with silver stains, in contrast to Leishman-Donovan bodies that are not argyrophilic. *H. capsulatum* and *S. schenckii* lack a kinetoplast and demonstrate narrow-necked budding.

References

1. Peeling RW, Hook 3rd EW. The pathogenesis of syphilis: the Great Mimicker, revisited. J Pathol. 2006;208: 224–32.
2. Schnirring-Judge M, Gustaferro C, Terol C. Vesiculobullous syphilis: a case involving an unusual cutaneous manifestation of secondary syphilis. J Foot Ankle Surg. 2011;50:96–101.
3. Avenel G, Goëb V, Abboud P, Ait-Abdesselam T, Vittecoq O. Atypical forms of syphilis: two cases. Joint Bone Spine. 2009;76:293–5.
4. Pournaras CC, Masouye I, Piletta P, Piguet V, Saurat J-H, French LE. Extensive annular verrucous late secondary syphilis. Br J Dermatol. 2005;152:1343–5.
5. Bari MM, Shulkin DJ, Abell E. Ulcerative syphilis in acquired immunodeficiency syndrome: a case of precocious tertiary syphilis in a patient infected with human immunodeficiency virus. J Am Acad Dermatol. 1989;21:1310–2.
6. Gregory N, Sanchez M, Buchness MR. The spectrum of syphilis in patients with human immunodeficiency virus infection. J Am Acad Dermatol. 1990;22:1061–7.
7. Buffet M, Grange PA, Gerhardt P, et al. Diagnosing *Treponema pallidum* in secondary syphilis by PCR and immunohistochemistry. J Invest Dermatol. 2007; 127:2345–50.
8. Jethwa HS, Schmitz JL, Dallabetta G, et al. Comparison of molecular and microscopic techniques for detection of *Treponema pallidum* in genital ulcers. J Clin Microbiol. 1995;33:180–3.
9. Carlson JA, Dabiri G, Cribier B, Sell S. The immunopathobiology of syphilis: the manifestations and course of syphilis are determined by the level of delayed-type hypersensitivity. Am J Dermatopathol. 2011;33:433–60.
10. Grimprel E, Sanchez PJ, Wendel GD, et al. Use of polymerase chain reaction and rabbit infectivity testing to detect *Treponema pallidum* in amniotic fluid, fetal and neonatal sera, and cerebrospinal fluid. J Clin Microbiol. 1991;29:1711–8.
11. Zinkernagel RM. Anti-infection immunity and autoimmunity. Ann N Y Acad Sci. 2002;958:3–6.
12. Smith G, Holman RP. The prozone phenomenon with syphilis and HIV-1 co-infection. South Med J. 2004;97:379–82.

13. Lynn WA, Lightman S. Syphilis and HIV: a dangerous combination. Lancet Infect Dis. 2004;4:456–66.
14. Don PC, Rubinstein R, Christie S. Malignant syphilis (lues maligna) and concurrent infection with HIV. Int J Dermatol. 1995;34:403–7.
15. Liotta EA, Turiansky GW, Berberian BJ, et al. Unusual presentation of secondary syphilis in 2 HIV-1 positive patients. Cutis. 2000;66:383–6.
16. Hook 3rd EW. Syphilis and HIV infection. J Infect Dis. 1989;160:530–4.
17. Lukehart SA, Hook 3rd EW, Baker-Zander SA, et al. Invasion of the central nervous system by *Treponema pallidum*: implications for diagnosis and treatment. Ann Intern Med. 1988;109:855–62.
18. Engelkens HJ, ten Kate FJ, Judanarso J, et al. The localisation of treponemes and characterisation of the inflammatory infiltrate in skin biopsies from patients with primary or secondary syphilis, or early infectious yaws. Genitourin Med. 1993;69:102–7.
19. Jeerapaet P, Ackerman AS. Histologic patterns of secondary syphilis. Arch Dermatol. 1973;107:373.
20. Martin-Ezquerra G, Fernandez-Casado A, Barco D, et al. *Treponema pallidum* distribution patterns in mucocutaneous lesions of primary and secondary syphilis: an immunohistochemical and ultrastructural study. Hum Pathol. 2009;40:624–30.
21. Hoang M, High W, Molberg K. Secondary syphilis: a histologic and immunohistochemical evaluation. J Cutan Pathol. 2004;31:595–9.
22. Lee WS, Lee MG, Chung KY, Lee JB. Detection of *Treponema pallidum* in tissue: a comparative study of the avidin-biotin-peroxidase complex, indirect immunoperoxidase. Yonsei Med J. 1991;32:335–41.
23. Gayet-Ageron A, Ninet B, Toutous-Trellu L, et al. Assessment of a real-time PCR test to diagnose syphilis from diverse biological samples. Sex Transm Infect. 2009;85:264–9.
24. Kouznetsov A, Prinz JC. Molecular diagnosis of syphilis: the Schaudinn-Hoffmann lymph-node biopsy. Lancet. 2002;360:388–9.
25. Wenhai L, Jianzhong Z, Cao Y. Detection of *Treponema pallidum* in skin lesions of secondary syphilis and characterization of the inflammatory infiltrate. Dermatology. 2004;208:94–7.
26. Sezer E, Luzar B, Calonje E. Secondary syphilis with an interstitial granuloma annulare-like histopathologic pattern. J Cutan Pathol. 2011;38:439–42.
27. Chudomirova K, Chapkanov A, Abadjieva T, Popov S. Gummatous cutaneous syphilis. Sex Transm Dis. 2009;36:239–40.
28. Mohammed TT, Olumide YM. Chancroid and human immunodeficiency virus infection – a review. Int J Dermatol. 2008;47:1–8.
29. Trees DL, Morse SA. Chancroid and *Haemophilus ducreyi*: an update. Clin Microbiol Rev. 1995;8:357–75.
30. Janowicz DM, Tenner-Racz K, Racz P, et al. Experimental infection with *Haemophilus ducreyi* in persons who are infected with HIV does not cause local or augment systemic viral replication. J Infect Dis. 2007;195:1443–51.
31. Morse SA. Chancroid and *Haemophilus ducreyi*. Clin Microbiol Rev. 1989;2:137–57.
32. Sehgal VN, Srivastava G. Chancroid: contemporary appraisal. Int J Dermatol. 2003;42:182–90.
33. Peel TN, Bhatti D, De Boer JC, Stratov I, Spelman DW. Chronic cutaneous ulcers secondary to *Haemophilus ducreyi* infection. Med J Aust. 2010;192: 348–50.
34. Janowicz DM, Li W, Bauer ME. Host-pathogen interplay of *Haemophilus ducreyi*. Curr Opin Infect Dis. 2010;23:64–9.
35. Freinkel AL. Histological aspects of sexually transmitted genital lesions. Histopathology. 1987;11:819–31.
36. Abeck D, Freinkel AL, Korting HC, Szeimis RM, Ballard RC. Immunohistochemical investigations of genital ulcers caused by *Haemophilus ducreyi*. Int J STD AIDS. 1997;8:585–8.
37. O'Farrell N. Donovanosis. Sex Transm Infect. 2002;78:452–7.
38. Wu JJ, Huang DB, Pang KR, Tyring SK. Selected sexually transmitted diseases and their relationship to HIV. Clin Dermatol. 2004;22:499–508.
39. Rashid RM, Janjua SA, Khachemoune A. Granuloma inguinale: a case report. Dermatol Online J. 2006; 12:14.
40. Sardana K, Garg VK, Arora P, Khurana N. Malignant transformation of donovanosis (granuloma inguinale) in a HIV-positive patient. Dermatol Online J. 2008;14:8.
41. Majmudar B. Granuloma inguinale (donovanosis). In: Connor DH, Chandler FW, Schwartz DA, Manz HJ, Lack EE, editors. Pathology of infectious diseases. Stamford: Appleton and Lange; 1997. p. 565–70.
42. Carter JS, Bowden FJ, Bastian I, Myers GM, Sriprakash KS, Kemp DJ. Phylogenetic evidence for reclassification of *Calymmatobacterium granulomatis* as *Klebsiella granulomatis* comb.nov. Int J Syst Bacteriol. 1999;49:1695–700.
43. Hinshaw M, Longley BJ. Fungal diseases. In: Elder DE, Elenitsas R, Johnson BL, Murphy GE, Xu G, editors. Lever's histopathology of the skin. Philadelphia: Lippincott Williams & Wilkins; 2009. p. 591–620.
44. Sellheyer K, Heneke E. Protozoan diseases and parasitic infestations. In: Elder DE, Elenitsas R, Johnson BL, Murphy GE, Xu G, editors. Lever's histopathology of the skin. Philadelphia: Lippincott Williams & Wilkins; 2009. p. 621–36.
45. Schwartz DA. Lymphogranuloma venereum. In: Connor DH, Chandler FW, Schwartz DA, Manz HJ, Lack EE, editors. Pathology of infectious diseases. Stamford: Appleton and Lange; 1997. p. 491–7.
46. Rosen T, Dhir A. Chancroid, granuloma inguinale, and lymphogranuloma venereum. In: Arndt KA, editor. Cutaneous medicine and surgery, an integrated program in dermatology. Philadelphia: WB Saunders; 1996. p. 973–82.
47. Schachter J. Chlamydial infections. N Engl J Med. 1978;298:428–35.
48. Schachter J, Osoba AO. Lymphogranuloma venereum. Br Med Bull. 1983;39:151–4.

49. Rönn MM, Ward H. The association between lymphogranuloma venereum and HIV among men who have sex with men: systematic review and meta-analysis. BMC Infect Dis. 2011;11:70.
50. Tchernev G, Costa MC, Nenoff P, Salaro C, Patterson JW. Lymphogranuloma venereum – "a clinical and histopathological chameleon?". An Bras Dermatol. 2010;85:525–30.
51. Joseph AK, Rosen T. Laboratory techniques used in the diagnosis of chancroid, granuloma inguinale, and lymphogranuloma venereum. Dermatol Clin. 1994;12: 1–8.
52. Rampf J, Essig A, Hinrichs R, Merkel M, Scharffetter-Kochanek K, Sunderkötter C. Lymphogranuloma venereum – a rare cause of genital ulcers in central Europe. Dermatology. 2004;209:230–2.
53. Whitley RJ, Roizman B. Herpes simplex virus infections. Lancet. 2001;357:1513–8.
54. Czelusta A, Yen-Moore A, Van Der Straten M, Carrasco D, Tyring SK. An overview of sexually transmitted diseases. Part III. Sexually transmitted diseases in HIV-infected patients. J Am Acad Dermatol. 2000;43:409–32.
55. Lowhagen GB, Bonde E, Forsgren-Brusk U, Runeman B, Tunback P. The microenvironment of vulvar skin in women with symptomatic and asymptomatic herpes simplex virus type 2 (HSV-2) infection. J Eur Acad Dermatol Venereol. 2006;20:1086–9.
56. Nader SN, Prober CG. Herpesvirus infections of the vulva. Semin Dermatol. 1996;15:266–8.
57. Palamaras L, Richardson D, Healy V, Lyons D, Byrne M, Lamba H. An atypical herpetic vulval ulcer in an African woman; an important lesson. Int J STD AIDS. 2006;17:427–8.
58. Reeves WC, Corey L, Adams HG, et al. Risk of recurrence after first episodes of genital herpes. Relation to HSV type and antibody response. N Engl J Med. 1981;305:15.
59. Gomes do Amaral RL, Giraldo PC, Cursino K, Goncalves AK, Eleuterio J, Giraldo H. Nodular vulvar herpes in an HIV-positive woman. Int J Gynaecol Obstet. 2009;107:255.
60. Ludwig RJ, Grundmann-Kollmann M, Holtmeier W, Wolter M, Glas J, Podda M, Kaufmann R, Zollner T. Herpes simplex virus type-2-associated eosinophilic cellulitis (Wells' syndrome). J Am Acad Dermatol. 2003;48:S60–1.
61. Adelson ME, Feola M, Trama J, Tilton RC, Mordechai E. Simultaneous detection of herpes simplex virus types 1 and 2 by real-time PCR and pyrosequencing. J Clin Virol. 2005;33:25–34.
62. Xu X, Erickson L, Chen L, Elder DE. Diseases caused by viruses. In: Elder DE, Elenitsas R, Johnson BL, Murphy GE, Xu G, editors. Lever's histopathology of the skin. Philadelphia: Lippincott Williams & Wilkins; 2009. p. 637–65.
63. Khalifa MA, Lack EE. Herpes simplex virus infection. In: Connor DH, Chandler FW, Schwartz DA, Manz HJ, Lack EE, editors. Pathology of infectious diseases, vol. 1. Stamford: Appleton and Lange; 1997. p. 147–52.
64. Choi SW, Yang JE, Kang SJ, Lee HR, Kim CW. Herpetic infection on the vulva associated with eccrine squamous syringometaplasia in malignant lymphoma. Acta Derm Venereol. 1999;79(6):500–1.
65. Muñoz E, Valks R, Fernández-Herrera J, Fraga J. Herpetic syringitis associated with eccrine squamous syringometaplasia in HIV-positive patients. J Cutan Pathol. 1997;24:425–8.
66. Frimer M, Chudnoff S, Hebert T, Shahabi S. Pseudoepitheliomatous hyperplasia mimicking vulvar cancer in a patient with AIDS. J Low Genit Tract Dis. 2011;15:66–8.
67. Maharaj R, Parboosing R, Moodley M, Naicker S, Ramdial PK. An unusual hypertrophic genital mass lesion – a diagnostic and treatment dilemma. J Clin Virol. 2009;46:303–4.
68. Hall CS, Klausner JD. Diagnostic tests for common STDs and HSV-2. Sex Transm Dis. 2004;36:10–21.
69. Leinweber B, Kerl H, Cerroni L. Histopathologic features of cutaneous herpes virus infections (Herpes simplex, Herpes varicella/zoster). A broad spectrum of presentations with common pseudolymphomatous aspects. Am J Surg Pathol. 2006;30:50–8.
70. Aroutcheva AA, Simoes JA, Behbakht K, Faro S. *Gardnerella vaginalis* isolated from patients with bacterial vaginosis and from patients with healthy vaginal ecosystems. Clin Infect Dis. 2001;33:1022–7.
71. Udayalaxmi J, Bhat GK, Kotigadde S. Biotypes and virulence factors of *Gardnerella vaginalis* isolated from cases of bacterial vaginosis. Indian J Med Microbiol. 2011;29:165–8.
72. Modak T, Arora P, Agnes C, Tay R, Goswami S, Ghosh P, Das NK. Diagnosis of bacterial vaginosis in cases of abnormal vaginal discharge: comparison of clinical and microbiological criteria. J Infect Dev Ctries. 2011;5:353–60.
73. Eady EA, Cove JH. Staphylococcal resistance revisited: community-acquired methicillin resistant *Staphylococcus aureus* – an emerging problem for the management of skin and soft tissue infections. Curr Opin Infect Dis. 2003;16:103–24.
74. Kilpatrick CC, Alagkiozidis I, Orejuela FJ, Chohan L, Hollier LM. Factors complicating surgical management of the vulvar abscess. J Reprod Med. 2010;55:139–42.
75. Reichman O, Sobel JD. MRSA infection of buttocks, vulva, and genital tract in women. Curr Infect Dis Rep. 2009;11:465–70.
76. Bleker OP, Smalbraak DJC, Schutte MF. Bartholin's abscess: the role of *Chlamydia trachomatis*. Genitourin Med. 1990;66:24–5.
77. Bora SA, Condous G. Bartholin's vulval and perineal abscesses. Best Pract Res Clin Obstet Gynaecol. 2009;23:661–6.
78. Pinsky BA, Baron EJ, Janda JM, Banaei N. Bartholin's abscess caused by hypermucoviscous *Klebsiella pneumoniae*. J Med Microbiol. 2009;58:671–3.

79. Rees E. Gonococcal bartholinitis. Br J Vener Dis. 1967;43:150–6.
80. Cabrera H, Skoczdopole L, Marini M, Giovanna PD, Saponaro A, Echeverría C. Necrotizing gangrene of the genitalia and perineum. Int J Dermatol. 2002;41: 847–51.
81. Martinelli G, Alessandrino EP, Bernasconi P, et al. Fournier's gangrene: a clinical presentation of necrotizing fasciitis after bone marrow transplantation. Bone Marrow Transplant. 1998;22:1023–6.
82. O'Dell ML. Skin and wound infections: an overview. Am Fam Physician. 1998;15:2424–32.
83. Karakatsanis G, Vakirlis E, Kastoridou C, Devliotou-Panagiotidou D. Co-existence of pityriasis versicolor and erythrasma. Mycoses. 2004;47:343–5.
84. Knox JM. Cutaneous inflammations and infections. Clin Obstet Gynecol. 1978;21:991–1005.
85. Sindhuphak W, MacDonald E, Smith EB. Erythrasma: overlooked or misdiagnosed. Int J Dermatol. 1985;24:95–6.
86. Kogulan PK, Smith M, Seidman J, et al. Malakoplakia involving the abdominal wall, urinary bladder, vagina and vulva: case report and discussion of malakoplakia-associated bacteria. Int J Gynecol Pathol. 2001;20:403–6.
87. Ramdial PK, Sing Y, Chotey NA, Bagratee JS. Concomitant malakoplakia and granuloma of the cervix in acquired immune deficiency syndrome. Int J Gynecol Pathol. 2008;27:282–7.
88. Lou TY, Teplitz C. Malacoplakia: pathogenesis and ultrastructural morphogenesis. A problem of altered macrophage (phagolysosomal) response. Hum Pathol. 1974;5:191–207.
89. van Crevel R, Curfs J, van der Ven AJAM, et al. Functional and morphological monocyte abnormalities in a patient with malakoplakia. Am J Med. 1998;105:74–7.
90. Yousef GM, Naghibi B. Malakoplakia outside the urinary tract. Arch Pathol Lab Med. 2007;131:297–300.
91. Achkar JM, Fries BC. Candida infections of the genitourinary tract. Clin Microbiol Rev. 2010;23: 253–73.
92. McClelland RS, Richardson BA, Hassan WM, et al. Prospective study of vaginal bacterial flora and other risk factors for vulvovaginal candidiasis. J Infect Dis. 2009;199:1883–90.
93. Jacobsen MD, Duncan AD, Bain J, et al. Mixed *Candida albicans* strain populations in colonized and infected mucosal tissues. FEMS Yeast Res. 2008;8: 1334–8.
94. Goswami RVD, Tejaswi S, Datta K, et al. Species-specific prevalence of vaginal candidiasis among patients with diabetes mellitus and its relation to their glycaemic status. J Infect. 2000;41:162–6.
95. Sobel JD. Vulvovaginal candidoses. Lancet. 2007;369:1961–71.
96. Galvin SR, Cohen MS. The role of sexually transmitted diseases in HIV transmission. Nat Rev Microbiol. 2004;2:33–42.
97. Laga M, Manoka A, Kivuvu M, et al. Non-ulcerative sexually transmitted diseases as risk factors for HIV-1 transmission in diseases as risk factors for HIV-transmission in women: results from a cohort study. AIDS. 1993;7:95–102.
98. Ryu JS, Min DY. Trichomonas vaginalis and trichomoniasis in the Republic of Korea. Korean J Parasitol. 2006;44:101–16.
99. Petrin D, Delgaty K, Bhatt R, Garber G. Clinical and microbiological aspects of *Trichomonas vaginalis*. Clin Microbiol Rev. 1998;11:300–17.
100. Wolner-Hanssen P, Krieger JN, Stevens CE, et al. Clinical manifestations of vaginal trichomoniasis. JAMA. 1989;27:571–6.
101. Schwebke JR, Burgess D. Trichomoniasis. Clin Microbiol Rev. 2004;17:794–803.
102. Ryu JS, Chung HL, Min DY, Cho YH, Ro YS, Kim SR. Diagnosis of trichomoniasis by polymerase chain reaction. Yonsei Med J. 1999;40:56–60.
103. Anderson AL, Chaney E. Pubic lice (*Phthirus pubis*): history, biology and treatment vs knowledge and beliefs of US college students. Int J Environ Res Public Health. 2009;6:592–600.
104. Ko SJ, Elston DM. Pediculosis. J Am Acad Dermatol. 2004;50:1–12.
105. Bakos I, Reusch MC, D'Elia P, Aquino V, Bakos RM. Crusted scabies of the vulva. J Eur Acad Dermatol Venereol. 2007;21:681–721.
106. Bumb RA, Mehta RD. Amoebiasis cutis in HIV positive patient. Indian J Dermatol Venereol Leprol. 2006;72:224–6.
107. Magaña M, Magaña ML, Alcántara A, Pérez-Martin M. Histopathology of cutaneous amebiasis. Am J Dermatopathol. 2004;26:280–4.
108. Parshad S, Grover PS, Sharma A, Verma DK, Sharma A. Primary cutaneous amoebiasis: case report with review of the literature. Int J Dermatol. 2002;41: 676–80.
109. Stanley Jr SL. Amoebiasis. Lancet. 2003;361:1025–34.
110. Leippe M. Amoebapores. Parasitol Today. 1997;13:178–83.
111. Seydel KB, Li E, Swanson PE, et al. Human intestinal epithelial cells produce pro-inflammatory cytokines in response to infection in a SCID mouse-human intestinal xenograft model of amebiasis. Infect Immun. 1997;65:1631–9.
112. Stenson WF, Zhang Z, Riehl T, et al. Amebic infection in the human colon induces cyclo-oxygenase-2. Infect Immun. 2001;69:3382–8.
113. Jarumilinta R, Kradolfer F. The toxic effect of *Entamoeba histolytica* on leucocytes. Ann Trop Med Parasitol. 1964;58:375–81.
114. Ramdial PK, Calonje E, Singh B, Bagratee JS, Singh SM, Sydney C. Amebiasis cutis revisited. J Cutan Pathol. 2007;34:620–8.
115. Avelar LGA, Nahum LA, Andrade LF, Oliveira G. Functional diversity of the *Schistosoma mansoni* tyrosine kinases. J Signal Transduct. 2011;2011: 603290.

116. Feldmeier H, Krantz I, Poggensee G. Female genital schistosomiasis as a risk-factor for the transmission of HIV. Int J STD AIDS. 1994;5:368–72.
117. Von Lichtenburg F. Schistosomiasis. In: Schwartz DA, Manz HJ, Lack EE, Connor DH, Chandler FW, editors. Pathology of infectious diseases, vol. 1. Stamford: Appleton and Lange; 1997. p. 1537–52.
118. Leslie TA, Goldsmith PC, Dowd PM. Vulval schistosomiasis. J R Soc Med. 1993;86:51.
119. Helling-Giese G, Sjaastad A, Poggensee G, et al. Female genital schistosomiasis (FGS): relationship between gynaecological and histopathological findings. Acta Trop. 1996;62:257–67.
120. Ismail M, Botros B, Metwally A, et al. Resistance to praziquantel: direct evidence from *Schistosoma mansoni* isolated from Egyptian villagers. Am J Trop Med Hyg. 1999;60:932–5.
121. Utzinger J, Keiser J, Shuhua X, Tanner M, Singer BH. Combination chemotherapy of schistosomiasis in laboratory studies and clinical trials. Antimicrob Agents Chemother. 2003;47:1487–95.
122. Zhou L, Tang J, Zhao Y, et al. A highly sensitive TaqMan real-time PCR assay for early detection of *Schistosoma* species. Acta Trop. 2011;120:88–94.
123. Ramdial PK. Transepithelial elimination of late cutaneous vulval schistosomiasis. Int J Gynecol Pathol. 2001;20:166–72.
124. Sinniah B. Enterobiasis. In: Connor DH, Chandler FW, Schwartz DA, Manz HJ, Lack EE, editors. Pathology of infectious diseases, vol. 1. Stamford: Appleton and Lange; 1997. p. 1415–8.
125. Konanahalli P, Menon P, Walsh MY, McCluggage WG. *Enterobius vermicularis* (pinworm) infestation of the vulva: report of 2 cases of a pseudoneoplastic lesion mimicking squamous carcinoma. Int J Gynecol Pathol. 2010;29:490–3.
126. McMahon JN, Connolly CE, Long SV, Meehan FP. Enterobius granulomas of the uterus, ovary and pelvic peritoneum. Two case reports. Br J Obstet Gynaecol. 1984;91:289–90.
127. Sun T, Schwartz NS, Sewell C, Lieberman P, Gross S. Enterobius egg granuloma of the vulva and peritoneum: review of the literature. Am J Trop Med Hyg. 1991;45:249–53.
128. Dutt AK. Epidemiology and host factors. In: Schlossberg D, editor. Tuberculosis and non-tuberculous mycobacterial infection. 5th ed. New York: McGraw-Hill; 2006. p. 1–17.
129. Lange C, Mori T. Advances in the diagnosis of tuberculosis. Respirology. 2010;15:220–40.
130. Shen HP, Chang WC, Hsieh CH, Yang TC, Hung YC. Vulvar tuberculosis. Taiwan J Obstet Gynecol. 2011;50:106–8.
131. Dhall K, Das SS, Dey P. Tuberculosis of Bartholin's gland. Int J Gynecol Obstet. 1995;48:223–4.
132. Brenner BN. Tuberculosis of the vulva. S Afr Med J. 1976;50:1798–800.
133. Manoj K, Soma M, Ajay L, Ashish A, Rakesh S, Paliwal RV. Tubercular sinus of labia majora: rare case report. Infect Dis Obstet Gynecol. 2008;2012;31:390–394. doi: 10.1155/2008/817515.
134. Mendiratta V, Harjai B, Sardana K. Tubercular lymphadenitis with lymphangiectasia of the vulva. J Eur Acad Dermatol Venereol. 2005;19:255–69.
135. Naik RPC, Srinivas CR, Balachandran C, Narayan PK, Ramnarayan K, Sahoo RC. Esthiomene resulting from cutaneous tuberculosis of external genitalia. Genitourin Med. 1987;63:133–4.
136. Talwar A, Puri N, Sandhu HPS. Vulval lymphoedema following pulmonary tuberculosis. Int J STD AIDS. 2009;20:437–9.
137. Trussell RR. Ulcerative and hypertrophic lesions of the vulva. Proc R Soc Med. 1968;61:363–5.
138. Millar JW, Holt S, Gilmour HM, Robertson DH. Vulvar tuberculosis. Tubercle. 1979;6:173–6.
139. Nogales-Ortiz F, Tarancon I, Nogales Jr FF. The pathology of female genital tuberculosis. A 31-year study of 1436 cases. Obstet Gynecol. 1979;53:422–8.
140. Ramdial PK, Mosam A, Mallett R, Aboobaker J. Papulonecrotic tuberculid in a 2-year-old girl: with emphasis on extent of disease and presence of leucocytoclastic vasculitis. Pediatr Dermatol. 1998;15:450–5.
141. Wong S, Rizvi H, Cerio R, O'Toole EA. An unusual case of vulval papulonecrotic tuberculid. Clin Exp Dermatol. 2010;36:277–80.
142. Pandhi D, Mehta S, Singal A. Genital tuberculid in a female child: a new entity (childhood vulval tuberculid). Pediatr Dermatol. 2007;24:573–5.
143. Amin I, Idrees M, Awan Z, Shahid M, Afzal S, Hussain A. PCR could be a method of choice for identification of both pulmonary and extrapulmonary tuberculosis. BMC Res Notes. 2011;4:332.
144. Amsbaugh S, Huiras E, Wang NS, et al. Bacillary angiomatosis associated with pseudoepitheliomatous hyperplasia. Am J Dermatopathol. 2006;28:32–5.
145. Chian CA, Arrese JE, Piérard GE. Skin manifestations of *Bartonella* infections. Int J Dermatol. 2002;41:461–6.
146. Weedon D. Vascular tumors. In: Weedon D, editor. Weedon's skin pathology. Philadelphia: Churchill Livingstone/Elsevier; 2010. p. 887–925.
147. Maguiña C, Guerra H, Ventosilla P. Bartonellosis. Clin Dermatol. 2009;27:271–80.
148. Minnick MF, Battisti JM. Pestilence, persistence and pathogenicity: infection strategies of *Bartonella*. Future Microbiol. 2009;4:743–58.
149. Long SR, Whitfeld MJ, Eades C, et al. Bacillary angiomatosis of the cervix and vulva in a patient with AIDS. Obstet Gynecol. 1996;88:709–11.
150. Ramdial PK, Sing Y, Ramburan A, Dlova NC, Bagratee JS, Calonje E. *Bartonella quintana*-induced vulval bacillary angiomatosis. Int J Gynecol Pathol (in press). 2012;31:390–394.
151. Tappero JW, Koehler JE, Berger TG, et al. Bacillary angiomatosis and bacillary splenitis in immunocompetent adults. Ann Intern Med. 1993;118:363–5.

152. Kaisar MO, Kirwan RM, Strutton GM, et al. Cutaneous manifestations of cytomegalovirus disease in renal transplant recipients: a case series. Transpl Infect Dis. 2008;10:209–13.
153. AbdullGaffar B, Raman LG, Muala AA. Cutaneous cytomegalovirus infection in a patient with acquired immunodeficiency syndrome. Int J Dermatol. 2008;47:944–6.
154. Pitarch G, Torrijos A, Garcia-Escriva D, Martinez-Menchon T. Eruptive pseudoangiomatosis associated to cytomegalovirus infection. Eur J Dermatol. 2007;17:455–6.
155. Ramdial PK, Dlova NC, Sydney C. Cytomegalovirus neuritis in perineal ulcers. J Cutan Pathol. 2002;29:439–44.
156. Choi YL, Kim JA, Jang KT, Kim DS, Kim WS, Lee JH, Yang JM, Lee ES, Lee DY. Characteristics of cutaneous cytomegalovirus infection in non-acquired immune deficiency syndrome, immunocompromised patients. Br J Dermatol. 2006;155:977–82.
157. Dauden E, Fernandez-Buezo G, Fraga J, Cardenoso L, Garcia-Diez A. Mucocutaneous presence of cytomegalovirus associated with human immunodeficiency virus infection. Arch Dermatol. 2001;137:443–8.
158. Ryan C, De Gascun CF, Powell C, Sheaban K, Mooney EE, McCormick A, Kirby B. Cytomegalovirus-induced cutaneous vasculopathy and perianal ulceration. J Am Acad Dermatol. 2011;64:1216–8.
159. Halvorsen JA, Brevig T, Aas T, Skar AG, Slevolden EM, Moi H. Genital ulcers as initial manifestation of Epstein-Barr virus infection: Two new cases and a review of the literature. Acta Derm Venereol. 2006;86:439–42.
160. Barnes CJ, Alió AB, Cunningham BB, Friedlander SF. Epstein-Barr virus-associated genital ulcers: an under-recognised disorder. Pediatr Dermatol. 2007;24:130–4.
161. O'Connell C, Oranje A, Van Gysel D, Silverberg NB. Congenital molluscum contagiosum: report of four cases and review of the literature. Pediatr Dermatol. 2008;25:553–6.
162. Lin HY, Linn G, Liu CB, Chen CJ, Yu KJ. An immunocompromised woman with severe molluscum contagiosum that responded well to topical imiquimod: a case report and literature review. Am Soc Colpos Cerv Pathol. 2010;14:134–5.
163. Palit A, Inamadar AC. Papulonodular genital growths in an HIV-infected woman. Clin Infect Dis. 2004;38:1585–633.
164. Fischer GO. Vulval disease in pre-pubertal girls. Australas J Dermatol. 2001;42:225–36.
165. Fischer G, Rogers M. Vulvar disease in children: a clinical audit of 130 cases. Pediatr Dermatol. 2000;17:1–6.
166. Chang SE, Lee DK, Choi JH, Moon KC, Koh JK. Majocchi's granuloma of the vulva caused by *Trichophyton* mentagrophytes. Mycoses. 2005;48:382–4.
167. Ashbee HR, Evans EGV. Immunology of diseases associated with *Malassezia* species. Clin Microbiol Rev. 2002;15:21–57.
168. Bonifaz A, Cansela R, Novales J, Montes de Oca G, Navarrete G, Romo J. Cutaneous histoplasmosis associated with acquired immunodeficiency syndrome (AIDS). Int J Dermatol. 2000;39:35–8.
169. Friedman A, Solomon G, Segal-Maurer S, Pereira F. Sudden onset of verrucous plaques to the face and trunk: a case of reactivation cutaneous histoplasmosis in the setting of HIV. Dermatol Online J. 2008;14:12.
170. Ramdial PK, Mosam A, Dlova NC, Satar NB, Aboobaker J, Singh S. Disseminated cutaneous histoplasmosis in patients infected with human immunodeficiency virus. J Cutan Pathol. 2002;29:215–25.
171. Isotalo PA, McCarthy AE, Eidus L. Ovarian histoplasmosis in systemic lupus erythematosus. Pathology. 2000;32:139–41.
172. Chandler FW, Watts JC. Histoplasmosis capsulati. In: Connor DH, Chandler FW, Schwartz DA, Manz HJ, Lack EE, editors. Pathology of infectious diseases. Stamford: Appleton and Lange; 1997. p. 1007–15.
173. Smith MB, Schnadig VJ, Zaharopoulos P, Van Hook C. Disseminated histoplasma capsulatum infection presenting as genital ulcerations. Obstet Gynecol. 1997;89:842–4.
174. Sills M, Schwartz A, Weg JG. Conjugal histoplasmosis. A consequence of progressive dissemination in the index case after steroid therapy. Ann Intern Med. 1973;79:221–4.
175. Bonifaz A, Chang P, Moreno K, et al. Disseminated cutaneous histoplasmosis in acquired immunodeficiency syndrome: report of 23 cases. Clin Exp Dermatol. 2008;34:481–6.
176. Eidbo J, Sanchez RL, Tschen JA, Ellner KM. Cutaneous manifestations of histoplasmosis in the acquired immune deficiency syndrome. Am J Surg Pathol. 1993;17:110–6.
177. Chandler FW, Watts JC. Cryptococcosis. In: Connor DH, Chandler FW, Schwartz DA, Manz HJ, Lack EE, editors. Pathology of infectious diseases. Stamford: Appleton and Lange; 1997. p. 989–97.
178. Durden FM, Elewski B. Cutaneous involvement with *Cryptococcus neoformans* in AIDS. J Am Acad Dermatol. 1994;30:844–8.
179. Manfredi R, Mazzoni A, Nanetti A, Mastroianni A, Coronado O, Chiodo F. Morphologic features and clinical significance of skin involvement in patients with AIDS-related cryptococcosis. Acta Derm Venereol (Stockh). 1996;76:72–4.
180. Christianson JC, Engber W, Andes D. Primary cutaneous cryptococcosis in immunocompetent and immunocompromised hosts. Med Mycol. 2003;41:177–88.
181. Ranganathan S, Moosa F, Kamarulzaman A, Looi LM. MRI and CT findings of cryptococcal vaginitis. Br J Radiol. 2005;78:353–4.

182. Sing Y, Ramdial PK, Ibrahim T. Cryptococcosis masquerading as a tuboovarian abscess. Int J Gynecol Pathol. 2007;27:37–40.
183. Blocher KS, Weeks JA, Noble RC. Cutaneous cryptococcal infection presenting as a vulvar lesion. Genitourin Med. 1987;63:341–3.
184. Chen CK, Chang DY, Chang SC, Lee EF, Huang SC, Chow SN. Cryptococcal infection of the vagina. Obstet Gynecol. 1993;81:867–9.
185. Cabello I, Caraballo A, Millan Y. Leishmaniasis in the genital area. Case report. Rev Inst Med Trop Sao Paulo. 2002;44:105–7.
186. Agostoni C, Migliorini D, Dorigoni N, Malfitano A, Scaglia M. Genital ulcer in an AIDS patient with disseminated leishmaniasis. Eur J Clin Microbiol Infect Dis. 1998;17:813–4.
187. Lindoso JAL, Barbosa RN, Posada-Vergara MP, Duarte MIS, Oyafuso LK, Amato VS, Goto H. Unusual manifestations of tegumentary leishmaniasis in AIDS patients from the New World. Br J Dermatol. 2009;160:311–8.
188. Rathi SK, Pandhi RK, Khanna N, Chopra P. Mucosal and peri-orificial involvement in Post-Kala-Azar dermal leishmaniasis. Indian J Dermatol Venereol Leprol. 2004;70:280–2.
189. Richens J. Genital manifestations of tropical diseases. Sex Transm Infect. 2004;80:12–7.

Noninfectious Dermatoses of the Vulva

3

Boštjan Luzar and Eduardo Calonje

Abstract

This chapter covers inflammatory dermatoses that affect the vulva primarily or secondarily in association with cutaneous or mucosal involvement elsewhere as well as the most common inflammatory systemic diseases that affect this organ. Each entity is outlined according to its definition, clinical features, most relevant epidemiological and demographical data, and pathogenesis where relevant. Defining histological features are detailed, with special emphasis given to the morphological diversity of the lesions at this particular location as a result of dampness, occlusion, and friction. Description of the entity is finally completed by the discussion of the most relevant differential diagnoses, whenever deemed necessary.

Infantile Gluteal Granuloma

Infantile gluteal granuloma, also called papuloerosive dermatitis of Jacquet and Sevestre, is a rare variant of diaper dermatitis, most commonly occurring in newborn and infants [1–5]. Clinically, well-demarcated papules or nodules with frequent erosions and ulcers develop on the genital skin but also perineal and sometimes perianal areas. Main etiological factors suggested in the development of infantile gluteal granuloma include urine and feces; however, infections by Candida and the use of corticosteroids have also been implicated [6]. Infantile gluteal granuloma in the majority of cases regresses spontaneously over the course of weeks after removing the offending agent, occasionally with scarring [7].

A similar condition has also been reported in children with Hirschsprung's disease following colo-anal anastomosis and subsequent chronic diarrhea and in adult, incontinent women [8–13]. With incontinent women, the labia majora are mostly involved.

Histological Features

The histological features are often entirely nonspecific, and the diagnosis relies heavily on

B. Luzar, M.D., Ph.D.
Medical Faculty, Institute of Pathology,
University of Ljubljana,
Ljubljana, Slovenia

E. Calonje, M.D., DipRCPath (✉)
Department of Dermatopathology,
St. John's Institute of Dermatology,
St. Thomas' Hospital, Westminster Bridge Road,
London SE1 7EH, UK
e-mail: jaime.calonje@kcl.ac.uk

L. Brown (ed.), *Pathology of the Vulva and Vagina*, Essentials of Diagnostic Gynecological Pathology,
DOI 10.1007/978-0-85729-757-0_3,

clinical presentation only. The surface epithelium is frequently ulcerated. In the dermis, there is a prominent inflammatory cell infiltrate composed of lymphocytes, plasma cells, and histiocytes. Areas of erythrocyte extravasation and deposition of hemosiderin pigment can also be seen. Formation of granulomas is rarely appreciated.

Genital Eczema

The term "eczema" is an expression used for a number of clinical conditions that have in common similar clinical and histological features but are frequently unrelated etiologically [14]. These conditions are frequently referred to as "eczematous dermatitides" or "eczema" and are characterized clinically by development of erythema with pruritic papules or papulovesicles that rupture easily with subsequent development of scale crust [14]. When severe, erosions and rarely ulcers can be seen [15]. Persistence of lesions is associated with formation of poorly delineated erythematous scaly plaques, and long-standing lesions frequently become lichenified, progressing to lichen simplex chronicus. The clinical features of "eczematous dermatitides" can vary according to the severity of the disease, site of presentation, duration of changes, individual predisposition, as well as secondary changes due to scratching, rubbing, and superimposed infection.

The exact prevalence of "eczematous dermatitides" of the vulva is not known. However, incidences from 20% to 30% and even as high as 64% have been reported in patients attending specialized clinics [16–22]. In a study of 89 patients with chronic vulvar pain, patients with genital eczema were usually diagnosed in their fifth decade of life (mean 43 years) [21]. Vulvar involvement can represent an isolated condition or be part of a more generalized dermatitis [16]. The main presenting symptom of genital eczema is pruritus, followed by irritation and burning [23].

Eczematous dermatitis has traditionally been classified as exogenous (irritant and allergic contact dermatitis) and endogenous (atopic and seborrheic) dermatitis [24]. While some studies have determined irritant contact dermatitis to be the most common type of genital dermatitis [23], others have demonstrated the predominance of atopic and/or seborrheic dermatitis [16]. Irritant contact dermatitis generally follows exposure to chemical, physical, or biological substances capable of direct skin damage. In the vulva, it can be attributed to diverse etiological factors, for example, urine, feces, deodorants, detergents, perfume, sanitary napkins, soap, antiseptics, disinfectants, as well as various solvents [20, 23, 25]. The lesions usually develop rapidly, depending on the length of exposure, and the type of triggering agent. Clinical presentation vary from mild erythema to ulceration and rarely, necrosis. Vesiculation can be seen in severe cases but is uncommon in the vulva due to the site-specific laxity of the tissue [26]. Allergic contact dermatitis represents a cell-mediated immunological reaction requiring previous sensitization with the particular antigen (allergen) and usually develops 12–48 h after the sensitization [27]. The most common allergens in the vulva include nickel, fragrances, latex, and particularly various drugs like antibiotics, corticosteroids, or topical anesthetics [20, 23, 24]. The lesions can spread outside of the exposed area. Mixed irritant and allergic contact dermatitis of the vulva are not uncommon [23]. Additional patch testing is often necessary to confirm the diagnosis of allergic contact dermatitis. Seborrheic dermatitis of the genital skin most commonly affects genitocrural folds and can be associated with similar lesions at other flexural sites. It is characterized by ill-defined scaly orange-red macules and papules with sticky crusts and fissures [26]. *Pityrosporum* ovale has been implicated in the pathogenesis of the disease elsewhere, although maceration of the skin at this particular site is also likely to play a role [28]. Patients with atopic dermatitis frequently have personal and/or family history of atopy, such as asthma, allergic conjunctivitis, or allergic rhinitis [24, 29]. Atopic dermatitis shows predilection for children and can begin in infancy [30]. A study on 130 prepubertal girls found atopic and irritant dermatitis to be as high as 33% [30]. Another study on vulvar dermatitides showed a history of atopic dermatitis in 78% of the patients [17]. Intractable pruritus can on occasion be present. Initial lesions

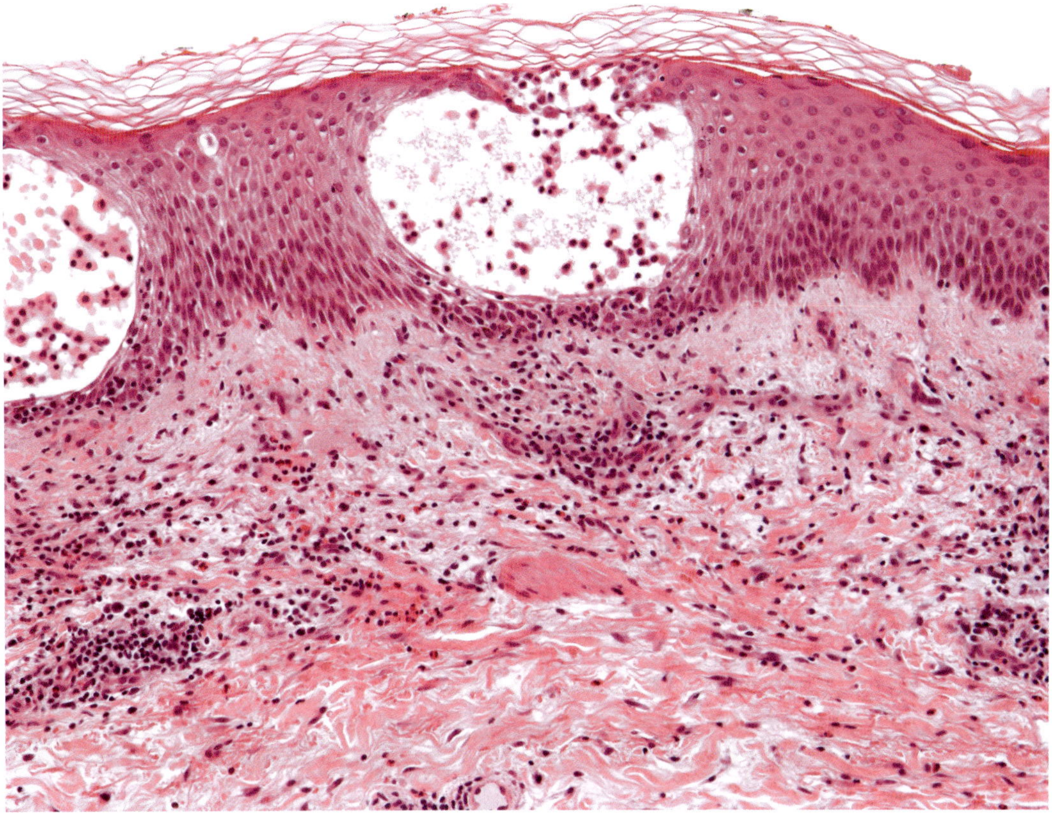

Fig. 3.1 Acute spongiotic dermatitis. Prominent spongiosis leads to intraepidermal vesicle formation and this is associated with exocytosis of inflammatory cells

present as erythema, with subsequent development of excoriated papules and vesicles, eventually becoming lichenified.

Histological Features

The microscopic features of spongiotic dermatitides of the vulva are identical to those seen in the skin elsewhere, but due to the special microenvironment of the area, particularly with regards to occlusion, secondary changes including crusting are more frequent. The common histological denominator of different "eczematous dermatitides" is the spongiotic reaction pattern, one of the most frequently encountered patterns in inflammatory skin diseases [31–33]. The primary feature of spongiotic dermatitis is the presence of epidermal spongiosis, which is defined as intercellular edema between keratinocytes due to the accumulation of edema fluid within the epidermis [31–33]. Spongiotic dermatitis is an inflammatory process that typically involves the epidermis and superficial dermis. However, the follicular infundibula, acrosyringia, and rarely, the deeper dermis can also be affected.

Three stages of spongiotic dermatitis can be separated, albeit arbitrarily, representing a continuum of changes as lesions evolve (1) acute, (2) subacute, and (3) chronic [14, 31–33]. Different stages of the lesions can coexist in the same patient. Acute spongiotic dermatitis is characterized by the normal thickness of the epidermis, which is usually covered by normal basket-weave stratum corneum. Keratinocytes are pale, the desmosomes are widened or disrupted, and this results in the formation of spongiotic microvesicles. These may enlarge with the formation of small blisters or larger vesicles (Fig. 3.1). The papillary dermis is edematous.

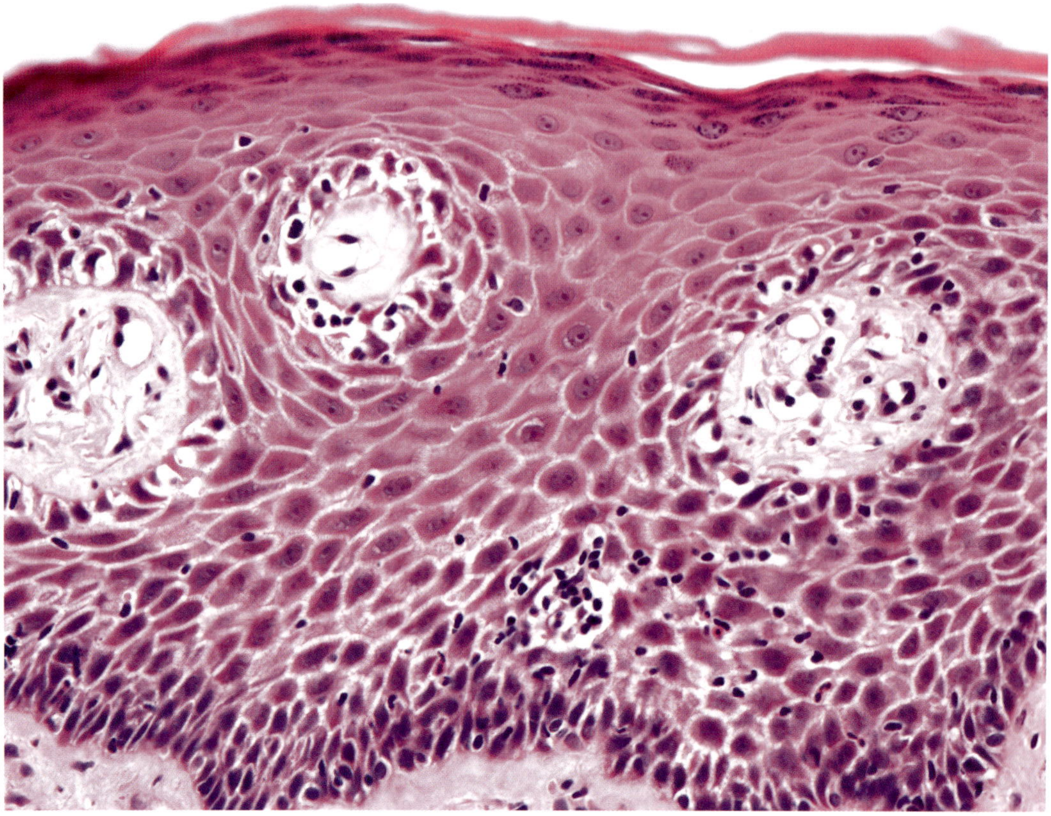

Fig. 3.2 Subacute spongiotic dermatitis. The epidermis becomes acanthotic, and spongiosis is focal and associated with exocytosis of lymphocytes

The inflammatory cell infiltrate in the dermis is usually superficial and perivascular but the distribution can be variable. The predominant inflammatory cells are lymphocytes and histiocytes, with frequent admixture of eosinophils and less often neutrophils. A scale crust consisting of proteinaceous material with fibrin, neutrophils, and parakeratotic cells frequently starts to evolve. Subacute spongiotic dermatitis is characterized by additional reactive changes of the epidermis, such as thickening (acanthosis) and the replacement of normal stratum corneum by parakeratosis. Some degree of psoriasiform hyperplasia is usually seen (Fig. 3.2). The granular layer can be diminished. Spongiosis is usually mild to moderate. The dermal inflammatory cell infiltrate and the papillary edema are less pronounced than in the acute phase. Scale crust can be seen. Chronic spongiotic dermatitis results from the persistence of the inflammatory process for a prolonged period of time. The epidermis is acanthotic, associated with compact orthokeratosis, decreasing parakeratosis, and hypergranulosis (Fig. 3.3). Spongiosis is usually minimal, and the inflammatory cell infiltrate in the dermis is often mild. Fibrosis of the dermis can be prominent. Changes secondary to excoriation are frequently present. In chronic cases, development of lichen simplex chronicus is often seen (see below).

Importantly, it is not possible to separate between different clinical variants of eczema on histological grounds alone, and clinical correlation is of utmost importance to assign a more specific diagnosis than spongiotic dermatitis. Langerhans cell microabscesses in the epidermis, when present, have been regarded as an important feature in the diagnosis of allergic contact

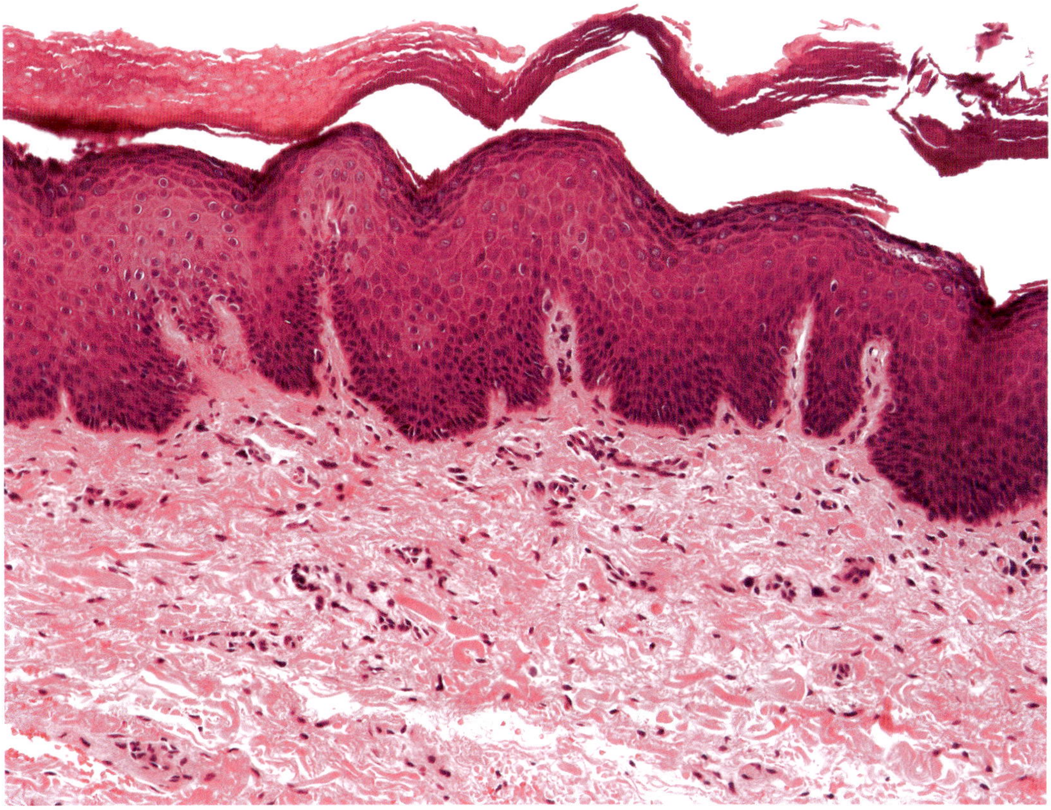

Fig. 3.3 Chronic spongiotic dermatitis. In chronic spongiotic processes, spongiosis is usually minimal or absent, and there is progressive psoriasiform hyperplasia of the epidermis with compact hyperkeratosis

dermatitis [26]. In our experience, however, this feature can be present in any type of spongiotic dermatitis (Fig. 3.4). Irritant contact dermatitis as any other type of spongiotic dermatitis can display a wide range of secondary changes including crusting. These changes are frequently associated with neutrophil exocytosis (Fig. 3.5). Eosinophilic spongiosis can be present in both allergic and irritant contact dermatitis. Although eosinophils have traditionally been regarded as characteristic or defining feature of contact dermatitis, they may on occasion be scarce or even absent. Contrarywise, the presence of eosinophils in an infiltrate does not imply a contact dermatitis as an etiological factor. The dermal inflammatory cell infiltrate is usually less pronounced in irritant contact dermatitis. Seborrheic dermatitis frequently demonstrates more prominent psoriasiform hyperplasia.

Differential Diagnosis

The differential diagnosis includes candidiasis and dermatophyte infections. Dermatophyte infections of the vulva are almost nonexistent but do occur on the groins. They are characterized clinically by annular erythema with scaling, frequently associated with maceration and bulla formation. Central clearing of the lesion is typical seen. Histologically, both candidiasis and dermatophyte infections have similar histological features. The epidermis is parakeratotic, and there are subcorneal and intraepidermal neutrophils or necrotic debris. Pustules may be seen. Fungal hyphae (dermatophytes) and spores and pseudohyphae (Candida) can usually be appreciated on sections stained with H&E but can additionally be highlighted by PAS or silver stains.

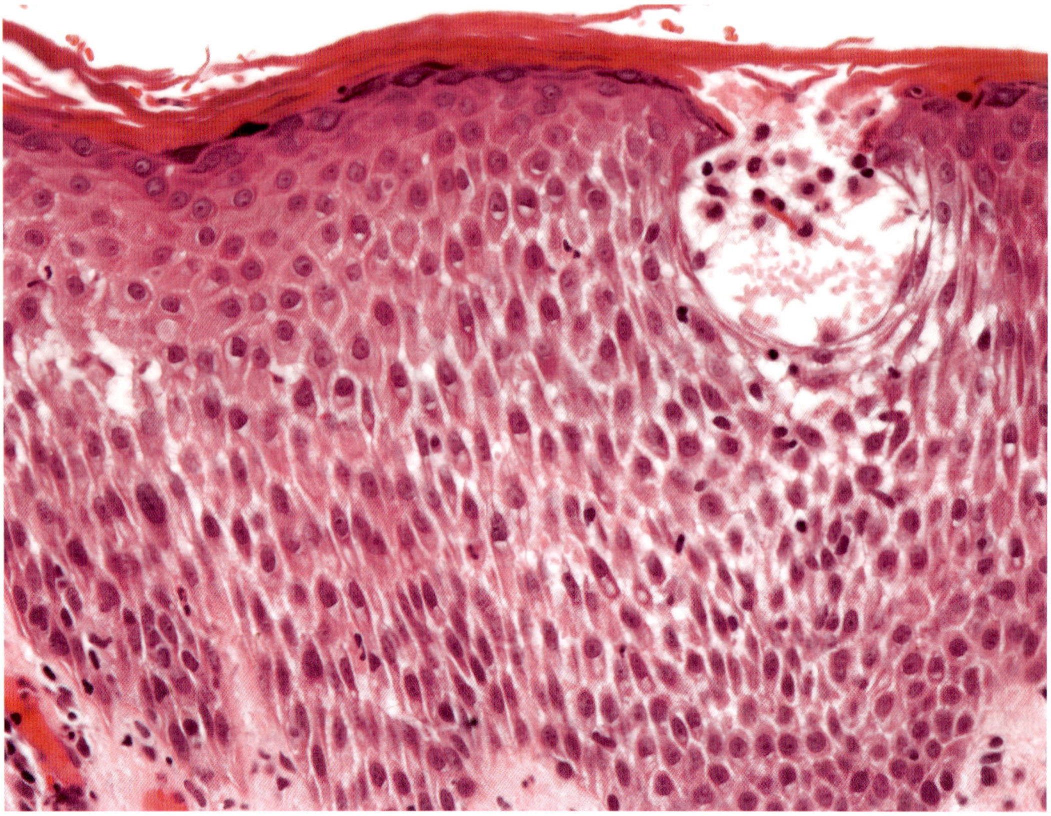

Fig. 3.4 Subacute spongiotic dermatitis. Note the presence of hyperplasia of Langerhans cells in the right upper hand corner, a feature common in spongiotic dermatitis

Lichen Simplex Chronicus and Prurigo Nodularis

Lichen simplex chronicus (previously termed squamous hyperplasia by gynecological pathologists) represents a well-defined clinicopathological entity resulting from chronic and persistent scratching and rubbing of skin [34]. When no underlying dermatological abnormality is present, the alternative designation of primary or de novo lichen simplex chronicus has also been used [35]. Lichenification represents a similar phenomenon occurring in the background of a pruritic preexisting dermatological condition, like eczema, dermatophyte infections, lichen planus, or lichen sclerosus. Such examples have also been labeled as a secondary lichen simplex chronicus [35].

The incidence of anogenital lichen simplex chronicus has been estimated to be about 0.5% in the Western European and American populations [35], while at specialized clinics, lichen simplex chronicus may be found in 10–35% of the patients [20, 22, 36]. Lichen simplex chronicus most commonly presents in the fifth decade of life (mean age, 42 years; range, 22–76 years) [22], with the vast majority of patients being older than 30 years [37]. The most common triggering factors include heat, sweat, irritation, and psychological stress [35]. The presenting symptom is pruritus, which can be intense and intractable. The labia majora are most commonly affected, followed by the vulvar vestibule, mons pubis, and perineum [35, 37]. Lichen simplex chronicus is characterized clinically by one or more erythematous lichenified plaque(s), with or without overlying excoriation. Follicular or perifollicular erythematous papules can frequently be seen at the periphery of lichenified plaques [35]. Linear fissures at sites of natural

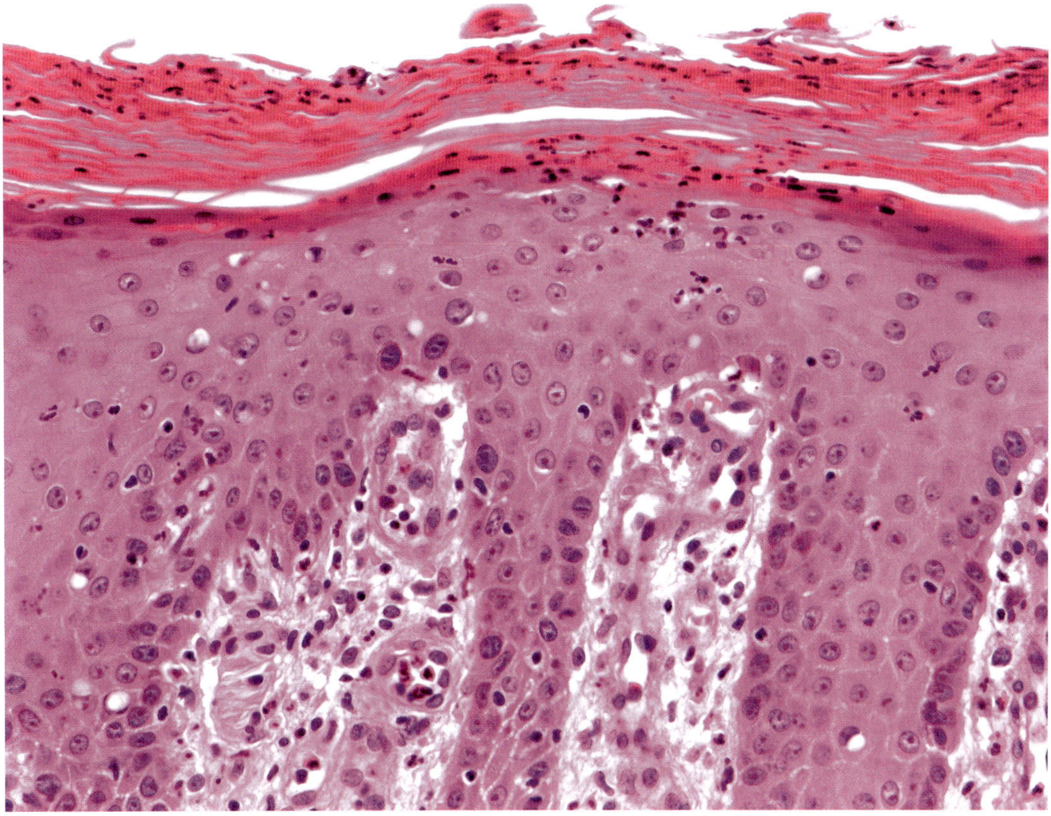

Fig. 3.5 Irritant contact dermatitis. The changes are identical to those of other spongiotic dermatitis, and eosinophils may or may not be present. In this example, there are secondary changes including crusting and exocytosis of neutrophils

skin folds are not uncommon and can be complicated by additional superinfection [35]. Bilateral distribution of the lesions is common, but more often, they are asymmetrical. Long-standing lesions can be either hyper- or hypopigmented [22, 35]. Prurigo nodularis (picker's nodule, chronic prurigo) represents a papular or nodular variant of lichen simplex chronicus and is often ulcerated on the surface [38].

Genital lichen simplex chronicus has also been reported in patients with celiac disease [39].

Histological Features

Lichen simplex chronicus can be recognized histologically by psoriasiform hyperplasia, compact orthokeratosis, variable parakeratosis, and hypergranulosis [38] (Fig. 3.6a). The rete ridges are elongated and unevenly thickened. Mild spongiosis is frequently seen. Vertically oriented thick collagen fibers (vertical streaking) and blood vessels are present within the papillary dermis (Fig. 3.6b). A mild superficial perivascular, predominantly mononuclear, inflammatory cell infiltrate is usually seen. Prurigo nodules which are very rare in the vulva are characterized by similar findings. Although the changes are more prominent, there is marked associated hyperplasia of the epidermis, and this is often pseudoepitheliomatous in nature. Dermal changes include proliferation and dilatation of blood vessels in the papillary and reticular dermis, fibrosis of the papillary dermis in a pattern in which the collagen is perpendicular to the epidermis, and in very rare cases, hypertrophy of dermal nerves [38].

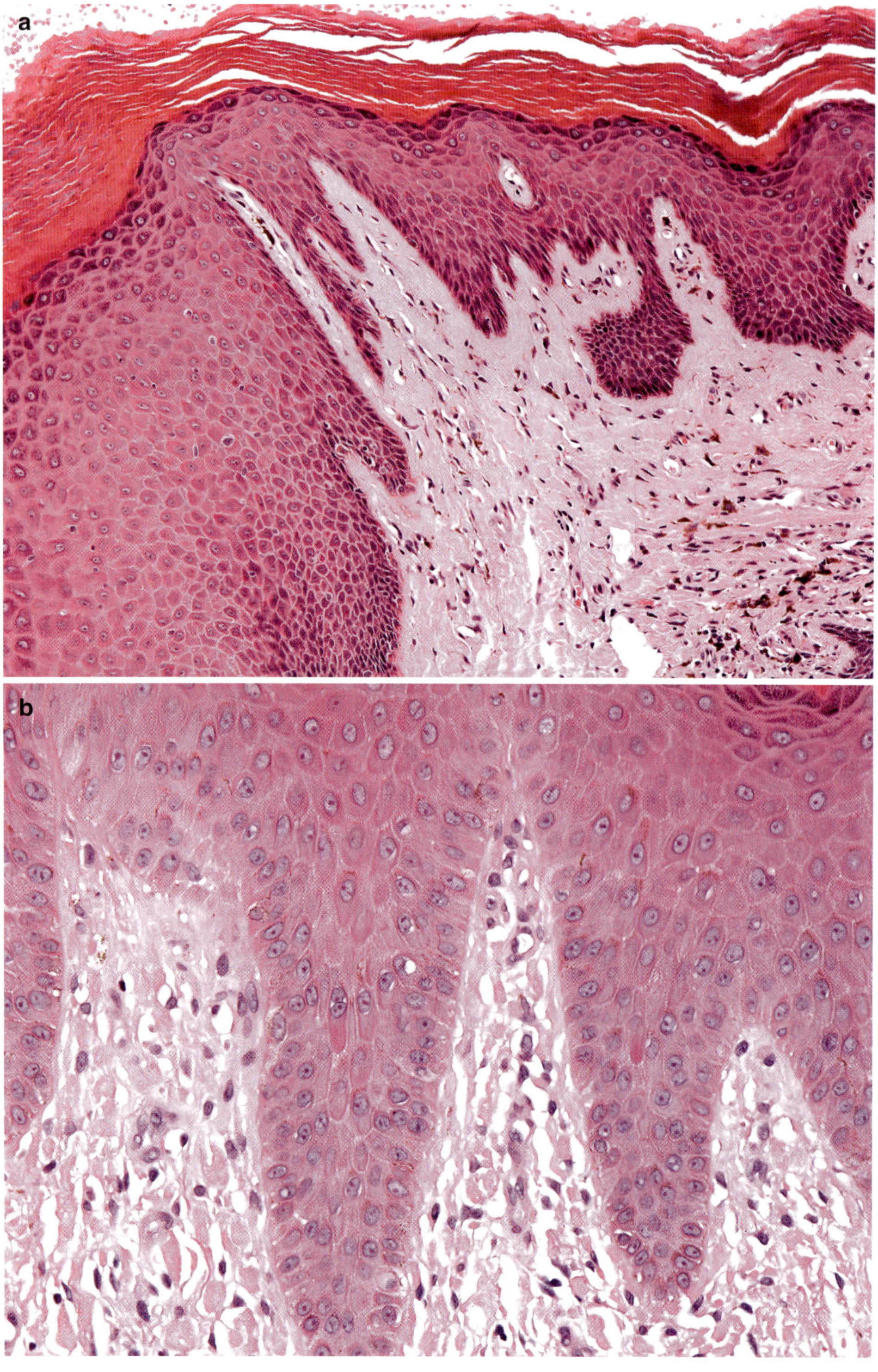

Fig. 3.6 (**a**) Lichen simplex chronicus. Prominent psoriasiform hyperplasia of the epidermis with compact hyperkeratosis and hypergranulosis mimicking the skin of palms or soles. (**b**) Lichen simplex chronicus. Fibrosis of the papillary dermis manifested as vertically oriented collagen bundles

Lichen Sclerosus

Lichen sclerosus is an acquired chronic inflammatory mucocutaneous disorder of unknown etiology, initially reported by Hallopeau as a variant of lichen planus, which he designated as lichen planus atrophicus [40]. Although genital and perianal involvement is by far the most common, extragenital lichen sclerosus can be observed in 15–20% of the patients [41]. Any extragenital cutaneous site can be affected, the most frequently upper trunk, neck, upper arms, flexor surfaces of the wrists, and lower extremities [41]. Exceptionally, lichen sclerosus develops on the lips, within the oral cavity, and on palms and soles [42–46].

Genital lichen sclerosus is characterized clinically by shiny ivory-white and/or red, intensely pruritic atrophic macules, papules, and plaques [47]. The distribution of anogenital changes is frequently bilateral and symmetrical. Vulvar lesions most commonly develop on the inner parts of labia majora, labia minora, clitoris, fossa navicularis, and the posterior commissure. Scarring can be prominent with the development of marked anatomical changes, including loss of labia minora, introital narrowing, and urethral periorificial stenosis [47, 48]. Development of bullae is rare and is more frequent at extragenital locations [43, 49, 50]. Extragenital lichen sclerosus is frequently asymptomatic, characterized by pink to ivory-white macules or plaques with well-defined border and the tendency to coalesce [41]. Genital lichen sclerosus is much more common in females (10:1), while extragenital lichen sclerosus shows more even gender distribution [41]. While the incidence of genital lichen sclerosus in females shows bimodal age distribution in premenarche girls and postmenopausal women, genital lesion in males show the tendency to develop in early childhood or between the ages 30 and 50 years [51].

A familial occurrence of lichen sclerosus is not uncommon. A recent study demonstrated the prevalence of lichen sclerosus as being 11% among the family member(s) of lichen sclerosus patients attending a specialized clinic, suggesting a genetic predisposition to the development of the disease [52]. An association between lichen sclerosus and several class II antigens, including HLA-DQ7, -DR4, -DR11, -DR12, -DQ2, and DQ8 has been determined [53–55]. Intrafamilial association between HLA-B*15-DRB1*04-DRB4* and antithyroid peroxidase autoantibodies has been found, confirming the strong association with autoimmune thyroid diseases [56]. Between 20% and 28% of patients with lichen sclerosus have associated autoimmune diseases, including autoimmune thyroiditis, alopecia areata, pernicious anemia, morphea, vitiligo, and diabetes mellitus [57–59]. Coexistence of vulvar lichen sclerosus and oral lichen planus has been detected in 0.6% of the patients, which is similar to the prevalence of oral lichen planus in the general population [46]. Lichen sclerosus has also been reported in a patient with Turner's syndrome [60]. Although a causative relationship between lichen sclerosus and infection by *Borrelia burgdorferi* has been suggested, recent PCR-based studies were unable to confirm this relationship [61].

Vulvar lichen sclerosus is associated with an increased risk of squamous cell carcinoma development, which has been estimated to be between 2% and 5% [62, 63]. A recent study has also found increased incidence of vulvar, but not perianal, lichen sclerosus and genital verrucous carcinoma [64]. An exceptional case of a squamous cell carcinoma developing in the background of extragenital lichen sclerosus has recently been reported [65].

Histological Features

Genital and extragenital lichen sclerosus are characterized by similar morphological features. Early lesions can be difficult to recognize and changes are often subtle. They include mild irregular acanthosis which can initially be seen in adnexal structures, thickening of the basement membrane, dilatation of blood vessels, homogenization of collagen, gradual loss of elastic fibers in the papillary dermis, and a mild, superficial inflammatory cell infiltrate in the dermis [66, 67] (Fig. 3.7). These inflammatory cell infiltrates display an interface pattern associated with hydropic degeneration of basal cells.

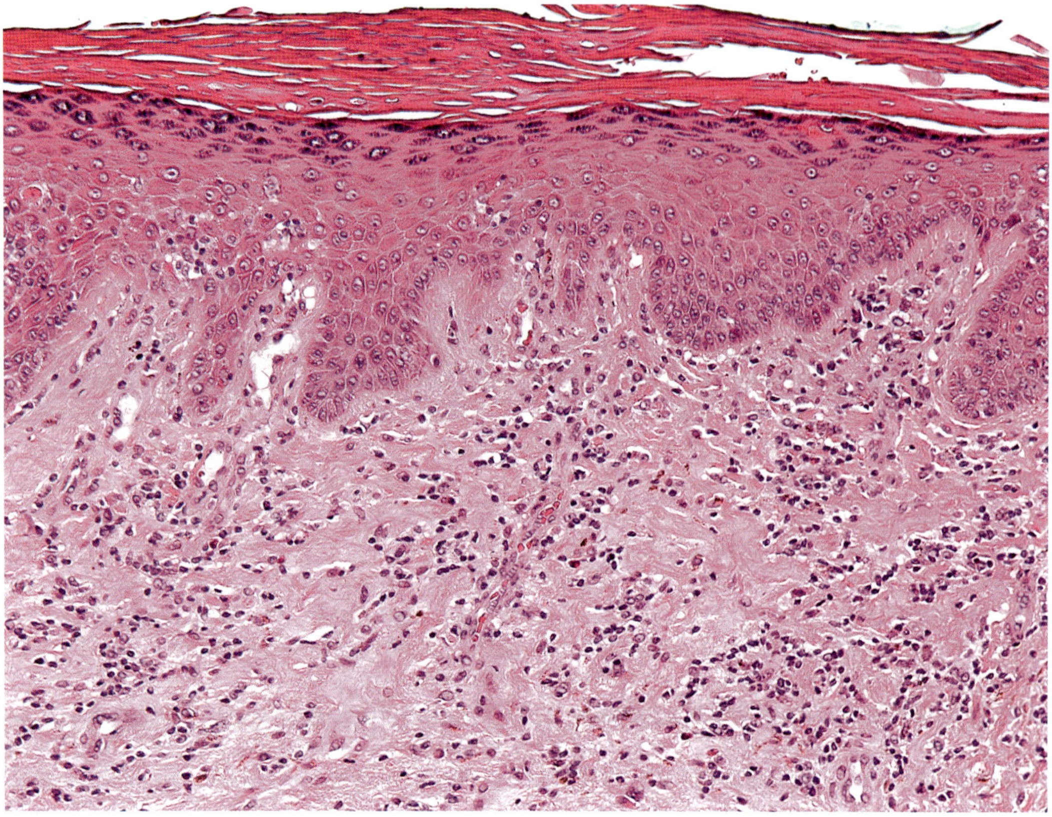

Fig. 3.7 Lichen sclerosus. Early changes are often subtle. This case is associated with thickening of the epidermis, and there is very focal interface dermatitis with hydropic degeneration of basal cells and mild thickening of the epidermal basal membrane

In established lesions, the epidermis becomes atrophic with loss of the normal rete ridge pattern (Fig. 3.8). Alternatively, the epidermis can be hyperplastic [63] (Fig. 3.9). Cases with persistent epidermal hyperplasia appear to be more often associated with development of squamous cell carcinoma. Additional changes in the epidermis include hyperkeratosis, follicular plugging, and vacuolar degeneration of basal keratinocytes [63, 66, 68]. Mucinous metaplasia has been reported in an exceptional case of genital lichen sclerosus but may be coincidental [69]. In the dermis, there is homogenization of the collagen just below the epidermis, and this is usually accompanied by a band-like dermal inflammatory cell infiltrate containing lymphocytes, histiocytes, and plasma cells. Prominent superficial dermal edema is not uncommon (Fig. 3.10). The latter may be associated with telangiectasia and hemorrhage (Fig. 3.11). Lesions in which these changes are prominent can mimic an angiokeratoma on clinical grounds. Clonal rearrangement of the T cell receptor gamma associated with low level of the clonal infiltrate has been detected in a minority of patients, suggesting a reactive proliferation of clonal T lymphocytes [70]. A lymphocytic vasculitis has been found in up to 50% of vulvar and penile lichen sclerosus [71]. Dilated, congested, and focally thrombosed vascular channels in close proximity to the epidermis, lined by flat endothelial cells, and mimicking an angiokeratoma have exceptionally been reported [72, 73]. Extravasation of red blood cells can occasionally be seen. Elastophagocytosis below or at the junction of homogenized collagen with normal reticular dermis has been observed in 20% of extragenital lichen sclerosus [74].

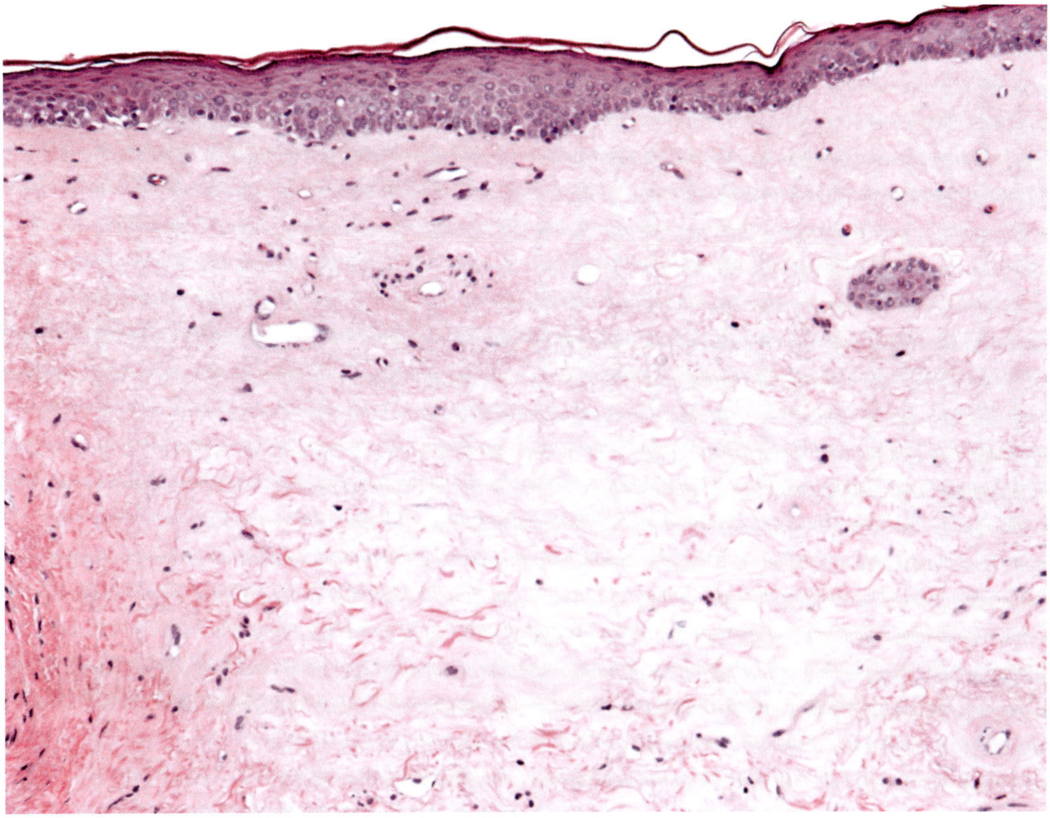

Fig. 3.8 Lichen sclerosus. Late lesion with atrophy of the epidermis, loss of rete ridges, and hyalinization of the upper dermis. Inflammation may be absent as in this case

Differential Diagnosis

Early changes of lichen sclerosus can mimic lichen planus. Irregular acanthosis of the epidermis, focal atrophy of the epidermis, as well as thickening of the basal membrane and loss of elastic fibers in the papillary dermis are features suggestive of lichen sclerosus [66, 67]. In lesions of chronic discoid lupus erythematosus, thickening of the basal membrane is characteristic; however, lupus erythematosus does not tend to involve the vulva. Focal epidermotropism by lymphocytes displaying mild cytological atypia and perinuclear halos can be present in lichen sclerosus, which in early lesions of the latter may raise the possibility of mycosis fungoides [75] (Fig. 3.12). Clonality studies are helpful to resolve diagnostic dilemmas as mycosis fungoides can present clinically with extragenital lichen sclerosus-like lesions [76]. Nevertheless, molecular studies in the early stages of mycosis fungoides can fail to detect T cell receptor rearrangements, and clinicopathological correlation is crucial in such cases. It is important to highlight that involvement of the vulva by mycosis fungoides is exceptional.

Genital Psoriasis

Genital involvement by psoriasis is present in up to 50% of patients with cutaneous psoriasis at some time during the course of the disease [77]. Alternatively, genital psoriasis can represent the first manifestation of the disease, roughly in about 20% of the patients [77]. Genital psoriasis as a sole manifestation of the disease is rare and occurs in 2–5% of the patients [78]. Although genital psoriasis has traditionally been grouped under the group of intertriginous or flexural (inverse) psoriasis, lack of

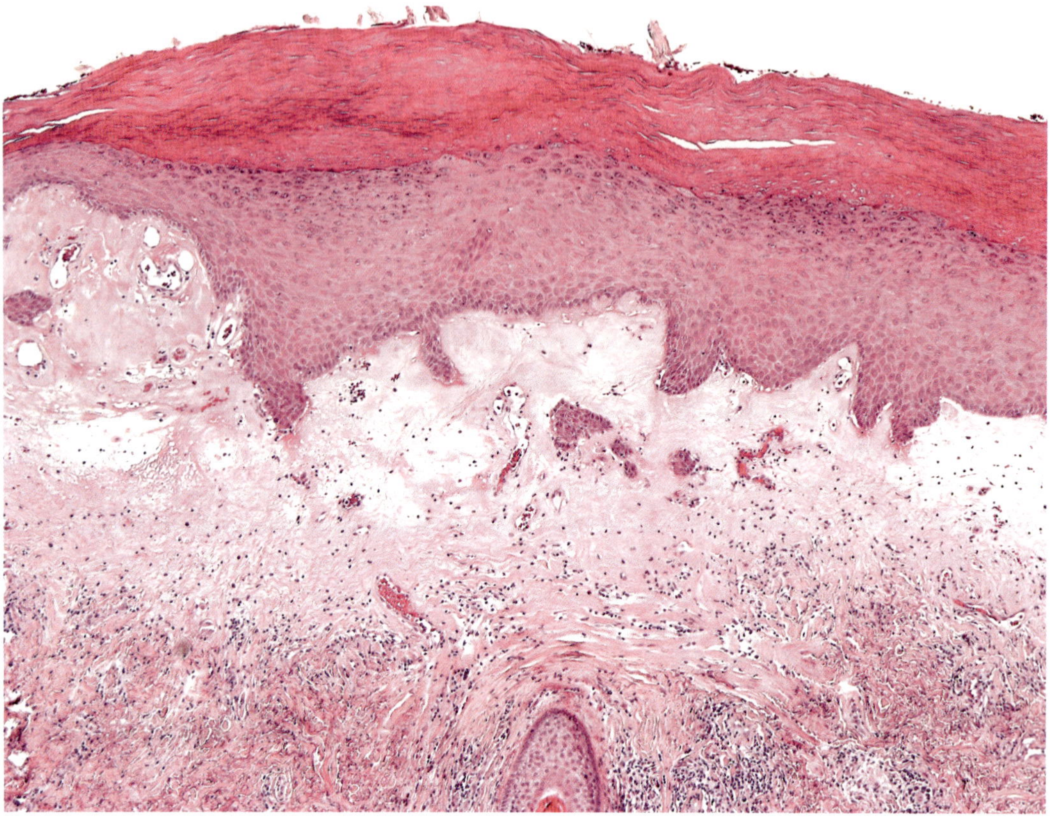

Fig. 3.9 Lichen sclerosus. This case is associated with hyperplasia of the epidermis. Note superficial dermal edema, telangiectasia, hyalinization, and a patchy inflammatory cell infiltrate below the area of hyalinized dermis

concurrent involvement of other intertriginous areas can be observed in up to 40% of patients with genital psoriasis [77]. Genital psoriasis is much more frequent in males [77, 79].

Genital psoriasis usually starts in the fourth decade of life (mean 35 years), but patients of any age can be affected (range 3–85 years) [77]. Clinically, vulval psoriasis is characterized by well-demarcated and frequently symmetrical erythematous plaques. Although the typical scale is generally lacking due to the moist local environment and maceration, scaling can, nevertheless, be seen at more external portions of the vulva. The most common presenting symptoms include vulvar discomfort, itching, and burning [80]. Complications include fissuring, rhagade formation, and secondary infections [81, 82]. Lesions are generally not associated with scarring [78].

Histological Features

The histological features of classical psoriasis, including uniform acanthosis of the epidermal ridges, diminution or loss of the granular cell layer, confluent parakeratosis, thinning of the suprapapillary plates, and formation of neutrophilic microabscesses within the stratum corneum (Munro microabscesses) and beneath the cornified layer (spongiform pustules of Kogoj), are frequently not seen in female genital skin, and the changes can be entirely nonspecific (Fig. 3.13). Spongiosis of the epidermis is common, leading to an overlap with the spongiotic process, such as eczema (see above). Close clinicopathological correlation is of utmost importance for the correct recognition of the underlying process. Although pustular psoriasis has exceptionally

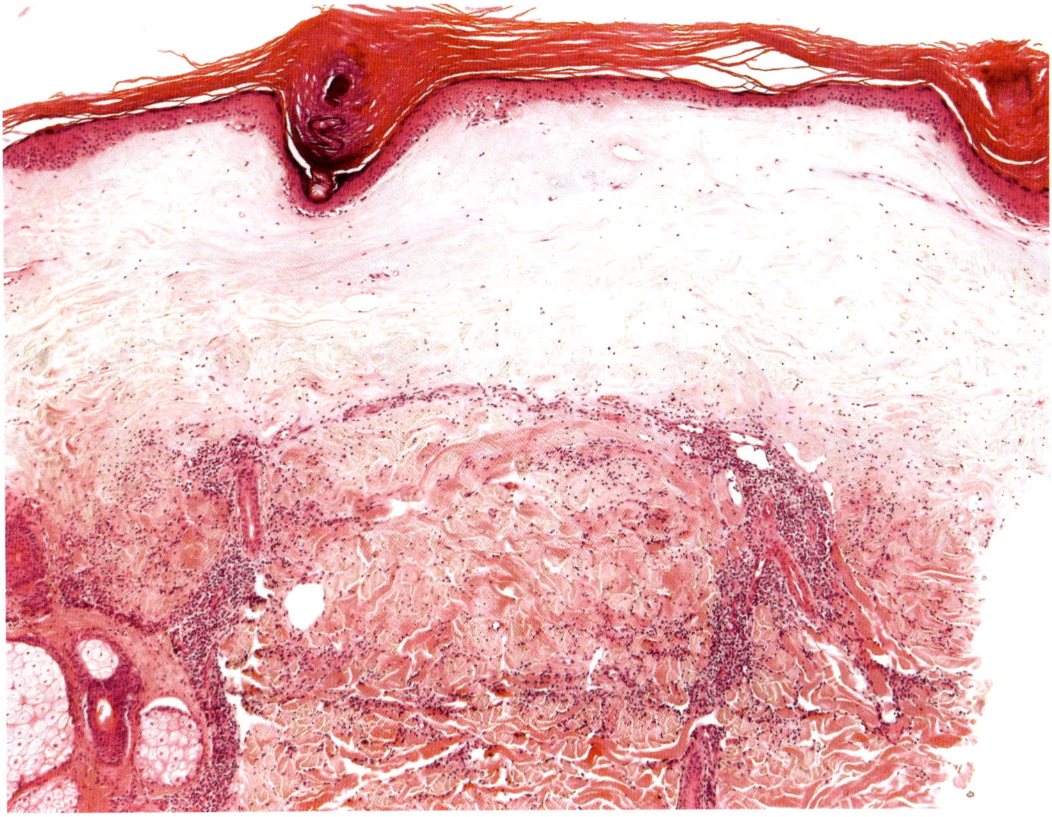

Fig. 3.10 Lichen sclerosus. Prominent hyperkeratosis, epidermal atrophy, and marked upper dermal edema

been described on male genital skin, this has not been reported in females [83, 84].

Genital Lichen Planus

Lichen planus is an inflammatory dermatosis, which can involve skin, oral, and genital mucous membranes, as well as different other sites like esophagus, stomach, anus, conjunctivae, larynx, or bladder [85, 86]. Lesions at diverse sites can occur either simultaneously or at different times [86, 87]. Genital lichen planus develops as a part of more widespread cutaneous disease in up to 50% of the patients or, more rarely, presents as an isolated condition [88]. The frequency of vulval lichen planus in the population of patients attending the vulval clinic has been reported to be 3,7% [89]. A recent study demonstrated the prevalence of vulval lichen planus in patients with oral lichen planus to be as high as 57% [86], which is much higher than previously estimated [90].

Several clinical variants of genital lichen planus have been described and include papulosquamous (classical), erosive/atrophic, hypertrophic, lichen planopilaris, and mixed type [62]. The most common clinical variant in genital skin is erosive lichen planus (85%), followed by papulosquamous (4%), and hypertrophic type of lichen planus (4%) as demonstrated by a study from a specialized clinic in the United Kingdom [62]. The vulvovaginogingival syndrome represents a distinctive variant of erosive lichen planus, characterized by the involvement of oral gingivae, vulval vestibule, and vagina [91]. Genital erosive lichen planus usually presents in the sixth decade of life [92, 93]. The sites most frequently affected are lower vagina, followed by upper vagina, and

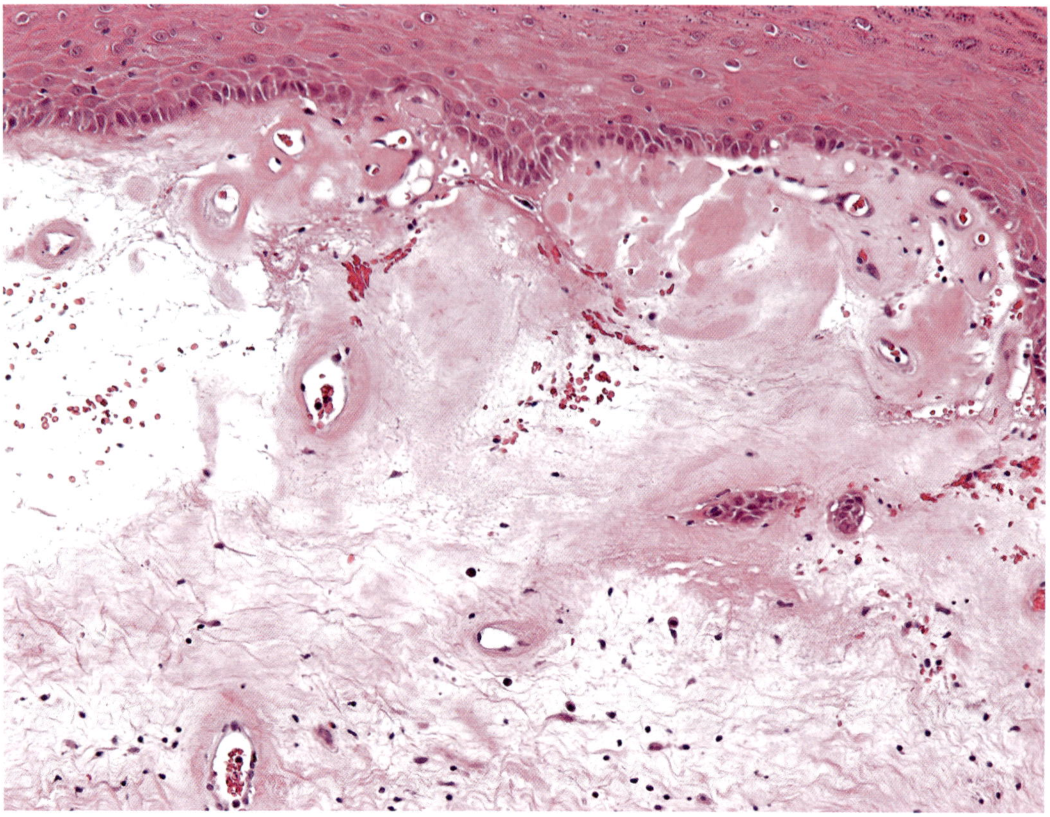

Fig. 3.11 Lichen sclerosus. Due to marked edema and telangiectasia, lesions may clinically mimic a blister or even an angiokeratoma

vulvar mucosa [62, 92]. Isolated lesions in the vagina are not uncommon [92]. An exceptional case of lichen planus affecting the uterine cervix has also been reported [94]. The presenting clinical symptoms generally include pain, itching, burning, dyspareunia, and abnormal vaginal discharge [86, 92, 93]. Genital erosive lichen planus is characterized clinically by prominent erythema with erosions, surrounded by lacy or reticulated white edge [62]. Classical or papulosquamous lichen planus is delineated clinically by flat-topped polygonal violaceous papules covered by scaly surface and delicate white lines, the so-called Wickham's striae. Hypertrophic lichen planus can be recognized clinically by hyperkeratotic papules and plaques. Lichen planopilaris affects hair-bearing parts of the vulva and is characterized by violaceous keratotic papules and plaques, perifollicular erythema, and scarring alopecia.

In contrast to cutaneous lichen planus, mucosal lichen planus usually follows a more chronic clinical course, frequently resulting in scarring and development of anatomical anomalies, such as absorption of labia, development of synechiae, stenosis of the introitus, and total obliteration of the vagina [92, 93, 95, 96]. Such complications are particularly common in erosive lichen planus and vulvovaginogingival syndrome.

Patients with vulvar lichen planus have an increased association with other autoimmune diseases, mostly autoimmune diseases of the thyroid, followed by alopecia areata, and celiac disease [97]. Different autoimmune diseases may coexist in an individual patient with vulvar lichen planus [97]. An exceptional case of vulvovaginal gingival lichen planus developing in a patient with Good's syndrome, representing an association of a combined B and T cell immunodeficiency and thymoma, has recently been reported [98].

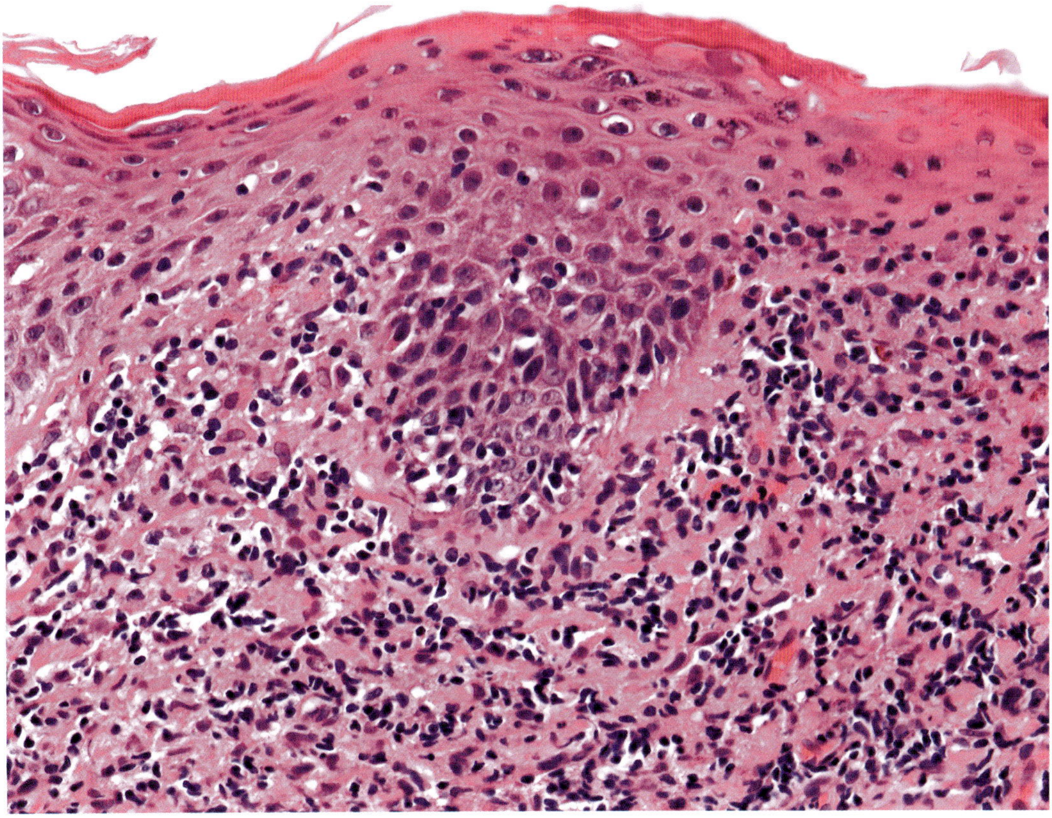

Fig. 3.12 Lichen sclerosus. Early inflammatory lesions may closely mimic cutaneous T cell lymphoma (mycosis fungoides)

Genital lichen planus is associated with an increased risk, albeit small, for the development of a squamous cell carcinoma [99–102]. Multifocal development of squamous cell carcinomas in the background of vulvovaginal lichen planus has also been reported [103].

Histological Features

The histological features of classical lichen planus, including hyperkeratosis, wedge-shaped hypergranulosis, and saw-toothed acanthosis may be seen (Fig. 3.14). However, these changes are often blurred in genital skin and particularly in mucosal surfaces. The epidermis in these instances frequently appears atrophic and ulcerated (see below, erosive lichen planus). Parakeratosis, alternating with hyperkeratosis, is not uncommon. Liquefaction degeneration of the basal cell layer is usually seen. In addition, the basal layer can display cytological and architectural abnormalities associated with limited maturation of keratinocytes. Cytoid bodies are usually not prominent. The band-like inflammatory cell infiltrate in addition to lymphocytes and histiocytes often contains plasma cells, which can be numerous, especially if accompanied by surface ulceration. Secondary spongiotic changes are frequently observed at mucosal sites and can be prominent. Rare cases are of the hypertrophic variant (Fig. 3.15). In erosive examples of the disease, the diagnosis is very difficult because of the presence of prominent superficial ulceration (Fig. 3.16a). More typical changes of lichen planus should be looked for at the edges of the ulceration (Fig. 3.16b). Long-standing lesions can be associated with a more sparse and patchy lichenoid inflammatory cell infiltrate (Fig. 3.17).

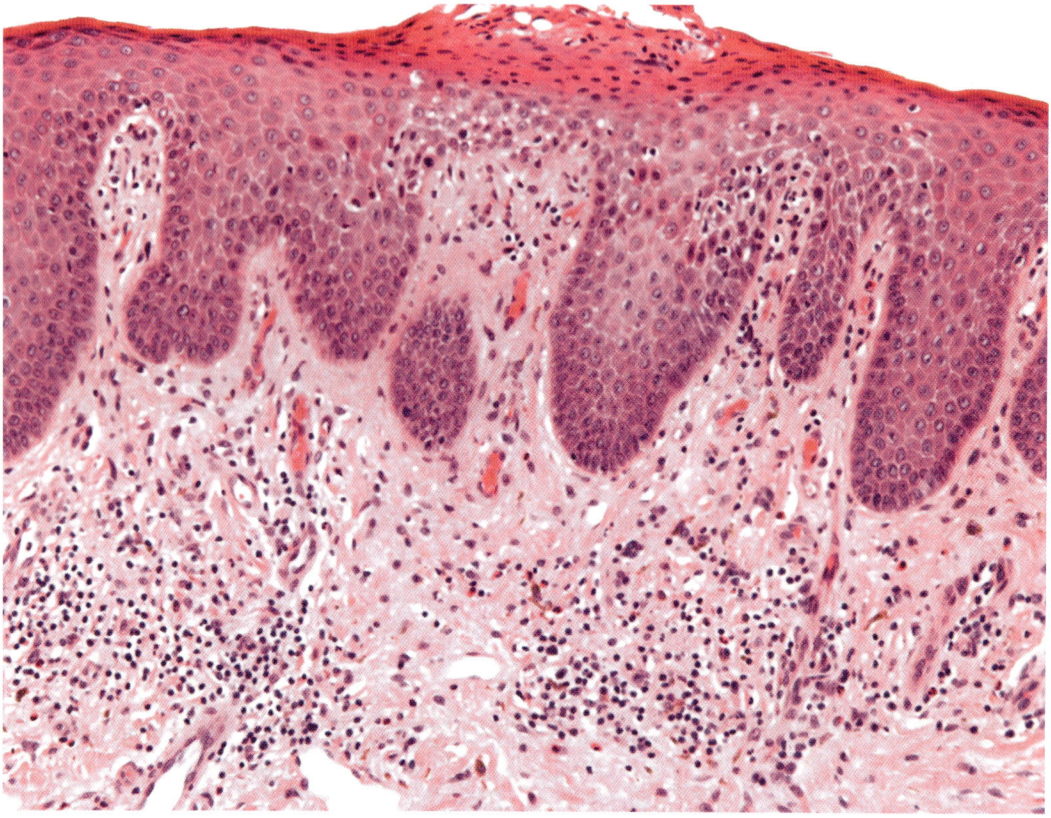

Fig. 3.13 Psoriasis. Classical histological changes of psoriasis are rare in vulval psoriasis. Note psoriasiform hyperplasia with hyperkeratosis and parakeratosis and a few neutrophils in the stratum corneum with secondary changes of crusting

Differential Diagnosis

The main differential diagnosis at genital sites includes lichen sclerosus, and the two diseases may coexist in the same patient. Lichen sclerosus can be recognized by prominent hyalinization of the papillary dermis or subepithelial stroma.

Zoon's Vulvitis

Originally described by Zoon in 1950 as a "chronic circumscribed balanitis with plasma cell infiltration" [104], similar lesions were reported in the vulva a few years later [105, 106]. Since the original description, less than 50 cases of Zoon's vulvitis have been published [107].

Zoon's vulvitis usually presents in the fifth decade of life (range 8–79 years, mean age 48 years) with one or several red or red-brown patches or plaques measuring up to 3 cm in diameter [107, 108]. The lesions are well demarcated, with irregular borders, often bilateral and symmetrical with the tendency to coalesce [109]. Several clinical variants have been described and include ecchymotic, telangiectatic, purpuric, erosive, and granulomatous [109]. The most frequent sites of involvement are the inner part of the labia minora, followed by the vestibule/introitus, urethral meatus, and clitoris [108]. The presenting symptoms include pruritus, which can be severe, burning sensation, spotting, pain, dyspareunia, irritation, dysuria, tenderness, discharge, and dryness in decreasing order of frequency [108]. The lesions can on occasion be asymptomatic.

Similar lesions to Zoon's vulvitis have also been described at other mucosal sites, including

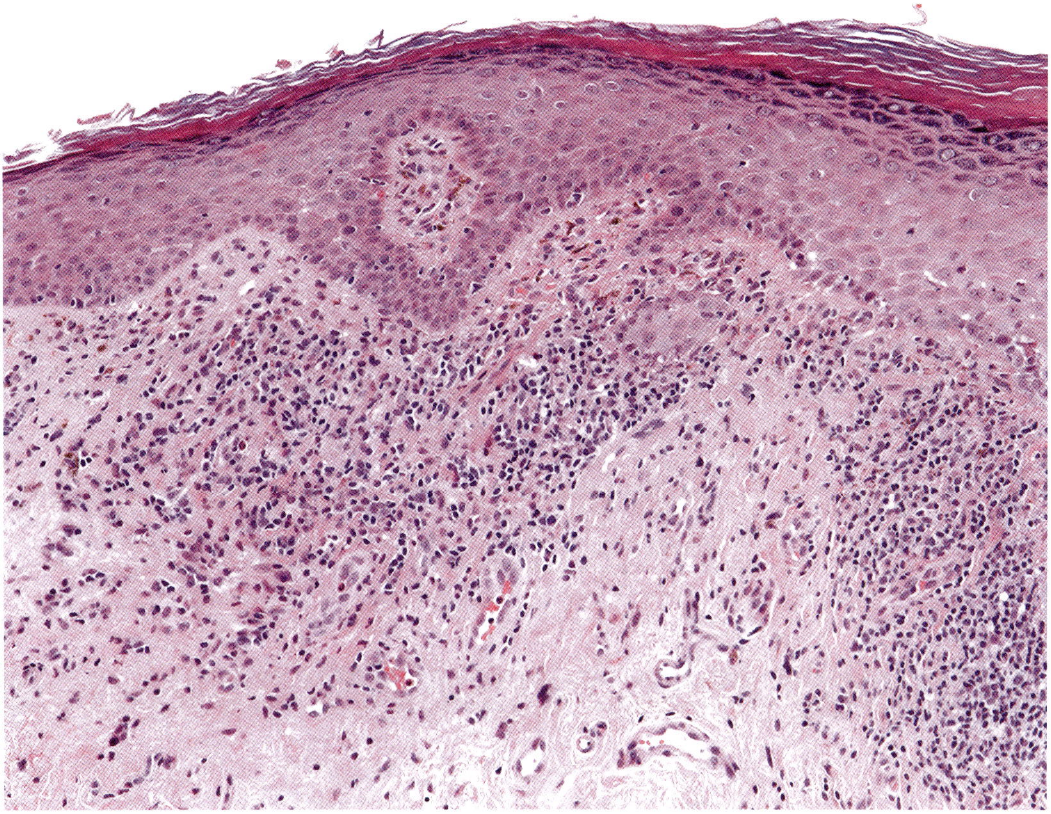

Fig. 3.14 Lichen planus. Classical appearance with acanthosis, hyperkeratosis, hypergranulosis, absence of spongiosis, saw toothing, a band-like mononuclear inflammatory cell infiltrate at the dermoepidermal junction, and hydropic degeneration of basal cells with colloid bodies

oral cavity, epiglottis, larynx, nasal cavity, and other orificial surfaces [110]. Different names have been used for such conditions, like plasma cell orificial mucositis or mucous membrane plasmacytosis [110, 111].

Zoon's vulvitis represents a chronic inflammatory condition of the vulva of unknown etiology. A site-specific mucosal reaction to various agents, including diverse inflammatory conditions and/or local trauma or chronic irritation, has been postulated as the pathogenesis of this condition [108].

Histological Features

The histological features are nonspecific and include a thinned epidermis with lozenge- or diamond-shaped keratinocytes associated with a dense band-like (lichenoid) inflammatory cell infiltrate in the dermis or subepithelial stroma containing numerous plasma cells. In addition to plasma cells, the inflammatory cell infiltrate can also contain lymphocytes, macrophages, and occasionally also neutrophils and eosinophils. Deposition of hemosiderin pigment and extravasation of erythrocytes can be present in 70% and 30% of cases, respectively [108], and is frequently associated with proliferation of capillaries and vascular dilatation. Therefore, an alternative designation for Zoon's vulvitis, namely, "chronic vulvar purpura," has been proposed [112]. Additional epithelial changes include spongiosis, decrease or absence of the granular cell layer and stratum corneum. Erosive changes are rare. Mucinous metaplasia has exceptionally been described and can be widespread [113, 114].

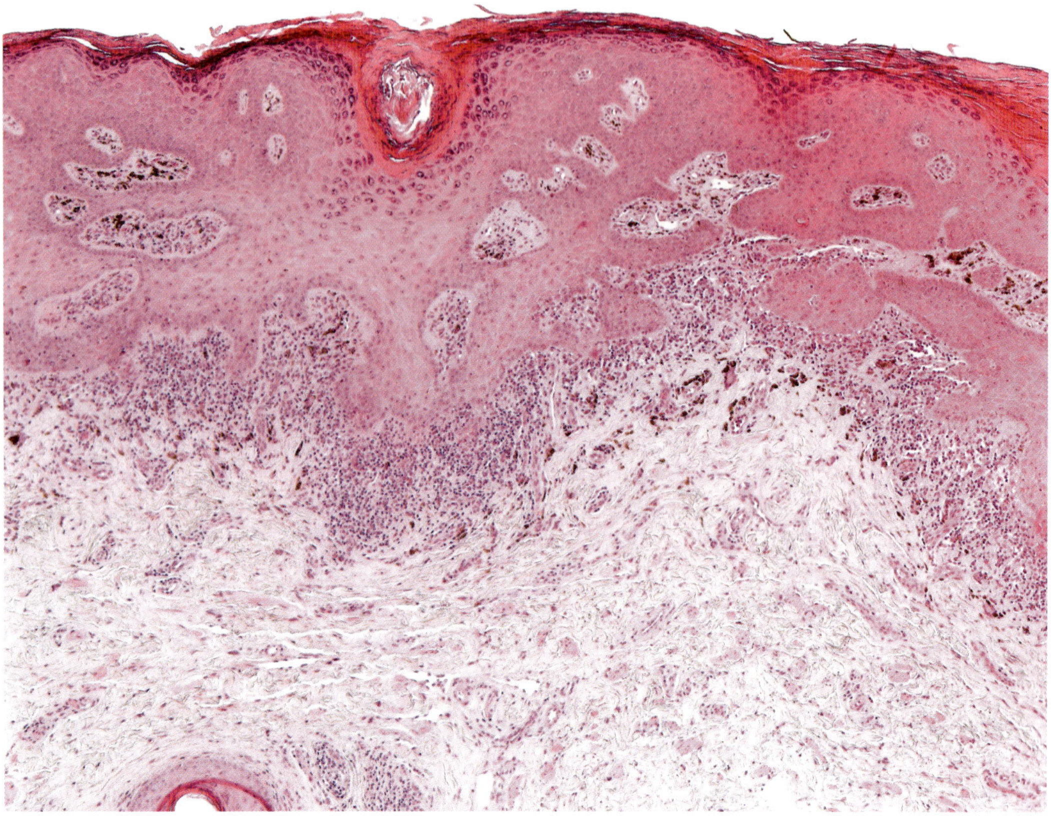

Fig. 3.15 Lichen planus. This case illustrates an example of vulval hypertrophic lichen planus. The epidermal changes mimic lichen simplex chronicus

Differential Diagnosis

Zoon's vulvitis is a diagnosis of exclusion, and the histological findings are usually nondiagnostic. Diverse other inflammatory dermatoses, in particular lichen planus, can be misdiagnosed as Zoon's vulvitis. Close clinicopathological correlation is necessary for the correct recognition of the underlying process.

Genital Crohn's Disease

Crohn's disease is an idiopathic chronic inflammatory granulomatous disease that can affect any part of the gastrointestinal tract, most often the terminal ileum [115]. Extraintestinal involvement by Crohn's disease has variably been reported between 22% and 75% of the patients and most commonly involves mucocutaneous sites [116–118]. Cutaneous Crohn's disease develops much more commonly in patients with colonic than with ileal disease [119, 120]. Anogenital lesions in Crohn's disease can result from direct extension of the disease from the gastrointestinal tract through fistulas or perianal spread [121]. Much more commonly, however, genital lesions are not in continuity with intestinal lesions; such lesions are generally referred to as "metastatic" Crohn's disease. About 90% of vulvar Crohn's disease represents metastatic disease [122].

Vulvar Crohn's disease usually affects premenopausal women (mean age 34 years, age range 12–64 years) [122]. Vulvar disease can represent the first manifestation of Crohn's disease in the absence of gastrointestinal symptoms in up to 25% of the patients [122, 123]. In children, however, metastatic Crohn's disease develops concurrently with the gastrointestinal Crohn's disease in about 50% of the patients [122, 124].

a

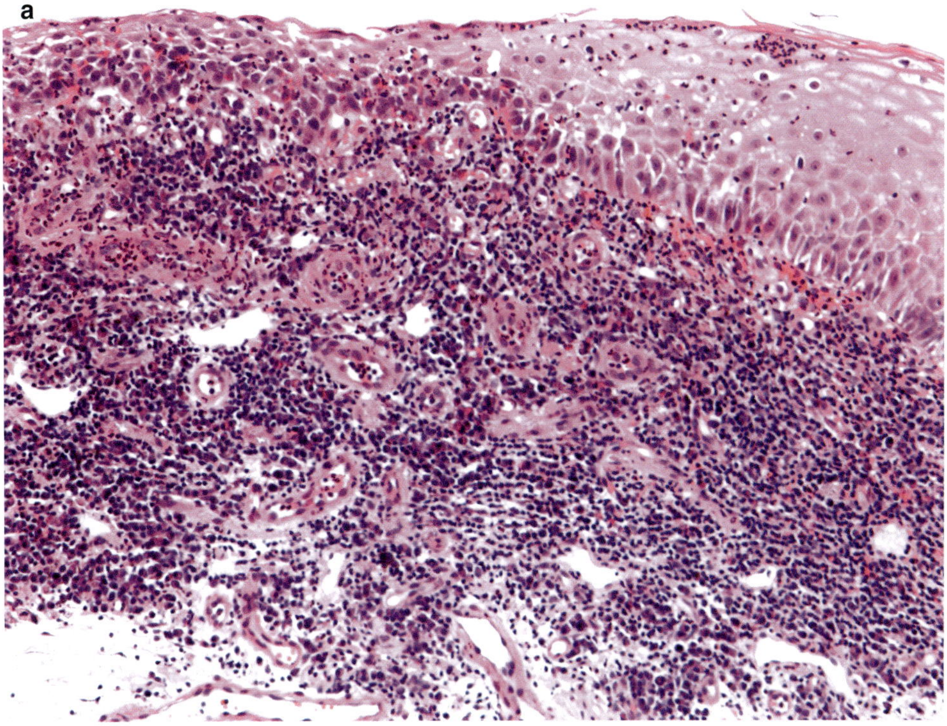

b

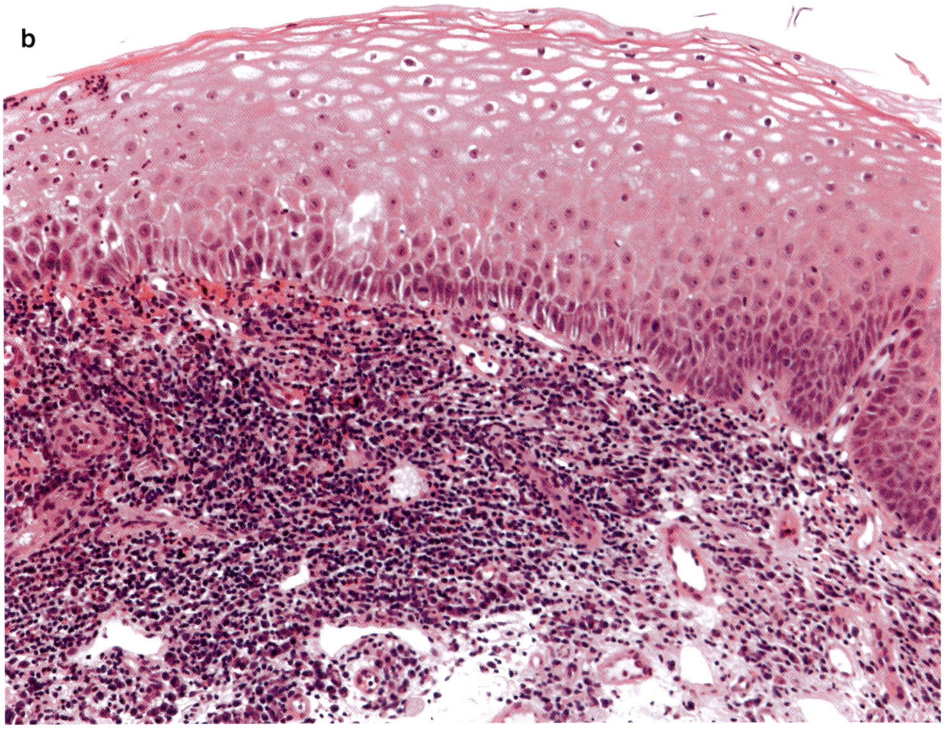

Fig. 3.16 (**a**) Erosive lichen planus. Note focal thinning of the epidermis that usually progresses to ulceration, spongiosis, and exocytosis of neutrophils. There is also a band-like inflammatory cell infiltrate and hemorrhage. (**b**) Erosive lichen planus. More typical changes in a biopsy taken from a non-eroded area. The epithelium is a mucosa, and therefore no hypergranulosis is seen

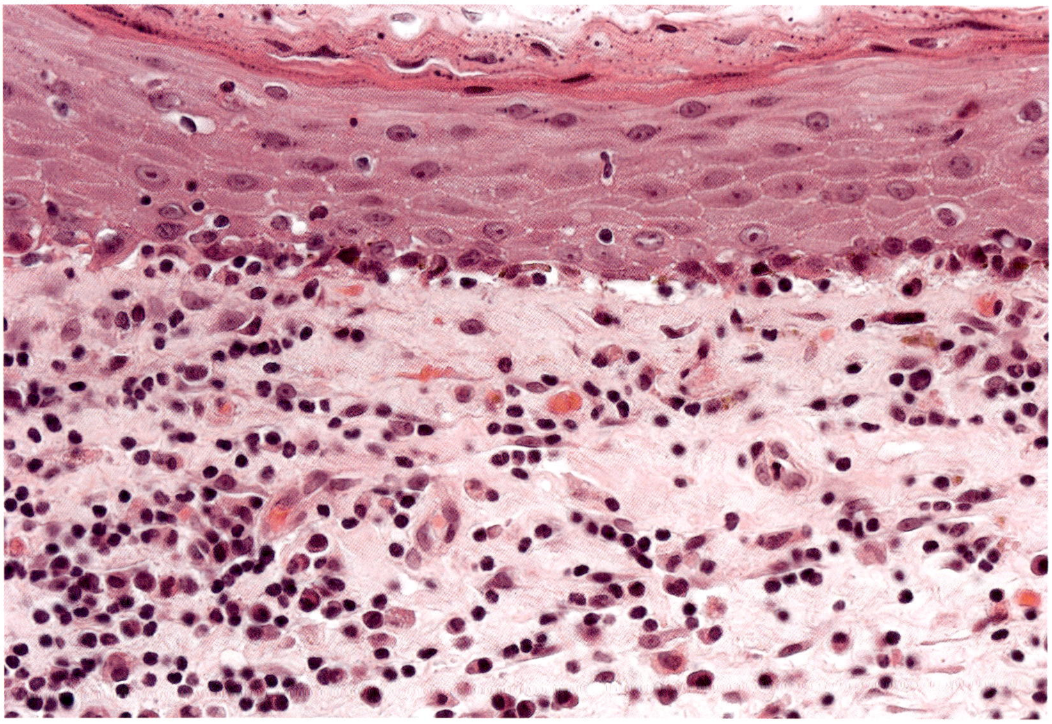

Fig. 3.17 Lichen planus. In late lesions, there band-like infiltrate may be absent and the interface change can be patchy. Note the abundance of plasma cells, a frequent feature in vulval lichen planus

The most common clinical presentation includes swelling and induration of the genitals with or without erythema, followed by ulceration, fissuring, and the formation of abscesses and fistulas [118, 122, 125, 126]. Deep fissures along the skin creases are typical. Pruritus can occasionally be present [122]. Papules and nodules can also develop, especially in the groin creases [127]. Unusual manifestations are unilateral hypertrophy of the vulva, condyloma-like lesions, and skin tags [128–130].

The incidence of perianal Crohn's disease varies, is more common in females, and can be present in up to 80% of the patients [131–133]. Concurrent or sequential involvement of gastrointestinal and perianal skin is seen in about two thirds of the patients [134, 135]. Mucinous adenocarcinoma can exceptionally develop in the background of persistent rectovaginal fistulas [136, 137].

Additional cutaneous manifestations of Crohn's disease include erythema nodosum, erythema multiforme, and pyoderma gangrenosum [138].

Histological Features

The hallmark of Crohn's disease is superficial and deep dermal noncaseating sarcoidal granulomas, associated with a mixed inflammatory cell infiltrate composed of lymphocytes, plasma cell, and occasionally also eosinophils [139]. Perivascular granulomas can be seen [139, 140]. Additional changes may include necrobiotic collagen with leukocytoclasis around granulomas [140]. The histological changes are frequently nonspecific, consisting mainly of edema, and dilated lymphatics.

Necrolytic Migratory Erythema

This peculiar cutaneous association with pancreatic endocrine malignancy was first reported by Becker et al. in 1942 [141], but it was not until 1971 when Wilkinson proposed the name "necrolytic migratory erythema" to refer to the cutaneous manifestations in a patient with pancreatic malignancy [142, 143].

Necrolytic migratory erythema is a distinctive dermatosis that usually develops in the background of glucagonoma syndrome, with about 70% of the patients presenting with skin changes during the course of the disease [144]. Glucagonomas represent about 10% of pancreatic endocrine tumors, usually develop in patients between 40 and 70 years of age, and are more common in males [144–146]. Most glucagonomas are malignant, and about 70% will already have metastasized to the regional lymph nodes and/or the liver by the time they are diagnosed [144, 145]. Extrapancreatic glucagonomas are extremely rare. Glucagonomas can be part of a multiple endocrine neoplasia syndrome 1, and such association has been reported in 13% of glucagonomas [147–149]. Glucagonoma syndrome consists of loss of weight, diabetes mellitus, stomatitis, anemia, venous thromboembolism, neuropsychiatric abnormalities, diarrhea, dilated cardiomyopathy, and necrolytic migratory erythema [146, 149]. Although it has been thought that glucagonoma syndrome is directly related to elevated serum levels of glucagon, no correlation could be detected between plasma glucagon levels and glucagonoma syndrome in some studies [146, 150]. These studies suggest the involvement of additional factors in the development of the glucagonoma syndrome, such as hypoaminoacidemia, zinc, fatty acid, and vitamin B deficiencies, which might be directly related to hyperglucagonemia [151–154].

Necrolytic migratory erythema is characterized clinically by intensely pruritic polycyclic migratory lesions with advancing borders and central clearing [144, 155]. Erythematous scaly lesion can progress to form papules or even flaccid bullae, with subsequent erosions and crusting. The skin changes have the propensity to resolve at one area and to develop in another, healing with postinflammatory hyperpigmentation [144, 155, 156]. The sites of predilection include genital areas, distal extremities, buttocks, and perioral areas. Patients are usually in their sixth decade of life [147, 155]. Skin changes can be the first manifestation of an underlying pancreatic malignancy [147, 157]. Normalization of glucagon levels following surgery of the primary neoplasm as well as treatment with somatostatin analogues is associated with a dramatic resolution of the skin changes [154].

Necrolytic migratory erythema has also been reported in association with other malignancies, including cholangiocarcinoma [158], small cell lung carcinoma [159], squamous cell carcinoma of the hypopharynx [160], jejunal adenocarcinoma [161], and myelodysplastic syndrome [162]. In addition, similar cutaneous lesions have also been described in patients with cystic fibrosis [163], celiac disease [164], heroin abuse [165], following methadone therapy due to the drug abuse [166], Waldmann's disease [167], zinc and essential fatty acid deficiency [168], hepatitis B infection [169], and following treatment with inhibitor of EGF-receptor due to non-small cell lung cancer [170].

Histological Features

The characteristic histological changes include pale, swollen, and vacuolated keratinocytes, associated with necrosis of the superficial epidermis and formation of intraepidermal vesicles (Fig. 3.18) [143, 155]. The epidermis usually displays irregular acanthosis, spongiosis, and confluent parakeratosis [171]. Subcorneal pustules can be present and can signify fungal or bacterial superinfection. Edema of the papillary dermis is usually seen, and there is a mild superficial inflammatory cell infiltrate composed of lymphocytes. Early changes are often nonspecific, consisting of mild spongiosis, scattered necrotic suprabasal keratinocytes, and a mild lymphocytic inflammatory cell infiltrate [172, 173].

Differential Diagnosis

Necrolytic migratory erythema displays histological overlap with acrodermatitis enteropathica, zinc and niacin deficiency, pellagra, and hepatitis C infection-related necrolytic acral erythema. In addition, an infectious etiology should also be excluded.

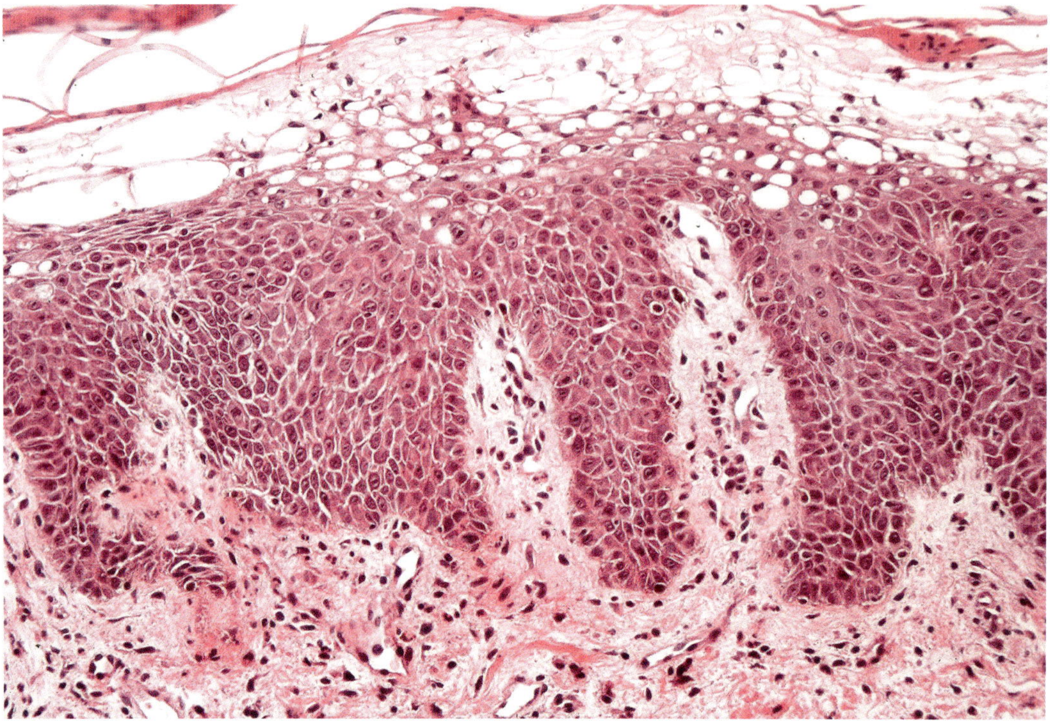

Fig. 3.18 Necrolytic migratory epidermis. Prominent pallor of the superficial epidermis associated with ballooning of keratinocytes

Reactive Arthritis (Reiter's Syndrome)

Reactive arthritis, previously called Reiter's syndrome, is characterized by a classical triad of nongonococcal urethritis and/or cervicitis, conjunctivitis, and arthritis, generally following bacterial infection of gastrointestinal or urogenital tract and much rarely, upper respiratory tract [174–176]. It has been suggested that the term reactive arthritis should be reserved for HLA-B27-positive patients with arthritis fulfilling also the criteria for the seronegative spondylarthropathy, while other arthritides causally related to infections should be called "infection-related" arthritides [176].

The incidence of the reactive arthritis has been estimated to be between 30 and 100/100,000 inhabitants but varies greatly between different geographic locations [177, 178]. Significant male predominance has been observed, with males being affected up to 15 times more often than females [176]. Reactive arthritis generally presents in young adults between the ages 20 and 40 years [179] but can also develop in children [180]. While adults more commonly develop reactive arthritis following venereal infections, epidemic or postdysenteric reactive arthritis predominates in children [181]. Familiar clustering of reactive arthritis has also been observed and is usually associated with HLA-B27 [182, 183]. HLA-B27 is present in about 10% of the normal population but has been detected in up to 80% of patients with reactive arthritis [184], suggesting its development in the background of a genetic predisposition. Possible association with HLA-B51 has also been proposed [185].

The classical clinical triad is present in only about one third of the patients [186]. The genitourinary tract is involved in 90% of the patients presenting clinically with urethritis, hemorrhagic cystitis, prostatitis, as well as inflammation of the seminal vesicles [187–189]. Arthritis is usually polyarticular, asymmetrical, and most commonly affects large joints of lower limbs [190]. Other joints, including sarcoiliacal, distal interphalangeal, and spinal can also be affected [190]. Conjunctivitis is the most frequent form of ocular involvement, followed by uveitis, keratitis, iritis, and iridocyclitis [187, 191]. Different other extra-articular manifestation has also been reported in reactive arthritis, including cardiovascular abnormalities, myelopathy, and IgA glomerulonephritis [187, 192, 193].

Mucocutaneous involvement in reactive arthritis is frequent and includes penile changes (circinate balanitis) in up to 50% of the patients, oral lesions in up to 40%, nail changes in 20–30%, involvement of palms and soles (keratoderma blennorhagicum) in about 10%, and ulcerative vulvitis [188]. Circinate balanitis in circumcised males presents as hyperkeratotic plaques on the glans penis. In noncircumcised males, however, vesicles and pustules are seen eventually progressing to superficial erosions with micropustules at the borders [188, 190]. Oral lesions most frequently include erosions or ulceration that can be painless. Nail changes are similar to psoriatic lesions (nail dystrophy, distal onycholysis, periungual pustule). The Terry's nail, which is characterized by white discoloration of the nail stopping 1–2 mm from the distal edge, has recently been reported [194]. Keratoderma blennorhagicum is characterized by the development of erythematous macules and vesicles, progressing in a course of a few days to pustules and waxy papules, covered by thick hyperkeratosis. Papules are usually numerous and show a tendency to coalesce, thus forming larger hyperkeratotic plaques. Although the lesions most commonly develop on the palms and soles, similar changes can also develop on the scalp, trunk, extremities, as well as at the back of the toes and fingers [188, 190]. Vulvar changes are the least frequent and include ulcerated plaques and papules, involving hair-bearing parts of the vulva, labia minora, and vestibule [188]. They can mimic mucocutaneous candidiasis.

Reactive arthritis develops in the background of urogenital, enteric, and upper respiratory tract infections. Microorganisms, associated with the development of reactive arthritis, include *Shigella flexneri*, *Salmonella enteritidis*, *Salmonella typhimurium*, *Chlamydia trachomatis*, *Chlamydia pneumoniae*, *Yersinia enterocolitica*, *Yersinia pseudotuberculosis*, *Campylobacter jejuni*, *Campylobacter fetus*, *Ureaplasma urealyticum* [176, 188, 195–198]. Less common microorganisms include *Escherichia coli*, *Clostridium difficile*, and *Streptococcus viridans* [199, 200]. The list is by no means complete. Reactive arthritis has also been reported following BCG therapy for bladder carcinoma [201, 202] as well as following treatment with adalimumab and leflunomide in a patient with Crohn's disease [203].

Histological Features

Histological changes in the skin and genital tract can closely mimic pustular psoriasis, and the distinction is very difficult, if not impossible, on histological grounds alone. The epidermis displays psoriasiform hyperplasia with elongated rete ridges and thinned suprapapillary plates. The epidermis is covered by a thickened horny layer including areas of parakeratosis. Exocytosis of neutrophils in the epidermis is seen, accompanied by the formation of spongiform pustules and microabscesses. The superficial dermis contains a predominantly mononuclear inflammatory cell infiltrate. Leukocytoclastic vasculitis involving the superficial vascular plexus can occasionally be present [204].

Differential Diagnosis

Close clinicopathological correlation is necessary to exclude pustular psoriasis due to the similar histological features. Additional staining is needed to exclude fungal infections.

Behçet's Disease

Behçet's disease represents a chronic, relapsing systemic vasculitis of unknown etiology with consequent multisystem and multiorgan involvement [205, 206]. The diagnosis of Behçet's disease is essentially a clinical one. According to the criteria proposed by the "International Study Group for Behçet's disease," Behçet's disease is diagnosed if the patient develops recurrent oral ulcer(s) at least three times in one 12-month period and, in addition, exhibits two of the four following criteria: recurrent genital ulceration(s), eye lesions, skin lesions, and positive pathergy test [205, 206]. A recent study on 661 patients with Behçet's disease found mucocutaneous lesions to be the most common manifestation of the disease, with oral ulcer(s), genital ulcer(s), and erythema nodosum-like changes being the presenting or initial manifestations in 88.7%, 14.2%, and 5.7%, respectively [207].

The typical oral lesions consist of exquisitely painful ulcers with necrotic yellowish base and erythematous borders, usually measuring up to 1 cm in diameter. Ulcers can be solitary or appear in crops. They normally regress spontaneously within the 14 days, but some can be fairly persistent. In addition to the oral cavity, ulcer(s) can also develop in the upper respiratory tract, including pharynx and larynx [208, 209]. Genital lesions are similar to the oral lesions. They most commonly develop on the scrotum, penis, and vulva. The frequency of genital involvement has been demonstrated to be significantly higher in patients with disease onset before the age of 40 years [207]. Erythema nodosum-like changes show predilection for lower extremities and are characterized by multiple painful subcutaneous nodules of different sizes. Additional cutaneous manifestation of Behçet's disease includes acneiform papules, pustules, furuncles, Sweet-like lesions, and pyoderma gangrenosum [205, 210, 211]. Papulopustular follicular and non-follicular acneiform lesions most frequently involve trunk, lower and upper extremities, and the face [211]. Other organ systems are also frequently involved, including ocular, vascular, articular, gastrointestinal, urogenital, pulmonary, cardiovascular, and neurological system [205, 206].

Behçet's disease shows worldwide distribution with the incidence differing significantly among countries. While the incidence in North America and United Kingdom is only 1–2/1,000,000 inhabitants, an incidence of up to 370/100,000 inhabitants has been observed in Turkey [212, 213]. Behçet's disease generally demonstrates a slight male predominance and usually starts in the third or fourth decade of life [212]. Children can also be affected [214]. The clinical course is characterized by exacerbations and remissions [214].

The underlying pathogenetic process in the development of the many clinical manifestations in Behçet's disease appears to vasculitis, triggered by yet unknown factor(s) [215]. Characteristically, the vasculitic process involves both veins and arteries of all sizes frequently leading to thromboses and formation of aneurysms without granuloma formation and without thickening of vessel walls [215]. Nevertheless, other pathogenetic factors have been suggested and include infectious triggers, heat shock proteins, gamma/delta T lymphocytes, neutrophilic hyperfunction, overproduction of pro-inflammatory cytokines (IL-1, IL-6, IL-8, and TNF-α), endothelial cell injury, increased levels of thrombomodulin, and genetic factors [216]. Several studies have demonstrated close association of HLA-B*51, HLA-B*15, HLA-A*26, and HLA-B*5701 with Behçet's disease confirming genetic predisposition for the development of the disease [217]. Familial clustering of Behçet's disease has also been observed [218].

Histological Features

The histological features in Behçet's disease are usually nonspecific. Oral and genital ulcers are characterized histologically by the ulceration of the epidermis or mucosa, associated with variably prominent mixed inflammatory cell infiltrate in the dermis and/or subepithelial stroma (Fig. 3.19). A lymphocytic vasculitis can occasionally be present.

In contrast to classical histological features of erythema nodosum, erythema nodosum-like lesions in patients with Behçet's disease are distinguished by both septal and lobular panniculitis with neutrophilic granulocytes being the predominant component of the inflammatory cell infiltrate, frequently associated with vasculitis [219–222]. The spectrum of vasculitic changes includes neutrophilic vasculitis, lymphocytic

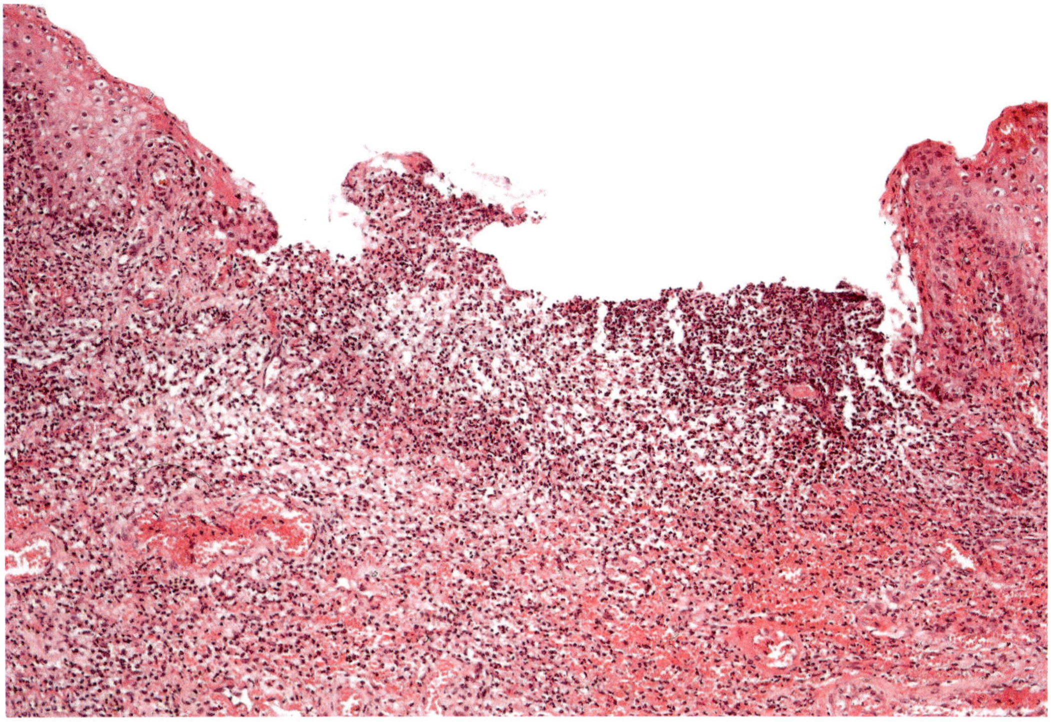

Fig. 3.19 Behcet's disease. Ulcers usually show a nonspecific histology with a prominent mixed inflammatory cell infiltrate rich in neutrophils. Granulation tissue and fibrin are also seen

vasculitis, leukocytoclastic vasculitis, as well as phlebitis and arteriolitis [219–222]. Necrotizing vasculitis involving small- and medium-sized arteries within the subcutaneous fat, similar to polyarteritis nodosa, has also been reported in patients with Behçet's disease [223–226].

Papulopustular lesions in Behçet's disease are characterized by perifollicular or follicular suppurative inflammation with concomitant vasculitis, either lymphocytic or leukocytoclastic [227–230]. The presence of vasculitis helps discriminate papulopustular lesions in Behçet's disease from acne [227, 228]. Superficial and/or deep perivascular and interstitial mixed inflammatory cell infiltrate composed of lymphocytes, macrophages, and neutrophils can also be seen [231].

Differential Diagnosis

The diagnosis of Behçet's disease is essentially a clinical one. Since histological features of mucocutaneous Behçet's disease are usually nonspecific, close clinicopathological correlation is essential. The histological differential diagnosis is broad and among others includes various infections, neutrophilic dermatoses, erythema nodosum, acne, and other systemic diseases.

Genital Bullous Pemphigoid

Bullous pemphigoid is an acquired autoimmune bullous disease characterized by the development of subepidermal blisters due to the IgG antibodies directed against 180- and 230-kDa proteins at the basement membrane [232]. The disease is distinguished clinically by the development of tense dome-shaped blisters on the normal or erythematous skin measuring up to several centimeters in diameter [232–234]. During the course of the disease, bullae eventually collapse with subsequent crust formation. The eruption can be localized or generalized. Sites of predilections include trunk, extremities, and intertriginous areas [232–234]. Mucosal sites can also be involved, with oral mucosa being predominantly affected [235, 236]. The incidence of oral mucosa involvement is highly variable and has been reported between 8% and 58% [235, 236].

Bullous pemphigoid most frequently develops after the age of 70 years and peeks after the age of 90 years [237]. A slight female predominance is observed before the age of 70 years and slight male predominance thereafter [237]. The incidence of bullous pemphigoid is about 10/1,000,000 inhabitants but can be as high as 40/100,000 inhabitants in the age group of over 90 years [234, 237]. Involvement of the vulva has been reported in 9% of adult women [238]. Bullous pemphigoid in children has traditionally been separated into infantile and childhood variant [238–241]. Infantile bullous pemphigoid generally develops in children up to the age of 1 year and typically develops on acral locations, particularly on palms and soles [238–241]. Genital involvement in this age group is exceedingly rare and is more common in boys [239]. Childhood bullous pemphigoid peeks at the age of 8 years, typically presents with genital involvement, almost exclusively in girls, and can represent localized genital involvement with the absence of other cutaneous manifestations [239, 240]. Genital involvement in childhood bullous pemphigoid is present in about 40% of the patients [239].

The two main target antigens involved in the pathogenesis of bullous pemphigoid are 230-kDa protein (BPAg1) and 180-kDa protein (BPAg2). The 230-kDa protein belongs to the plakin family and localizes to the hemidesmosomes [242, 243]. The 180-kDa protein is an adhesion molecule composed of an intracytoplasmic N-terminal fragment, a transmembrane fragment, and a collagenous extracellular C-terminal, extending to the lamina lucida [244]. Up to 90% of patients with generalized bullous pemphigoid have antibodies targeting the 230-kDa protein and up to 50% also have antibodies against 180-kDa protein [245]. Other antigens, much rarely involved in the pathogenesis of bullous pemphigoid, include 105-kDa protein and 200-kDa protein [246, 247]. In children, antibodies against 120-kDa protein have rarely been detected, thus overlapping with the linear IgA disease [248, 249].

Histological Features

Histological changes depend on the stage of the disease at which the biopsy is performed. Early lesions are characterized by absence of blistering and eosinophilic spongiosis (spongiosis with eosinophils) and edema in the papillary dermis and superficial, predominantly perivascular, inflammatory cell infiltrate containing lymphocytes, histiocytes, and usually abundant eosinophils. Established lesions are those of a cell-rich subepidermal blister covered by a thin layer of the epidermis. The blister cavity in cell-rich variant typically contains fibrin, serum, and numerous eosinophils (Fig. 3.20). The dermal papillae are generally well preserved, forming projections into the blister cavity. The papillary dermis is edematous and contains numerous eosinophils in perivascular and interstitial distribution. Very rare cases are inflammatory cell poor.

Direct immunofluorescence on frozen tissue sections typically demonstrates linear deposition of IgG and C3 along the basement membrane [250]. More rarely, linear deposition of IgA, IgM, and IgE can also be seen [251, 252]. Split skin indirect immunofluorescence against 180- and 230-kDa protein characteristically labels the roof of the vesicle, while anti-p105-kDa antibody typically demonstrates positivity at the dermal site of the blister [246].

Differential Diagnosis

Other types of subepidermal blistering dermatoses, including linear IgA dermatosis, dermatitis herpetiformis, epidermolysis bullosa acquisita, as well as bullous systemic lupus erythematosus should be considered in the differential diagnosis of an inflammatory cell-rich subepidermal blister. Close clinicopathological correlation, supplemented by immunofluorescence analysis, is crucial for correct recognition of the lesions.

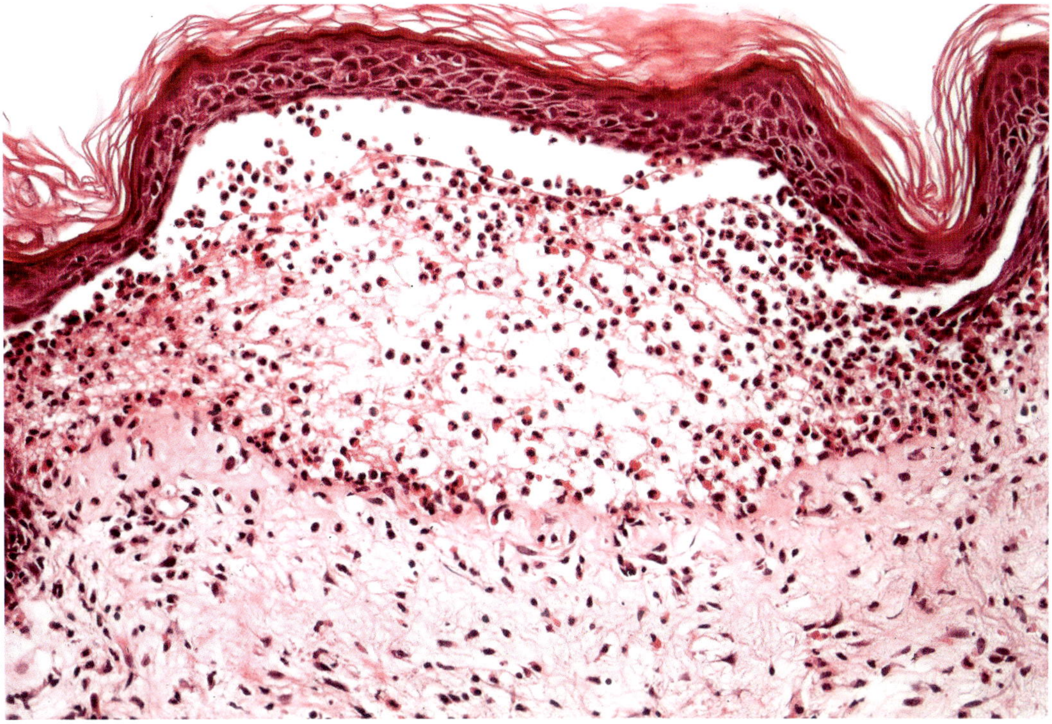

Fig. 3.20 Bullous pemphigoid. Eosinophil-rich subepidermal blister

Differential diagnosis of cell-pure subepidermal blisters mainly includes epidermolysis bullosa and porphyria cutanea tarda.

Genital Mucous Membrane Pemphigoid (Cicatricial Pemphigoid)

Mucous membrane pemphigoid, previously designated as cicatricial pemphigoid is an autoimmune bullous disease affecting mucous membranes of the urogenital tract, oral cavity, eye, esophagus, nasal cavity, nasopharynx, and larynx [253, 254]. Involvement of the skin is present in about 30% of the patients [255]. Involvement of the vulva is seen in about 50% of adult patients [256].

The incidence of mucous membrane pemphigoid has been estimated to be about 1/1,000,000 inhabitants [257]. The disease most frequently presents in the sixth or seventh decade of life and is about twice as common in females than in males [253].

Mucous membrane pemphigoid is characterized clinically by the development of blisters and bullae that rupture easily with subsequent erosions. The genital lesions typical appear most commonly on the labia majora and minora as well as on the prepuce and glans penis. Frequently, however, synechiae of the labia majora and minora develop due to the extensive fibrosis and scarring, eventually leading to the narrowing of the vaginal orifice and stenosis of the urethral ostium [253, 255]. Sclerotic lesion of mucus membrane pemphigoid can closely mimic lichen sclerosus on clinical examination [258]. In children, mucous membrane pemphigoid is extremely rare and most commonly involves the oral cavity followed by the vulva [259–261]. Vulvar changes can represent the only manifestation of the disease in children [259].

Bullous pemphigoid of 180-kDa protein is the most frequently involved antigen in the pathogenesis of the mucous membrane pemphigoid [262]. Other target antigens include the $\alpha 3$ chain of laminin 5, $\beta 4$ integrin, 230-kDa protein, 168-kDa protein, and 45-kDa protein [263–267].

Histological Features

Histological features of mucous membrane pemphigoid closely mimic those in bullous pemphigoid. A subepidermal cell-rich blister is seen, frequently extending along the adnexal structures. The blister cavity contains fibrin, serum, and a mixed inflammatory cell infiltrate consisting of neutrophils and eosinophils. In the dermis, a perivascular and/or interstitial mixed inflammatory cell infiltrate with eosinophils, neutrophils, lymphocytes, and histiocytes is identified. Occasionally, plasma cells can be prominent. Eosinophils within the blister cavity and in the dermis are not usually as prominent as in bullous pemphigoid. Scarring is invariably present, especially in older or recurring lesions.

Direct immunofluorescence findings are similar to bullous pemphigoid. A linear and continuous band along the basement membrane of IgG (and sometimes IgA) and/or complement component C3 is present in about 80–100% of patients with mucous membrane pemphigoid [268]. The best results are generally obtained from the perilesional tissue. Diagnostic sensitivity can be increased by indirect immunofluorescence on normal salt-split mucosa. Circulating anti-p180-kDa protein IgG antibodies are the most common and can be detected in about 50% of the patients [269].

Genital Pemphigus Vulgaris

Pemphigus vulgaris is an autoimmune bullous disorder involving mucous membranes and the skin. The incidence of pemphigus vulgaris has been estimated to be 1–5/1000,000 inhabitants [270, 271]. The disease usually presents between the 40 and 60 years and affects man and women equally [271]. The oral cavity is the initial site of occurrence in up to 70% of the patients [272]. Other mucosal sites include the eye, pharynx, larynx, esophagus, urethra, and anal mucosa [273]. Genital involvement in pemphigus vulgaris generally occurs in patients with extensive involvement of other sites [274]. Genital pemphigus vulgaris most commonly develops on labia majora and labia minora, followed by vagina [275]. Involvement of the uterine cervix is not uncommon [275]. Exceptionally, the genital area can be the sole presentation of pemphigus vulgaris, particularly in children [276, 277]. Nevertheless, Initial presentation in childhood is rare. In children, mucosal involvement is more common than skin involvement, the frequencies being 97% and 84% in altogether 33 children, respectively [277]. Two clinical variants of pemphigus vulgaris are recognized in children: a childhood and juvenile variant, both associated with a higher incidence of genital pemphigus vulgaris than in adults [277].

Mucosal changes in pemphigus vulgaris are characterized clinically by erosions and ulcers, while intact blisters are rarely seen. Cutaneous lesions develop in the background of normal or erythematous skin and include round to oval vesicles and bullae that easily rupture with subsequent painful erosions, bleeding, and crusting [271]. The lesions are generally nonpruritic but can be associated with significant burning and pain. Cutaneous lesions show predilection for the scalp, face, axillae, and groins. Healing is accompanied by postinflammatory hyperpigmentations, while scarring is not a feature of pemphigus vulgaris [278]. Pemphigus vegetans is a distinctive variant of pemphigus vulgaris characterized by vegetating skin lesions in fold areas, including inguinal, perianal, umbilical, mammary, axillary, as well as on the scalp [279].

The main target antigens involved in the pathogenesis of pemphigus vulgaris include desmoglein 3 and in many patients, also desmoglein 1 [280, 281]. While desmoglein 3 is generally expressed in the oral mucosa, the expression of desmoglein 1 is limited to the skin [282]. Direct immunofluorescence of the perilesional skin typically reveals IgG antibodies and C3 fraction of the complement in the intercellular part of the epidermis, characteristically forming a honeycombing pattern throughout the epidermis [250, 283]. Circulating IgG antibodies in the serum appear to reflect the disease activity are present in about 90% of the patients and can be detected by indirect immunofluorescence [284–286].

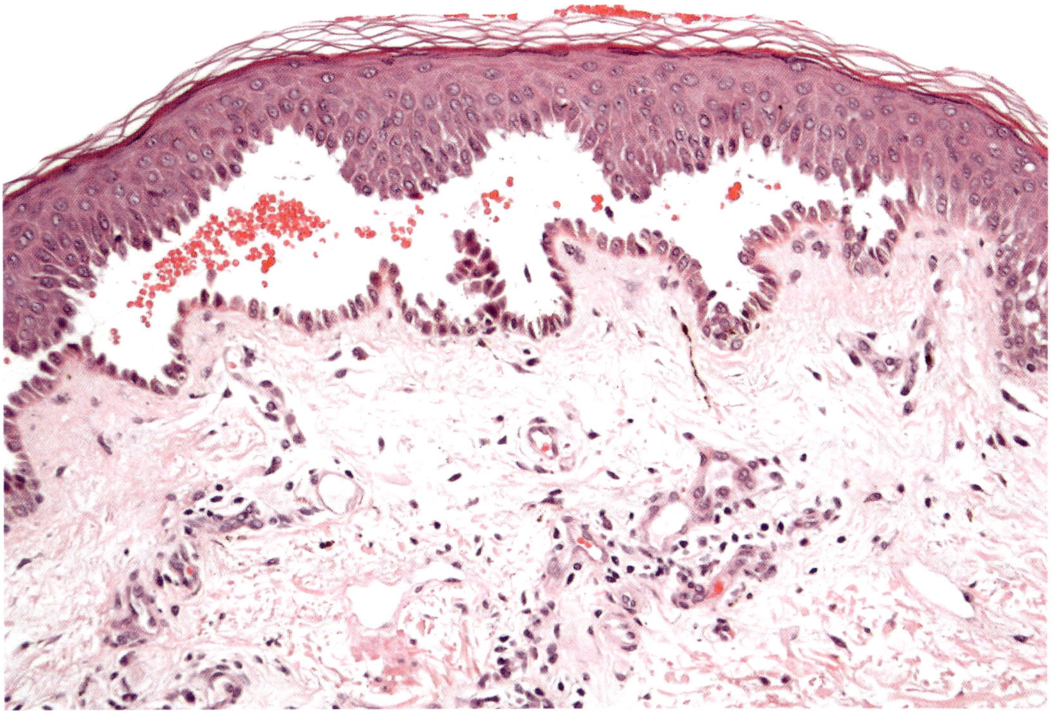

Fig. 3.21 Pemphigus. Early lesion with hardly any inflammation, suprabasal clefting, acantholysis, and tombstoning

Histological Features

Pemphigus vulgaris is characterized histologically by acantholysis, involving both the epidermis and adnexal epithelium. Early lesions typically demonstrate a suprabasal cleft or vesicle (Fig. 3.21). The floor of the blister is lined by a single layer of basal cells. Dermal papillae frequently protrude into the base of the blister. The blister cavity contains occasional rounded and intensely basophilic acantholytic cells, admixed with scarce inflammatory cells, usually eosinophils. In the dermis, a mixed inflammatory cell infiltrate composed of lymphocytes, histiocytes, and variable number of eosinophils is usually seen.

Differential Diagnosis

The differential diagnosis of pemphigus vulgaris includes other bullous disorders, mainly Darier's disease, Hailey-Hailey disease, and transient acantholytic dermatosis. Distinction may be impossible without clinicopathological correlation and additional use of immunofluorescence studies.

Hailey-Hailey Disease

Hailey-Hailey disease (benign familial pemphigus) is an autosomal dominant disease caused by mutations in the *ATP2C1* gene located on the chromosome 3q21–24, which encodes the human secretory pathway Ca^{2+}/Mn^{2+} ATPase protein 1 (hSPCA1) [287–289]. The hSPCA1 is part of an adhesion complex between desmosomal proteins and tonofilaments [287, 288]. Mutations of the *ATP2C1* gene result in skin fragility [287, 288].

The exact prevalence of the Hailey-Hailey disease is unknown. The disease usually develops in the second to fourth decade of life [290, 291]. Hailey-Hailey typically presents with vesicles and bullae on normal or erythematous skin, which are rapidly replaced by eroded and crusted plaques with cracks and fissures [290]. Vegetating hypertrophic lesions can also be seen [290]. The lesions show predilection for flexural sites, including nape of the neck, axillae, submammary region, inguinal folds, perianal region, and genital area [290]. Bacterial, fungal, or viral superinfection is not uncommon [292, 293]. Although in the majority of the patients the lesions are limited to a few flexural areas, a generalized variant of the disease may occur [294]. Isolated involvement of a particular region, including the vulva, can also be seen [295]. Anogenital lesions in Hailey-Hailey disease can, especially in women, occasionally present with distinctive warty papules measuring 3–5 mm in diameter [296]. Such lesions show overlap with papular acantholytic dyskeratosis of the vulva (see below). The course of the Hailey-Hailey disease is characterized by frequent remissions and relapses. Precipitating factors include mechanical trauma, stress, as well as ultraviolet radiation, and the disease usually worsens during the summer months [290]. The lesions generally heal without scarring.

Development of an invasive squamous cell carcinoma in the background of vulval Hailey-Hailey disease has exceptionally been reported [297, 298].

Histological Features

The main histological feature of Hailey-Hailey disease is incomplete acantholysis with the cells retaining some connections to neighboring cells, resulting in a characteristic "dilapidated brick wall" appearance. Focal formation of "corps ronds" and "grains" can be seen, but this phenomenon is generally not prominent. The adnexal epithelium is not involved.

Differential Diagnosis

Differential diagnosis of Hailey-Hailey disease mainly includes Darier's disease and pemphigus vulgaris. Darier's disease is characterized by involvement of adnexal epithelium with frequent formation of corps ronds and grains. Pemphigus vulgaris, in addition to typical immunofluorescence findings, displays suprabasal acantholysis, which is not of the dilapidated wall type and usually extends into the adnexal epithelium. An overlap with papular acantholytic dyskeratosis is discussed below.

Papular Acantholytic Dyskeratosis of the Vulva

Papular acantholytic dyskeratosis of the vulva, originally reported in 1984 by Chorzelski et al. is characterized by multiple dome-shaped skin to white-colored papules developing on the vulva and perianal area, with occasional extension to perineum and the thigh [299–307]. Similar changes have also been described in males on the penis, scrotum, thigh, perianal region, and within the anal canal [308–310]. Confluence of the lesions and formation of plaques can be seen [307]. Papular acantholytic dyskeratosis of the vulva is usually asymptomatic, but pruritus and burning sensation can sometimes be present [300]. No similar lesions are present outside the anogenital area [311]. Furthermore, family history for other vesiculobullous dermatoses is, as a rule, negative.

Histology

Papular acantholytic dyskeratosis is characterized by suprabasal acantholysis accompanied by prominent hyperkeratosis, parakeratosis, and acanthosis [299]. Acantholysis and dyskeratotic cells can involve the entire thickness of the epidermis, with formation of the corps ronds and grains, similar to those seen in Darier's disease.

Differential Diagnosis

Differential diagnosis mainly includes Hailey-Hailey disease, Darier's disease, Grover's disease, and warty dyskeratoma. The absence of a family history of bullous diseases and the absence of lesions outside the genital area help establish the correct diagnosis. Warty dyskeratoma is characterized by a cup-shaped invagination with a central keratotic plug and occurs predominantly on the head.

References

1. Tappeiner J, Pfleger L. Granuloma gluteale infantum. Hautarzt. 1971;22:383–8.
2. Bazex A, Dupre A, Christol B, et al. Infantile gluteal granuloma (Tappeiner and Pfleger). Should it be considered as 'contact vegetating fluorides' or as 'infant halogenosis'. Ann Dermatol Syphiligr (Paris). 1972; 99:121–33.
3. Strögmann W. Gluteal granuloma of infants. A new (detergent-induced?) infantile dermatosis. Monatsschr Kinderheilkd. 1974;122:665–6.
4. Lovell CR, Atherton DJ. Infantile gluteal granuloma – case report. Clin Exp Dermatol. 1984;9:522–5.
5. Valli F, Della Morte MA, Meschi V, et al. Infantile gluteal granuloma. Case report. Pediatr Med Chir. 1985;7:137–9.
6. Delacretaz J, Grigoriu D, de Crousaz H, et al. Nodular candidiasis of the inguino-genital and gluteal region (granuloma gluteale infantum). Dermatologica. 1972;144:143–55.
7. Bonifazi E, Garofalo L, Lospalluti M, et al. Granuloma gluteale infantum with atrophic scars: clinical and histological observations in eleven cases. Clin Exp Dermatol. 1981;6:23–9.
8. Bourrat E, Vaquin C, Prigent F, et al. Perianal papulonodular dermatitis in Hirschsprung disease. Ann Dermatol Venereol. 1996;123:549–51.
9. Rodriguez-Poblador J, Gonzalez-Castro U, Herranz-Martinez S, et al. Jacquet erosive dermatitis after surgery for Hirschsprung disease. Pediatr Dermatol. 1998;15:46–7.
10. Virgili A, Corazza M. Sevestre et Jacquet. Ann Dermatol Venereol. 1992;119:744–5.
11. Virgili A, Corazza M, Califono A. Diaper dermatitis in an adult. A case of erythema papuloerosive of Sevestre and Jacquet. J Reprod Med. 1998;43:949–51.
12. Fujita M, Ohno S, Danno K, et al. Two cases of diaper area granuloma of the adult. J Dermatol. 1991;18: 671–5.
13. Maekawa Y, Sakazaki Y, Hayashibara T. Diaper area granuloma of the aged. Arch Dermatol. 1978;114: 382–3.
14. McKee PH, Calonje E, Granter SR. Spongiotic, psoriasiform and pustular dermatoses. In: McKee PH, Calonje E, Granter SR, editors. Pathology of the skin with clinical correlations. 3rd ed. Philadelphia: Elsevier Mosby; 2005. p. 171–216.
15. Fischer GO. The commonest causes of symptomatic vulvar disease: a dermatologist's perspective. Australas J Dermatol. 1996;37:12–8.
16. Crone AM, Stewart EJC, Wojnarowska F, et al. Aetiological factors in vulvar dermatitis. J Eur Acad Dermatol Venereol. 2000;14:181–6.
17. Fisher G, Spurret B, Fisher A. The chronically symptomatic vulva: aetiology and management. Br J Obstet Gynaecol. 1995;102:773–9.
18. Niamh L, Naveen S, Hazel B. Diagnosis of vulval inflammatory dermatoses: a pathological study with clinical correlation. Int J Gynecol Pathol. 2009;28: 554–8.
19. Cheung ST, Gach JE, Lewis FM. A retrospective study of the referral patterns to a vulval clinic: highlighting educational needs in this subspecialty. J Obstet Gynaecol. 2006;26:435–7.
20. Ball SB, Wojnarowska F. Vulvar dermatoses: lichen sclerosus, lichen planus, and vulval dermatitis/lichen simplex chronicus. Semin Cutan Med Surg. 1998;17: 182–8.
21. Bowen AR, Vester A, Marsden L, et al. The role of vulvar skin biopsy in the evaluation of chronic vulvar pain. Am J Obstet Gynecol. 2008;199:467.e1–e6.
22. O'Keefe RJ, Scurry JP, Dennerstein G, et al. Audit of 114 non-neoplastic vulvar biopsies. Br J Obstet Gynaecol. 1995;102:780–6.
23. Margesson LJ. Contact dermatitis of the vulva. Dermatol Ther. 2004;17:20–7.
24. Johansson SGO, Bieber T, Dahl R, et al. Revised nomenclature for allergy for global use: report of the nomenclature review committee of the World Allergy Organization, October 2003. J Allergy Clin Immunol. 2004;113:832–6.
25. Wakashin K. Sanitary napkin contact dermatitis of the vulva: location-dependent differences in skin surface conditions may play a role in negative patch test results. J Dermatol. 2007;34:834–7.
26. Hammock LA, Barret TL. Inflammatory dermatoses of the vulva. J Cutan Pathol. 2005;32:604–11.
27. Eiermann HJ, Larsen W, Maibach HI, et al. Prospective study of cosmetic reactions: 1977–1980. North American Contact Dermatitis Group. J Am Acad Dermatol. 1982;6:909–17.
28. Faergemann J, Bergbrant IM, Dohsé M, et al. Seborrhoeic dermatitis and Pityrosporum (Malassezia) folliculitis: characterization of inflammatory cells and mediators in the skin by immunohistochemistry. Br J Dermatol. 2001;144:549–56.
29. Williams HC. Diagnostic criteria for atopic dermatitis. Where do we go from here? Arch Dermatol. 1999;135:583–6.
30. Fischer G, Rogers M. Vulvar disease in children: a clinical audit of 130 children. Pediatr Dermatol. 2000;17:1–6.
31. Taylor RM. Histopathology of contact dermatitis. Clin Dermatol. 1986;4:18–22.
32. White Jr CR. Histopathology of atopic dermatitis. Semin Dermatol. 1983;2:234–8.
33. White CR. Histopathology of exogenous and systemic contact dermatitis. Semin Dermatol. 1990;9:226–9.
34. Shaffer B, Beerman H. Lichen simplex chronicus and its variants: discussion of certain psychodynamic

mechanisms and clinical and histopathologic correlations. AMA Arch Derm Syphilol. 1951;64:340–51.
35. Lynch PJ. Lichen simplex chronicus (atopic/neurodermatitis) of the anogenital region. Dermatol Ther. 2004;17:8–19.
36. Sullivan AK, Straughair GJ, Marwood RP, et al. A multidisciplinary vulva clinic: the role of genito-urinary medicine. J Eur Acad Dermatol Venereol. 1999;13:36–40.
37. Rajalakshmi R, Trappa DM, Jainsankar TJ, et al. Lichen simplex chronicus of anogenital region: a clinic-etiological study. Indian J Dermatol Venereol Leprol. 2011;77:28–36.
38. Rowland Payne CM, Wilkinson JD, McKee PH, et al. Nodular prurigo – a clinicopathological study of 46 patients. Br J Dermatol. 1985;113:431–9.
39. Gach JE, Seddon HF. Gluten-sensitive enteropathy associated with genital lichen simplex chronicus. JRSM Short Rep. 2010;1:43–6.
40. Hallopeau H. Lichen plan sclereux. Ann Dermatol Syph (2nd Ser). 1889;20:447–9.
41. Meffert JJ, Davis BM, Grimwood RE. Lichen sclerosus. J Am Acad Dermatol. 1995;32:393–416.
42. Attili VR, Attili SK. Lichen sclerosus of lips: a clinical and histopathological study of 27 cases. Int J Dermatol. 2010;49:520–5.
43. Ballester I, Banuls J, Perez-Crespo M, et al. Extragenital bullous lichen sclerosus atrophicus. Dermatol Online J. 2009;1:6.
44. Aggarwal K, Jain VK, Brahma D. Palmo-plantar lichen sclerosus et atrophicus. Indian J Dermatol Venereol Leprol. 2003;69:43–4.
45. Sherlin HJ, Ramalingam K, Natesan A, et al. Lichen sclerosus of the oral cavity. Case report and review of the literature. J Dermatol Case Rep. 2010;3:38–43.
46. Saunders H, Buchanan JAG, Cooper S, et al. The period prevalence of oral lichen planus in a cohort of patients with wulvar lichen sclerosus. J Eur Acad Dermatol Venereol. 2009;24:18–21.
47. Powell JJ, Wojnarowska F. Lichen sclerosus. Lancet. 1999;353:1777–83.
48. Barbagli G, Mirri F, Gallucci M, et al. Histological evidence of urethral involvement in male patients with genital lichen sclerosus: a preliminary report. J Urol. 2011;185:2171–6.
49. Kimura A, Kambe N, Satoh T, et al. Follicular keratosis and bullous formation are typical signs of extragenital lichen sclerosus. J Dermatol. 2010;38:834–6.
50. Ristić B, Divic J, Belic LJ, et al. Bullous lichen sclerosus atrophicus. J Eur Acad Dermatol Venereol. 2004;18:99–117.
51. Tasker GL, Wojnarowska F. Lichen sclerosus. Clin Exp Dermatol. 2003;28:128–33.
52. Sherman V, McPherson T, Baldo M, et al. The high rate of familial lichen sclerosus suggests a genetic contribution: an observational cohort study. J Eur Acad Dermatol Venereol. 2010;24:1031–4.
53. Powel JJ, Wojnarowska F, Winsey S, et al. Lichen sclerosus premenarche: autoimmunity and immunogenetics. Br J Dermatol. 2000;142:481–4.
54. Marren P, Yell J, Charnock FM, et al. The association between lichen sclerosus and the HLA system. Br J Dermatol. 1995;132:197–203.
55. Azurdia RM, Luzzi GA, Byren I, et al. Lichen sclerosus in adult men: a study of HLA associations and susceptibility to autoimmune disease. Br J Dermatol. 1999;140:79–83.
56. Aslanian FMNP, Marques MTQ, Matos HJ, et al. HLA markers in familial lichen sclerosus. J Dtsch Dermatol Ges. 2006;4:842–7.
57. Meyrick Thomas RH, Ridley CM, McGibbon DH, et al. Lichen sclerosus et atrophicus and autoimmunity: a study of 350 women. Br J Dermatol. 1988;118:41–6.
58. Cooper S, Ali I, Baldo M, Wojnarowska F. The association of lichen sclerosus and erosive lichen planus of the vulva with autoimmune disease. A case-control study. Arch Dermatol. 2008;144:1432–5.
59. Kim DH, Lee KR, Kim TY, et al. Coexistence of lichen sclerosus with morphea showing bilateral symmetry. Clin Exp Dermatol. 2009;34:416–8.
60. Goolamali SI, Neill SM. A first case of lichen sclerosus with Turner's syndrome. Clin Exp Dermatol. 2009;34:419–20.
61. Zollinger T, Mertz KD, Schmid M, et al. Borrelia in granuloma annulare, morphea and lichen sclerosus: a PCR-based study and review of the literature. J Cutan Pathol. 2010;37:571–7.
62. McPherson T, Cooper S. Vulvar lichen sclerosus and lichen planus. Dermatol Ther. 2010;523:532.
63. Carlson JA, Ambros R, Malfetano J, et al. Vulvar lichen sclerosus and squamous cell carcinoma: a cohort, case control, and investigational study with historical perspective; implications for chronic inflammation and sclerosis in the development of neoplasia. Hum Pathol. 1998;29:239–48.
64. Wang S-H, Chi C-C, Wong YW, et al. Genital verrucous carcinoma is associated with lichen sclerosus: a retrospective study and review of the literature. J Eur Acad Dermatol Venereol. 2010;24:815–9.
65. Serheant A, Vernall N, Mackintosh LJ, et al. Squamous cell carcinoma arising in extragenital lichen sclerosus. Clin Exp Dermatol. 2009;34:278–9.
66. Regauer S, Liegl B, Reich O. Early vulvar lichen sclerosus: a histopathological challenge. Histopathology. 2005;47:340–7.
67. Slater DN, Wagner BE. Early vulvar lichen sclerosus: a histopathological challenge. Histopathology. 2007;50:388–9.
68. Uitto J, Santa Cruz DJ, Bauer EA, et al. Morphea and liche sclerosus et atrophicus. Clinical and histologic studies in patients with combined features. J Am Acad Dermatol. 1980;3:271–9.
69. Rakha E, Mayne C, Brown L. Mucinous metaplasia of the vulva in a case of lichen sclerosus. A case report. J Clin Pathol. 2005;58:1217–8.
70. Regauer S, Beham-Schmid C. Detailed analysis of the T-cell lymphocytic infiltrate in penile lichen sclerosus: an immunohistochemical and molecular investigation. Histopathology. 2006;48:730–5.

71. Regauer S, Liegl B, Reich O, et al. Vasculitis in lichen sclerosus: an under recognized feature? Histopathology. 2004;45:237–44.
72. Luzar B, Neil SM, Calonje E. Angiokeratoma-like changes in extragenital and genital lichen sclerosus. J Cutan Pathol. 2009;36:540–2.
73. Dargent J-L. Acquired lymphangiectasias in genital lichen sclerosus. Am J Dermatopathol. 2011;33: 200–2.
74. Abbas O, Chatrath V, Goldberg LJ. Elastophagocytosis in extragenital lichen sclerosus. J Cutan Pathol. 2010;37:1032–7.
75. Suchak R, Verdolini R, Robson A, et al. Extragenital lichen sclerosus et atrophicus mimicking cutaneous T-cell lymphoma: report of a case. J Cutan Pathol. 2010;37:982–6.
76. Perera E, Toll A, Gallardo F, et al. Lichen sclerosus et atrophicus-like lesions in mycosis fungoides. Br J Dermatol. 2007;157:411–3.
77. Meeuwis KA, De Hullu JA, de Jager MEA, et al. Genital psoriasis: a questionnaire-based survey on a concealed skin disease in the Netherlands. J Eur Acad Dermatol Venereol. 2010;24:1425–30.
78. Meeuwis KA, de Hullu JA, Massuger LF, et al. Genital psoriasis: a systematic review on this hidden skin disease. Acta Derm Venereol. 2011;91:5–11.
79. Farber EM, Nall ML. The natural history of psoriasis in 5600 patients. Dermatologica. 1974;148:1–18.
80. Zamirska A, Reich A, Berny-Moreno J, et al. Vulvar pruritus and burning sensation in women with psoriasis. Acta Derm Venereol. 2008;88:132–5.
81. Gross G. Dermatologische befunde an Mamma und Genitale. Der Gynakologe. 2001;34:940–8.
82. Porter WM, Bunker CB. The dysfunctional foreskin. Int J STD AIDS. 2001;12:216–20.
83. Quan MB, Ruben BS. Pustular psoriasis limited to the penis. Int J Dermatol. 1996;35:202–4.
84. Singh N, Thappa DM. Circinate pustular psoriasis localized to glans penis mimicking 'circinate balanitis' and responsive to dapsone. Indian J Dermatol Venereol Leprol. 2008;74:388–9.
85. Scully G, El-Kom M. Lichen planus: review and update on pathogenesis. J Oral Pathol. 1985;14: 431–58.
86. Belifore P, Di Fede O, Cabibi D, et al. Prevalence of vulval lichen planus in a cohort of women with oral lichen planus: an interdisciplinary study. Br J Dermatol. 2006;155:994–8.
87. Eisen D. The clinical manifestations and treatment of oral lichen planus. Dermatol Clin. 2003;21:79–89.
88. Lewis FM, Shah M, Harrington CI. Vulval involvement in lichen planus: a study of 37 women. Br J Dermatol. 1996;135:89–91.
89. Micheletti L, Preti M, Bogliatto F, et al. Vulval lichen planus in the practice of vulval clinic. Br J Dermatol. 2000;143:1349–50.
90. Eisen D. The clinical features, malignant potential and systemic association of oral lichen planus: a study of 723 patients. J Am Acad Dermatol. 2002;46: 207–14.
91. Pelisse M, Leibowitch M, Sedel D, et al. Un nouveau syndrome vulvo-vaginal gingival: lichen planus erosive plurimuqueux. Ann Dermatol Venereol. 1982;109: 797–8.
92. Helgersen ALO, Gjersvik P, Jebsen P, et al. Vaginal involvement in genital erosive lichen planus. Acta Obstet Gynecol Scand. 2010;89:966–70.
93. Kennedy CM, Galask RP. Erosive vulvar lichen planus: retrospective review of characteristics and outcomes in 113 patients seen in a vulvar specialty clinic. J Reprod Med. 2007;52:43–7.
94. Gupta R, Bansal B, Singh S, et al. Lichen planus of the uterine cervix – the first report of a novel site of occurrence: a case report. Cases J. 2009;2:9306–8.
95. Goldstein AT, Metz A. Vulvar lichen planus. Clin Obstet Gynecol. 2005;48:818–23.
96. Cooper SM. Influence of treatment of erosive lichen planus of the vulva and its prognosis. Arch Dermatol. 2006;142:289–94.
97. Cooper SM, Ali I, Baldo M, et al. The association of lichen sclerosus and erosive lichen planus of the vulva with autoimmune disease. Arch Dermatol. 2008;144:1432–5.
98. Moutasim KA, Poate TWJ, Setterfield JF, et al. A case of vulvovaginal gingival lichen planus in association with Good's syndrome. Oral Surg Oral Med Oral Pathol Oral Radiol Endod. 2008;105:57–60.
99. Lewis FM. Vulval lichen planus. Br J Dermatol. 1998;138:569–75.
100. Dwyer CM, Kerr REI, Millan DWM. Squamous carcinoma following lichen planus of the vulva. Clin Exp Dermatol. 1995;20:171–2.
101. Franck JM, Young AW. Squamous cell carcinoma arising within lichen planus of the vulva. Dermatol Surg. 1995;21:890–4.
102. Jones RW, Rowan DM, Kirker J, et al. Vulval lichen planus: progression of pseudoepitheliomatous hyperplasia to invasive vulval carcinomas. BJOG. 2001;108:665–6.
103. Chiu TL, Jones RW. Multicentric multifocal squamous cell carcinomas arising in vulvovaginal lichen planus. J Low Genit Tract Dis. 2011;15:246–7.
104. Zoon JJ. Chronic circumscribed balanitis with plasma cells infiltration. Ned Tijdschr Geneeskd. 1950;94:1529–30.
105. Garnier G. Vulvite erythemateuse circonscrite benigne a type erythroplasique. Bull Soc Fr Dermatol Syphiligr. 1954;61:102–4.
106. Zoon JJ. Balanitis and vulvitis plasmacellularis. Dermatologica. 1955;11:157.
107. Fernandez-Aceñero MJ, Cordova S. Zoon's vulvitis (vulvitis circumscripta plasmacellularis). Arch Gynecol Obstet. 2010;282:351–2.
108. Li Q, Leopold K, Carlson JA. Chronic vulvar purpura: persistent pigmented purpuric dermatitis (lichen aureus) of the vulva or plasma cell (Zoon's) vulvitis? J Cutan Pathol. 2003;30:572–6.
109. Neri I, Patrizi A, Marzaduri S, et al. Vulvitis plasmacellularis: two new cases. Genitourin Med. 1995;71: 311–3.

110. Bharti R, Smith DR. Mucous membrane plasmacytosis: a case report and review of the literature. Dermatol Online J. 2003;9:15.
111. White Jr JW, Olsen KD, Banks PM. Plasma cell orificial mucositis. Report of a case and review of the literature. Arch Dermatol. 1986;122:1321–4.
112. Kato T, Kuramoto Y, Tadaki T, et al. Chronic vulvar purpura. Dermatologica. 1990;180:174–6.
113. Thomson MA, Carr RA, Ganesan R, et al. Extensive mucinous metaplasia of the vulva arising in Zoon's vulvitis. Br J Dermatol. 2007;156:750–2.
114. Coghill SB, Tyler X, Shaxted EJ. Benign mucinous metaplasia of the vulva. Histopathology. 1990;17: 373–5.
115. Crohn BB, Ginzburg L, Oppenheimer GD. Regional ileitis. JAMA. 1932;99:1323–9.
116. Burgdorf W. Cutaneous manifestations of Crohn's disease. J Am Acad Dermatol. 1981;5:689–95.
117. Schrodt BJ, Callen JP. Metastatic Crohn's disease presenting as chronic perivulvar and perirectal ulcerations in an adolescent patient. Pediatrics. 1999;103:500–2.
118. Palamaras I, El-Jabbour J, Pietropaolo N, et al. Metastatic Crohn's disease: a review. J Eur Acad Dermatol Venereol. 2008;22:1033–43.
119. Greenstein AJ, Janowitz HD, Sachar DB. The extraintestinal complications of Crohn's disease and ulcerative colitis: a study of 700 patients. Medicine (Baltimore). 1976;55:401–12.
120. Rankin GB, Watts HD, Melnyk CS, et al. National cooperative Crohn's disease study: extraintestinal manifestations and perianal complications. Gastroenterology. 1979;77:914–20.
121. De la Poza G, Lopez-Sanroman A, Taxonera C, et al. Genital fistulas in female Crohn's disease patients. Clinical characteristics and response to therapy. J Crohns Colitis. 2012;6:276–80.
122. Andreani SM, Ratnasingham K, Dang HH, et al. Crohn's disease of the vulva. Int J Surg. 2010;8:2–5.
123. Galbraith SS, Drolet BA, Kugathasan S, et al. Asymptomatic inflammatory bowel disease presenting with mucocutaneous findings. Pediatrics. 2005; 116:439–44.
124. Vaid RM, Cohen BA. Cutaneous Crohn's disease in the pediatric population. Pediatr Dermatol. 2010;27: 279–81.
125. Ploysangam T, Heubi JE, Eisen D, et al. Cutaneous Crohn's disease in children. J Am Acad Dermatol. 1997;36:697–704.
126. Savino A, Pelliccia P, Breda L, et al. Genital swelling in an adolescent patient. Eur J Pediatr. 2006; 165:76–9.
127. Guest MB, Fink RL. Metastatic Crohn's disease. Dis Colon Rectum. 2000;43:1764–6.
128. Günthert AR, Hinney B, Nesselhut K, et al. Vulvitis granulomatosa and unilateral hypertrophy of the vulva related to Crohn's disease: a case report. Am J Obstet Gynecol. 2004;191:1719–20.
129. Paradisi A, Diociaiuti A, Marchesi A, et al. Cutaneous Crohn disease mimicking anal condyloma in a child. J Am Acad Dermatol. 2010;63:165–6.
130. Lestre S, Ramos J, Joao A, et al. Cutaneous Crohn's disease presenting as genital warts: successful treatment with adalimumab. Eur J Dermatol. 2010;20:504–5.
131. Lockhart-Mummery HE. Symposium. Crohn's disease: anal lesions. Dis Colon Rectum. 1975;18: 200–2.
132. Fielding JF. Perianal lesions in Crohn's disease. J R Coll Surg Edinb. 1972;17:32–7.
133. McClane SJ, Rombeau JL. Anorectal Crohn's disease. Surg Clin North Am. 2001;81:169–83.
134. Williams DR, Coller JA, Corman ML, et al. Anal complications of Crohn's disease. Dis Colon Rectum. 1981;34:22–4.
135. Keighley MR, Allan RN. Current status and influence of operation on perianal Crohn's disease. Int J Colorectal Dis. 1986;1:104–7.
136. Buchmann P, Allan R, Thompson H, et al. Carcinoma in rectovaginal fistula in a patient with Crohn's disease. Am J Surg. 1980;140:462–3.
137. Moore-Maxwell CA, Robboy SJ. Mucinous adenocarcinoma arising in rectovaginal fistulas associated with Crohn's disease. Gynecol Oncol. 2004;93:266–8.
138. McCallum DI, Gray WM. Metastatic Crohn's disease. Br J Dermatol. 1976;95:551–4.
139. Acker SM, Sahn EE, Rogers HC, et al. Genital cutaneous Crohn disease. Am J Dermatopathol. 2000;22: 443–6.
140. Hackzell-Bradely M, Hedblad MA, Stephansson EA. Metastatic Crohn's disease. Report of 3 cases with special reference to histopathologic findings. Arch Dermatol. 1996;132:928–32.
141. Becker SW, Kahn D, Rothman S. Cutaneous manifestations of internal malignant tumors. Arch Dermatol. 1942;45:1069–80.
142. Wilkinson DS. Necrolytic migratory erythema with pancreatic carcinoma. Proc R Soc Med. 1971;64: 1197–8.
143. Wilkinson DS. Necrolytic migratory erythema with carcinoma of the pancreas. Trans St Johns Hosp Dermatol Soc. 1973;59:244–50.
144. Wermers RA, Fatourechi V, Wynne AG, et al. The glucagonoma syndrome. Clinical and pathological features in 21 patients. Medicine (Baltimore). 1996;75:53–63.
145. Lack EE. Pancreatic endocrine neoplasms. In: Lack EE, editor. Pathology of the pancreas, gallbladder, extrahepatic biliary tract and ampullary region. Oxford: Oxford University Press Inc.; 2003. p. 323–72.
146. Eldor R, Glaser B, Fraenkel M, et al. Glucagonoma and the glucagonoma syndrome – cumulative experience with en elusive tumour. Clin Endocrinol (Oxf). 2011;74:593–8.
147. Soga J, Yakuwa Y. Glucagonomas/diabetic-dermatogenic syndrome (DS): a statistical evaluation of 407 reported cases. J Hepatobiliary Pancreat Surg. 1998;5:312–9.
148. Castro PG, de Leon AM, Trancon JG, et al. Glucagonoma syndrome: a case report. J Med Case Reports. 2011;5:402.

149. Boden G, Owen OE. Familial hyperglucagonemia: an autosomal dominant disorder. N Engl J Med. 1977;296:534–8.
150. Kindmark H, Sundin A, Granberg D, et al. Endocrine pancreatic tumors with glucagon hypersecretion: a retrospective study of 23 cases during 20 years. Med Oncol. 2007;24:330–7.
151. Mallinson CN, Bloom SR, Warin AP, et al. A glucagonoma syndrome. Lancet. 1974;2:1–5.
152. Miller SJ. Nutritional deficiency and the skin. J Am Acad Dermatol. 1989;21:1–30.
153. Paterson LL, Shaw JC, Acott KM, et al. Glucagonoma syndrome: in vitro evidence that glucagon increases epidermal arachidonic acid. J Am Acad Dermatol. 1984;11:468–73.
154. Van Beek AP, de Haas ERM, van Vloten WA, et al. The glucagonoma syndrome and necrolytic migratory erythema: a clinical review. Eur J Endocrinol. 2004;151:531–7.
155. Pujol RM, Wang C-YE, el Azhary RA, et al. Necrolytic migratory erythema. Int J Dermatol. 2004;43:12–8.
156. Luzar B, Koser-Kola N, Ferlan-Marolt V, et al. A 47-year-old woman with refractory migratory erythema. Clin Exp Dermatol. 2008;33:533–5.
157. El Rassi Z, Partensky C, Valette PJ, et al. Necrolytic migratory erythema, first symptom of a malignant glucagonoma: treatment by long-acting somatostatin and surgical resection. Report of three cases. Eur J Surg Oncol. 1998;24:562–7.
158. Chiyomaru K, Takai T, Ohashi A, et al. Necrolytic migratory erythema with cholangiocarcinoma: pseudoglucagonoma syndrome. Eur J Dermatol. 2010;20:238–9.
159. Mignogna MD, Fortuna G. Small-cell lung cancer and necrolytic migratory erythema. N Engl J Med. 2008;359:2731–2.
160. Möhrenschlager M, Köhler LD, Bruckbauer H, et al. Plattenepithelkarcinom-assoziiertes nekrolytisches migratorisches Erythem. Hautarzt. 1999;50:198–202.
161. Walker NPJ. Atypical necrolytic migratory erythema in association with a jejunal adenocarcinoma. J R Soc Med. 1982;75:134–5.
162. Technau K, Renkl A, Norgauer J, et al. Necrolytic migratory erythema with myelodysplastic syndrome without glucagonoma. Eur J Dermatol. 2005;15:110–2.
163. Koch LH, Lewis DW, Williams JV. Necrolytic migratory erythema-like presentation for cystic fibrosis. J Am Acad Dermatol. 2008;58:29–30.
164. Kelly CP, Johnston CF, Nolan N, et al. Necrolytic migratory erythema with elevated plasma enteroglucagon in celiac disease. Gastroenterology. 1989;96:1350–3.
165. Bencini PL, Vigo GP, Caputo R. Necrolytic migratory erythema without glucagonoma in a heroin-dependent patient. Dermatology. 1994;189:72–4.
166. Muller FM, Arseculerante G, Evans A, et al. Necrolytic migratory erythema in an opiate-dependent patient. Clin Exp Dermatol. 2007;33:40–2.
167. Baricault S, Soubrane JC, Courville P, et al. Necrolytic migratory erythema in Waldmann's disease. Ann Dermatol Venereol. 2006;133:693–6.
168. Topham EJ, Child FJ. Exfoliative erythema of malnutrition with zinc and essential amino acid deficiency. Clin Exp Dermatol. 2005;30:235–7.
169. Kitamura Y, Sato M, Hatamochi A, et al. Necrolytic migratory erythema without glucagonoma associated with hepatitis B. Eur J Dermatol. 2005;15:49–51.
170. Trojan A, Jacky E, Follath F, et al. Necrolytic migratory erythema (glucagonoma) – like skin lesions induced by EGF-receptor inhibition. Swiss Med Wkly. 2003;133:22–3.
171. Kheir SM, Omura EF, Grizzle WE, et al. Histological variations in the skin lesions of the glucagonoma syndrome. Am J Surg Pathol. 1996;10:445–53.
172. Hunt SJ, Narus VT, Abell E. Necrolytic migratory erythema: dyskeratotic dermatitis, a clue to early diagnosis. J Am Acad Dermatol. 1991;24:473–7.
173. Macbeth AE, James A, Rhodes M, et al. Necrolytic migratory erythema with the absence of necrolysis. Clin Exp Dermatol. 2010;35:810–1.
174. Reiter H. Über eine bisher unerkannte Spirochaeteninfektion (Spirochaetosis arthritica). Dtsch Med Wochenschr. 1916;42:1535–6.
175. Gottlieb NL, Altman RD. An ethical dilemma in rheumatology: should the eponym Reiter's syndrome be discharged? Semin Arthritis Rheum. 2003;32:207.
176. Kwiatkowska B, Filipowicz-Sosnowska A. Reactive arthritis. Pol Arch Med Wewn. 2009;119:60–5.
177. Aho K. Bowel infection predisposing to reactive arthritis. Baillieres Clin Rheumatol. 1989;3:303–19.
178. Edmonds J. Reactive arthritis. Aust N Z J Med. 1984;14:81–8.
179. Humdulay SS, Glynne SJ, Keat A. When is arthritis reactive? Postgrad Med J. 2006;82:446–53.
180. Li CW, Ma JJ, Yin J, et al. Reiter's syndrome in children (abstract). Zhonghua Er Ke Za Zhi. 2010;48:212–5.
181. Bauman C, Cron RQ, Sherry DD, et al. Reiter's syndrome initially misdiagnosed as Kawasaki disease. J Pediatr. 1996;128:366–9.
182. Gladman DD. Clinical aspects of the spondyloarthropathies. Am J Med Sci. 1998;316:234–8.
183. Keat A. Reiter's syndrome and reactive arthritis in perspective. N Engl J Med. 1983;309:1606–15.
184. Sampaio-Barros PD, Conde RA, Donadi EA, et al. Frequency of HLA-B27 and its alleles in patients with Reiter syndrome: comparison with frequencies in other spondyloarthropathies and a healthy control population. Rheumatol Int. 2008;28:483–6.
185. Taniguchi Y, Yorioka N, Kyuden Y, et al. Reiter's syndrome associated with HLA-B51: a case report. J Int Med Res. 2003;31:55–7.
186. Rothe MJ, Kerdel FA. Reiter syndrome. Int J Dermatol. 1991;30:173–80.
187. Callen JP, Mahl CF. Oculocutaneous manifestations observed in multisystem disorders. Dermatol Clin. 1992;10:709–16.

188. Wu IB, Schwartz R. Reiter's syndrome: the classic triad and more. J Am Acad Dermatol. 2008;59:113–21.
189. Amor B. Reiter's syndrome: diagnosis and clinical features. Rheum Dis Clin North Am. 1998;24: 677–95.
190. Willkens RF, Arnett FC, Bitter T, et al. Reiter's syndrome. Evaluation of preliminary criteria for definite disease. Bull Rheum Dis. 1982;32:31–4.
191. Kozeis N, Trachana M, Tyradellis S. Keratitis in reactive arthritis (Reiter syndrome) in childhood. Cornea. 2011;30:924–5.
192. Kim SK, Young J, Park MS, et al. A case of Reiter's syndrome with progressive myelopathy. J Clin Neurol. 2007;3:215–8.
193. Sako SG, Iskander SS, Appel RG. IgA nephropathy and Reiter's syndrome: report of two cases and review of the literature. Nephron. 2000;84:177–82.
194. Coskun BK, Saral Y, Ozturk P, et al. Reiter syndrome accompanied by Terry nail. J Eur Acad Dermatol Venereol. 2005;19:87–9.
195. Hannu T, Mattila L, Siitonen A, et al. Reactive arthritis attributable to Shigella infection: a clinical and epidemiological nationwide study. Ann Rheum Dis. 2005;64:594–8.
196. Uotila T, Antonen J, Laine J, for the Pirkanmaa Waterborne Outbreak Study Group, et al. Reactive arthritis in a population exposed to an extensive waterborne gastroenteritis outbreak after sewage contamination in Pirkanmaa, Finland. Scand J Rheumatol. 2011;40(5):358–62.
197. Carter JD, Inman RD, Whittum-Hudson J, et al. Chlamydia and chronic arthritis. Ann Med. 2011; Epub ahead of print.
198. Renou F, Wartel G, Raffray L, et al. Reactive arthritis due to *Escherichia coli* urinary tract infection. Rev Med Interne. 2011;32:4–5.
199. Chou YS, Horng CT, Huang HS, et al. Reactive arthritis following *Streptococcus viridans* urinary tract infection. Ocul Immunol Inflamm. 2010;18:52–3.
200. Birnbaum J, Bartlett JG, Gelber AC. Clostridium difficile: an under-recognized cause of reactive arthritis. Clin Rheumatol. 2008;27:253–5.
201. Tektonidou MG. Reiter's syndrome during intravesical BCG therapy for bladder carcinoma. Clin Rheumatol. 2007;26:1368–9.
202. Murata H, Adachi Y, Ebitsuka T, et al. Reiter's syndrome following intravesical bacille Calmette-Guerin treatment for superficial bladder carcinoma: report of six cases. Mod Rheumatol. 2004;14:82–6.
203. Thielen AM, Barde C, Janer V, et al. Reiter syndrome triggered by adalimumab (Humira®) and leflunomide (Arava®) in a patient with ankylosing spondylarthropathy and Crohn's disease. Br J Dermatol. 2007;156:188–9.
204. Magro CM, Crowson AN, Peeling R. Vasculitis as the basis of cutaneous lesions in Reiter's disease. Hum Pathol. 1995;26:633–8.
205. International Study Group on Behçet's Disease. Criteria for diagnosis of Behçet's disease. Lancet. 1990;335:1078–80.
206. O'Neill TW, Rigby AS, Silman AJ, et al. Validation of the International Study Group criteria for Behçet's disease. Br J Rheumatol. 1994;33:115–7.
207. Alpsoy E, Donmez L, Onder M, et al. Clinical features and natural course of Behçet's disease in 661 cases: a multicentric study. Br J Dermatol. 2007;157: 901–6.
208. Yiğit O, Alkan S, Başak T, et al. Behçet's disease presenting with a hypopharyngeal ulcer. Eur Arch Otorhinolaryngol. 2005;262:151–3.
209. Webb CJ, Moots RJ, Swift AC. Ear, nose and throat manifestations of Behçet's disease: a review. J Laryngol Otol. 2008;122:1279–83.
210. Jorizzo JL, Abernethy JJ, White WL, et al. Mucocutaneous criteria for the diagnosis of Behçet's disease: an analysis of clinicopathologic data from multiple international centers. J Am Acad Dermatol. 1995;32:968–76.
211. Alpsoy E, Aktekin M, Er H, et al. A randomized, controlled and blinded study of papulopustular lesions in Turkish Behçet's patients. Int J Dermatol. 1998;17:333–41.
212. Davatchi F, Davatchi F, Shahram F, et al. Behçet's disease: from east to west. Clin Rheumatol. 2010; 29:823–33.
213. Mendoza-Pinto C, García-Carrasco M, Jiménez-Hernández M, et al. Etiopathogenesis of Behcet's disease. Autoimmun Rev. 2010;9:241–5.
214. Özen S. Pediatric onset Behcet's disease. Curr Opin Rheumatol. 2010;22:585–9.
215. Calamia KT, Schmirer M, Melikoglu M. Major vessel involvement in Behçet's disease: an update. Curr Opin Rheumatol. 2011;23:24–31.
216. Kapsimali VD, Kanakis MA, Vaiopoulos GA, et al. Etiopathogenesis of Behçet's disease with emphasis on the role of immunological aberrations. Clin Rheumatol. 2010;29:1211–6.
217. Piga M, Mathieu A. Genetic susceptibility to Behçet's disease: role of genes belonging to the MHC region. Rheumatology. 2011;50:299–310.
218. Kone-Paut I, Geisler I, Wechsler B, et al. Familial aggregation in Behçet's disease: high frequency in siblings and parents of pediatric probands. J Pediatr. 1999;135:89–93.
219. Kim B, LeBoit PE. Histopathologic features of erythema nodosum-like lesions in Behçet's disease: comparison with erythema nodosum, focusing on the role of vasculitis. Am J Dermatopathol. 2000;22: 379–90.
220. Demirkesen C, Tüzüner N, Mat C, et al. Clinicopathologic evaluation of nodular cutaneous lesions of Behçet's syndrome. Am J Clin Pathol. 2001;116:341–6.
221. Chen K, Kawahara Y, Miyakava S, et al. Cutaneous vasculitis in Behçet's disease: a clinical and histopathologic study of 20 patients. J Am Acad Dermatol. 1997;36:689–96.
222. Chun SI, Su WPD, Lee S. Histopathologic study of cutaneous lesions in Behçet's disease. J Dermatol. 1990;17:333–41.

223. Serra-Guillen C, Llombart B, Alfaro-Rubio A, et al. Behçet's disease and periarteritis nodosa with cutaneous lesions. Actas Dermosifiliogr. 2007;98:217–8.
224. Liao YH, Hsiao GH, Hsiao CH. Behçet's disease with cutaneous changes resembling polyarteritis nodosa. Br J Dermatol. 1999;140:368–9.
225. Vikas A, Atul S, Singh R, et al. Behçet's disease with relapsing cutaneous polyarteritis nodosa-like lesions, responsive to oral cyclosporine therapy. Dermatol Online J. 2003;9:9.
226. Heller M. Behçet's disease (incomplete) and cutaneous polyarteritis nodosa. Dermatol Online J. 2005;11:25.
227. Kalkan G, Karadag AS, Astarci HM, et al. A histopathological approach: when papulopustular lesions should be in the diagnostic criteria of Behçet's disease? J Eur Acad Dermatol Venereol. 2009;23: 1056–60.
228. Ergun T, Gürbüz O, Dogusoy G, et al. Histopathologic features of the spontaneous pustular lesions of Behçet's syndrome. Int J Dermatol. 1998;37:194–6.
229. Magro CM, Crowson AN. Sterile neutrophilic folliculitis with perifollicular vasculopathy: a distinctive cutaneous reaction pattern reflecting systemic disease. J Cutan Pathol. 1998;25:215–21.
230. Alpsoy E, Uzun S, Akman A, et al. Histological and immunofluorescence findings in non-follicular papulopustular lesions in patients with Behçet's disease. J Eur Acad Dermatol Venereol. 2003;17:521–4.
231. Ilknur T, Pabuççuoglu U, Akin C, et al. Histopathologic and direct immunofluorescence findings of the papulopustular lesions in Behçet's disease. Eur J Dermatol. 2006;16:146–50.
232. Korman NJ. Bullous pemphigoid: the latest in diagnosis, prognosis and therapy. Arch Dermatol. 1998; 134:1137–41.
233. Ahmed AR, Newcomer VD. Bullous pemphigoid: clinical features. Clin Dermatol. 1987;5:6–12.
234. Kneisel A, Hertl M. Autoimmune bullous skin diseases. Part 1: clinical manifestations. J Dtsch Dermatol Des. 2011;9:844–57.
235. Venning VA, Frith PA, Bron AJ, et al. Mucosal involvement in bullous and cicatricial pemphigoid. A clinical and immunopathological study. Br J Dermatol. 1988;118:7–15.
236. Kippes W, Schmidt E, Roth A, et al. Immunopathologic changes in 115 patients with bullous pemphigoid. Hautarzt. 1999;50:866–72.
237. Marazza G, Pham HC, Schärer L, for the Autoimmune Bullous Disease Swiss Study Group, et al. Incidence of bullous pemphigoid and pemphigus in Switzerland: a 2-year prospective study. Br J Dermatol. 2009;16: 861–8.
238. Farrell AM, Kirtschig G, Dalziel KL, et al. Childhood genital pemphigoid: a clinical and immunopathological study of five patients. Br J Dermatol. 1999; 140:308–12.
239. Waisbourd-Zinman O, Ben-Amitai D, Cohen AD, et al. Bullous pemphigoid in infancy: clinical and epidemiological characteristics. J Am Acad Dermatol. 2008;58:41–8.
240. Fisler RE, Saeb M, Liang MG, et al. Childhood bullous pemphigoid. A clinicopathologic study and review of the literature. Am J Dermatopathol. 2003;25:183–9.
241. Nemeth AJ, Klein AD, Gould EW, et al. Childhood bullous pemphigoid: clinical and immunologic features, treatment and prognosis. Arch Dermatol. 1991;127:378–86.
242. Mueller S, Klaus-Kovtum V, Stanley JR. A 230-kD basic protein is the major bullous pemphigoid antigen. J Invest Dermatol. 1989;9:33–8.
243. Sawamura D, Li KH, Nomura K, et al. Bullous pemphigoid antigen: cDNA cloning, cellular expression, and evidence for polymorphism of the human gene. J Invest Dermatol. 1991;96:908–15.
244. Zillikens D, Giudice GJ. BP180/type XVII collagen: its role in acquired and inherited disorders or the dermal-epidermal junction. Arch Dermatol Res. 1999;291:187–94.
245. Kawahara Y, Matsumura K, Hashimoto T, et al. Immunoblot analysis of autoantigens in localized pemphigoid and pemphigoid nodularis. Acta Derm Venereol. 1997;77:187–90.
246. Chan LS, Fine JD, Briggaman RA, et al. Identification and partial characterization of a novel 105-kDalton lower lamina lucida autoantigen associated with a novel immune-mediated subepidermal blistering disease. J Invest Dermatol. 1993;101:262–7.
247. Mascaró Jr JM, Zillikens D, Giudice GJ, et al. A subepidermal bullous eruption associated with IgG autoantibodies to a 200 kd dermal antigen: the first case report from the United States. J Am Acad Dermatol. 2000;42:309–15.
248. Arechalde A, Braun RP, Calza AM, et al. Childhood bullous pemphigoid associated with IgA antibodies against BP180 or BP230 antigens. Br J Dermatol. 1999;140:112–8.
249. Collier P, Wojnarowska F, Allen J, et al. Molecular overlap of the IgA target antigens in the subepidermal blistering diseases. Dermatology. 1994;189:105–7.
250. Beutner EH, Jordon RE, Chorzelski TP. The immunopathology of pemphigus and pemphigoid. J Invest Dermatol. 1968;51:63–80.
251. Imber MJ, Murphy GF, Jordon RE. The immunopathology of bullous pemphigoid. Clin Dermatol. 1987;5:81–92.
252. Provost TT, Tomasi TB. Immunopathology of bullous pemphigoid: basement membrane deposition of IgE, alternative pathway component and fibrin. Clin Exp Immunol. 1974;18:193–200.
253. Ahmed AR, Hombal SM. Cicatricial pemphigoid. Int J Dermatol. 1986;25:90–6.
254. Trimarchi M, Bellini C, Fabiano B, et al. Multiple mucosal involvement in cicatricial pemphigoid. Acta Otorhinolaryngol Ital. 2009;29:222–5.
255. Eschle-Meniconi ME, Ahmad SR, Foster CS. Mucous membrane pemphigoid: an update. Curr Opin Ophthalmol. 2005;16:303–7.
256. Marran P, Wojnarowska F, Venning V, et al. Vulval involvement in autoimmune bullous disease. J Reprod Med. 1993;38:101–7.

257. Bernard P, Vaillant L, Labeille B, et al. Incidence and distribution of subepidermal autoimmune bullous skin diseases in three French regions. Bullous disease French Studying Group. Arch Dermatol. 1995;131:48–52.
258. Marren P, Walkden V, Mallon E, et al. Vulval cicatricial pemphigoid may mimic lichen sclerosus. Br J Dermatol. 1996;134:522–4.
259. Kharfi M, Khaled A, Anane R, et al. Early onset childhood cicatricial pemphigoid: a case report and review of the literature. Pediatr Dermatol. 2010;27:119–24.
260. Schoeffler A, Roth B, Causeret A, et al. Vulvar cicatricial pemphigoid of childhood. Pediatr Dermatol. 2004;21:51–3.
261. Hoque SR, Patel M, Farrell AM. Childhood cicatricial pemphigoid confined to the vulva. Clin Exp Dermatol. 2006;31:63–4.
262. Bernard P, Prost C, Durepaire N, et al. The major cicatricial pemphigoid antigen is a 180-kD protein that shows immunologic cross-reactivities with the bullous pemphigoid antigen. J Invest Dermatol. 1992;99:174–9.
263. Leverkus M, Bhol K, Hirako Y, et al. Cicatricial pemphigoid with circulating autoantibodies to β4 integrin, bullous pemphigoid 180 and bullous pemphigoid 230. Br J Dermatol. 2001;145:998–1004.
264. Tyagi S, Bhol K, Natarajan K, et al. Ocular cicatricial pemphigoid antigen: partial sequence and biochemical characterization. Proc Natl Acad Sci USA. 1996;93:14714–9.
265. Ghohestani RF, Nicolas JF, Rouselle P, et al. Identification of a 168-kDa mucosal antigen in a subset of patients with cicatricial pemphigoid. J Invest Dermatol. 1996;107:136–9.
266. Smith EP, Taylor TB, Meyer LJ, et al. Identification of a basement membrane zone antigen reactive with circulating IgA antibody in ocular cicatricial pemphigoid. J Invest Dermatol. 1993;101:619–23.
267. Setterfield J, Theron J, Vaughan RW, et al. Mucous membrane pemphigoid: HLD-DQ*0301 is associated with all clinical sites of involvement and may be linked to antibasement membrane IgG production. Br J Dermatol. 2001;145:406–14.
268. Bruch-Gerharz D, Hertl M, Ruzicka T. Mucous membrane pemphigoid: clinical aspects, immunopathological features and therapy. Eur J Dermatol. 2007;17:191–200.
269. Kelly SE, Wojnarowska F. The use of chemically split tissue in the detection of circulating anti-basement membrane zone antibodies in bullous pemphigoid and cicatricial pemphigoid. Br J Dermatol. 1988;118:31–40.
270. Bastuji-Garin S, Souissi R, Blum L, et al. Comparative epidemiology of pemphigus in Tunisia and France: unusual incidence of pemphigus foliaceus in young Tunisian women. J Invest Dermatol. 1995;104:302–5.
271. Joly P, Litrowski N. Pemphigus group (vulgaris, vegetans, foliaceus, herpetiformis, brasiliensis). Clin Dermatol. 2011;29:432–6.
272. Meurer M, Millns JL, Rogers RS, et al. Oral pemphigus vulgaris. Arch Dermatol. 1977;113:1520–4.
273. Korman NJ. Pemphigus. Dermatol Clin. 1990;8: 689–700.
274. Lim HW, Bystryn J. Bullous diseases. Clin Obstet Gynecol. 1978;21:1007–22.
275. Akhyani M, Chams-Davatchi C, Naragi Z, et al. Cevicovaginal involvement in pemphigus vulgaris. Br J Dermatol. 2007;158:478–82.
276. Batta K, Munday PE, Tatnall FM. Pemphigus vulgaris localized to the vagina presenting as chronic vulval discharge. Br J Dermatol. 1999; 140:945–7.
277. Mabrouk D, Razzaque Ahmed A. Analysis of current therapy and clinical outcome in childhood pemphigus vulgaris. Pediatr Dermatol. 2011;28:485–93.
278. Becker BA, Gaspari AA. Pemphigus vulgaris and vegetans. Dermatol Clin. 1993;11:429–52.
279. Zaraa I, Sellami A, Bouguerra C, et al. Pemphigus vegetans: a clinical, histological, immunopathological and prognostic study. J Eur Acad Dermatol Venereol. 2011;25:1160–7.
280. Amagai M, Karpati S, Prussick R, et al. Autoantibodies against the amino-terminal cadherin-like binding domain of pemphigus vulgaris antigen are pathogenic. J Clin Invest. 1992;90:919–26.
281. Ding X, Diaz LA, Fairley JA, et al. The anti-desmoglein 1 autoantibodies in pemphigus vulgaris sera are pathogenic. J Invest Dermatol. 1999;112:739–43.
282. Mahoney MG, Wang Z, Rothenberger K, et al. Explanations for the clinical and microscopic localization of lesions in pemphigus foliaceus and vulgaris. J Clin Invest. 1999;103:461–8.
283. Hashimoto T. Recent advances in the study of the pathophysiology of pemphigus. Arch Dermatol Res. 2003;295:2–11.
284. Sabolinski ML, Beutner EH, Krasny S, et al. Substrate specificity of anti-epithelial antibodies of pemphigus vulgaris and pemphigus foliaceus sera in immunofluorescence tests on monkey and guinea pig esophagus sections. J Invest Dermatol. 1987;88: 545–9.
285. Sabolinski ML, Beutner EH, Chorzelski TP, et al. Differentiation of pemphigus antibodies of the vulgaris and foliaceus types on monkey and guinea pig esophagus sections. Autoimmunity. 1990;5:229–32.
286. Tremeau-Martinage C, Oksman F, Bazex J. Immunoglobulin G subclass distribution of anti-intercellular substance antibodies in pemphigus. Ann Dermatol Venereol. 1995;122:409–11.
287. Hu Z, Bonifas JM, Beech J, et al. Mutations in ATP2C1, encoding a calcium pump, cause Hailey-Hailey disease. Nat Genet. 2000;24:61–5.
288. Sudbrak R, Brown J, Dobson-Stone C, et al. Hailey-Hailey disease is caused by mutations in ATP2C1 encoding a novel Ca(2+) pump. Hum Mol Genet. 2000;9:1131–40.
289. Richard G, Korge BP, Wright AR. Hailey-Hailey disease maps to a 5cM interval on chromosome 2q21-q24. J Invest Dermatol. 1995;105:357–60.

290. Burge SM. Hailey-Hailey disease: the clinical features, response to treatment and prognosis. Br J Dermatol. 1992;126:275–82.
291. Cheng TS, Ho KM, Lam CW. Heterogeneous mutations of the ATP2C1 gene causing Hailey-Hailey disease in Hong Kong Chinese. J Eur Acad Dermatol Venereol. 2010;24:1202–6.
292. Schirren H, Schirren CG, Schlüpen EM, et al. Exacerbation of Hailey-Hailey disease by infection with herpes simplex virus. Detection with polymerase chain reaction. Hautarzt. 1995;46:494–7.
293. Leyden JJ, Marples RR. Superinfection induced by antibiotics in familial benign chronic pemphigus. Acta Derm Venereol. 1973;53:61–4.
294. Marsch WC, Stuttgen G. Generalized Hailey-Hailey disease. Br J Dermatol. 1978;99:553–60.
295. Lyle TW, Knox JM, Richardson JB. Atypical features in benign chronic pemphigus. Arch Dermatol. 1958;78:446–53.
296. Denis J, Ganansia R, Puy-Montbrun T. Rare anorectal pathologic conditions. Curr Opin Gen Surg. 1994;103–7.
297. Cockayne SE, Rassl DM, Thomas SE. Squamous cell carcinoma arising in Hailey-Hailey disease of the vulva. Br J Dermatol. 1992;142:540–2.
298. Ochiai T, Honda A, Morishima T, et al. Human papillomavirus types 16 and 39 in a vulval carcinoma occurring in a woman with Hailey-Hailey disease. Br J Dermatol. 1999;140:509–13.
299. Chorzelski TP, Kudejko J, Jablonska S. Is papular acantholytic dyskeratosis of the vulva a new entity? Am J Dermatopathol. 1984;6:557–9.
300. Coppola G, Muscardin LM, Piazza P. Papular acantholytic dyskeratosis. Am J Dermatopathol. 1986;8:364–5.
301. Lee SH, Jang JG. Papular acantholytic dyskeratosis of the genitalia. J Dermatol. 1989;16:312–4.
302. Van Joost TH, Vuzevski VD, Tank B, et al. Benign persistent papular acantholytic and dyskeratotic eruption of vulva. A case report and review of the literature. Br J Dermatol. 1991;124:92–5.
303. Bell HK, Farrar CW, Curley RK. Papular acantholytic dermatosis of the vulva. Clin Exp Dermatol. 2001;26:386–8.
304. Sáenz AM, Cirocco A, Avendaño M, et al. Papular acantholytic dyskeratosis of the vulva. Pediatr Dermatol. 2005;22:237–9.
305. Browne F, Keane H, Walsh M, et al. Papular acantholytic dyskeratosis presenting as genital warts. Int J STD AIDS. 2007;18:867–8.
306. Dittmer CJ, Hornemann A, Rose C, et al. Successful laser therapy of a papular acantholytic dyskeratosis of the vulva: case report and review of the literature. Arch Gynecol Obstet. 2010;281:723–5.
307. Roh MR, Choi YJ, Lee KG. Papular acantholytic dyskeratosis of the vulva. J Dermatol. 2009;36:427–9.
308. Van der Putte SCJ, Oey HB. Papular acantholytic dyskeratosis of the penis. Am J Dermatopathol. 1986;8:365–6.
309. Wong TY, Mihm Jr MC. Acantholytic dermatosis localized to the genitalia and crural areas of male patients: a report of three cases. J Cutan Pathol. 1994;21:27–32.
310. Warkel RL, Jager RM. Focal acantholytic dyskeratosis of the anal canal. Am J Dermatopathol. 1986;8:362–3.
311. Cooper PH. Acantholytic disorders localized to vulvocrural area. J Cutan Pathol. 1998;16:81–4.

Cysts, Non neoplastic Glandular Lesions, and Glandular Neoplasms of the Vulva and Vagina

4

Asma Zaman Faruqi

Abstract

This chapter gives an overview of neoplastic and non neoplastic glandular lesions in the vulva and vagina. The topics covered include benign vulvovaginal cysts, prostatic-type lesions, non neoplastic glandular lesions, benign and malignant glandular neoplasms, and lesions arising in Bartholin's gland.

Benign Vulvovaginal Cysts

Table 4.1 lists and compares the common vulvovaginal cysts discussed below.

Mullerian (Paramesonephric) Cysts

As the name indicates, these cysts arise from the Mullerian ducts and can therefore be located at any site in the upper part of the vagina. They are commonly found in the anterolateral wall of the vagina and are variable in size, ranging from 1 to 7 cm. Reflecting its Mullerian origin, the epithelial lining can resemble any part of the female genital tract and so can be endocervical, endometrial, or tubal in type. Endocervical-type epithelium is the commonest, comprising basally located nuclei with apically dispersed mucin as seen in normal endocervical glands. Endometrioid epithelium consists of columnar cells with stratified nuclei that may or may not show mitotic activity. Tubal epithelium on the other hand is simple columnar epithelium which includes ciliated, secretory, and intercalated (peg) cells with basal T lymphocytes. Mixed epithelial types can be seen in the same cyst and may undergo squamous metaplasia. If the entire epithelial lining is affected by squamous metaplastic change, it may then be impossible to differentiate from an epithelial inclusion cyst [1, 2] (Fig. 4.1).

Mucous Cyst of Vulva and Vestibule

This usually occurs in the vestibule; however it may also present at other sites within the vulva. The minor vestibular glands form a ring round the vestibule, extending from the frenulum, around the base of the hymen, to the fourchette posteriorly. They are located within 2–3 mm of the surface epithelium and consist of acini lined by simple mucinous epithelium that communicates

A.Z. Faruqi, MBBS, LMCK, FRCPath
Department of Cellular Pathology,
The Royal London and St. Bartholomew's Hospitals,
80 Newark Street, London E1 2ES, UK
e-mail: asma.faruqi@bartshealth.nhs.uk

L. Brown (ed.), *Pathology of the Vulva and Vagina*, Essentials of Diagnostic Gynecological Pathology,
DOI 10.1007/978-0-85729-757-0_4, © Springer-Verlag London 2013

Table 4.1 Common vulvovaginal cysts

Lining		Site	Origin
Mucinous	Mullerian cyst	Upper vagina, usually anterolateral wall	Mullerian duct
	Mucous cyst of vestibule	Usually vestibule, may occur at other sites	Minor vestibular glands
	Bartholin's cyst	Posterolateral vagina	Bartholin's gland/duct
Non mucinous, non ciliated, cuboidal	Gartner's cyst	Lateral wall of vagina	Wolffian remnants
Columnar endometrial type (may be ciliated)	Mullerian cyst	Upper vagina, usually anterolateral wall	Mullerian duct
	Endometriotic cyst	Vulvovaginal endometrosis	Site of trauma/scars
			Vault or posterior fornix
Transitional	Bartholin's cyst	Posterolateral vagina	Bartholin's duct
	Skene's cyst	Close to urethral meatus	Skene's duct

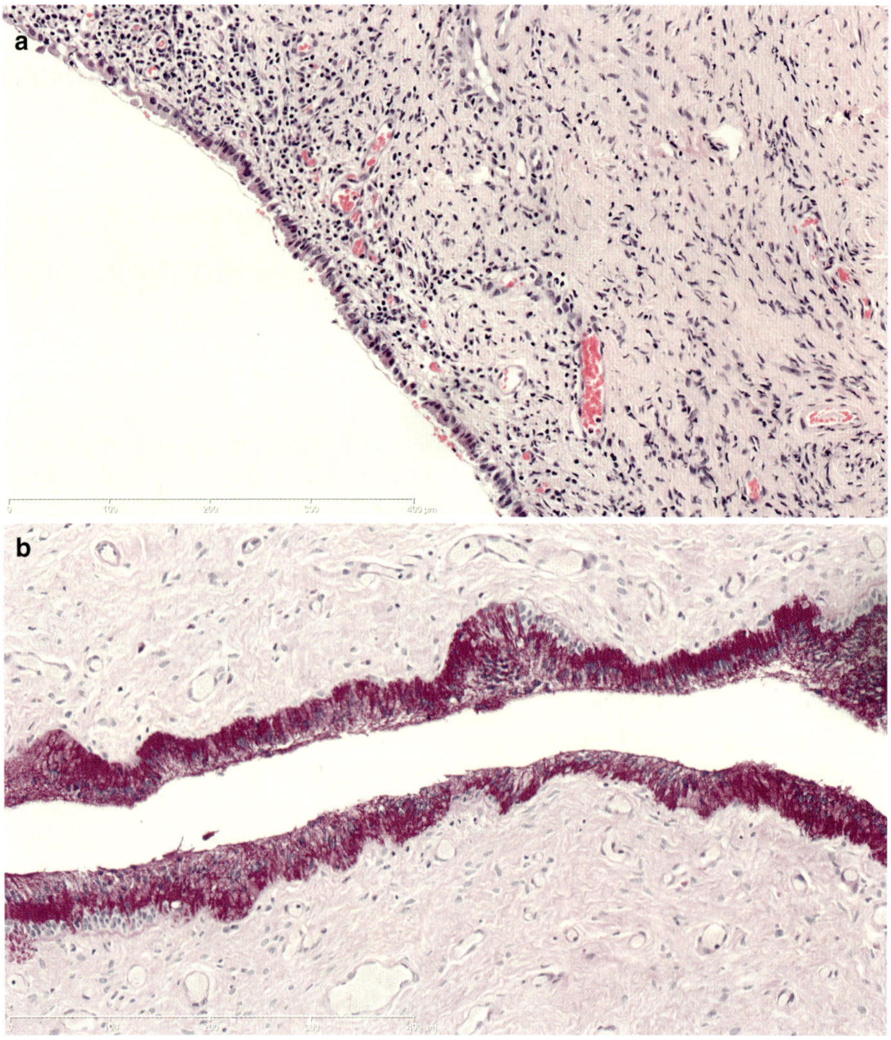

Fig. 4.1 (**a**) Mullerian cyst; (**b**) Mullerian cyst demonstrating mucinous epithelium, PASD

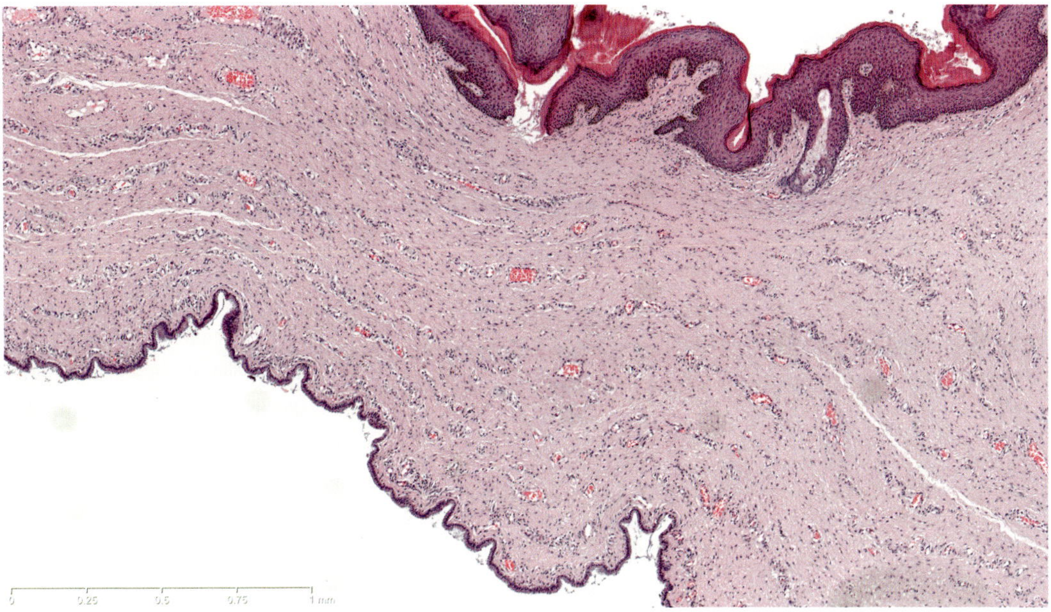

Fig. 4.2 Mucous cyst of vestibule

with the surface of the vaginal vestibule. The cyst is thought to arise from occlusion of these glands and is thus lined by a single layer of columnar to cuboidal endocervical-type mucinous epithelium. (Skeletal muscle is not typically found in the cyst wall. As at all other sites, these cysts may undergo squamous metaplasia [1, 3] Fig. 4.2).

Ciliated Cyst of Vulva/Vestibular Adenosis

This is a rare lesion that has been reported in association with chronic inflammation, Stevens-Johnson syndrome, and 5FU therapy [3–7]. The cyst is lined by tubal or endometrial-type epithelium and is thought to be an acquired lesion. The Mullerian lining of these cysts is difficult to explain as the vulval vestibule is not Mullerian in origin. It is possible that the lining epithelium occurs as a result of metaplasia. These cysts can be distinguished from endometriosis by the absence of endometrial-type stroma and an appropriate clinical scenario.

Gartner's Duct (Mesonephric/Wolffian) Cysts

These are always in a lateral location in the vagina and arise from the remnants of the Wolffian duct. They are lined by nonciliated cuboidal or columnar epithelium which may become flattened. Unlike Mullerian cysts, the lining epithelium is non mucinous and smooth muscle may be seen within the cyst wall. It is unusual for the epithelium to undergo squamous metaplasia. The cysts may be accompanied by small or hyperplastic duct remnants. A deeply eosinophilic secretion may be present in the cyst or in the lumina of the duct remnants. Gartner's duct cysts may be associated with developmental abnormalities in the urinary system, such as ectopic ureter, unilateral renal hypoplasia, and renal agenesis [1, 2, 4, 8, 9] (Fig. 4.3a, b).

Skene's Duct Cysts and Urothelial Cysts

These are rare lesions which generally arise due to obstruction of the duct. The Skene's glands

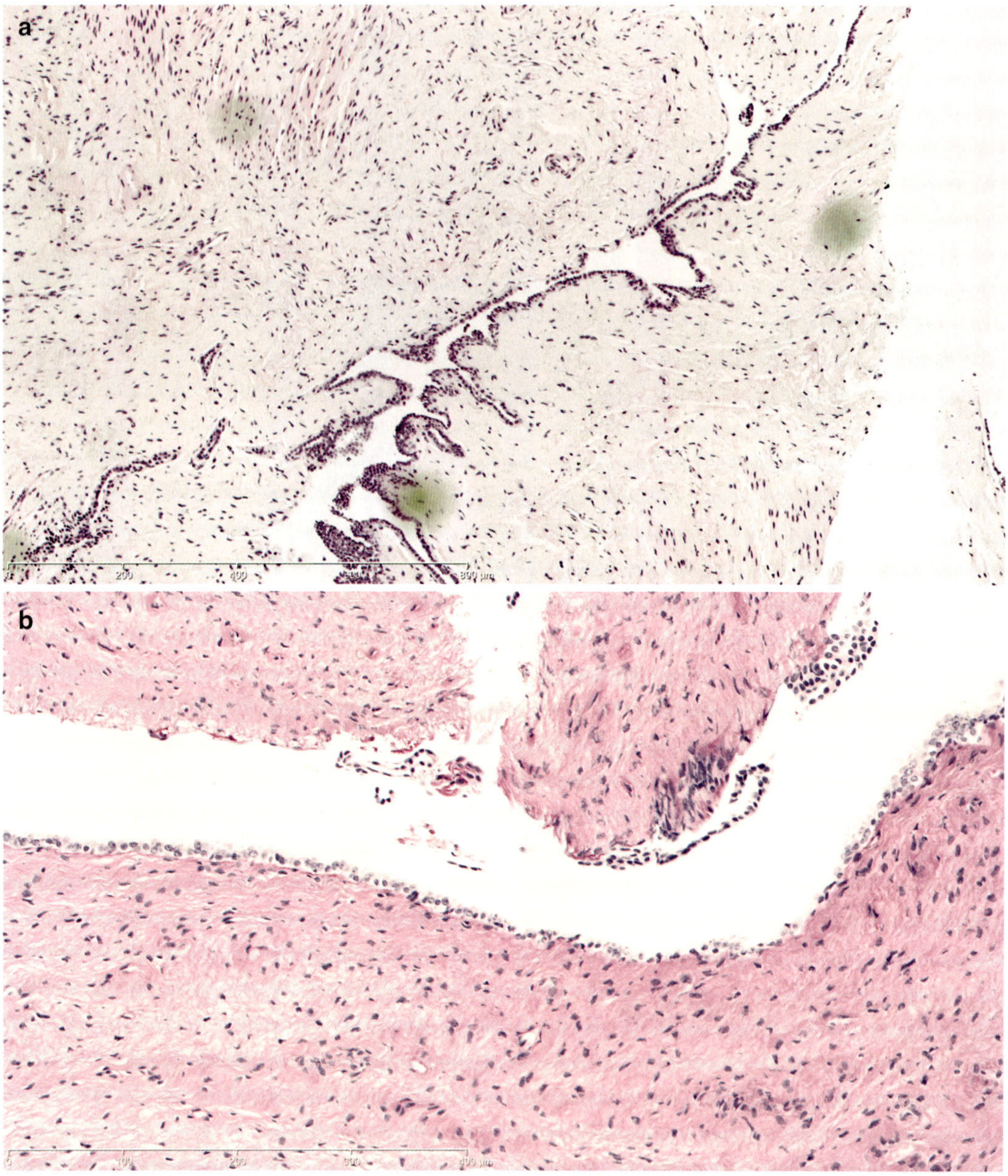

Fig. 4.3 (**a**) Gartner's duct cyst; (**b**) Gartner's duct cyst, nonmucinous epithelium, PASD

are homologous to the male prostate and lie on either side of the urethra. Their ducts drain into the urethra. Cysts arising from these structures therefore present at or near the urethral meatus and are lined by transitional epithelium. They should be differentiated from other periurethral lesions such as urethral diverticula which have a similar lining and may also arise from the lower urethra. Clinical findings and imaging are usually necessary in order to distinguish the two lesions.

Urothelial cysts are seen in infants. They are lined by transitional epithelium and usually occur in the lower vagina. They are usually 1 cm or less in size and are thought to originate in Skene's duct [2, 4, 8].

Cyst of the Canal of Nuck

The round ligaments pass through the internal and external inguinal rings and insert into the labia majora. The canal of Nuck is a protrusion of the parietal peritoneum which accompanies the round ligament and extends through the inguinal canal. When filled with fluid, it can form a cystic swelling which is the equivalent of a hydrocele in males. It usually presents as lesion in the labium majus or the inguinal canal and has mesothelial lining [3, 10].

Epithelial Inclusion Cysts

These are commonly located in labium majus, the clitoris and vagina. They often occur as a result of trauma [11], including ritual genital mutilation [12, 13] or surgery leading to burial of the overlying epithelium. It is possible for these cysts to occur many years after the initial injury and attain large sizes [13, 14]. Rarely an epidermoid cyst may present as clitoromegaly [15]. The cysts are lined by squamous epithelium and the contents usually consist of laminated keratin. Not all cysts are associated with trauma and some may occur due to obstruction of sebaceous ducts which then undergo squamous metaplasia [1–4].

Vaginitis Emphysematosa

This is a rare condition of unknown etiology that has been reported in association with pregnancy, lowered immunity, circulatory disturbances, and infections such as *T. vaginalis*. The presentation includes vaginal discharge, pruritis, and a popping sound during sexual intercourse. There are gas filled cysts present in the lamina propria which are devoid of lining epithelium but may be surrounded by a giant cell reaction [16–22].

Bartholin's Cyst

See below in section "Lesions of Bartholin's Gland."

Non neoplastic Glandular Lesions

Endometriosis

Endometriosis of the lower female genital is not uncommon. It is more often seen in the cervix but may also occur in the vulva and the vagina [23]. There is a particular tendency for endometriosis to develop at the sites of trauma such as episiotomy scars or following obstetric injury and it is thought that the lesions arise as a result of implantation. Cyclical bleeding may occur within these foci in which case they present as hemorrhagic nodules. Vaginal lesions can give rise to abnormal glandular cells in cervical smears. Both vulval and vaginal endometriosis occurs in the superficial lamina propria and may not necessarily be associated with pelvic endometriosis; deep vaginal endometriosis on the other hand is generally associated with pelvic disease [24]. The histological appearances are similar to endometriosis at other sites in the body, featuring endometrial-type glands and stroma, hemosiderin-laden macrophages and fibrosis. Mitotic activity and secretory changes within the glandular cells can occur as the foci may be hormonally responsive. It is important to bear this entity in mind and not confuse glands with stratified nuclei for dysplasia or adenocarcinoma. The absence of significant nuclear atypia or abnormal mitoses, the presence of endometrial-type stroma around the glands, features of old hemorrhage in the form of hemosiderin-laden macrophages, and fibrosis should indicate that the lesion is endometriosis rather than adenocarcinoma. There may also be pseudodecidual alteration of endometrial stromal cells, especially if the woman is undergoing treatment with progestogenic agents. The endometriotic focus may then consist of an island of cells with abundant eosinophilic cytoplasm and tiny, inconspicuous glands which could give rise to a mistaken diagnosis of squamous cell carcinoma on superficial microscopic examination. Alternatively, during pregnancy or treatment with exogenous progestogens, endometrial glands may undergo Arias-Stella reaction and be mistaken for clear cell carcinoma. Once again, decidualized endometrial stroma around the glands and correlation with the patient's history should prevent misdiagnosis. Inflammation and degeneration can produce reactive nuclear changes, but in such cases the presence of inflammatory cells, relative lack of mitoses, and the sometimes smudged appearance of the nuclear chromatin assist in recognizing the appearances as reactive rather than neoplastic (Fig. 4.4a, b).

Prolapse of the Fallopian Tubes

The Fallopian tubes may prolapse into the vault of the vagina following hysterectomy. The condition may come to light due to abnormal glandular cells in cervical smears raising a suspicion of cervical intraepithelial glandular neoplasia (CGIN) or the presentation may be as a nodule or polyp with a clinical suspicion of malignancy. Prolapsed Fallopian tubes are an important differential diagnosis of possible vaginal adenocarcinoma in women with a history of vaginal or abdominal hysterectomy. As this vital clinical information may not always be included on the pathology request form, the entity should always be borne in mind when faced with a relatively bland glandular lesion in the upper vagina.

On microscopic examination, Fallopian tube-type epithelium with ciliated and nonciliated cells is observed. Unlike adenocarcinoma the epithelial cells are regular in size and lack significant nuclear atypia, but at low power the heterogeneity of the normal cell types in tubal epithelium may give a misleading impression of pleomorphism. If marked inflammation is present, the epithelial cells may exhibit reactive atypia (Fig. 4.5a, b). Immunohistochemistry using WT1 may be helpful as most primary vaginal adenocarcinomas are WT1 negative whereas Fallopian tube epithelium is WT1 positive (Fig. 4.6). Metastatic ovarian serous carcinoma also expresses WT1, but this tumor has high-grade nuclear features. Endometriotic foci may contain ciliated cells but they can be differentiated from a prolapsed Fallopian tube by the presence of the other features associated with endometriosis (see section "Endometriosis") and the epithelial cells are negative for WT1.

Adenosis

The vagina is lined by squamous epithelium and normally there are no glands present within the stroma. Vaginal adenosis is a condition whereby there is abnormal persistence of Mullerian epithelium of the cervical or endometrial type within the vagina. It usually occurs in women who have been exposed to diethylstilboestrol (DES) in utero. DES is a synthetic estrogen which was first manufactured in 1938 [25]. Between 1938 and 1971, it was prescribed to pregnant women in order to prevent miscarriage or preterm labor. Although there was evidence that the drug was ineffective at preventing either of these complications, it continued to be used until a study found it to be associated with clear cell adenocarcinoma of the vagina [26]. Following this study, the FDA warned that it was unsafe for use in pregnancy. It is thought that DES prevents the normal upgrowth of squamous epithelium derived from the urogenital sinus [4, 27, 28]. This results in persistence of embryonic Mullerian epithelium within the vagina, which then gives rise to adenosis. With the cessation of DES use in pregnancy, cases of vaginal adenosis are becoming rare. Nevertheless spontaneous adenosis is still reported although some cases may be associated with prolonged intake of oral contraceptives or tamoxifen [4, 29, 30]. Microscopic examination of the lesions reveals glands in the vaginal mucosa which may or may not show cystic dilatation. The glands may be lined by any type of Mullerian epithelium – mucinous, columnar, ciliated, or nonciliated. Squamous metaplasia is not uncommon in which case the squamous epithelium is usually non glycogenated unlike normal vaginal epithelium (Fig. 4.7). Although there is an association between clear cell carcinoma of the vagina and DES-associated adenosis, spontaneous adenosis is much less likely to give rise to malignant lesions.

Endocervicosis

This is a rare condition that has been reported in the urinary bladder, pelvic peritoneum, and

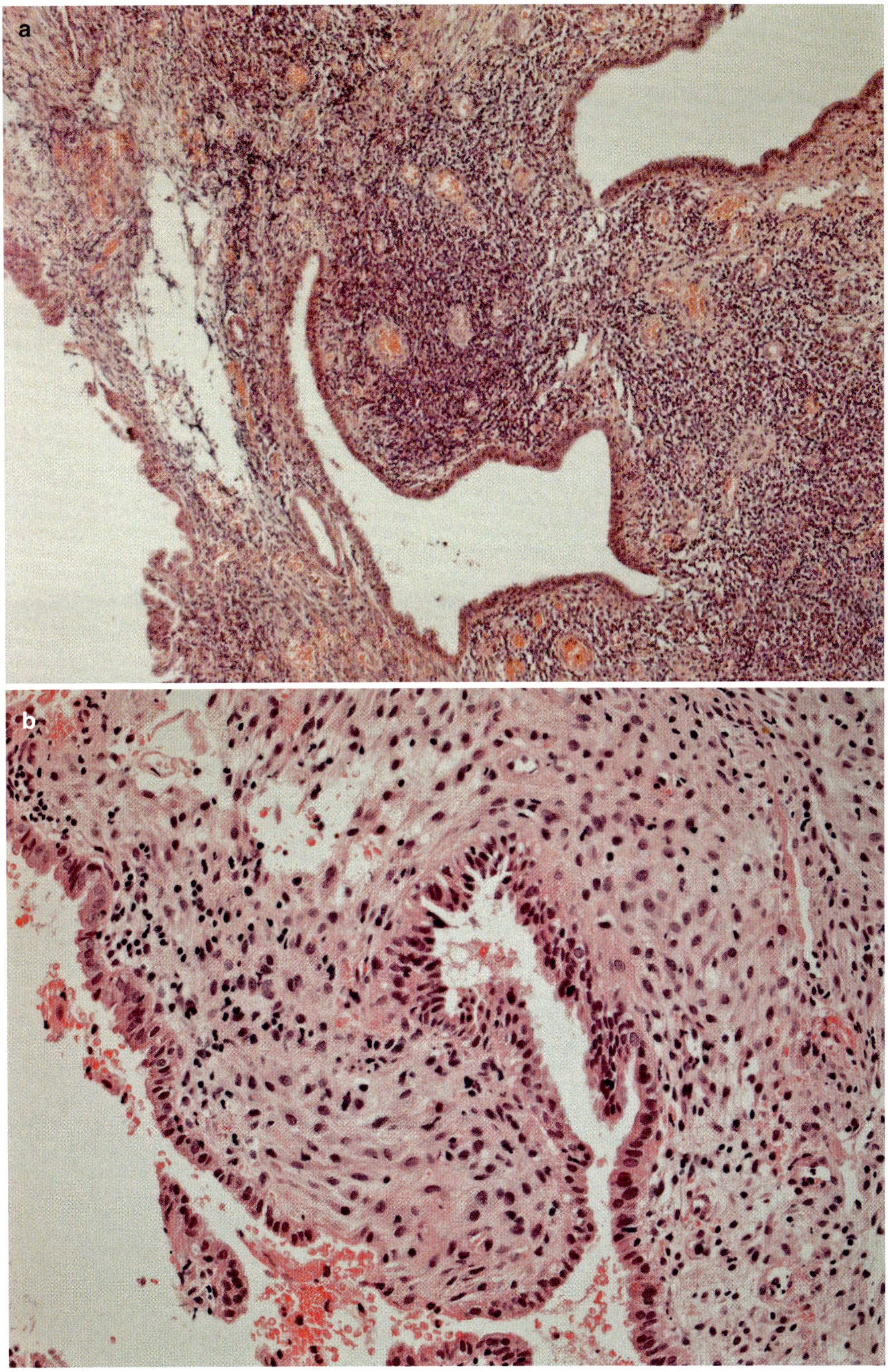

Fig. 4.4 (**a**) Vaginal endometriosis; (**b**) Vaginal endometriosis, decidual alteration of the stroma

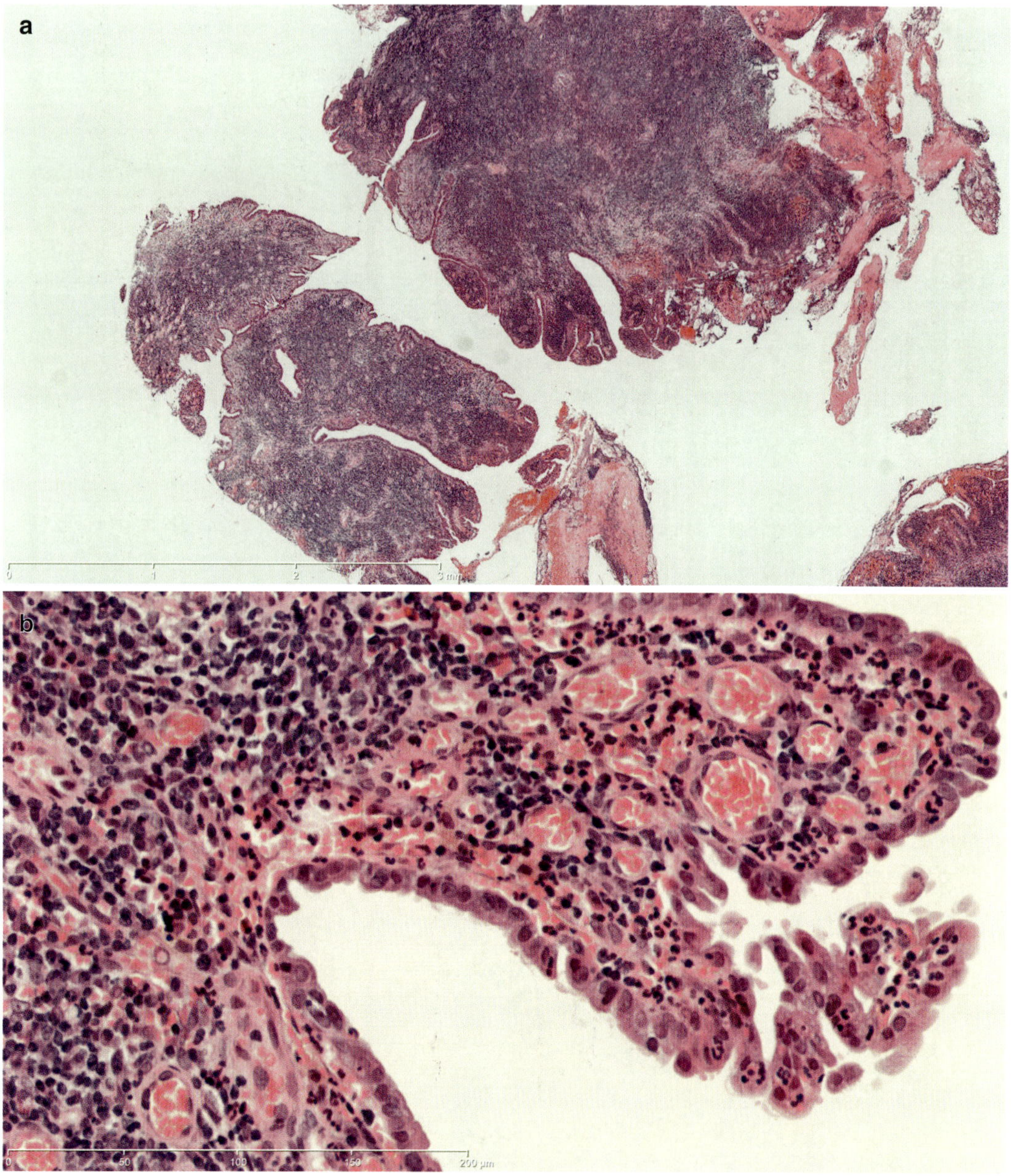

Fig. 4.5 (**a**) Prolapsed Fallopian tube. This presented with a clinical suspicion of carcinoma. Note dense inflammation. (**b**) Prolapsed Fallopian tube. Inflammatory atypia but there is no mitotic activity and nuclei appear smudged. Ciliated and nonciliated cells present

lymph nodes. The lesions are thought to arise as part of the secondary Mullerian system [31–33]. There has been one reported case of endocervicosis occurring in the vagina [34]. As the vagina does not possess a Mullerian lining, the source of the benign mucinous glands is postulated as being from the serosal surface of the uterus, which is close to the anterolateral wall of the vagina, the site where the lesion was reported. Alternatively the source of endocervicosis could have been implantation at the time of hysterectomy. The presentation was as

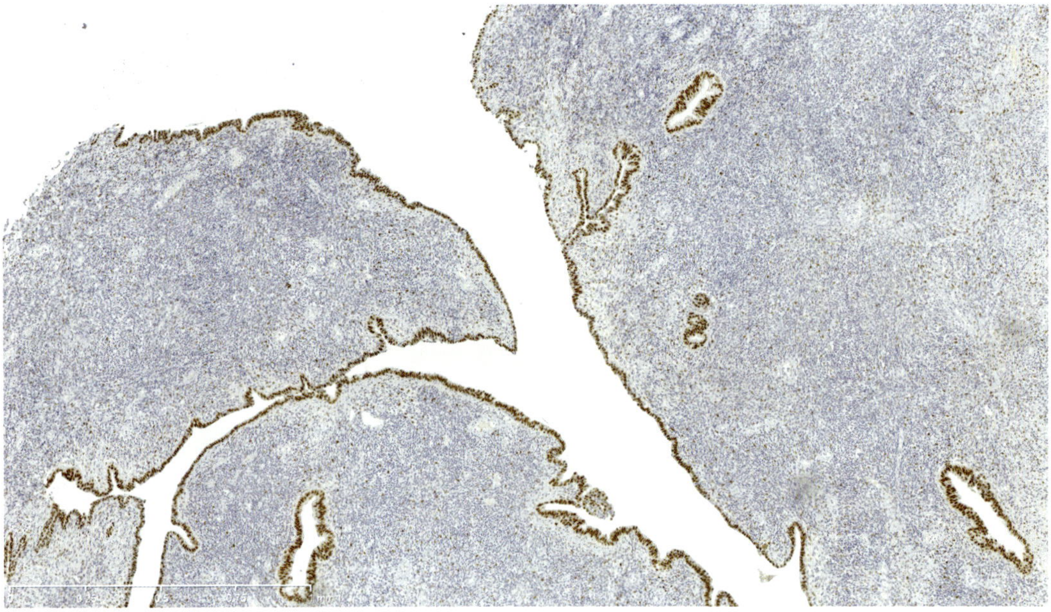

Fig. 4.6 Prolapsed Fallopian tube. WT1 highlights the lining epithelial cells

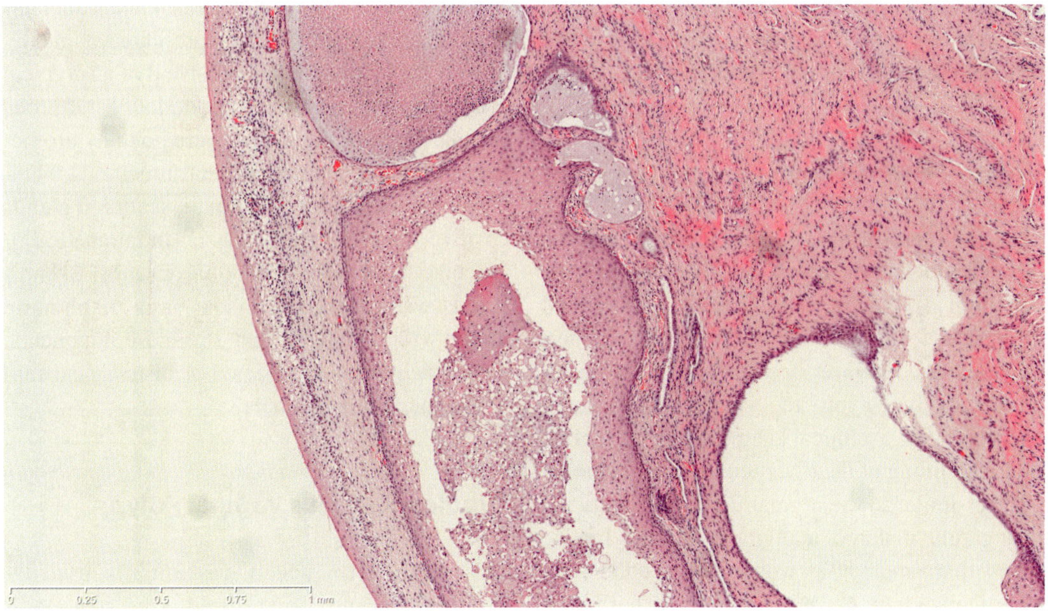

Fig. 4.7 Vaginal adenosis. There was no history of exposure to DES in utero. Mucinous cysts with squamous metaplasia

a tumor-like mass; although the glands had an infiltrative growth pattern, the lining epithelium which was of the mucinous endocervical type did not exhibit cytological atypia or mitotic activity. There has been one report of adenocarcinoma arising in endocervicosis (see below in section on mucinous and intestinal-type neoplasms).

Urethral Lesions

Prolapse and Urethral Caruncle

Prolapse of the urethral mucosa occurs in children, postmenopausal women, or following lower genital tract surgery [35–37]. Weakness of the surrounding supportive connective tissue is postulated as one of the causes. The urethral mucosa protrudes through the meatus and can lead to bleeding and a clinical suspicion of neoplasia. Histologically, congested and dilated blood vessels are present in the lamina propria with accompanying inflammation and possible ulceration.

Urethral caruncles arise from prolapsed urethral mucosa. On histological examination, the submucosa contains dilated blood vessels, eosinophils, and chronic inflammatory cells accompanied by edema and myxoid change in the stroma.

Although neither of these lesions is glandular in origin, inclusions of surface epithelium and the presence of plump endothelial cells may lead to a mistaken diagnosis of abnormal glands.

Urethral Diverticulum

This is a protrusion of the urethral mucosa through the wall of the urethra [38]. Usually the condition is recognized by clinical symptoms and on imaging. The first line of treatment is generally medical. However occasionally the diverticulum may bulge into the vagina and undergo excision with a clinical diagnosis of a vaginal cyst. The lining of the diverticulum is transitional in type similar to the normal urethra. Diverticula may rarely undergo malignant change. In one series that studied 90 women who underwent diverticulectomy, 6 were reported as harboring invasive adenocarcinoma [39].

Prostatic-Type Lesions in the Female Genital Tract

The presence of prostatic-type tissue has been reported in the lower female genital tract [40–43] (Fig. 4.8). These are rare lesions and the key to recognition is knowledge of their existence. Prostatic-type tissue may be found in the cervical stroma, beneath the surface epithelium and less commonly in the vagina and vulva. It is postulated that the likely histiogenesis is from misplaced Skene's glands, which are homologous to the male prostate. In one series, the presence of prostate-like glands was described in the dermis of the vulva [40]. These glands had Paneth cell-like changes, which can also occur in the normal male prostate. Both benign and malignant lesions have been reported.

Skene's gland hyperplasia (analogous to benign prostatic hyperplasia in the male) and adenocarcinoma of Skene's gland have been described [44–47]. The adenocarcinomas presented as periurethral masses. In cases where PSA was measured, preoperative elevation was found. The neoplastic glandular cells were also reactive for PSA on immunohistochemistry.

One case of adenofibroma of Skene's duct has been documented [48]. This presented clinically as a urethral caruncle and consisted of an atypical glandular proliferation surrounded by fibrous stroma. Some of the glands were lined by urothelial epithelium with occasional mucinous metaplasia but there were also small, scattered glands positive for PSA. There was no inflammation or vascular dilatation. Adenofibroma of Skene's glands was diagnosed on the basis of biphasic tumor with glandular and stromal components, PSA reactivity, and absence of histological features typical of a caruncle.

Tubulosquamous Vaginal Polyps

This was a term which was initially used by McCluggage and Young to describe a series of ten vaginal polyps [49]. Apart from two cases, the rest occurred in women who were postmenopausal and over the age of 50. Most of the polyps were located in the upper vagina and consisted of islands of squamous epithelium in a hypocellular fibrous stroma. Apart from one case, there was no apparent connection between these islands and the overlying vaginal squamous

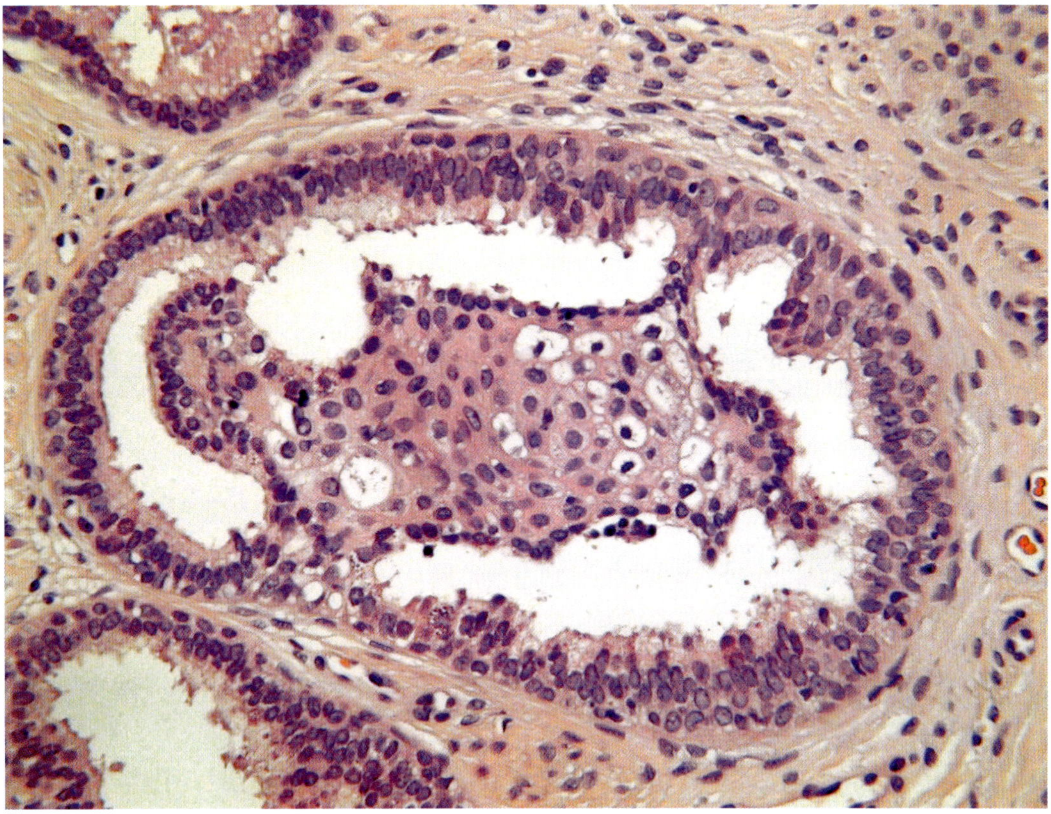

Fig. 4.8 Prostatic tissue in vagina. Glandular and squamous elements are present. A double epithelial layer is evident in the glandular component (Courtesy of Professor Glenn McCluggage)

epithelium. There was no obvious uninvolved Grenz zone, and the epithelial islands showed peripheral palisading with some of the nests containing necrotic keratinous debris. All ten cases had small tubules, mostly located around squamous nests. Squamous metaplasia was common, affecting the entire acinus with only a rim of identifiable epithelium at the periphery (Fig. 4.9a). Some of the tubules exhibited a double lining of glandular epithelium with cuboidal luminal cells and a basal layer. Four of the cases were examined by immunohistochemistry, revealing that the squamous epithelium as well as the tubular glands expressed broad-spectrum cytokeratins AE1/3 and also CK7; in addition the squamous elements expressed high-molecular-weight cytokeratins (LP34 and the 34(beta) β E12). There was no cytokeratin reaction in the lesional stroma. Focal CD10 reactivity was noted in the squamous elements whereas the tubules exhibited luminal reactivity only. ER was diffusely and strongly positive in the stroma as well as the epithelial islands. Three out of the four cases examined by immunohistochemistry revealed PrAP reactivity in tubules and two of these cases were also positive for PSA (Fig. 4.9b). The authors discuss various theories regarding histiogenesis of these lesions. These include origin from the Mullerian or Wolffian ducts, mesonephric glands, and ectopic Skene's glands. The fact that some but not all the lesions stain for PSA and PrAP raises the possibility that they are derived from other glands which are not necessarily prostatic in origin. Since the original paper, there have been a handful of reports of tubulosquamous vaginal polyps, some of which were reported to show mucinous and basaloid features [50, 51]. Although follow-up is limited, the MIB 1 proliferation index in these lesions was low and it is likely that the behavior would be benign

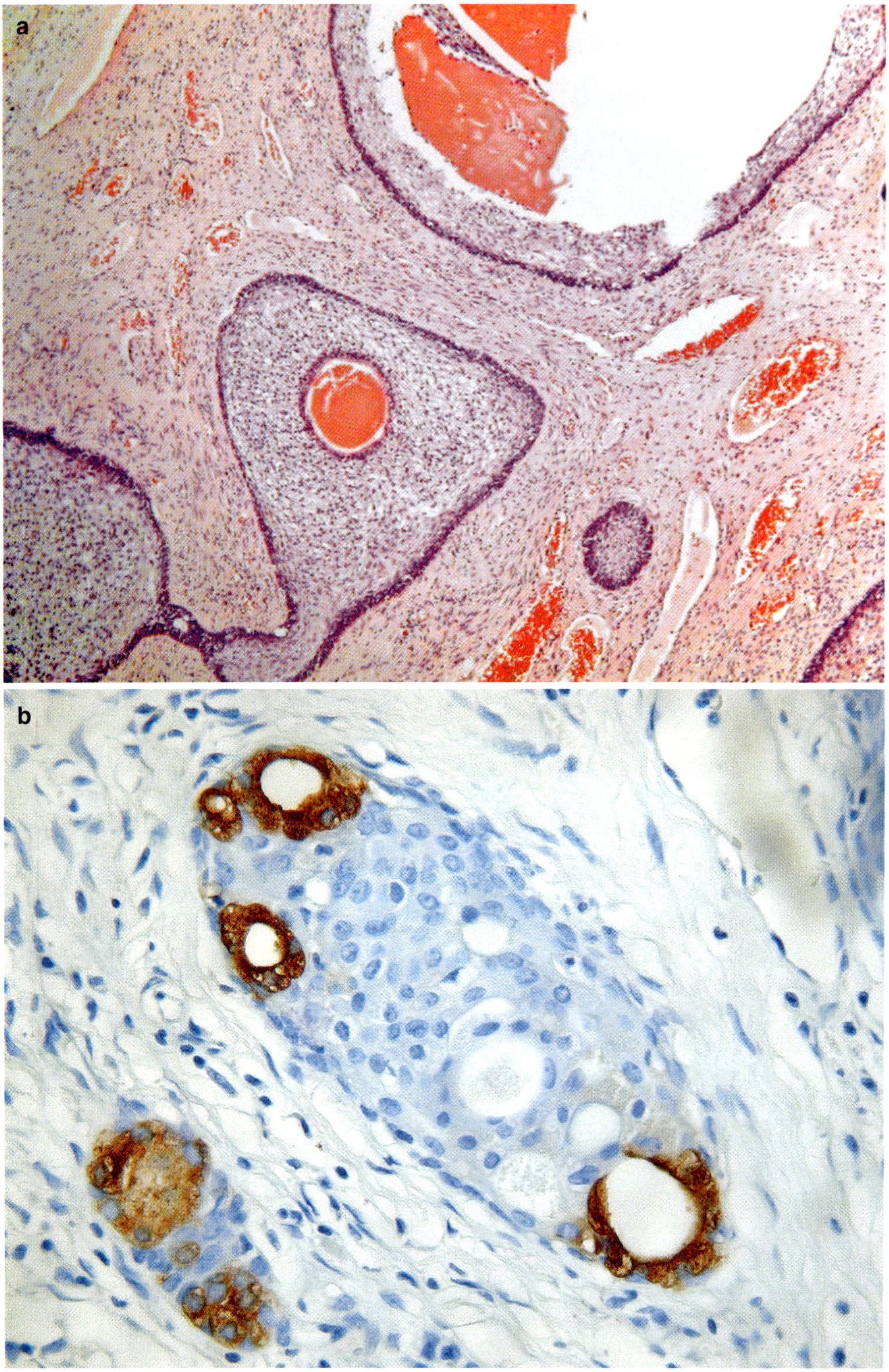

Fig. 4.9 (**a**) Tubulosquamous vaginal polyp. Squamous nests in a hypocellular stroma. (**b**) Tubulosquamous vaginal polyp. PSA highlights the glandular epithelium (Courtesy of Professor Glenn McCluggage)

although the possibility of local recurrence exists. The differential diagnoses discussed by the authors include benign mixed tumor of the vagina, Brenner tumor, fibroepithelial stromal polyp, vaginal adenosis with florid squamous metaplasia, adenoid basal carcinoma, and synovial sarcoma. Benign mixed tumor of the vagina has a predominant spindle cell component which usually stains positively with cytokeratin markers. Brenner tumors have characteristic nuclei and transitional rather than squamous epithelium. Fibroepithelial stromal polyps do not feature tubules within the stroma. Vaginal adenosis also occurs in the upper vagina but does not usually form polyps; furthermore the epithelial elements of vaginal adenosis are present beneath the surface epithelium rather than deep within the stroma. Adenoid basal carcinoma is associated with surface dysplasia, and the cells are basaloid rather than squamous. Synovial sarcoma is a far more cellular tumor with features of malignancy in both epithelial and spindle components.

Neoplasms

Benign Tumors

Benign glandular tumors may arise from the vulval skin adnexa or mammary-type tissue. These include nodular (clear cell) hidradenoma, benign mixed tumor (pleomorphic adenoma), and papillary hidradenoma. These will be dealt with in detail in Chap. 9.

Adenoma of the Minor Vestibular Glands

Hyperplasia of the minor vestibular glands has been reported in association with vulval vestibulitis [52]. There have also been rare reports of adenoma arising in these glands. The neoplasm can be up to 2 cm in size and consists of clusters of mucin-secreting glands. It is usually an incidental finding and it is debatable whether it represents a true neoplasm or nodular hyperplasia [4, 53].

Mullerian Papilloma

This is a benign tumor that occurs in the upper vagina, which is formed from fusion of the Mullerian ducts. It usually presents in infancy or childhood and rarely in young women. The neoplasm has a papillary architecture and is composed of fibrovascular cores covered by cuboidal or mucinous epithelial cells. Occasionally a clear cell or hobnail morphology may be identified [54–57]. The lesion may be differentiated from clear cell carcinoma by the absence of nuclear atypia or mitotic activity. There has been one reported case of borderline changes occurring in a 49-year-old female with a history of recurrent Mullerian papillomas [2, 4, 58].

Malignant Tumors

Adenocarcinoma of the vulva and vagina is rare as the majority of malignant tumors at this site are usually squamous. Vaginal adenocarcinoma commonly arises in foci of adenosis or endometriosis and there is one reported case of origin in endocervicosis. Intestinal-type tumors arising in cloacogenic remnants and adenocarcinoma of the Bartholin's glands may present as vulval or vaginal masses. Before diagnosing primary vulvovaginal adenocarcinoma, it is essential to exclude metastatic disease. This includes full clinical details, imaging, and appropriate immunohistochemistry.

Clear Cell Carcinoma

Clear cell carcinoma of the vagina has an association with DES use during pregnancy. It is becoming increasingly rare and most cases are now sporadic with no relationship to DES [4]. Clear cell carcinoma in women who have been exposed to DES has a bimodal distribution with two age peaks – one in the 20s and the other in the 70s [2]. Vaginal tumors are more common in the younger age group whereas older women are more likely to get cervical tumors. The neoplasm usually presents as a polypoid or hemorrhagic nodule. Microscopically the appearance is similar to clear cell carcinomas of other sites. Hobnail cells are common and may be more numerous than the classical clear cells which have prominent thick, plant-like cell membranes and optically clear or pale pink cytoplasm with large irregular nuclei and prominent nucleoli. The cytoplasmic clearing is due to the presence of glycogen which can be demonstrated with periodic acid Schiff (PAS) stain. Before diagnosing primary vaginal clear cell carcinoma, metastatic disease from other sites should be excluded. Primary clear cell carcinoma of the female genital tract is far more common in the endometrium or the ovaries, with vaginal lesions occurring as a result of metastatic spread. The differential diagnosis also includes other tumors which may have a clear cell morphology. These include mesonephric carcinoma (see below), dysgerminoma (PLAP and CD117 positive), yolk sac tumor (AFP positive), trophoblastic tumors (β (beta) HCG, HPL and CK7 positive), smooth muscle tumors (SMA and h-caldesmon positive), steroid cell tumors (inhibin positive and EMA negative), and benign conditions such as Arias-Stella reaction occurring in a focus of endometriosis. An appropriate panel of immunohistochemistry may prove useful in difficult cases.

Endometrioid Adenocarcinoma

Foci of endometriosis in the vulva or vagina may undergo any of the pathological changes that occur in uterine endometrium. These include hyperplasia, atypia, and carcinoma. Primary vaginal endometrioid adenocarcinoma is indistinguishable from primary endometrial and ovarian endometrioid carcinoma. When such a tumor is encountered in the vagina or the vulva, metastatic disease from the uterus or the ovary should always be excluded (Figs. 4.10a, b, 4.11 and 4.12).

Mucinous and Intestinal-Type Neoplasms

Carcinomas with mucin-containing epithelial cells may arise within preexisting developmental cysts of the Mullerian type.

There is one case report of primary adenocarcinoma arising in endocervicosis [59]. This presented as a vaginal nodule which on histological examination was a mucin-secreting adenocarcinoma. Benign mucin-secreting endocervical-type glands were observed deep in the tumor. The neoplastic cells were positive for PAS after diastase digestion. Unlike cloacogenic intestinal-type adenocarcinoma, there was no dysplasia of the overlying vaginal epithelium which was squamous rather than columnar. The immunoprofile was Mullerian in type, being CA125 and CK7 positive and CK20 and CEA negative.

Enteric-Type Neoplasms, Adenocarcinoma of Cloacogenic Origin

Gastrointestinal-type neoplasms in the vagina and vulva are extremely rare with about 17 cases reported in literature [60–74]. Developmentally the lower vagina arises from the cloaca when it is partitioned by the urorectal septum into the urogenital sinus anteriorly and the rectal canal posteriorly. The urogenital sinus then divides into the bladder, the pelvic urethra, and the vestibule of the vagina (Chap. 1). Thus cloacal remnants in the vaginal wall could give rise to enteric lesions [60, 63, 68]. Alternatively, the process could be one of intestinal metaplasia arising in vulval skin adnexa [60], Skene's glands, the minor vestibular glands, or Bartholin's glands. Other theories regarding the development of these rare neoplasms include origin in foci of adenosis, heterotopic gastrointestinal epithelium, and mesonephric remnants. Most of the reported cases have occurred in the lower vagina and two cases have been reported in a periurethral location [65]. One case describes a tubulovillous vulval adenoma associated with a villous adenoma of the rectum which had been resected 6 months previously [72].

In the majority of cases, the tumor arises in continuity with the surface epithelium of the vulva and may be confined to epithelium (Fig. 4.13a, b). It has a villoglandular architecture and in some cases small mucin-containing glands are present in the subjacent stroma. The

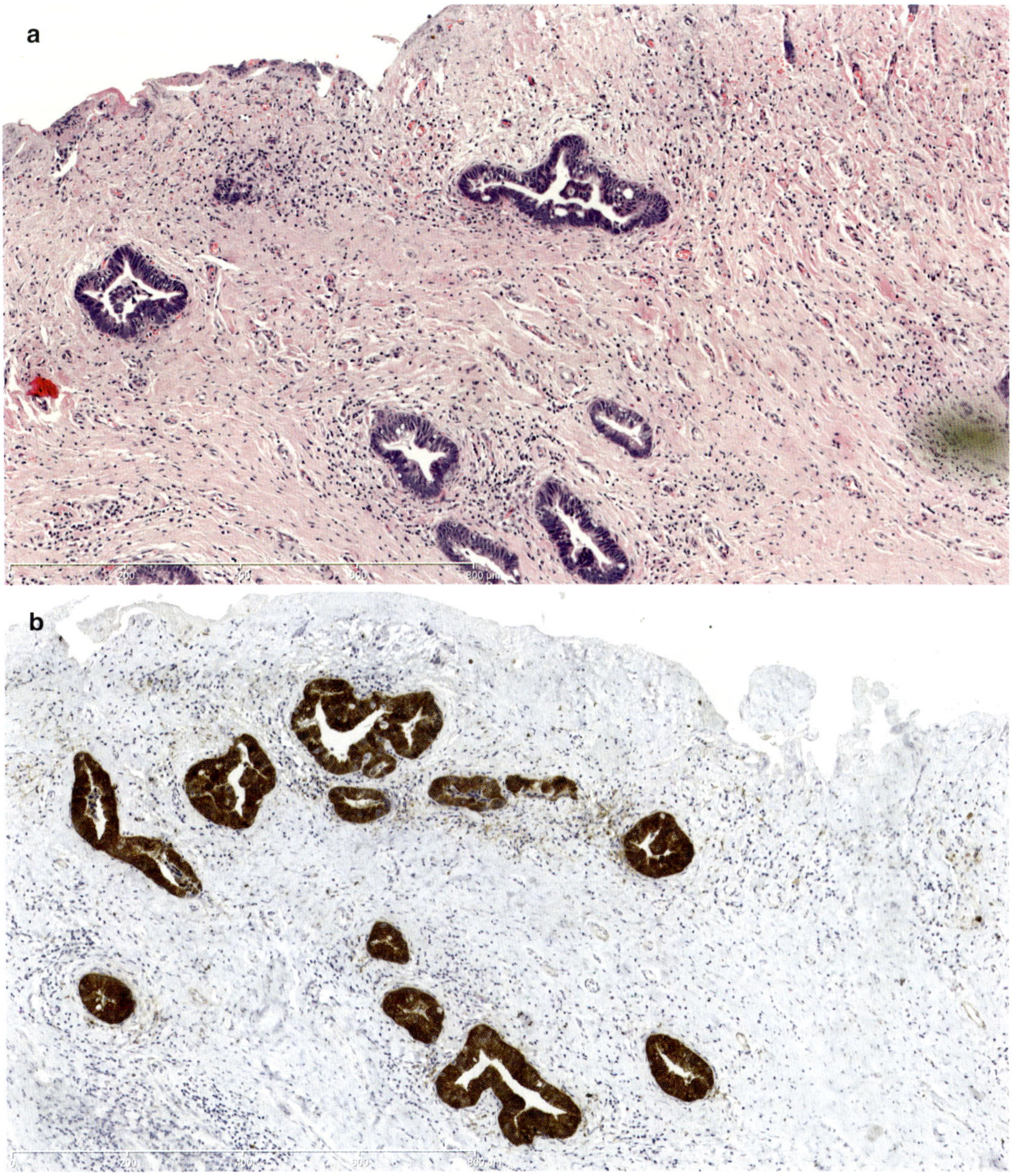

Fig. 4.10 (**a**) Cervical carcinoma, metastatic to the vagina. (**b**) Cervical carcinoma, metastatic to the vagina. The epithelial cells are strongly positive for p16

epithelium is columnar with intracytoplasmic mucin and goblet cells. O-acetylated sialomucin which is specific for large intestinal differentiation has been identified and neuroendocrine-type cells may be present [65, 66]. On immunohistochemistry, the cells have been reported to be positive for polyclonal CEA, Cam 5.2, CK7, and p53. Strong reactivity for CDX2 has also been reported. The epithelial cells are negative for monoclonal CEA, ER, and PR. Focal CK20, S100, and chromogranin reactivity may occur.

Morphologically these intestinal-type tumors may resemble endometrioid carcinomas which can also contain focal intracytoplasmic mucin.

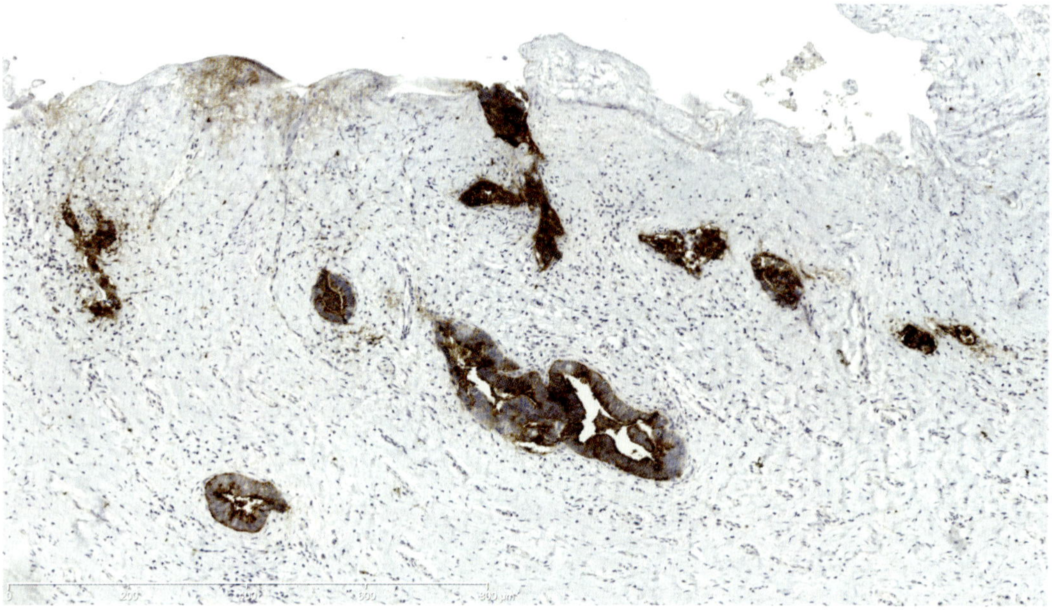

Fig. 4.11 Cervical carcinoma, metastatic to the vagina. Positivity for CEA

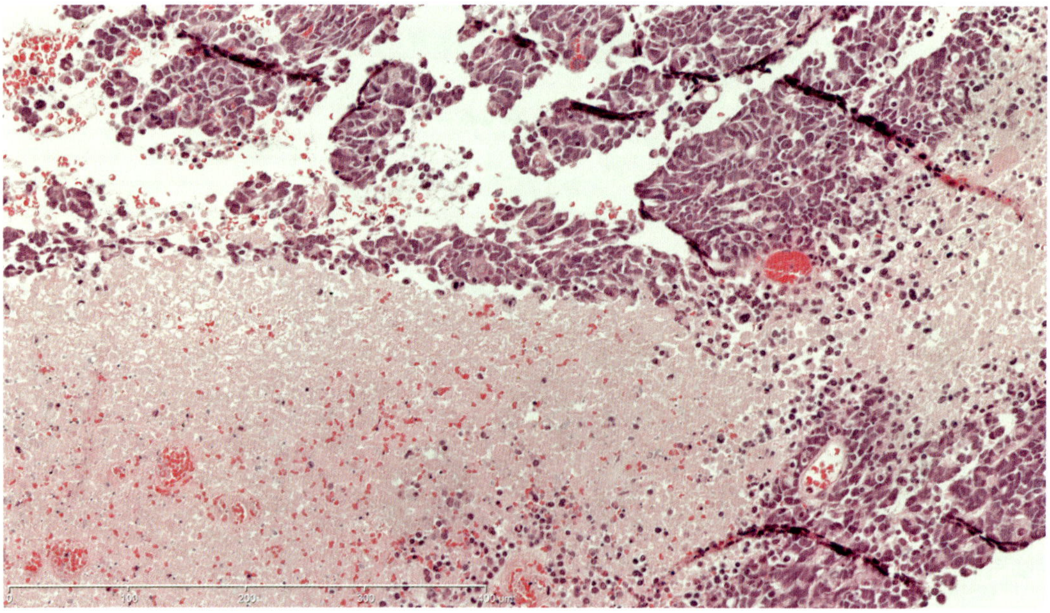

Fig. 4.12 Vaginal nodule. Metastatic serous ovarian carcinoma

However, unlike enteric carcinomas, most endometrioid carcinomas express ER and PR and are negative for markers of intestinal differentiation such as CK20 and CDX2. Cloacogenic carcinoma is rare; therefore when confronted with a vaginal adenocarcinoma that consists of glands lined by pseudostratified, columnar epithelium with focal mucin, there is a higher likelihood that it represents endometrioid carcinoma (primary or secondary) rather than enteric-type carcinoma.

Synchronous and multifocal mucinous lesions with a gastric phenotype have been described in

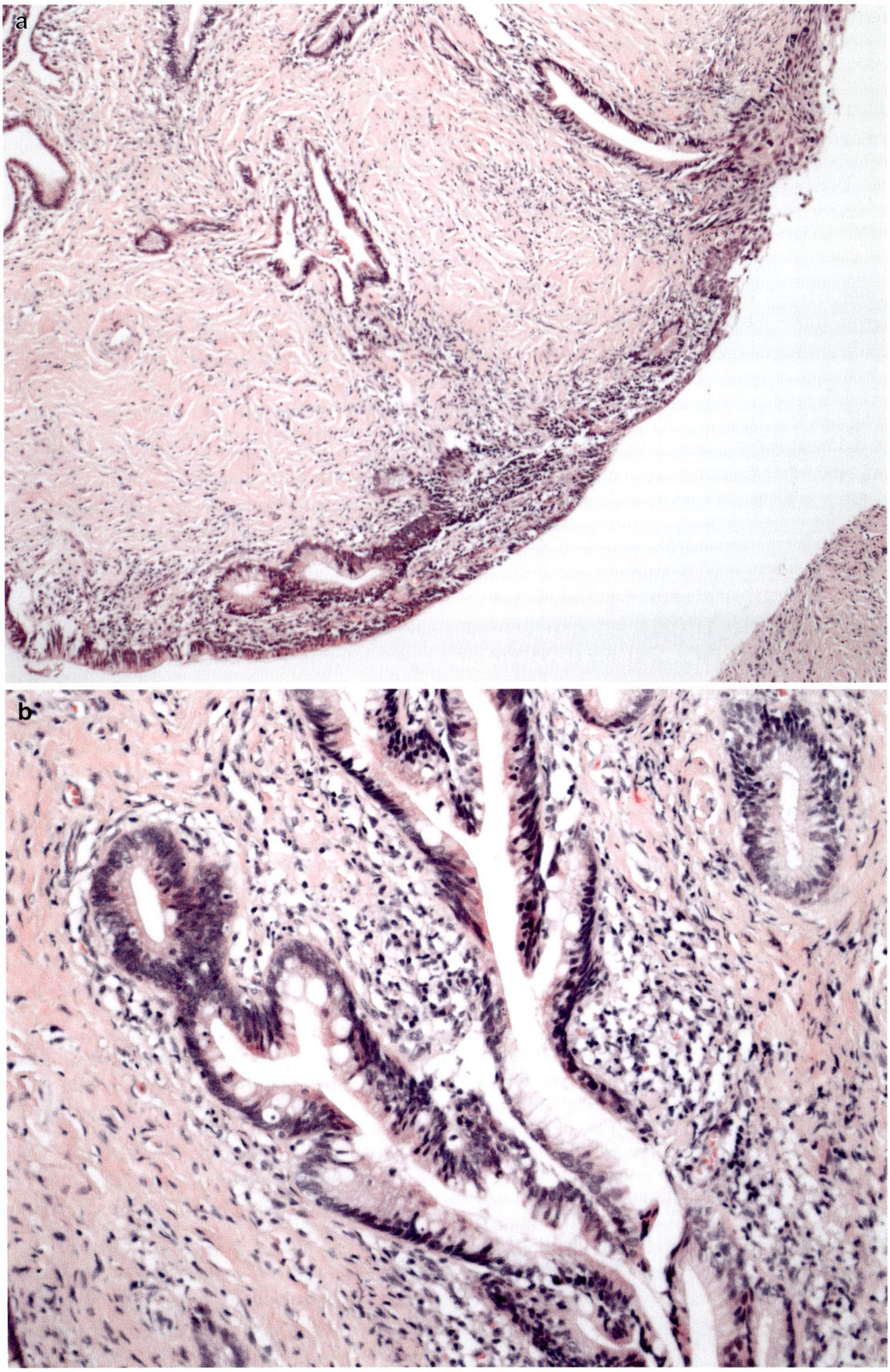

Fig. 4.13 (**a**) Cloacogenic carcinoma. Presented as a vulval lump. The glandular epithelium is in continuity with the surface squamous epithelium. (**b**) Cloacogenic carcinoma. The neoplastic glands are of the intestinal in type (Courtesy of Dr. Ray Lonsdale)

the female genital tract [75]. However these tend to occur in the cervix, uterine corpus, Fallopian tubes, and ovary. To date there has been no report of mucinous neoplasia in the vulva or the vagina associated with this condition (Fig. 4.13).

Mesonephric Adenocarcinoma

The majority of these occur within the cervix. However there have been rare cases of mesonephric carcinoma presenting as a primary tumor in the vagina [76–78]. Mesonephric remnants in the vagina can give rise to cysts (e.g., Gartner's cyst) and neoplastic lesions. As adenocarcinoma arising from mesonephric remnants may contain clear cells, it needs to be differentiated from primary or metastatic clear cell carcinoma. Immunohistochemistry may help in these circumstances. The typical immunoprofile of mesonephric carcinoma is CD10, CK 5/6, and calretinin positive whereas ER, PR, CEA, and CK20 are all negative. Other malignant tumors included in the differential diagnosis are carcinosarcoma (malignant mixed Mullerian tumor), yolk sac tumor, and rarely endometrioid adenocarcinoma.

Lesions of Bartholin's Gland

Bartholin's Cyst

The commonest lesions of Bartholin's gland are cysts. Large examples present as a classical S-shaped deformity of the vulval labia. The cysts may vary from a few to several centimeters in size, and very large cysts can extend upward into the labium majus. In such a case, the clinical differential includes an inguinal hernia or a cyst of the canal of Nuck. Cyst formation usually occurs due to occlusion of Bartholin's duct. The lining epithelium is therefore transitional, squamous, or mucinous in type. The typical mucinous acini of Bartholin's gland may persist in the adjacent tissue. Cysts originating in the glandular acini are lined by mucinous epithelium. Treatment is usually by marsupialization (Fig. 4.14).

Hyperplasia

Lobular hyperplasia of Bartholin's gland is a little recognized entity but is probably commoner than might be expected due to underreporting [79–81]. Careful examination of a Bartholin's cyst may reveal hyperplastic acini with a lobular architecture within the cyst wall. Alternatively the lesion may present as a cystic or solid vulval mass which is usually painless unless there is superimposed inflammation. The normal Bartholin's gland has a lobular arrangement of acini and ductules around a large central duct (Fig. 4.15). In lobular hyperplasia, there is proliferation of mucinous acini and ducts in which the normal lobular architecture of the gland is maintained. The lesion is non encapsulated and has an irregular edge (Fig. 4.16a, b). The epithelial cells are positive for broad-spectrum cytokeratins, AE1/3, low-molecular-weight cytokeratin Cam 5.2, EMA, and CEA. A basal layer of myoepithelial cells can sometimes be identified using antibodies against SMA.

Neoplasms of Bartholin's Gland

Adenoma

This is a rare lesion which presents as a mass in the posterolateral vulva. It is well circumscribed and usually encapsulated. It is composed of mucinous acini with loss of the normal lobular architecture [79].

The main differential diagnosis microscopically is from lobular hyperplasia of the gland. Table 4.2 highlights the main differentiating features as proposed by Koenig and Tavassoli [79].

A study of 72 lesions of Bartholin's gland published in 2006 showed that approximately 64% were cysts arising from Bartholin's ducts, 22% were abscesses, and 14% were diagnosed as nodular hyperplasia [81]. There were no neoplastic lesions, thus demonstrating the rarity of neoplasia in Bartholin's glands. There has been some debate as to whether lesions reported as adenomas are neoplastic or whether they represent hamartomas or merely focal hyperplasia. In Koenig and

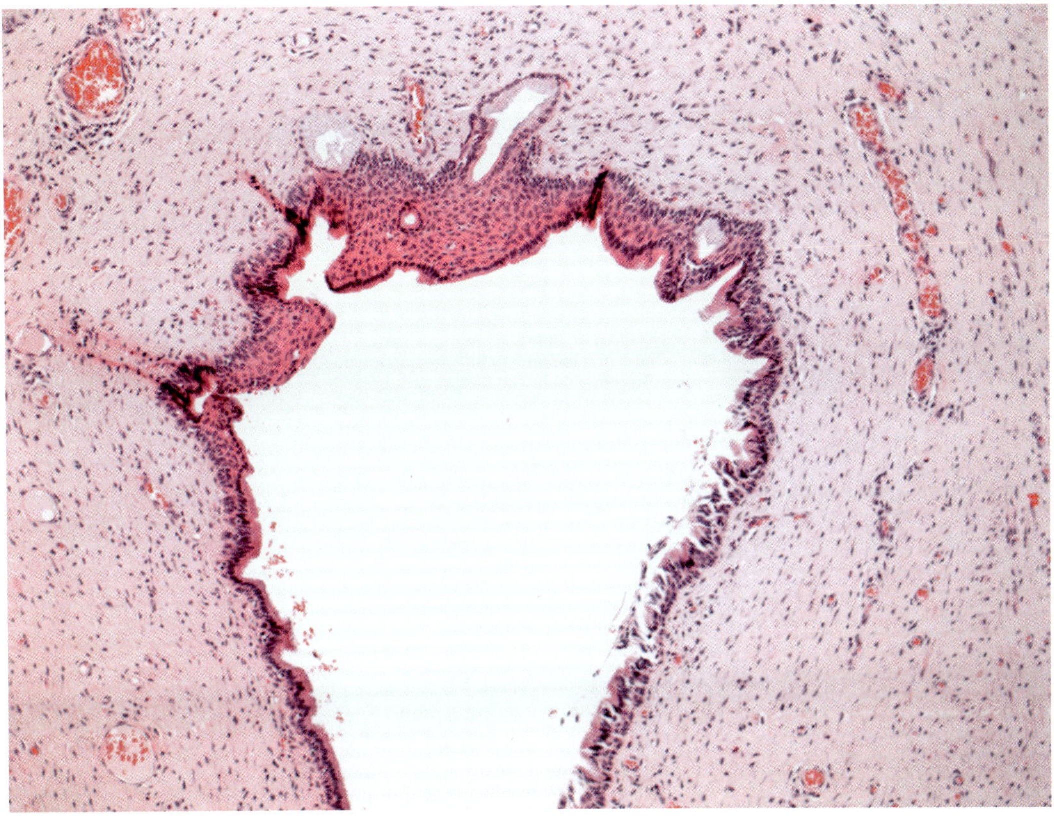

Fig. 4.14 Bartholin's cyst

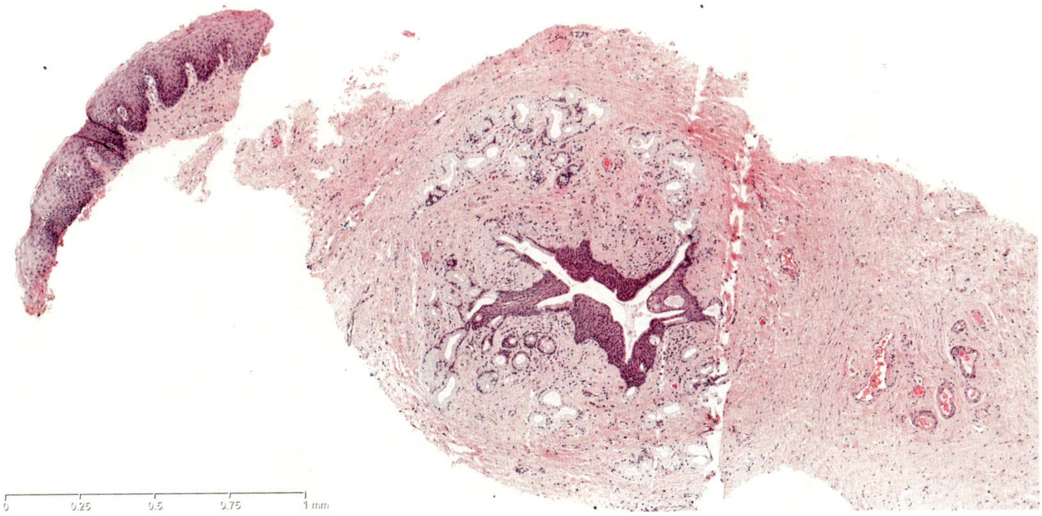

Fig. 4.15 Normal Bartholin's gland

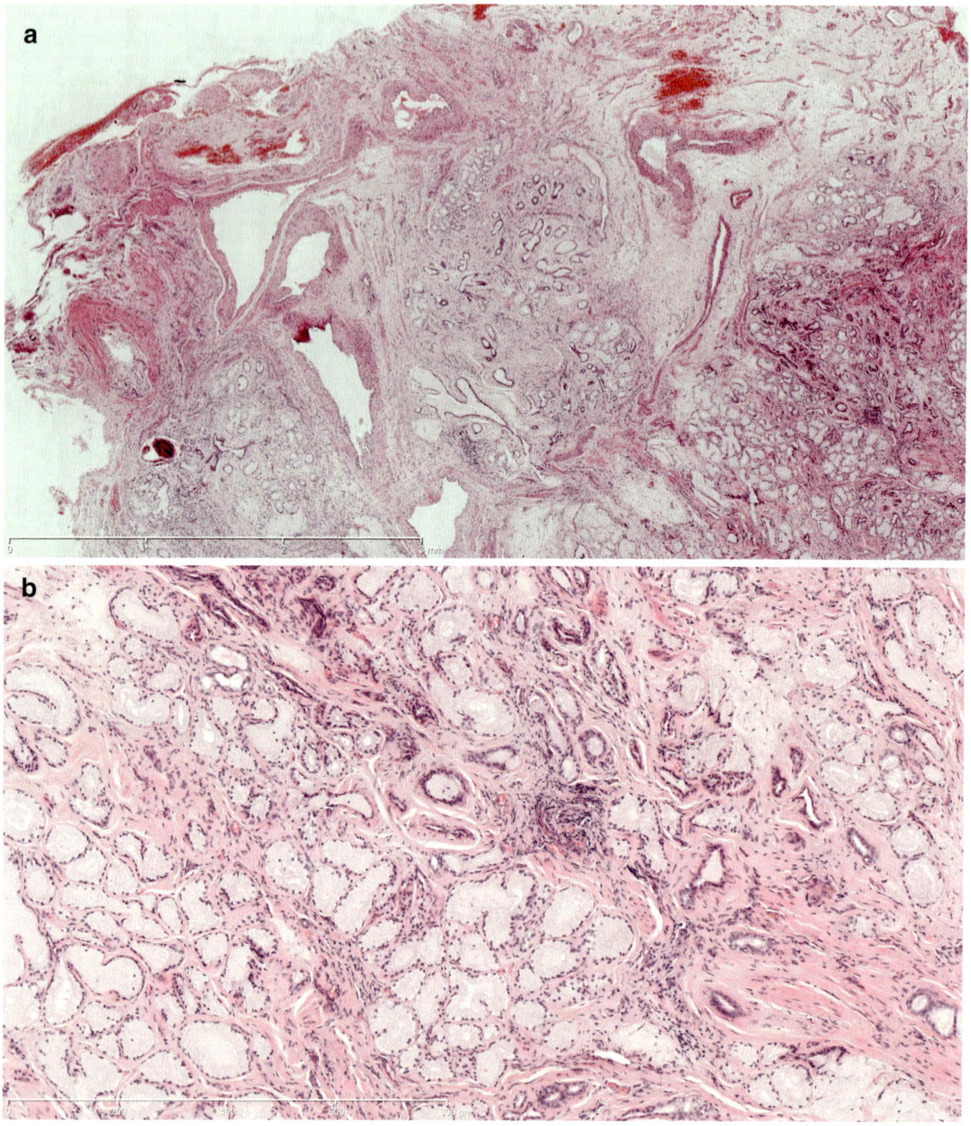

Fig. 4.16 (**a**) Bartholin's gland lobular hyperplasia. The lesion is nonencapsulated with an irregular periphery. (**b**) Proliferation of acini and ducts with maintenance of the lobular architecture

Table 4.2 Differentiating features between hyperplasia and adenoma of Bartholin's gland

Nodular hyperplasia	Adenoma
Proliferation of acini	Haphazard/diffuse proliferation of glands and tubules
Lobular architecture	Loss of lobular architecture
Maintenance of duct-acinar relationship	Loss of duct-acinar relationship
Unencapsulated/irregular outline	Sharply circumscribed/encapsulated
Mucin present	Loss/decrease of intracellular mucin

Tavassoli's series which looked at AFIP files over a 50-year period for cases with a diagnosis of Bartholin's gland adenoma or hyperplasia, one of nineteen cases was diagnosed as adenoma and one as an adenomyoma. In a report investigating clonality in two cases of nodular hyperplasia of Bartholin's gland diagnosed by the criteria of Koenig and Tavassoli [80], one was monoclonal. The authors question whether this actually represents true neoplasia as monoclonality does not necessarily equate with neoplasia.

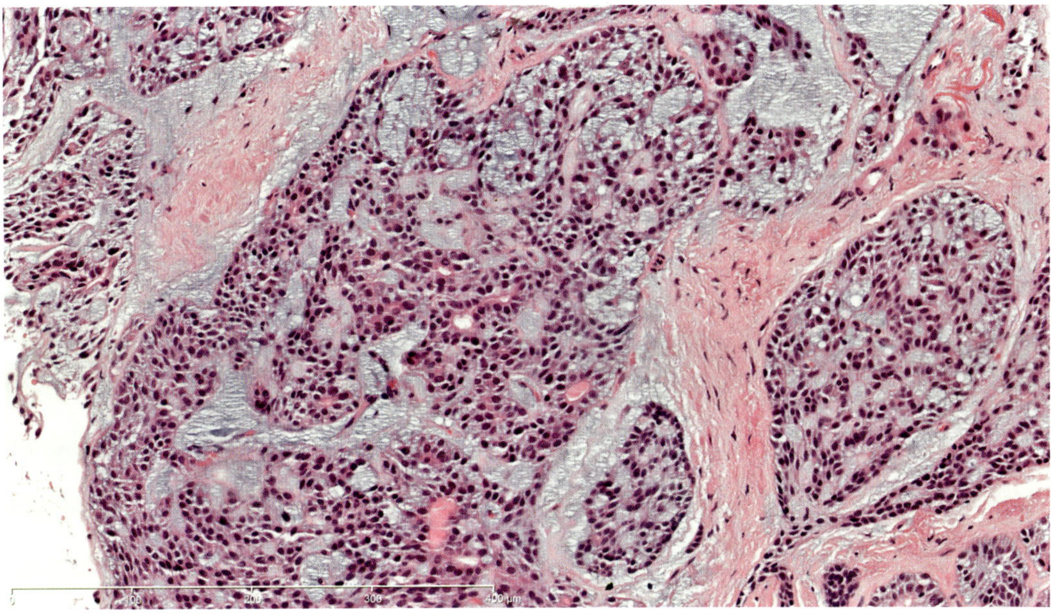

Fig. 4.17 Adenoid cystic carcinoma of Bartholin's gland. H&E, ×20 (Courtesy of Dr Eric Sumithran). Bartholin's gland lobular hyperplasia

Adenomyoma

One example of this was included in Koenig and Tavassoli's series. It was well circumscribed and sharply demarcated from the surrounding tissue. The tumor had a prominent fibromuscular stroma with a haphazard proliferation of small acini lined by epithelial cells with bland nuclei and cytoplasmic mucin [79].

Carcinoma of Bartholin's Glands

The criteria for diagnosing carcinoma of Bartholin's glands include an appropriate anatomical location, transition between normal and neoplastic tissue, exclusion of metastatic tumor, and histological features compatible with origin from Bartholin's gland [4, 82]. It has been suggested that these criteria may be somewhat restrictive as the entire gland could have been replaced by neoplasia. In up to 80% of cases, the tumor type is either adenocarcinoma or squamous cell carcinoma. Adenocarcinomas are usually non specific in type; however reports of specific types of adenocarcinoma include salivary gland-type carcinomas such as adenoid cystic carcinoma [66–69] epithelial-myoepithelial carcinoma [83], basal cell carcinoma [84], and low-grade polymorphous adenocarcinoma [85]. Other rare tumors that have been encountered at this site are lymphoepithelioma-like tumors [86], small cell carcinoma [87], and Merkel cell carcinoma [88] (Figs. 4.17 and 4.18).

Salivary Gland-Type Carcinomas

The most commonly reported are adenoid cystic carcinomas [89–92] consisting of trabeculae and cribriform tubules containing densely eosinophilic basement membrane-like material (Fig. 4.17). The tumor cells express CEA and S100. The basement membrane-like material reacts for type IV collagen and may be admixed with mucin. The tumor is similar to the prototype in the salivary gland and is poorly circumscribed and with a tendency to perineurial invasion. Due to this feature, complete resection is difficult to achieve and the neoplasm is prone to recurrences.

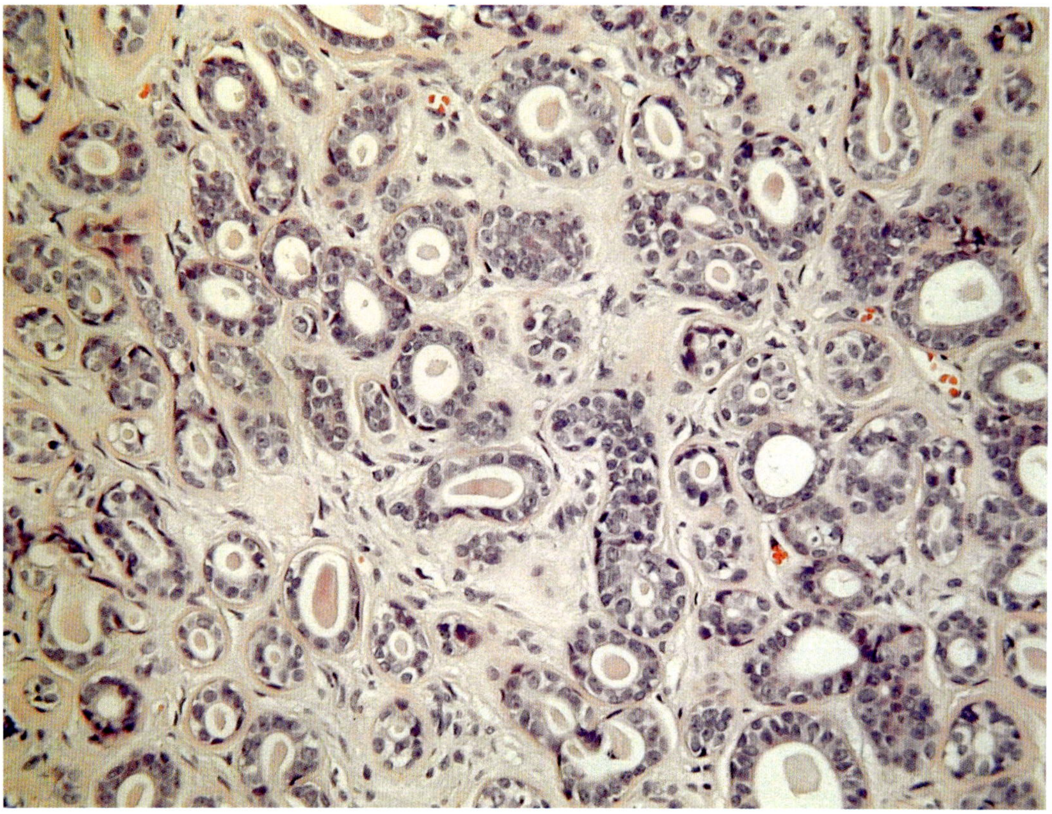

Fig. 4.18 Epithelial-myoepithelial carcinoma of Bartholin's gland (Courtesy of Professor Glenn McCluggage)

Basal cell carcinoma is thought to be derived from myoepithelial cells. It consists of nests of cells with a tendency to peripheral palisading. The cells at the periphery have scanty cytoplasm and ovoid nuclei whereas the central cells have more abundant amphophilic cytoplasm. They lack the cystic spaces and basement membrane material that are present in adenoid cystic carcinoma. The epithelial cells stain with Cam 5.2 and LP 34 while the myoepithelial components are positive for S100, SMA, and calponin [84].

Epithelial-myoepithelial carcinoma has also been reported [83]. The tumor had an insular, tubular, and trabecular architecture (Fig. 4.18). The lesions were mitotically active with an infiltrative border. Two morphologically distinct types of cells were identified in the tubules – an outer layer of myoepithelial type cells that stained positively for p63, calponin, and SMA and an inner layer of cuboidal to low columnar cells which stained with broad-spectrum cytokeratins and epithelial membrane antigen. Membranous c-kit (CD117) reactivity was noted in the epithelial cells. Eosinophilic basement membrane-like material was identified, and as there were also cribriform glands present, the differential diagnosis was with adenoid cystic carcinoma. The authors concluded that this was more likely to represent a low-grade epithelial-myoepithelial neoplasm as the characteristic perineurial infiltration of adenoid cystic carcinoma was lacking.

References

1. Anderson SR. Benign vulvovaginal cysts. Diagn Histopathol. 2010;16(11):495–9.
2. Zaino RNM, Kurman RJ. Diseases of the vagina. In: Kurman RJ, HE Lora, Ronnett BM, editors. Blaustein's pathology of the female genital tract. 6th ed. New York: Springer; 2011, p. 127.
3. Wilkinson EM, Nicole AM. Benign diseases of the vagina. In: Kurman RJ, Lora HE, Brigitte MR, editors.

Blaustein's pathology of the female genital tract. 6th ed. New York: Springer; 2011, p. 126.
4. Kurman RJ, Ronnett BM, Sherman ME, Wilkinson EJ. Tumours of the cervix, vagina and vulva, Fascicle 13. Washington, DC: ARP Press; 2010. p 431.
5. Hamada M, Kiryu H, Ohta T, Furue M. Ciliated cyst of the vulva. Eur J Dermatol. 2004;14(5):347–9. Epub 2004/09/11.
6. Marquette GP, Su B, Woodruff JD. Introital adenosis associated with Stevens-Johnson syndrome. Obstet Gynecol. 1985;66(1):143–5. Epub 1985/07/01.
7. Sedlacek TV, Riva JM, Magen AB, Mangan CE, Cunnane MF. Vaginal and vulvar adenosis. An unsuspected side effect of CO_2 laser vaporization. J Reprod Med. 1990;35(11):995–1001. Epub 1990/11/01.
8. Eilber KS, Raz S. Benign cystic lesions of the vagina: a literature review. J Urol. 2003;170(3):717–22. Epub 2003/08/13.
9. Currarino G. Single vaginal ectopic ureter and Gartner's duct cyst with ipsilateral renal hypoplasia and dysplasia (or agenesis). J Urol. 1982;128(5):988–93. Epub 1982/11/01.
10. Schneider CA, Festa S, Spillert CR, Bruce CJ, Lazaro EJ. Hydrocele of the canal of Nuck. N J Med. 1994;91(1):37–8. Epub 1994/01/01.
11. Celik N, Yalcin S, Gucer S, Karnak I. Clitoral epidermoid cyst secondary to blunt trauma in a 9-year-old child. Turk J Pediatr. 2011;53(1):108–10. Epub 2011/05/04.
12. Osifo OD. Post genital mutilation giant clitoral epidermoid inclusion cyst in Benin City, Nigeria. J Pediatr Adolesc Gynecol. 2010;23(6):336–40. Epub 2010/08/06.
13. Hamoudi A, Shier M. Late complications of childhood female genital mutilation. J Obstet Gynaecol Can. 2010;32(6):587–9. Epub 2010/06/24.
14. Asante A, Omurtag K, Roberts C. Epidermal inclusion cyst of the clitoris 30 years after female genital mutilation. Fertil Steril. 2010;94(3):1097e1–3. Epub 2010/03/20.
15. Mueller BE, Laudenschlager MD, Hansen KA. Epidermoid cyst of the clitoris: an unusual cause of clitoromegaly in a patient without history of previous female circumcision. J Pediatr Adolesc Gynecol. 2009;22(5):e130–2. Epub 2009/07/07.
16. Tjugum J, Jonassen F, Olsson JH. Vaginitis emphysematosa in a renal transplant patient. Acta Obstet Gynecol Scand. 1986;65(4):377–8. Epub 1986/01/01.
17. Rowland R, Inman SE. A case of vaginitis emphysematosa. J Obstet Gynaecol Br Commonw. 1968;75(1): 97–9. Epub 1968/01/01.
18. Mautner LS. Vaginitis emphysematosa. Can Med Assoc J. 1958;80(8):643–7. Epub 1958/04/15.
19. Leder RA, Paulson EK. Vaginitis emphysematosa: CT and review of the literature. AJR Am J Roentgenol. 2001;176(3):623–5. Epub 2001/02/27.
20. Josey WE, Campbell Jr WG. Vaginitis emphysematosa. A report of four cases. J Reprod Med. 1990;35(10):974–7. Epub 1990/10/01.
21. Gardner HL, Fernet P. Etiology of vaginitis emphysematosa: report of ten cases and review of literature. Am J Obstet Gynecol. 1964;88:680–94. Epub 1964/03/01.
22. Daino JA, Girerd RJ, Tchertkoff V. Nonpuerperal vaginitis emphysematosa. Obstet Gynecol. 1968;31(1): 128–31. Epub 1968/01/01.
23. Stern RC, Dash R, Bentley RC, Snyder MJ, Haney AF, Robboy SJ. Malignancy in endometriosis: frequency and comparison of ovarian and extraovarian types. Int J Gynecol Pathol. 2001;20(2):133–9. Epub 2001/04/11.
24. Gardner HL. Cervical and vaginal endometriosis. Clin Obstet Gynecol. 1966;9(2):358–72. Epub 1966/06/01.
25. Dodds E, Goldberg L, Lawson W, Robinson R. Estrogenic activity of certain synthetic compounds. Nature. 1938;141:247–8.
26. Herbst AL, Ulfelder H, Poskanzer DC. Adenocarcinoma of the vagina. Association of maternal stilbestrol therapy with tumor appearance in young women. N Engl J Med. 1971;284(15):878–81. Epub 1971/04/15.
27. Robboy SJ, Taguchi O, Cunha GR. Normal development of the human female reproductive tract and alterations resulting from experimental exposure to diethylstilbestrol. Hum Pathol. 1982;13(3):190–8. Epub 1982/03/01.
28. Robboy SJ, Kaufman RH, Prat J, Welch WR, Gaffey T, Scully RE, et al. Pathologic findings in young women enrolled in the National Cooperative Diethylstilbestrol Adenosis (DESAD) project. Obstet Gynecol. 1979;53(3):309–17. Epub 1979/03/01.
29. Kranl C, Zelger B, Kofler H, Heim K, Sepp N, Fritsch P. Vulval and vaginal adenosis. Br J Dermatol. 1998;139(1):128–31. Epub 1998/10/09.
30. Ganesan R, Ferryman SR, Waddell CA. Vaginal adenosis in a patient on Tamoxifen therapy: a case report. Cytopathology. 1999;10(2):127–30; discussion 31. Epub 1999/04/22.
31. Clement PB, Young RH. Endocervicosis of the urinary bladder. A report of six cases of a benign Mullerian lesion that may mimic adenocarcinoma. Am J Surg Pathol. 1992;16(6):533–42. Epub 1992/06/01.
32. Young RH, Clement PB. Mullerianosis of the urinary bladder. Mod Pathol. 1996;9(7):731–7. Epub 1996/07/01.
33. Nazeer T, Ro JY, Tornos C, Ordonez NG, Ayala AG. Endocervical type glands in urinary bladder: a clinicopathologic study of six cases. Hum Pathol. 1996;27(8):816–20. Epub 1996/08/01.
34. Martinka M, Allaire C, Clement PB. Endocervicosis presenting as a painful vaginal mass: a case report. Int J Gynecol Pathol. 1999;18(3):274–6. Epub 2002/07/02.
35. Rudin JE, Geldt VG, Alecseev EB. Prolapse of urethral mucosa in white female children: experience with 58 cases. J Pediatr Surg. 1997;32(3):423–5. Epub 1997/03/01.
36. Richardson DA, Hajj SN, Herbst AL. Medical treatment of urethral prolapse in children. Obstet Gynecol. 1982;59(1):69–74. Epub 1982/01/01.

37. Valerie E, Gilchrist BF, Frischer J, Scriven R, Klotz DH, Ramenofsky ML. Diagnosis and treatment of urethral prolapse in children. Urology. 1999;54(6): 1082–4. Epub 1999/12/22.
38. Lee JW, Fynes MM. Female urethral diverticula. Best Pract Res Clin Obstet Gynaecol. 2005;19(6):875–93. Epub 2005/09/27.
39. Thomas AA, Rackley RR, Lee U, Goldman HB, Vasavada SP, Hansel DE. Urethral diverticula in 90 female patients: a study with emphasis on neoplastic alterations. J Urol. 2008;180(6):2463–7.
40. Kazakov DV, Stewart CJ, Kacerovska D, Leake R, Kreuzberg B, Chudacek Z, et al. Prostatic-type tissue in the lower female genital tract: a morphologic spectrum, including vaginal tubulosquamous polyp, adenomyomatous hyperplasia of paraurethral Skene glands (female prostate), and ectopic lesion in the vulva. Am J Surg Pathol. 2010;34(7):950–5. Epub 2010/05/28.
41. McCluggage WG, Ganesan R, Hirschowitz L, Miller K, Rollason TP. Ectopic prostatic tissue in the uterine cervix and vagina: report of a series with a detailed immunohistochemical analysis. Am J Surg Pathol. 2006;30(2):209–15. Epub 2006/01/26.
42. Larraza-Hernandez O, Molberg KH, Lindberg G, Albores-Saavedra J. Ectopic prostatic tissue in the uterine cervix. Int J Gynecol Pathol. 1997;16(3):291–3. Epub 1997/07/01.
43. Nucci MR, Ferry JA, Young RH. Ectopic prostatic tissue in the uterine cervix: a report of four cases and review of ectopic prostatic tissue. Am J Surg Pathol. 2000;24(9):1224–30. Epub 2000/09/08.
44. Korytko TP, Lowe GJ, Jimenez RE, Pohar KS, Martin DD. Prostate-specific antigen response after definitive radiotherapy for Skene's gland adenocarcinoma resembling prostate adenocarcinoma. Urol Oncol. 2010. Epub 2010/09/28.
45. Pongtippan A, Malpica A, Levenback C, Deavers MT, Silva EG. Skene's gland adenocarcinoma resembling prostatic adenocarcinoma. Int J Gynecol Pathol. 2004;23(1):71–4. Epub 2003/12/12.
46. Dodson MK, Cliby WA, Keeney GL, Peterson MF, Podratz KC. Skene's gland adenocarcinoma with increased serum level of prostate-specific antigen. Gynecol Oncol. 1994;55(2):304–7. Epub 1994/11/01.
47. Zaviacic M, Sidlo J, Borovsky M. Prostate specific antigen and prostate specific acid phosphatase in adenocarcinoma of Skene's paraurethral glands and ducts. Virchows Arch A Pathol Anat Histopathol. 1993;423(6):503–5. Epub 1993/01/01.
48. Chong Y, Eom M, Park KH, Chung HC, Ro JY. Adenofibroma of Skene's duct: a case report. Pathol Res Int. 2010;2010:318973. Epub 2010/12/15.
49. McCluggage WG, Young RH. Tubulo-squamous polyp: a report of ten cases of a distinctive hitherto uncharacterized vaginal polyp. Am J Surg Pathol. 2007;31(7):1013–9. Epub 2007/06/27.
50. Tong B, Clarke BA, Ghazarian D. Tubulo-squamous polyp with mucinous and goblet cell differentiation: a unique morphologic variant. Int J Gynecol Pathol. 2011;30(5):518–9. Epub 2011/08/02.
51. Stewart CJ. Tubulo-squamous vaginal polyp with basaloid epithelial differentiation. Int J Gynecol Pathol. 2009;28(6):563–6. Epub 2009/10/24.
52. Prayson RA, Stoler MH, Hart WR. Vulvar vestibulitis. A histopathologic study of 36 cases, including human papillomavirus in situ hybridization analysis. Am J Surg Pathol. 1995;19(2):154–60. Epub 1995/02/01.
53. Punia RP, Bal A, Jain P, Mohan H. Minor vestibular gland adenoma: a case report. Aust N Z J Obstet Gynaecol. 2003;43(4):322–3. Epub 2004/01/13.
54. Ulbright TM, Alexander RW, Kraus FT. Intramural papilloma of the vagina: evidence of Mullerian histogenesis. Cancer. 1981;48(10):2260–6. Epub 1981/11/15.
55. McCluggage WG, Nirmala V, Radhakumari K. Intramural Mullerian papilloma of the vagina. Int J Gynecol Pathol. 1999;18(1):94–5. Epub 1999/01/19.
56. Cohen M, Pedemonte L, Drut R. Pigmented Mullerian papilloma of the vagina. Histopathology. 2001;39(5): 541–3. Epub 2001/12/12.
57. Arbo E, dos Reis R, Uchoa D, Acetta SG, Rivoire WA, Capp E. Vaginal Mullerian papilloma in a 2-year-old child. Gynecol Obstet Invest. 2004;58(1):55–6. Epub 2004/05/19.
58. Dobbs SP, Shaw PA, Brown LJ, Ireland D. Borderline malignant change in recurrent Mullerian papilloma of the vagina. J Clin Pathol. 1998;51(11):875–7. Epub 1999/04/08.
59. McCluggage WG, Price JH, Dobbs SP. Primary adenocarcinoma of the vagina arising in endocervicosis. Int J Gynecol Pathol. 2001;20(4):399–402. Epub 2001/10/18.
60. Fox HW M, Harris M, McWilliam LJ, Anderson GS. Enteric tumours of the lower female genital tract: a report of three cases. Histopathology. 1998;12(2):167–76.
61. Yaghsezian H, Palazzo JP, Finkel GC, Carlson Jr JA, Talerman A. Primary vaginal adenocarcinoma of the intestinal type associated with adenosis. Gynecol Oncol. 1992;45(1):62–5. Epub 1992/04/11.
62. Tjalma WA, Colpaert CG. Primary vaginal adenocarcinoma of intestinal type arising from a tubulovillous adenoma. Int J Gynecol Cancer. 2006;16(3):1461–5. Epub 2006/06/29.
63. Nagar HA, McKinney KA, Price JH, McClelland HR, Biggart JD. Enteric epithelium progressing through dysplasia to adenocarcinoma within the vagina. Eur J Surg Oncol. 1999;25(1):106–7. Epub 1999/04/03.
64. Mudhar HS, Smith JH, Tidy J. Primary vaginal adenocarcinoma of intestinal type arising from an adenoma: case report and review of the literature. Int J Gynecol Pathol. 2001;20(2):204–9. Epub 2001/04/11.
65. Heller DS, Merrell M, Sama J, Anderson J, Cracchiolo B. Periurethral vaginal adenocarcinoma of the intestinal type: report of two cases and review of the literature. Gynecol Oncol. 2000;77(3):478–81. Epub 2000/06/01.
66. Fukushima M, Twiggs LB, Okagaki T. Mixed intestinal adenocarcinoma-argentaffin carcinoma of the vagina. Gynecol Oncol. 1986;23(3):387–94.

67. Ditto A, Martinelli F, Carcangiu ML, Hanozet F, Solima E, Barisella M, et al. Incidental diagnosis of primary vaginal adenocarcinoma of intestinal type: a case report and review of the literature. Int J Gynecol Pathol. 2007;26(4):490–3. Epub 2007/09/22.
68. Kennedy JC, Majmudar B. Primary adenocarcinoma of the vulva, possibly cloacogenic. A report of two cases. J Reprod Med. 1993;38(2):113–6. Epub 1993/02/01.
69. Zaidi SN, Conner MG. Primary vulvar adenocarcinoma of cloacogenic origin. South Med J. 2001;94(7): 744–6. Epub 2001/09/04.
70. Rodriguez A, Isaac MA, Hidalgo E, Marquez B, Nogales FF. Villoglandular adenocarcinoma of the vulva. Gynecol Oncol. 2001;83(2):409–11. Epub 2001/10/19.
71. Dube V, Veilleux C, Plante M, Tetu B. Primary villoglandular adenocarcinoma of cloacogenic origin of the vulva. Hum Pathol. 2004;35(3):377–9. Epub 2004/03/16.
72. Vitrey D, Frachon S, Balme B, Golfier F. Tubulovillous adenoma of the vulva. Obstet Gynecol. 2003;102(5 Pt 2):1160–3. Epub 2003/11/11.
73. Willen R, Carlen B, Bozoky B, Cajander S, Bekassy AN. Cloacogenic adenocarcinoma of the vulva. Gynecol Oncol. 1999;74(2):298–301. Epub 1999/07/27.
74. Ghamande SA, Kasznica J, Griffiths CT, Finkler NJ, Hamid AM. Mucinous adenocarcinomas of the vulva. Gynecol Oncol. 1995;57(1):117–20. Epub 1995/04/01.
75. Mikami Y, Kiyokawa T, Sasajima Y, Teramoto N, Wakasa T, Wakasa K, et al. Reappraisal of synchronous and multifocal mucinous lesions of the female genital tract: a close association with gastric metaplasia. Histopathology. 2009;54(2):184–91. Epub 2009/02/12.
76. Bifulco G, Mandato VD, Mignogna C, Giampaolino P, Di Spiezio Sardo A, DeCecio R, et al. A case of mesonephric adenocarcinoma of the vagina with a 1-year follow-up. Int J Gynecol Cancer. 2008;18(5): 1127–31. Epub 2007/11/22.
77. Bague S, Rodriguez IM, Prat J. Malignant mesonephric tumors of the female genital tract: a clinicopathologic study of 9 cases. Am J Surg Pathol. 2004;28(5):601–7. Epub 2004/04/24.
78. Ersahin C, Huang M, Potkul RK, Hammadeh R, Salhadar A. Mesonephric adenocarcinoma of the vagina with a 3-year follow-up. Gynecol Oncol. 2005;99(3):757–60. Epub 2005/09/03.
79. Koenig C, Tavassoli FA. Nodular hyperplasia, adenoma, and adenomyoma of Bartholin's gland. Int J Gynecol Pathol. 1998;17(4):289–94. Epub 1998/10/24.
80. Kazakov DV, Curik R, Vanecek T, Mukensnabl P, Michal M. Nodular hyperplasia of the Bartholin gland: a clinicopathological study of two cases, including detection of clonality by HUMARA. Am J Dermatopathol. 2007;29(4):385–7. Epub 2007/08/02.
81. Santos LD, Kennerson AR, Killingsworth MC. Nodular hyperplasia of Bartholin's gland. Pathology. 2006;38(3):223–8. Epub 2006/06/07.
82. Cardosi RJ, Speights A, Fiorica JV, Grendys Jr EC, Hakam A, Hoffman MS. Bartholin's gland carcinoma: a 15-year experience. Gynecol Oncol. 2001;82(2):247–51. Epub 2001/09/05.
83. McCluggage WG, Aydin NE, Wong NA, Cooper K. Low-grade epithelial-myoepithelial carcinoma of Bartholin gland: report of 2 cases of a distinctive neoplasm arising in the vulvovaginal region. Int J Gynecol Pathol. 2009;28(3):286–91. Epub 2009/07/22.
84. Felix A, Moura Nunes JF, Soares J. Salivary gland-type basal cell adenocarcinoma of presumed Bartholin's gland origin: a case report. Int J Gynecol Pathol. 2002;21(2):194–7. Epub 2002/03/28.
85. Young S, Leon M, Talerman A, Teresi M, Emmadi R. Polymorphous low-grade adenocarcinoma of the vulva and vagina: a tumor resembling adenoid cystic carcinoma. Int J Surg Pathol. 2003;11(1):43–9. Epub 2003/02/25.
86. Kacerovska D, Nemcova J, Petrik R, Michal M, Kazakov DV. Lymphoepithelioma-like carcinoma of the Bartholin gland. Am J Dermatopathol. 2008;30(6):586–9. Epub 2008/11/27.
87. Mirhashemi R, Kratz A, Weir MM, Molpus KL, Goodman AK. Vaginal small cell carcinoma mimicking a Bartholin's gland abscess: a case report. Gynecol Oncol. 1998;68(3):297–300. Epub 1998/05/08.
88. Khoury-Collado F, Elliott KS, Lee YC, Chen PC, Abulafia O. Merkel cell carcinoma of the Bartholin's gland. Gynecol Oncol. 2005;97(3):928–31. Epub 2005/05/12.
89. Wahlstrom T, Vesterinen E, Saksela E. Primary carcinoma of Bartholin's glands: a morphological and clinical study of six cases including a transitional cell carcinoma. Gynecol Oncol. 1978;6(4):354–62. Epub 1978/08/01.
90. Nasu K, Kawano Y, Takai N, Kashima K, Miyakawa I. Adenoid cystic carcinoma of Bartholin's gland. Case report with review of the literature. Gynecol Obstet Invest. 2005;59(1):54–8. Epub 2004/10/14.
91. Woida FM, Ribeiro-Silva A. Adenoid cystic carcinoma of the Bartholin gland: an overview. Arch Pathol Lab Med. 2007;131(5):796–8. Epub 2007/05/10.
92. Morita Y, Hikage S, Ogino M. Adenoid cystic carcinoma of Bartholin's gland. Int J Gynaecol Obstet. 1996;54(3):279–80. Epub 1996/09/01.

Melanoctyic Lesions of the Vulva and Vagina

5

Thomas Brenn and Eduardo Calonje

Abstract

Pigmentary abnormalities of the lower female genital tract most commonly affect the vulva and only rarely the vagina. They are identified in about 10% of patients at routine gynecological examination and encompass melanocytic proliferations as well as non-melanocytic disorders including squamous lesions and inflammatory and reactive conditions. Only the true melanocytic proliferations as well as disorders characterized by hyperpigmentation are discussed in this chapter. The vast majority of pigmented lesions are benign, most frequently presenting as common acquired melanocytic nevi and genital lentigines/melanosis. In contrast, genital melanoma is a rare disease but early detection is crucial due to its poor prognosis at advanced stage. Its correct diagnosis may be challenging due to significant clinical and histological overlap with a subset of benign nevi, in particular the dysplastic and the atypical genital nevi. The salient clinical and histological features of these important entities are discussed in the appropriate context and with a particular focus on differential diagnosis.

Genital Melanosis (Genital Melanotic Macule)

Clinical Findings

Genital melanosis is among the most frequently encountered pigmentary abnormalities of the female genital tract [1–4]. It is closely related to mucosal melanosis at other sites such as the lip, i.e., the labial melanotic macule. Both cutaneous as well as mucosal surfaces are involved and the vulva is the most frequently affected site [3, 5].

T. Brenn, M.D., Ph.D., FRCPath
Department of Pathology, Western General Hospital and The University of Edinburgh,
Edinburgh, UK

E. Calonje, M.D., DipRCPath (✉)
Department of Dermatopathology, St. John's Institute of Dermatology, St. Thomas' Hospital,
Westminster Bridge Road, London SE1 7EH, UK
e-mail: jaime.calonje@kcl.ac.uk

L. Brown (ed.), *Pathology of the Vulva and Vagina*, Essentials of Diagnostic Gynecological Pathology,
DOI 10.1007/978-0-85729-757-0_5, © Springer-Verlag London 2013

Presentation is in adulthood at around 40 years of age [3, 6]. The clinical manifestation is of solitary or multiple and sometimes confluent macules and patches with tan to dark brown or bluish-black hyperpigmentation ranging in size from 0.5 to 2 cm [3, 6, 7]. Irregular borders, variable pigmentation, and the large size are clinically alarming features which may be easily mistaken for melanoma [3, 7, 8]. The behavior of genital melanosis is however entirely benign with only rare reports documenting the development of melanoma on a background of genital melanosis [9, 10].

While most cases of genital melanosis are sporadic, they may also be part of an underlying clinical syndrome. The Laugier-Hunziker syndrome (idiopathic lenticular mucocutaneous pigmentation) is a benign, acquired disease characterized by mucocutaneous hyperpigmentation affecting in particular the oral and labial mucosae as well as the fingernails in the form of longitudinal melanotic streaks [6, 11–14]. The Peutz-Jeghers syndrome shows a similar clinical presentation characterized by mucocutaneous hyperpigmentation predominantly of the lip and oral mucosa. It shows however an autosomal-dominant inheritance pattern and may be complicated by gastrointestinal polyposis with risk for malignant transformation [6, 14]. Finally, mucocutaneous hyperpigmentation is also a hallmark of the Carney complex [15]. Additional signs include epithelioid blue nevi; multiple myxomas of the skin, breast, and cardiac atrium; multiple endocrine tumors of the thyroid, pituitary, and adrenal gland with endocrine hyperactivity; and the psammomatous melanotic schwannoma. Early recognition of the syndrome is important to prevent complications in particular due to embolization from the cardiac myxomas.

Histological Findings

The histological hallmark of genital melanosis is hyperpigmentation of basal cell layer keratinocytes (Fig. 5.1a, b). This is accompanied by mild epithelial acanthosis and pigmentary incontinence with melanin deposition and melanin-laden histiocytes within the papillary dermis or lamina propria (Fig. 5.2) [6–8, 16, 17]. Slight melanocyte hyperplasia may rarely be an additional feature but melanocyte confluence or atypia is not observed (Fig. 5.2) [7, 8].

Differential Diagnosis

Genital melanosis may show clinically atypical features concerning for a diagnosis of genital melanoma. The increased pigmentation is however largely due to hyperpigmentation of the basal cell layer of the epidermis and associated superficial dermal pigmentary incontinence. There is no significant proliferation of melanocytes. In particular, there is no confluent growth of melanocytes and cytological atypia is not a feature. In difficult cases, immunohistochemistry for Melan A and HMB-45 is useful to highlight melanocyte density.

Genital Melanocytic Nevi

Melanocytic nevi only rarely affect the lower genital female tract. On routine gynecological screening examination, melanocytic nevi are present in only 2.3% of patients only [2]. The vulva and perineum are most commonly affected, while vaginal involvement is exceptional with only scattered reports of common or cellular blue nevi affecting the vaginal wall [18–20].

Fig. 5.1 Genital melanosis. This diffuse process is characterized by epithelial hyperplasia and hyperpigmentation of basal cell layer keratinocytes (**a**). Higher magnification (**b**)

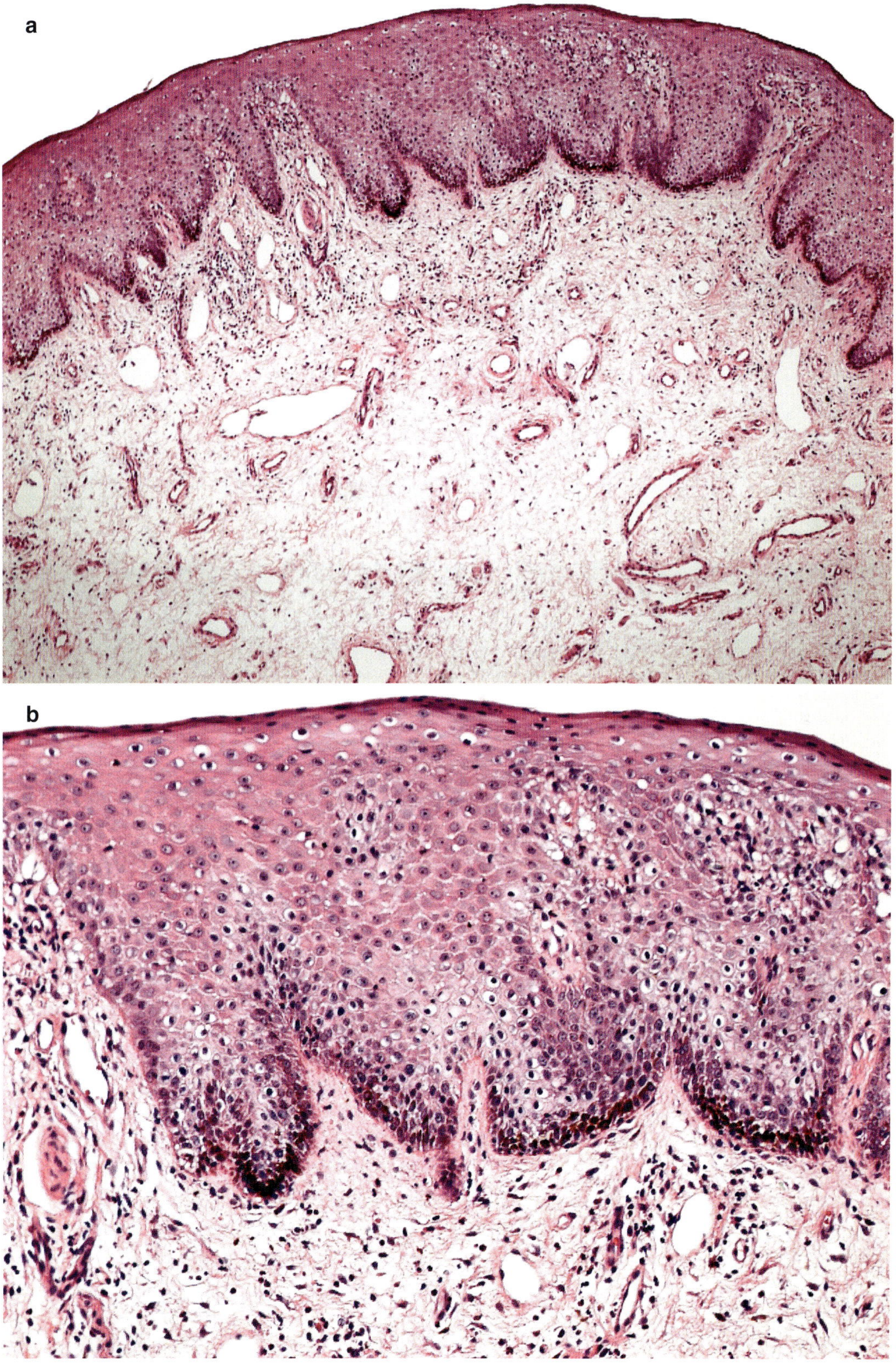
a
b

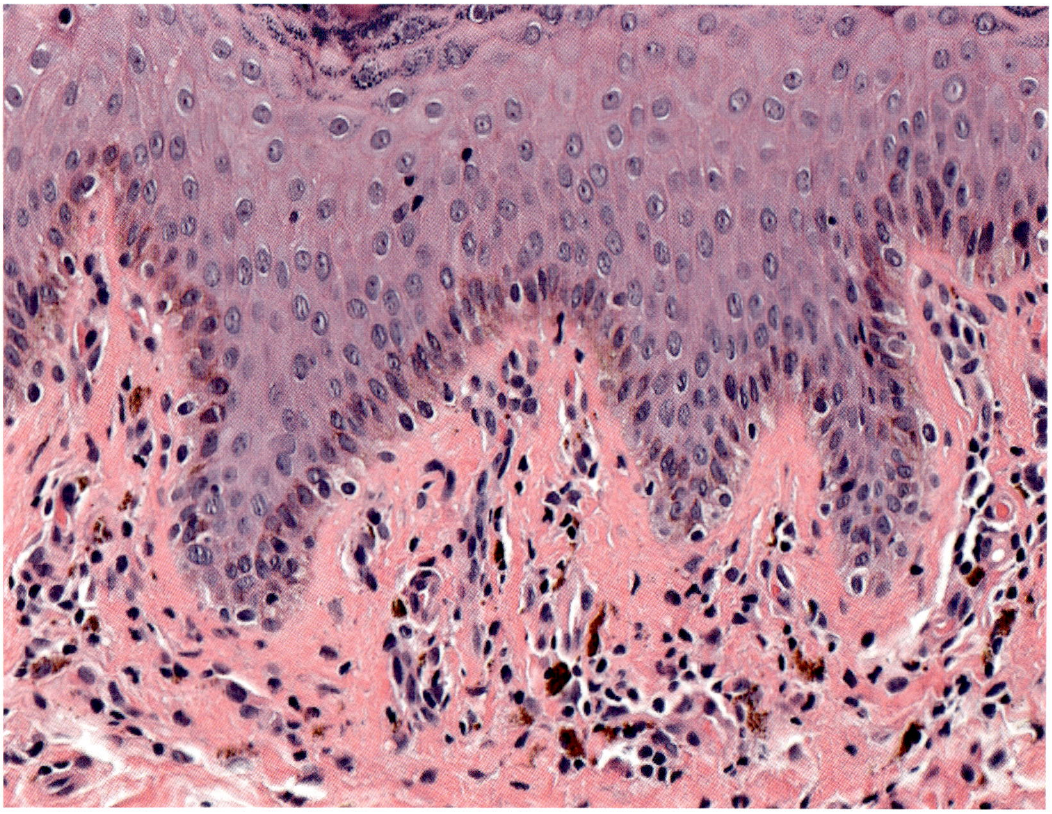

Fig. 5.2 Additional findings include a mild chronic inflammatory infiltrate and pigmentary incontinence within the superficial dermis or lamina propria. A background of mild lentiginous melanocyte hyperplasia may be present, but melanocyte atypia and a confluent growth pattern are not seen

Common acquired nevi comprise the large majority of melanocytic nevi of the vulva [21]. They affect both labia majora and minora and present in young females [21]. They are only rarely biopsied as they show no worrying clinical features. Their histological presentation is identical to that at other sites including junctional, dermal, or compound nevi [21].

Congenital, blue and Spitz nevi are particularly rare and have been documented in isolated reports only [22, 23]. Their clinical and histological findings are identical to their cutaneous counterparts.

Dysplastic nevi affect a wide range of anatomical locations, but presentation on the trunk and the extremities is most commonly seen. The genital area is only rarely affected with preferential involvement of the hair-bearing skin of the labia majora or the perineum [24].

Clinical Findings

Presentation is in young adulthood at around 30 years of age [21]. Like dysplastic nevi at other sites, they are biopsied because of their atypical clinical features with increased lesional size greater than 0.5-cm, "fuzzy" irregular borders and a variegated pattern of tan-brown pigmentation [24, 25]. Dysplastic nevi are slightly elevated in the center and are surrounded by a macular tan to erythematous rim corresponding to the histological "shoulder" phenomenon where the junctional component extends significantly beyond the dermal aspect. Patients may have multiple dysplastic nevi ranging from few to hundreds. They may be familial (dysplastic nevus syndrome) or more commonly sporadic. Despite their atypical features, the clinical behavior of dysplastic nevi is entirely benign. Their recognition is however important as the presence of multiple dysplastic nevi confers an increased relative risk for the subsequent development of melanoma [26]. This increased risk is particularly pronounced in patients with a positive family or personal history of melanoma or in those with the dysplastic nevus syndrome [27]. Appropriate treatment is complete excision in particular of those nevi showing moderate to severe atypia as reliable distinction from melanoma may be challenging, especially on partial samples. Complete excision at time of initial presentation is therefore the preferred method of biopsy as it reduces the need for subsequent procedures and allows for a more definitive diagnosis.

Histological Findings

Histologically, dysplastic nevi on the vulva are identical to those at other locations [21, 24]. They are characterized by atypical cytological and architectural disorder as well as a host response. The lesional outlines are slightly ill-defined and asymmetrical (Fig. 5.3a). The junctional component is broad, extending significantly beyond the small dermal aspect in a lentiginous and nested growth pattern (shoulder phenomenon). Melanocytic nests are irregularly distributed across the epidermis and nest confluence is present often involving more than one rete ridge, also known as bridging (Fig. 5.3b). Melanocytes are epithelioid and display at least some degree of cytological atypia (Fig. 5.4a). Atypia is expressed as mild, moderate, and severe and is measured by comparison of nuclear size with that of midspinous layer keratinocytes and by the presence of nucleoli. Cytological atypia is however random and scattered rather than confluent and pagetoid spread is not a feature. Melanocytes often contain finely dispersed cytoplasmic melanin giving rise to a characteristic “dusky” appearance (Fig. 5.4b). The dermal component is small and shallow and cytological atypia is not a feature. Papillary dermal pigmentary incontinence and a lymphohistiocytic inflammatory infiltrate in addition to mild vascular ectasia and eosinophilic lamellar fibrosis surrounding the characteristically extended epidermal rete ridges are additional features (Fig. 5.5).

Differential Diagnosis

Reliable separation of dysplastic nevi with marked atypia form superficial spreading melanoma is notoriously difficult, and both diseases certainly show overlapping histological features (Table 5.1). Findings arguing in favor of a diagnosis of melanoma are confluent rather than random cytological atypia, effacement of the overlying epidermis, and epidermal atrophy with lack of the pronounced rete ridge pattern characteristic of dysplastic nevi, pagetoid spread, expansile dermal growth showing melanocyte atypia, and dermal mitotic activity.

Atypical Genital Nevus

The so-called *atypical genital nevus* (*atypical melanocytic nevus of genital type*) is a distinctive variant of melanocytic nevi with a strong predilection for the vulva and perineum. It was originally reported by Friedman and Ackerman in 1981 and it is characterized by atypical and concerning histological features [28]. It is currently best regarded within the spectrum of melanocytic nevi of special sites [29].

Clinical Findings

The atypical genital nevus comprises approximately 5–14% of all melanocytic nevi on the vulva [21, 30]. It affects premenopausal women with a strong predilection for adolescents and young adults and childhood presentation is not infrequent [21, 31–33]. The vulva is preferentially involved followed by the perineum and the mons pubis [31, 32]. The labia majora, minora, and the clitoris are all affected with a roughly equal distribution between mucosal surfaces and hair-bearing skin [29, 31–33]. Only in childhood does there appear to be a strong predilection for mucosal sites [32, 33]. The clinical presentation is often atypical and concerning due to lesional hyperpigmentation and increased size of up to 2 cm (median = 0.5 cm) in diameter [31, 32]. Presentation on a background of lichen sclerosus may appear particularly alarming [34]. Despite the worrying clinical and histological appearances, the clinical behavior of atypical genital nevi is entirely benign with only rare local recurrence after incomplete excision [32]. In a recent study, 22% of patients with atypical genital nevi were found to have a personal or family history of dysplastic nevi or melanoma [32]. This increased incidence may be a reflection of surveillance in this patient population, and no true link between atypical genital nevi and increased risk for the development of melanoma has been established as yet.

Histological Findings

The low-power magnification appearances of atypical genital nevi are quite characteristic and striking. The nevi are large and appear nodular with increased cellularity (Fig. 5.6a). Intense and variable melanin pigmentation may be an additional concerning low-power feature (Fig. 5.6b). Lesional circumscription and symmetry are however largely preserved. Atypical genital nevi are compound melanocytic lesions with a florid junctional component composed of irregularly distributed melanocytic nests along the epidermis (Fig. 5.7a). The nests vary in shape and size. They may be large and prominent and often show a fusiform or ovoid appearance with parallel alignment to the dermo-epidermal junction. Nest confluence and retraction artifact are often noted, and extension along skin adnexal structures is an additional feature (Fig. 5.7b, 5.8a). A lentiginous growth pattern of melanocytes is occasionally identified, but it represents only a minor aspect and it is limited to the central aspect of the lesion (Fig. 5.8b). Similarly, pagetoid spread of single melanocytes into the granular cell layer may be a rare and focal finding confined to the lesional center. Individual melanocytes are epithelioid to ovoid with abundant cytoplasm and vesicular nuclei containing small eosinophilic nucleoli (Fig. 5.9a). More polygonal melanocytes with reduced amounts of cytoplasm and hyperchromatic nuclei as well as multinucleated forms may also be present. Coarse cytoplasmic melanin pigmentation is frequently encountered and may be marked in areas. In general, atypical genital nevi display mild to moderate degrees of cytological atypia, but even severe atypia may be seen in a subset of cases (Fig. 5.9b). Cytological atypia is uniform rather than random and scattered raising further cause for concern. The adjacent epidermis is slightly hyperplastic but areas of epidermal atrophy may also be present. The pronounced rete ridge pattern, typical of dysplastic nevi, is not present.

The dermal component is often prominent and cellular with nodular outlines, sometimes referred to as mushroom-shaped. In the superficial aspects, it is composed of melanocytes reminiscent of those seen in the junctional component. These are

Fig. 5.3 (**a**) Dysplastic nevus. This subgroup of nevi is characterized by poor margination and slight lesional asymmetry containing broad junctional and shallow dermal components. (**b**) Dysplastic nevus. The junctional component is composed of irregularly shaped and distributed melanocytic nests occasionally involving more than one epidermal rete ridge (bridging)

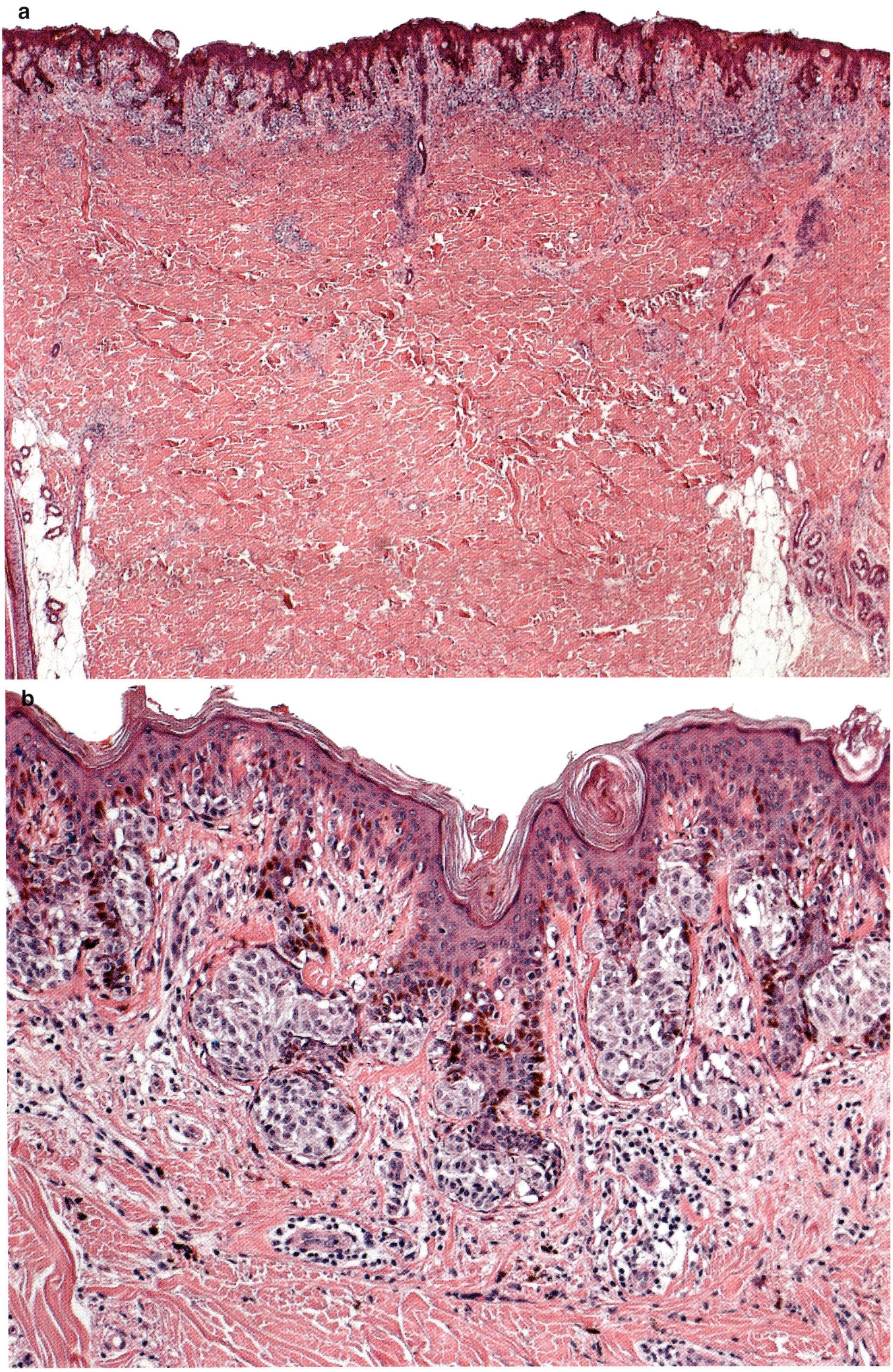

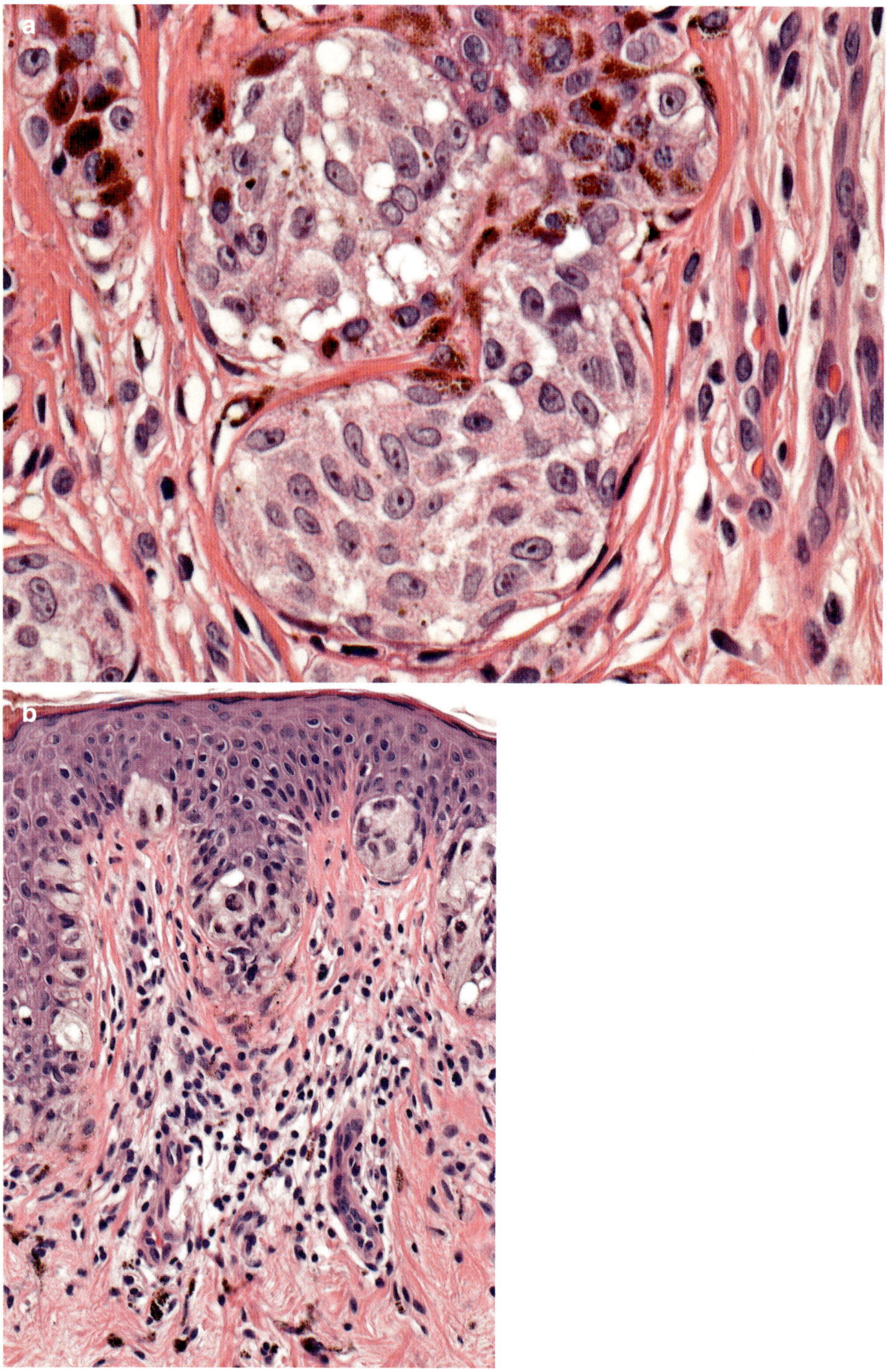

Fig. 5.4 (**a**) Dysplastic nevus. Junctional melanocytes display at least some degree of cytological atypia characterized by nuclear enlargement and the presence of small eosinophilic nucleoli. (**b**) Dysplastic nevus. Scattered bur significant cytological atypia and finely dispersed ("dusky") cytoplasmic melanin pigmentation are distinctive cytological features. Also note the host response with a superficial dermal chronic inflammatory infiltrate, pigmentary incontinence, and vertically orientated vessels

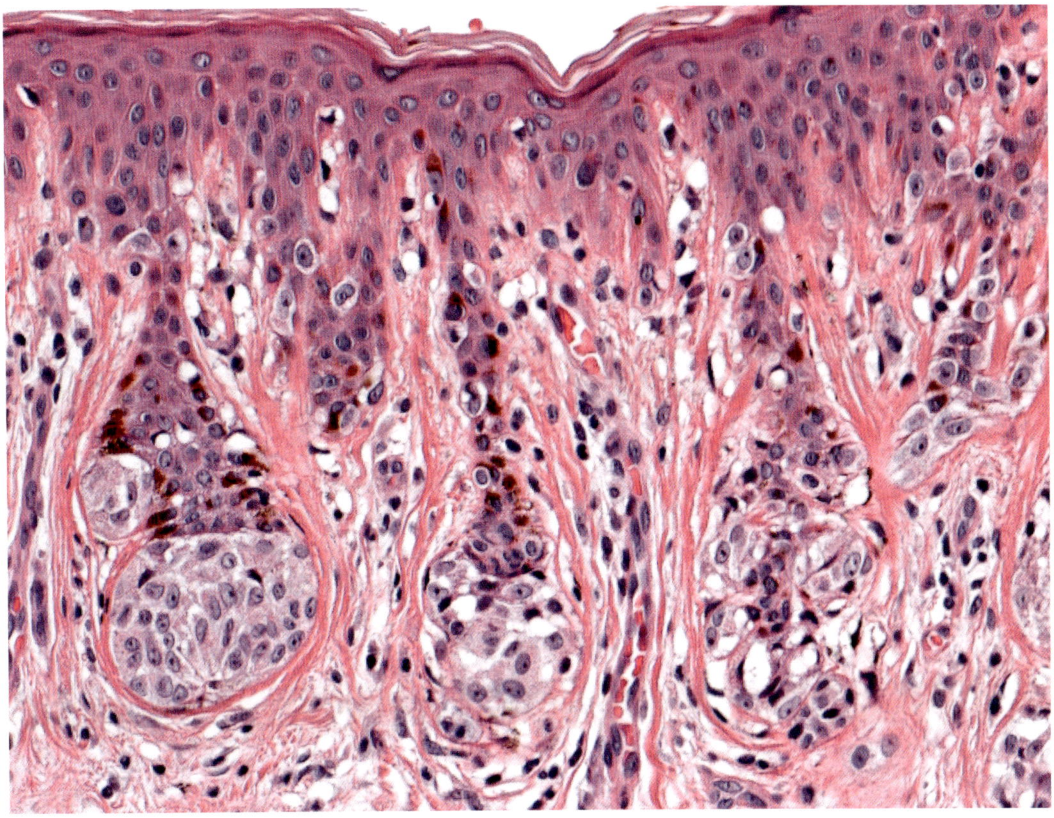

Fig. 5.5 Dysplastic nevus. Elongated rete ridges with surrounding eosinophilic lamellar fibrosis are typical findings

Table 5.1 Comparison of the clinical and histological features of atypical genital nevi, dysplastic nevi, and vulval melanoma

Clinical and histological finding	Atypical genital nevus	Dysplastic nevus	Vulval melanoma
Age	Premenopausal	Premenopausal	Postmenopausal
Size, cm	<1	<1	>1
Lesional symmetry	Preserved	Slight asymmetry	Absent
Lesional contours	Well defined and circumscribed	Indistinct	Ill-defined and indistinct
Shoulder	Absent	Present	Extensive
Lentiginous growth pattern	Minor component	Present	Major component
Pagetoid invasion	Focal and rare, confined to lesional center	Absent	Extensive and randomly distributed across the lesion
Epidermal hyperplasia	Present	Pronounced rete ridge pattern	Absent
Ulceration	Absent	Absent	Present in majority of cases
Dermal melanocyte atypia	Limited to the superficial dermal aspect	Absent	Prominent
Dermal growth	Non-expansile	Non-expansile	Expansile
Dermal maturation with depth	Preserved	Preserved	Absent
Dermal mitotic activity	Rare and limited to superficial dermal aspect	Absent	Brisk throughout the tumor
Necrosis	Absent	Absent	May be present
Lymphovascular invasion	Absent	Absent	May be present

arranged in enlarged and somewhat prominent nests showing variable but in areas intense melanin pigmentation. Furthermore, melanocyte atypia and rare mitotic activity may be identified (Fig. 5.10a, b). These features are limited to the most superficial aspects of the dermal component. Architectural and cytological maturation is preserved with depth and no deep or atypical mitoses are present (Fig. 5.11a). An additional finding is the presence of a characteristic band-like pattern of fibrosis affecting the superficial dermis (Fig. 5.11b).

Pathogenesis

As in ordinary nevi and a subset of melanomas at other anatomic locations, the BRAF V600E mutation has also been detected in a significant number of ordinary and atypical genital nevi. Enhanced expression of the tumor suppressor IGFBP7 has also been identified in these cases in support of their benign behavior [35].

Differential Diagnosis

The atypical genital nevus may appear clinically concerning due to its large size and prominent and variable pigmentation. It can be distinguished from dysplastic nevi by the absence of a radial shoulder and lack of a significant lentiginous growth pattern and prominent rete ridge pattern associated with the characteristic eosinophilic lamellar fibrosis. Furthermore, the prominent dermal component and confluent rather than random and scattered cytological atypia are findings in favor of atypical genital nevi. More important however is separation from invasive melanoma. The most important distinguishing features are also summarized in Table 5.1. Atypical genital nevi occur predominantly in younger premenopausal women, an age group in which genital melanoma is only rarely encountered. Despite the atypical architectural and cytological features of atypical genital nevi, the histological differences are quite pronounced. In genital melanoma, there is an extensive radial growth phase composed of a predominantly lentiginous melanocyte growth pattern and an invasive component with expansile growth, lack of maturation, nuclear pleomorphism, and brisk mitotic activity.

Genital Melanoma

Melanoma of the lower female genital tract is rare. The vulva is most commonly affected and vaginal presentation is particularly uncommon. It is a disease of postmenopausal women and the mucosal surfaces are most commonly affected. The disease differs significantly from cutaneous melanoma both histologically as well as on a molecular basis as UV irradiation is not a causative factor. Mucosal melanomas of the female genital tract show an aggressive course with poor survival rates compared to its cutaneous counterpart largely due to its advanced tumor thickness and stage at presentation.

Vulval Melanoma

Vulval melanoma is a rare disease with an estimated incidence ranging of 0.1–0.19/100,000 [36, 37]. It is however the second most common

Fig. 5.6 (**a** and **b**) Atypical genital nevus. On low-power examination, this type is large with a nodular growth pattern and a prominent dermal component, also referred to as "mushroom"-shaped (**a**). Prominent and irregularly distributed melanin pigmentation is an additional concerning low-power feature (**b**)

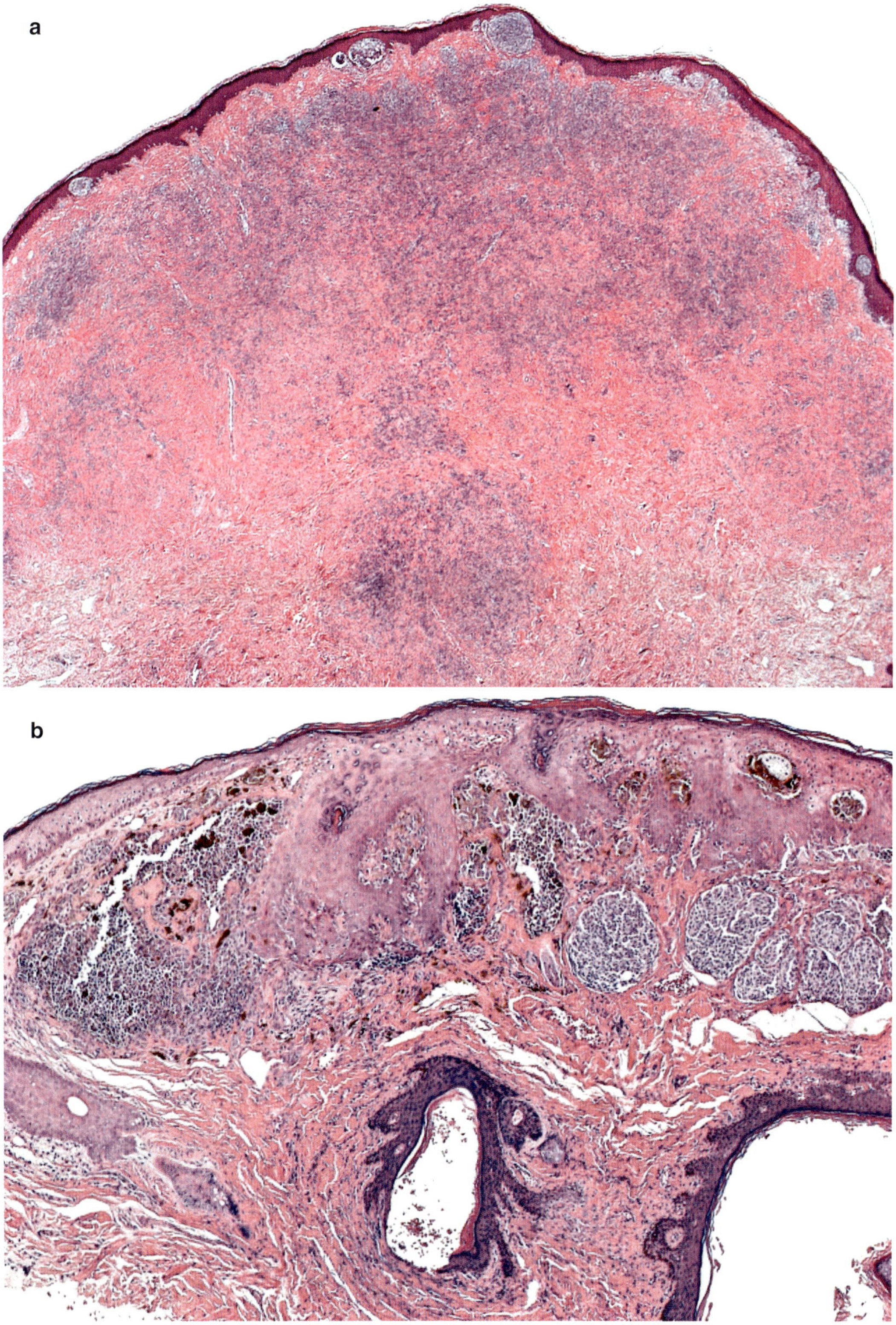

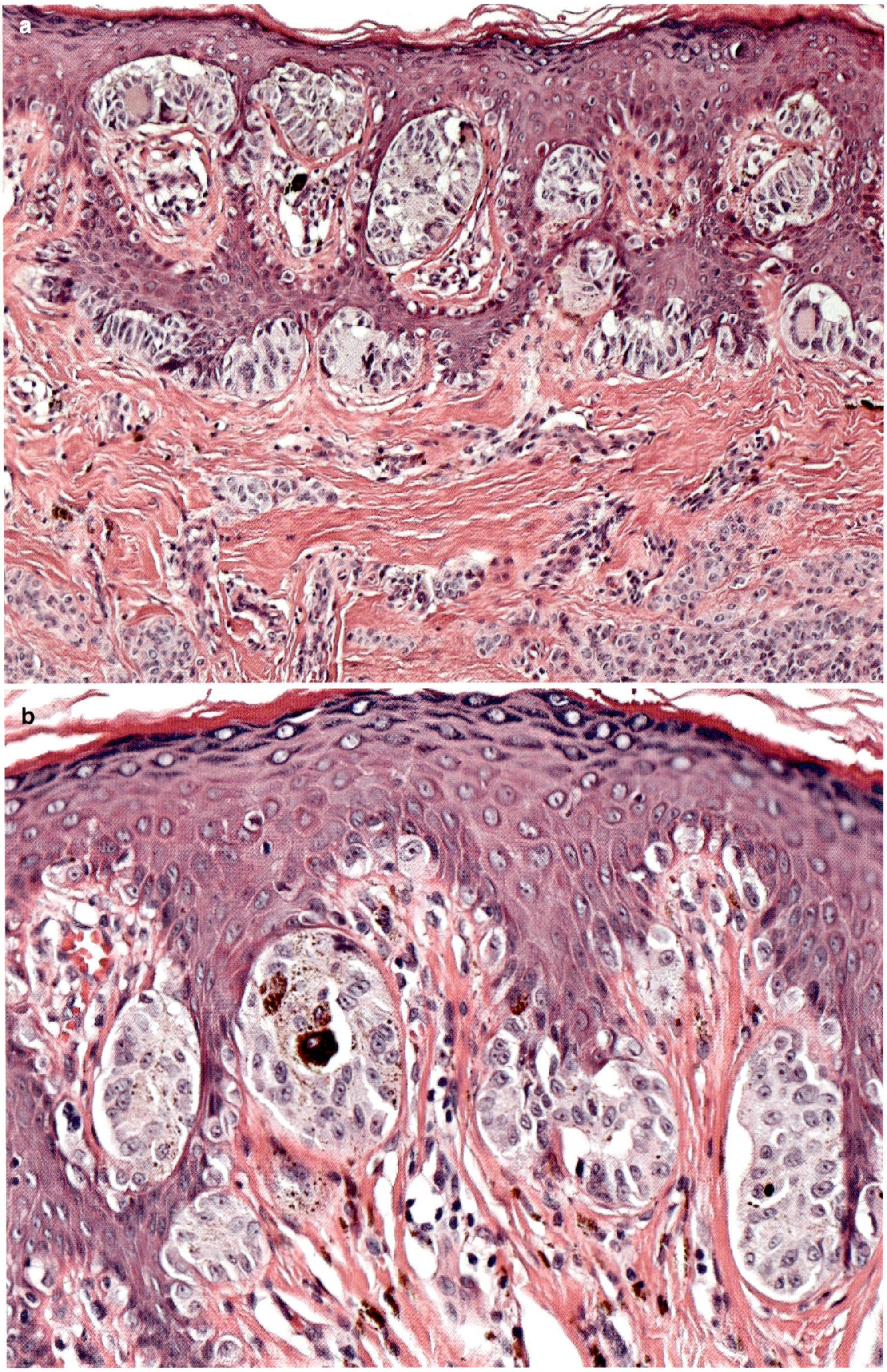

Fig. 5.7 (**a**) Atypical genital nevus. The junctional component is composed of ovoid nests often showing separation artifact form the surrounding epidermis. The nests are irregularly shaped and randomly distributed along the epidermis. (**b**) Atypical genital nevus. Melanocytes are epithelioid to ovoid and coarse cytoplasmic melanin pigmentation is often identified

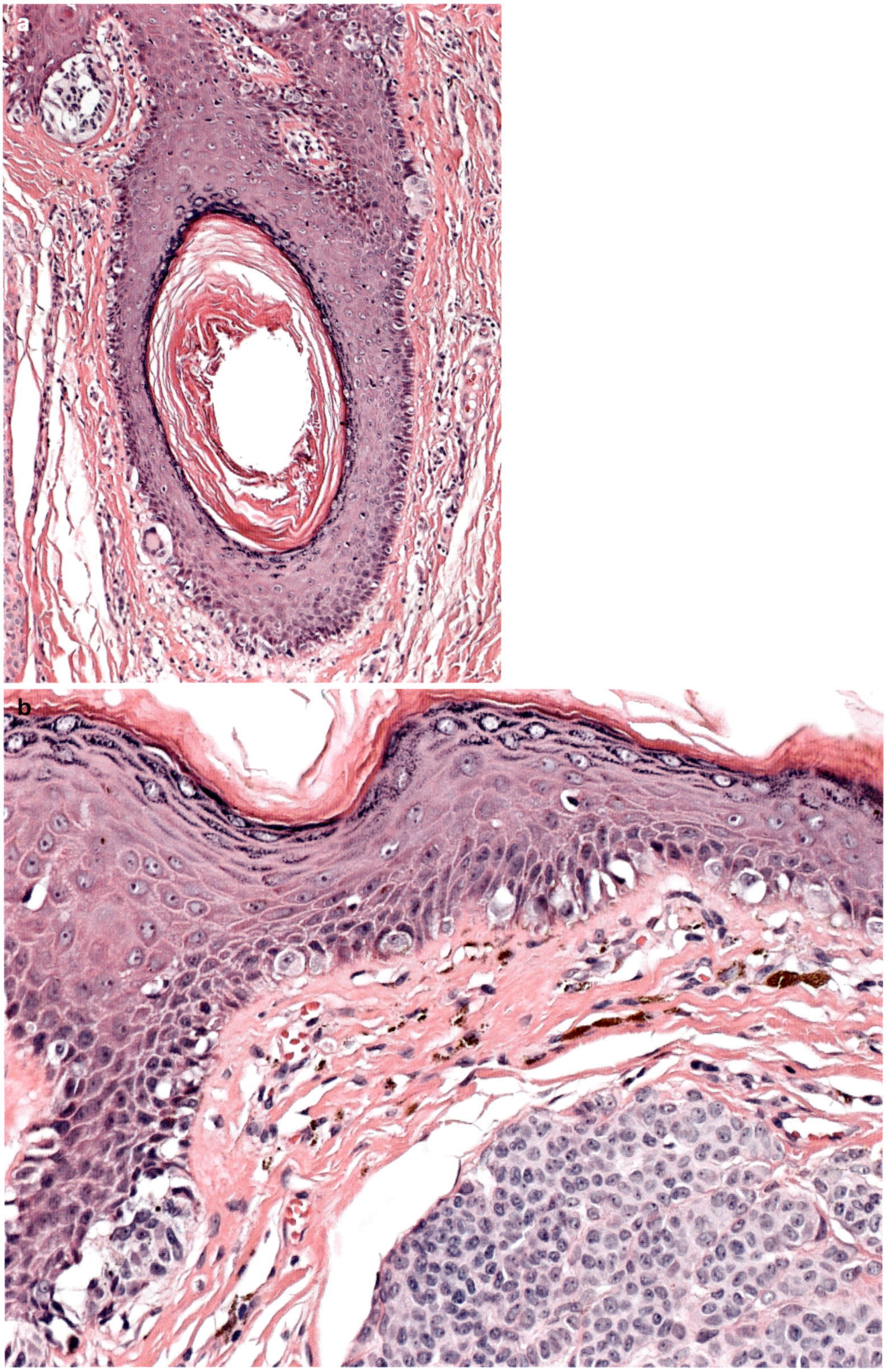

Fig. 5.8 (**a**) Atypical genital nevus. Melanocyte spread in single cells or nest along hair follicular structures is a frequently observed feature. (**b**) Atypical genital nevus. A lentiginous growth pattern of melanocytes is a minor component in atypical genital nevi

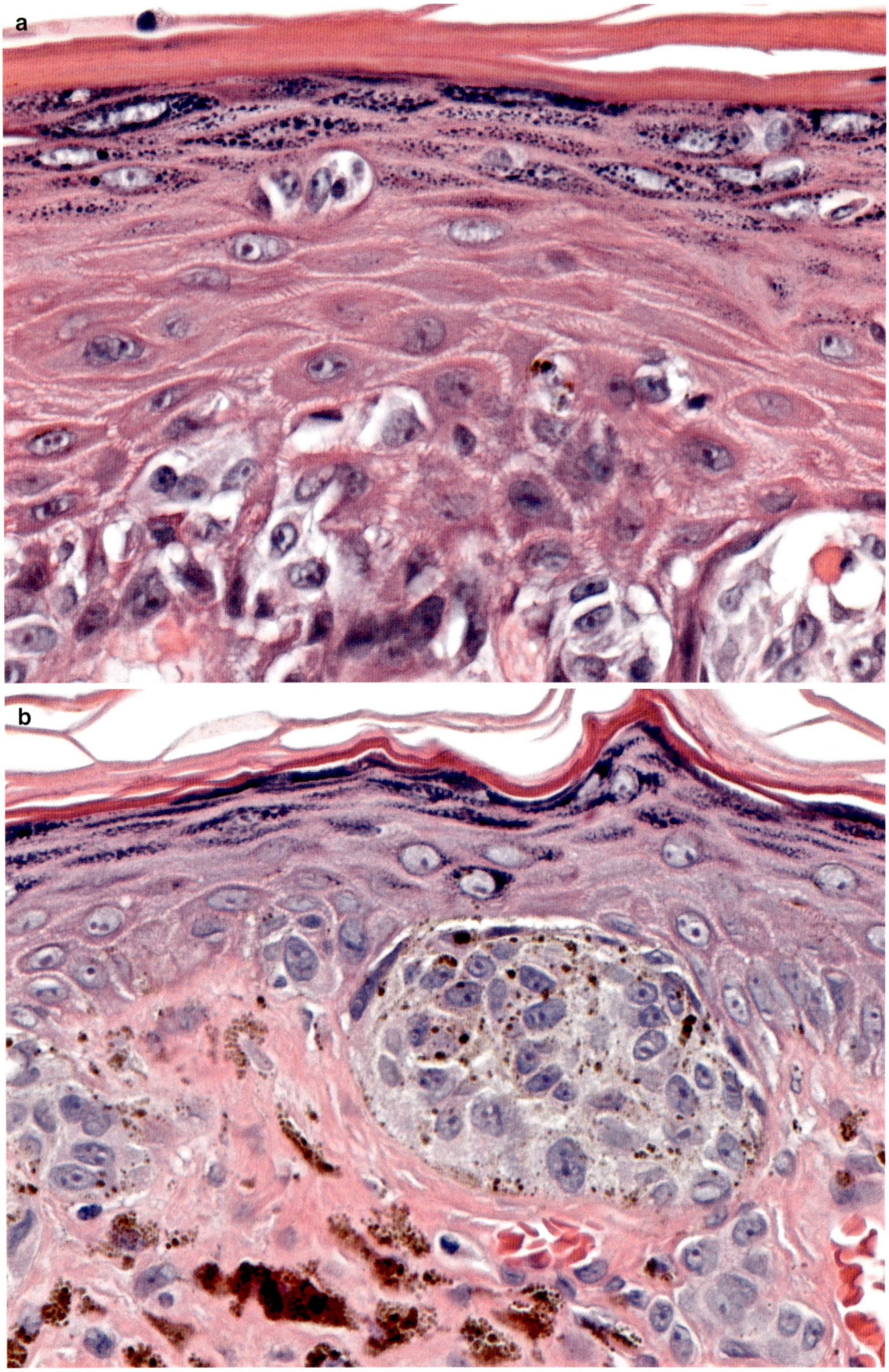

Fig. 5.9 (**a**) Atypical genital nevus. Focal pagetoid spread may be appreciated. It is however confined to the center of the lesion. (**b**) (**5.10a b, 5.11**) Significant atypia of junctional melanocytes may be present (**b**)

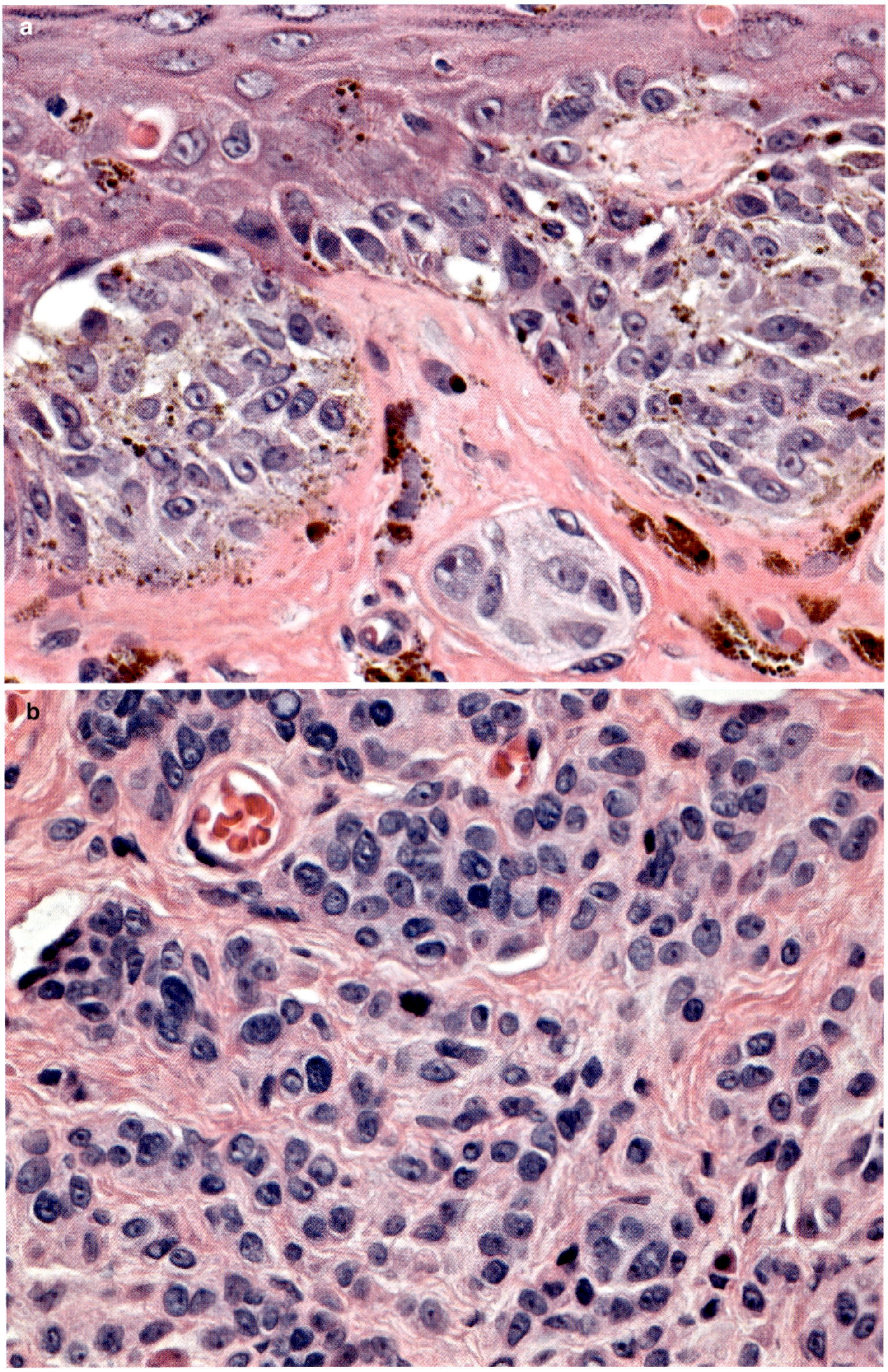

Fig. 5.10 Significant atypia of junctional melanocytes may occasionally also affect the superficial dermal component (**a**) In addition, rare mitotic activity may be present within the superficial dermal aspect (**b**)

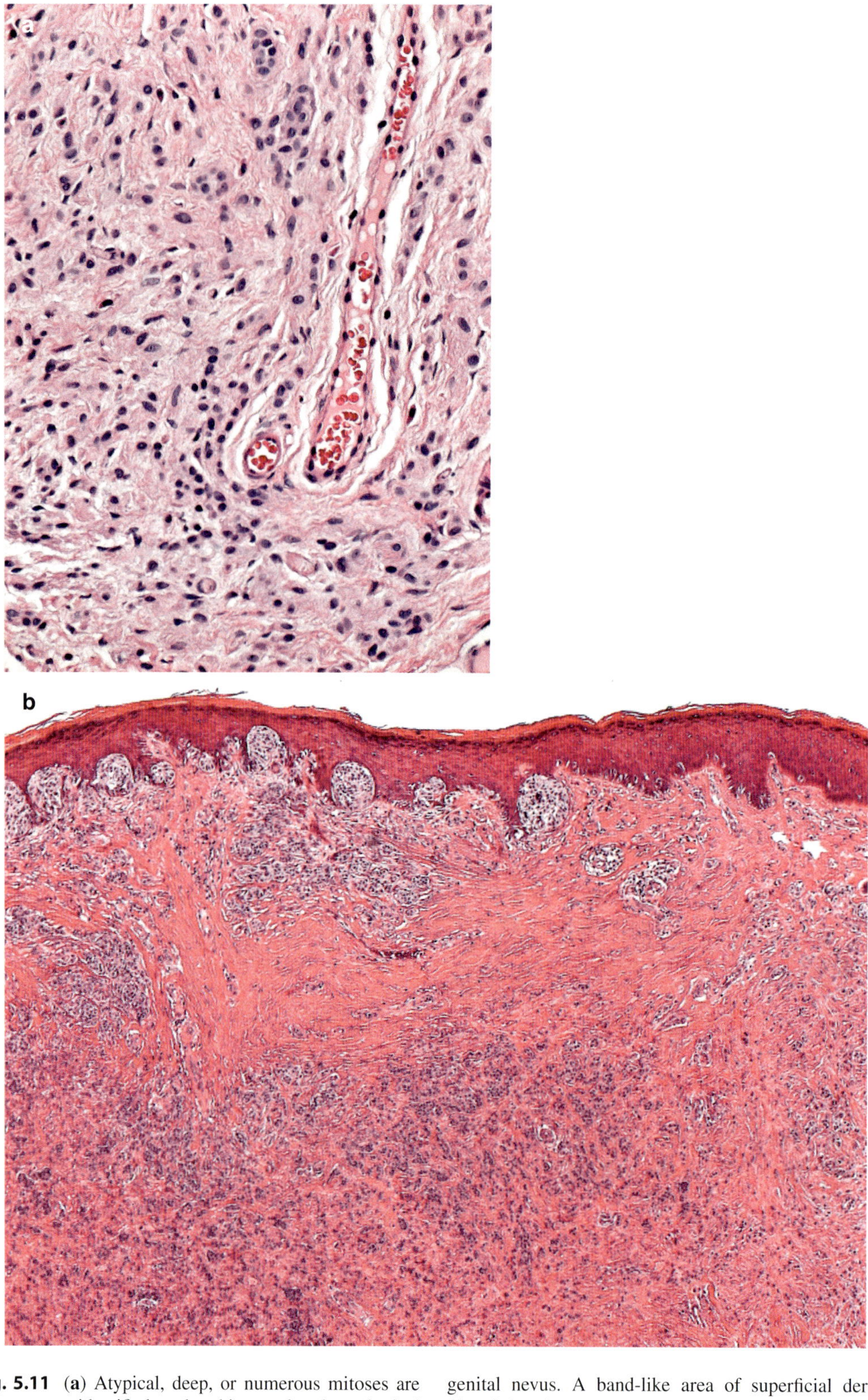

Fig. 5.11 (**a**) Atypical, deep, or numerous mitoses are however not identified, and architectural and cytological maturation is however preserved with depth. (**b**) Atypical genital nevus. A band-like area of superficial dermal fibrosis is a frequently observed finding

malignancy of the vulva accounting for 2–4% of all melanomas in women and between 3% and 10% of mucosal melanomas.

Clinical Findings

Vulval melanoma is a disease of postmenopausal women with a peak in the sixth and seventh decade [38–41]. Approximately 20% of vulval melanomas present before the age of 50 years and childhood presentation are exceptional [42]. All ethnic groups are affected but there is a predilections for patients of Caucasian descent with a relative risk of 2.6 [37]. As UV exposure is not a causative factor for the development of vulval melanoma, ethnic differences are less pronounced than in cutaneous melanoma [43, 44]. A positive family history for melanoma was identified in 15% of patients in one study [45]. The large majority of tumors involve the mucosal aspects, and the labia majora followed by the clitoris and labia minora are most commonly affected [37, 40, 46]. The clinical presentation is of an enlarged, flat, or raised and often nodular or polypoid tumor measuring around 2 cm (Fig. 5.4a) [47]. The lesional contours are irregular with variable pigmentation, and ulceration is a frequent finding [40]. Clinically detectable satellites are present in around 20% of patients (Fig. 5.4b). Other presenting signs include pain, pruritus, and bleeding [47]. Amelanotic presentation was reported in up to 27% of patients in a Swedish series representing a particular diagnostic pitfall. A preexisting nevus has been identified in only 5% of cases arguing that most mucosal melanomas of the vulva arise de novo [46].

Staging, Prognosis, and Treatment

Vulval melanoma is an aggressive disease with a documented 5-year disease-specific survival rate ranging from 27% to 61% in more recent studies [36, 37, 40, 41, 47–49]. 73% of patients present with Stage I/II disease [38]. Overall, the prognosis appears to be worse compared with cutaneous melanoma largely due to advanced tumor thickness and stage at presentation. Favorable outcome is associated with younger age at presentation, localized disease, and lack of lymph node involvement. The 5-year disease-specific survival is 75.5% for localized, 38.7% for regional, and 22.1% for distant disease [41]. Breslow thickness appears to be an independent predictor of recurrence, and the 2002 AJCC staging criteria as developed for melanoma presenting in the skin elsewhere has also been validated as the best predictor of outcome for vulval disease [38]. In addition, Breslow thickness appears to be the most significant prognostic factor in Stage 1 disease, and amelanotic presentation and ulceration are associated with reduced survival rates in this setting [50]. Surgical excision is the mainstay of treatment with recent data showing no improvement of radical vulvectomy over wide local excision [38, 51, 52]. In addition, sentinel lymph node biopsy may be beneficial in identifying early metastatic disease [45, 53]. Adjuvant options include radiation, chemotherapy, and more recently targeted therapies such as imatinib for mucosal melanoma showing activating mutation of the receptor tyrosine kinase c-kit.

Histological Findings

The documented histological spectrum of vulval melanoma is wide and includes conventional variants such as superficial spreading and nodular melanoma as well as a distinctive subtype unique to mucosal surfaces, the mucosal lentiginous melanoma (Fig. 5.13a). In a review of the histological features of 219 vulval melanomas, mucosal lentiginous melanoma was found to be the most frequent subtype (56%) followed by nodular melanoma (22%) [46]. While a significant subset of tumors is unclassifiable, pure superficial spreading melanoma and tumors showing overlapping features of superficial spreading and mucosal lentiginous melanoma are rare [46]. Desmoplastic melanomas affecting the vulva are an exceptional finding [54]. Independent of subtype, vulval melanoma is characterized by increased tumor thickness at presentation (Fig. 5.4c). The reported median tumor thickness ranges from 2.8 to 4.4 mm and the majority of melanomas are over 4 mm in thickness, even in Stage 1 disease [46, 47]. Most tumors are in the vertical growth phase and in situ tumors are rare. A preexisting nevus is only rarely identified. If present, it is most commonly associated with the superficial spreading variant affecting hair-bearing skin.

Fig. 5.12 (**a** and **b**) Vulval melanoma. This large and ulcerated tumor shows variable bluish-black to brown coloration (**a**). Multiple satellites are present affecting surrounding skin

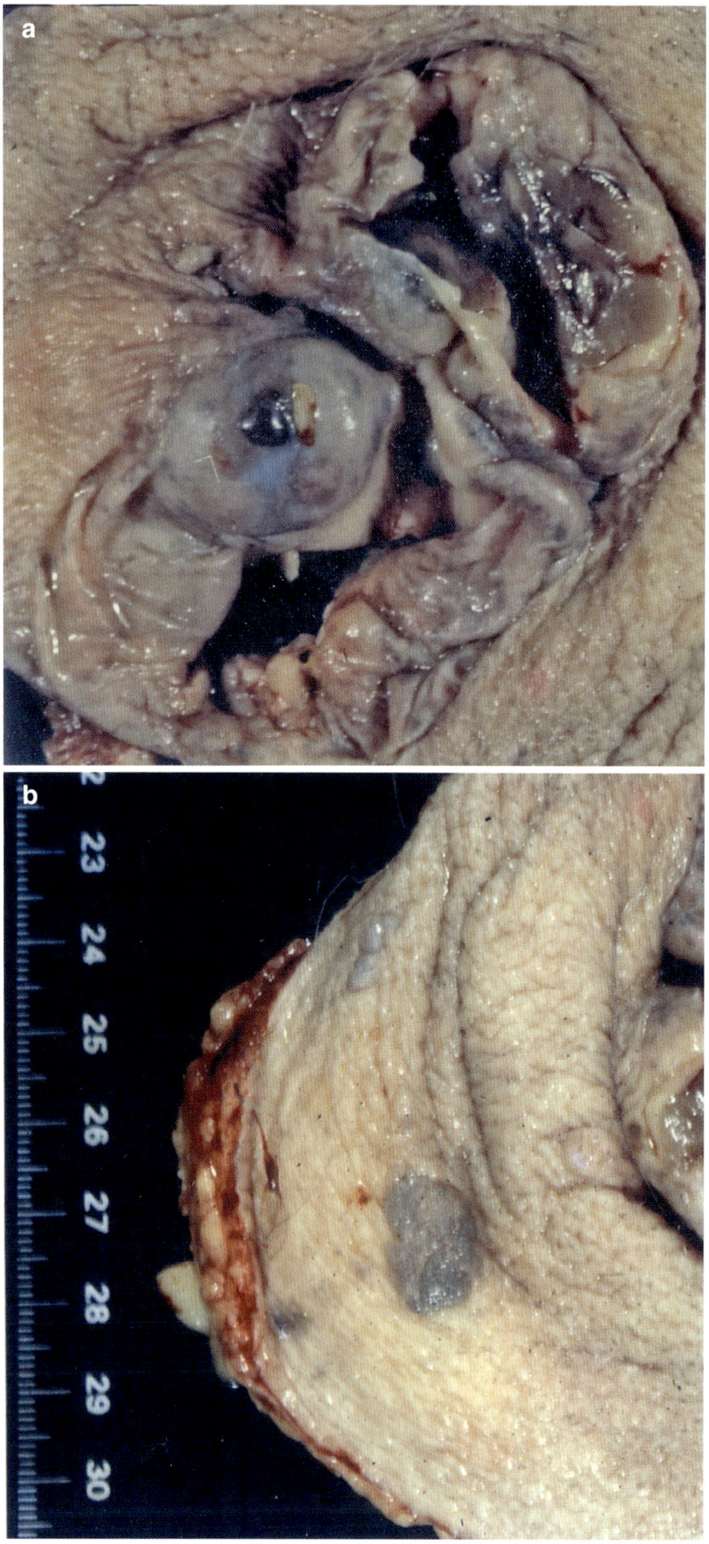

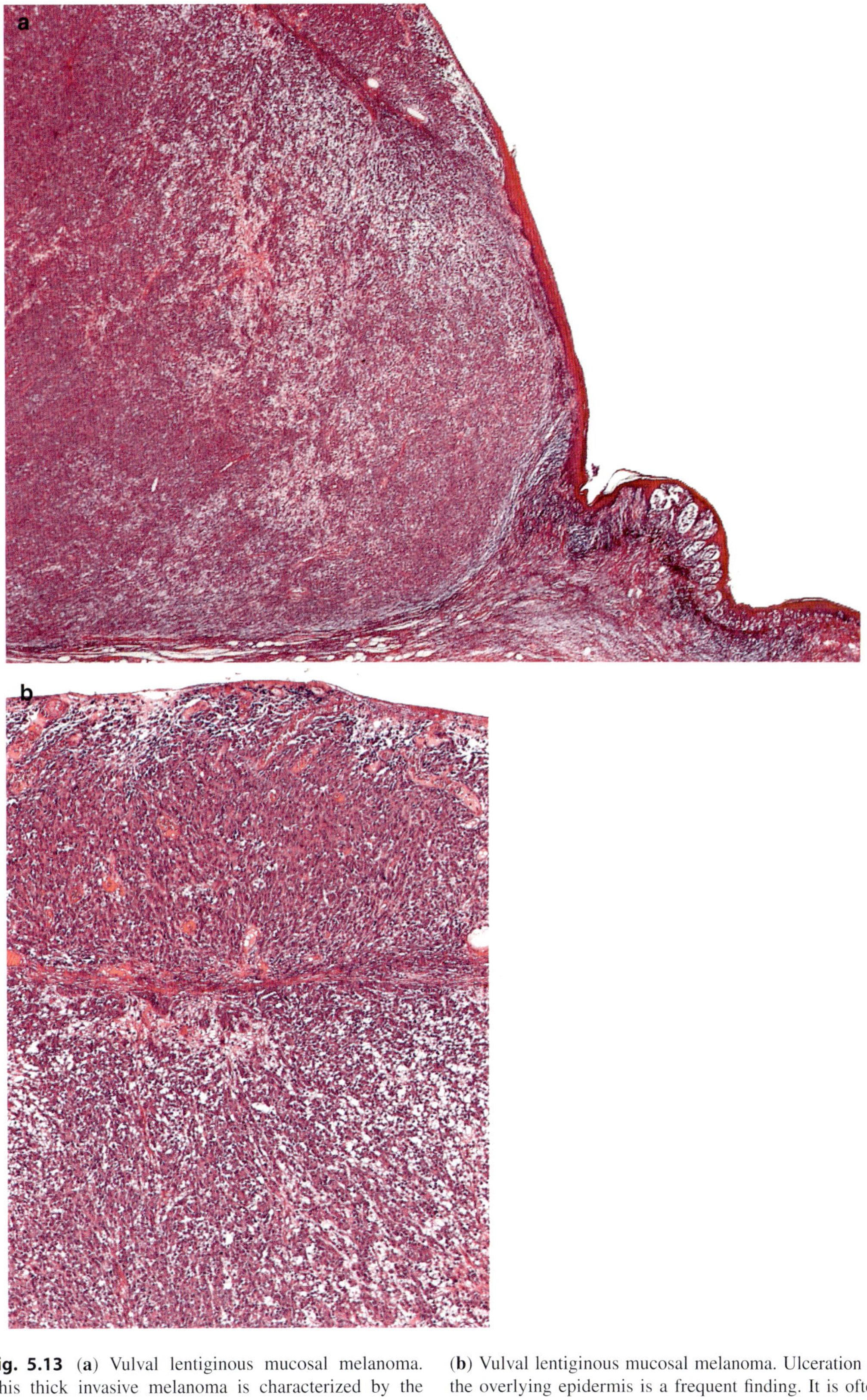

Fig. 5.13 (**a**) Vulval lentiginous mucosal melanoma. This thick invasive melanoma is characterized by the presence of an extensive adjacent in in situ component. (**b**) Vulval lentiginous mucosal melanoma. Ulceration of the overlying epidermis is a frequent finding. It is often extensive

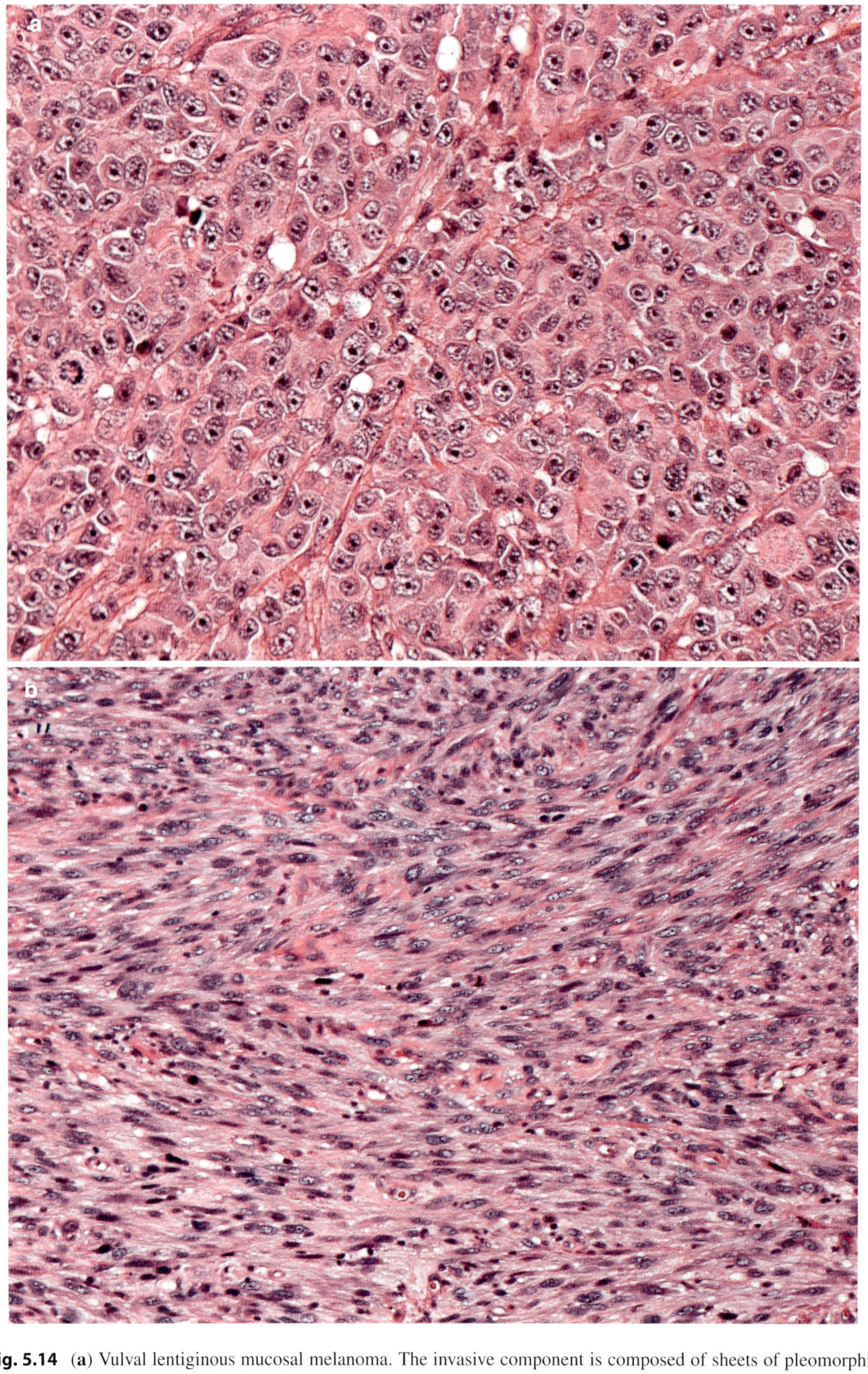

Fig. 5.14 (**a**) Vulval lentiginous mucosal melanoma. The invasive component is composed of sheets of pleomorphic epithelioid melanocytes. (**b, Figs 5.15, 5.16**) Spindle cell differentiation (**b**)

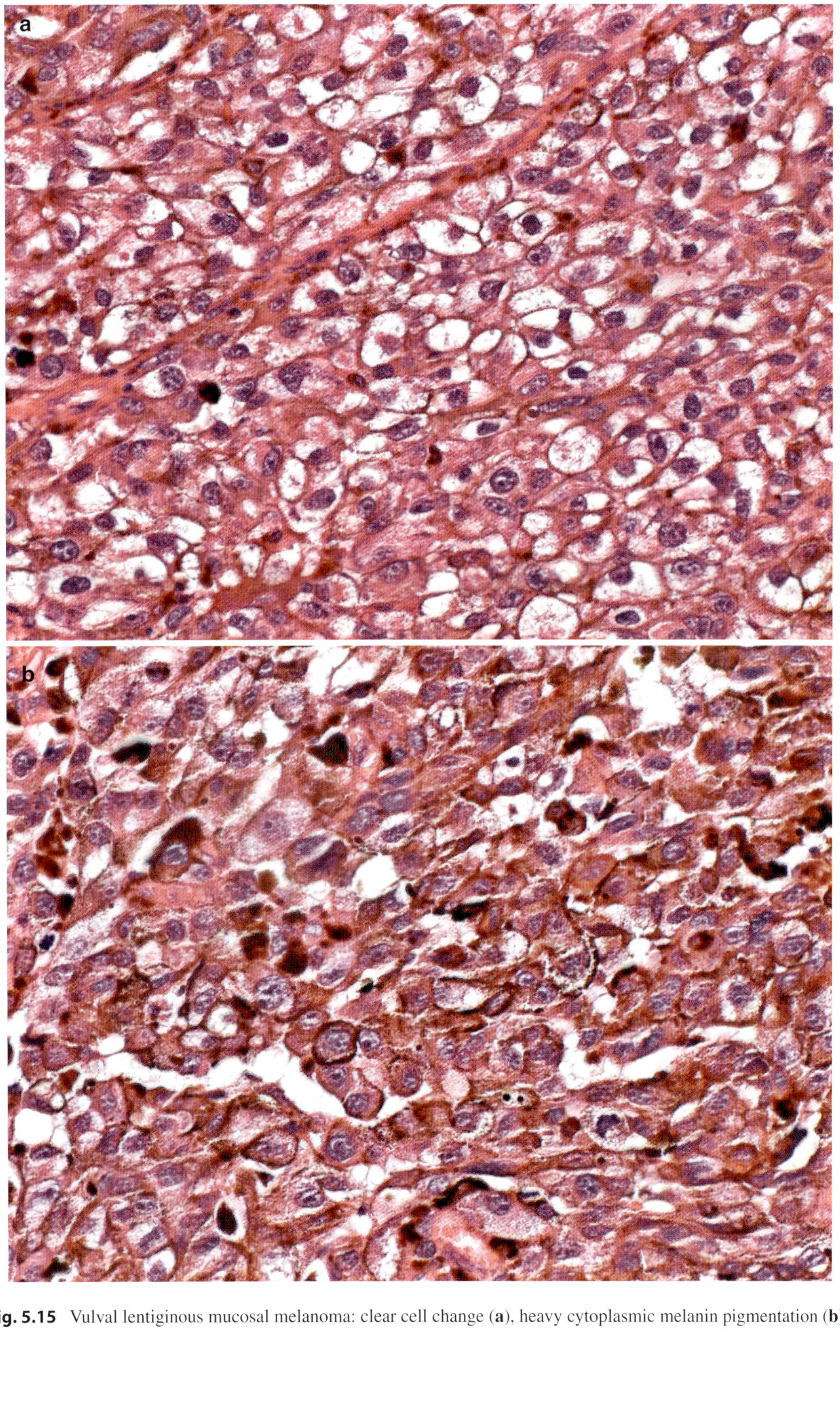

Fig. 5.15 Vulval lentiginous mucosal melanoma: clear cell change (**a**), heavy cytoplasmic melanin pigmentation (**b**)

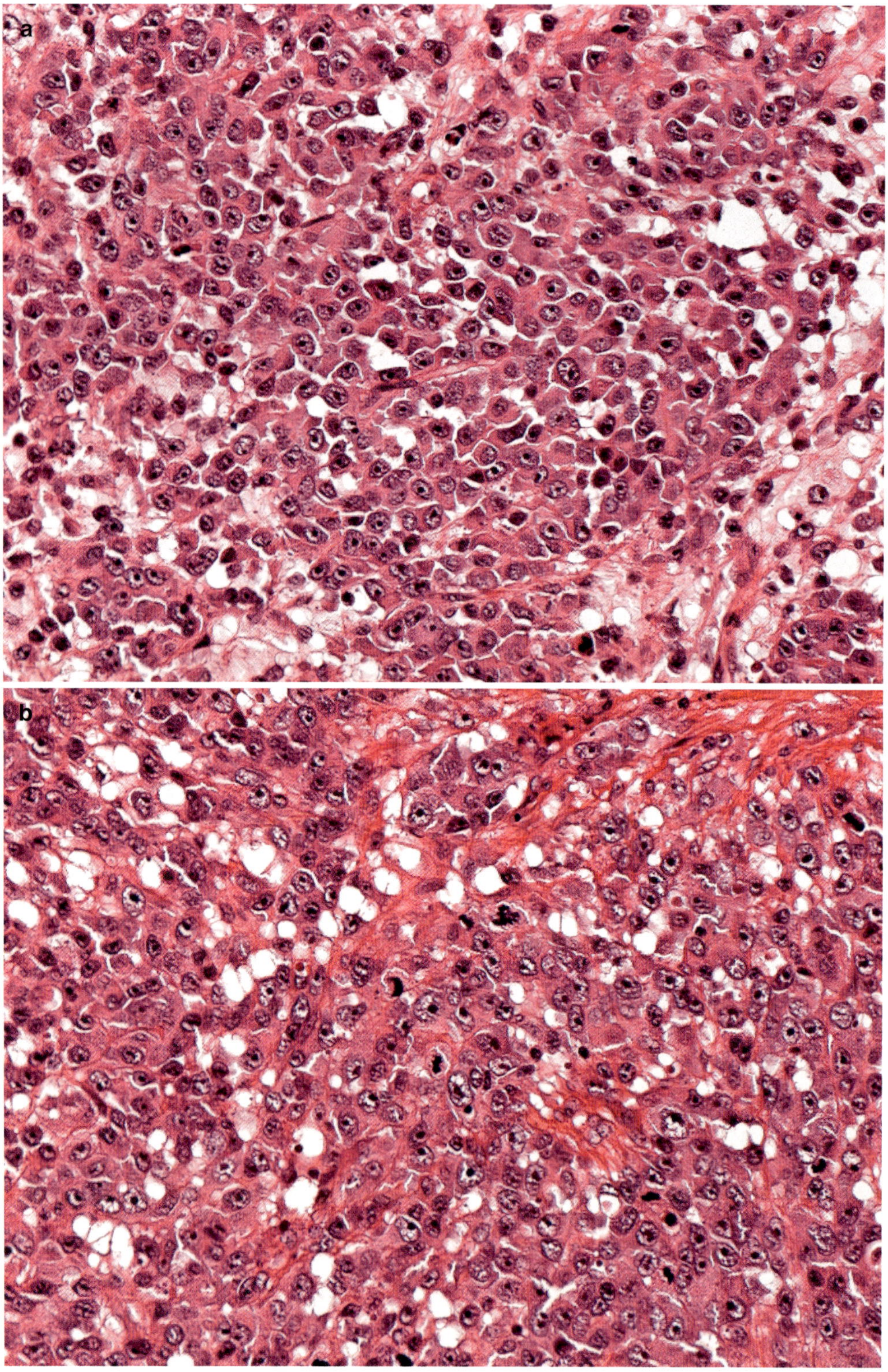

Fig. 5.16 Vulval lentiginous mucosal melanoma: rhabdoid features (**a**) are additional findings seen in particular in deeply invasive tumors. (**b** and **5.17a**). Mitotic activity is brisk (**b**)

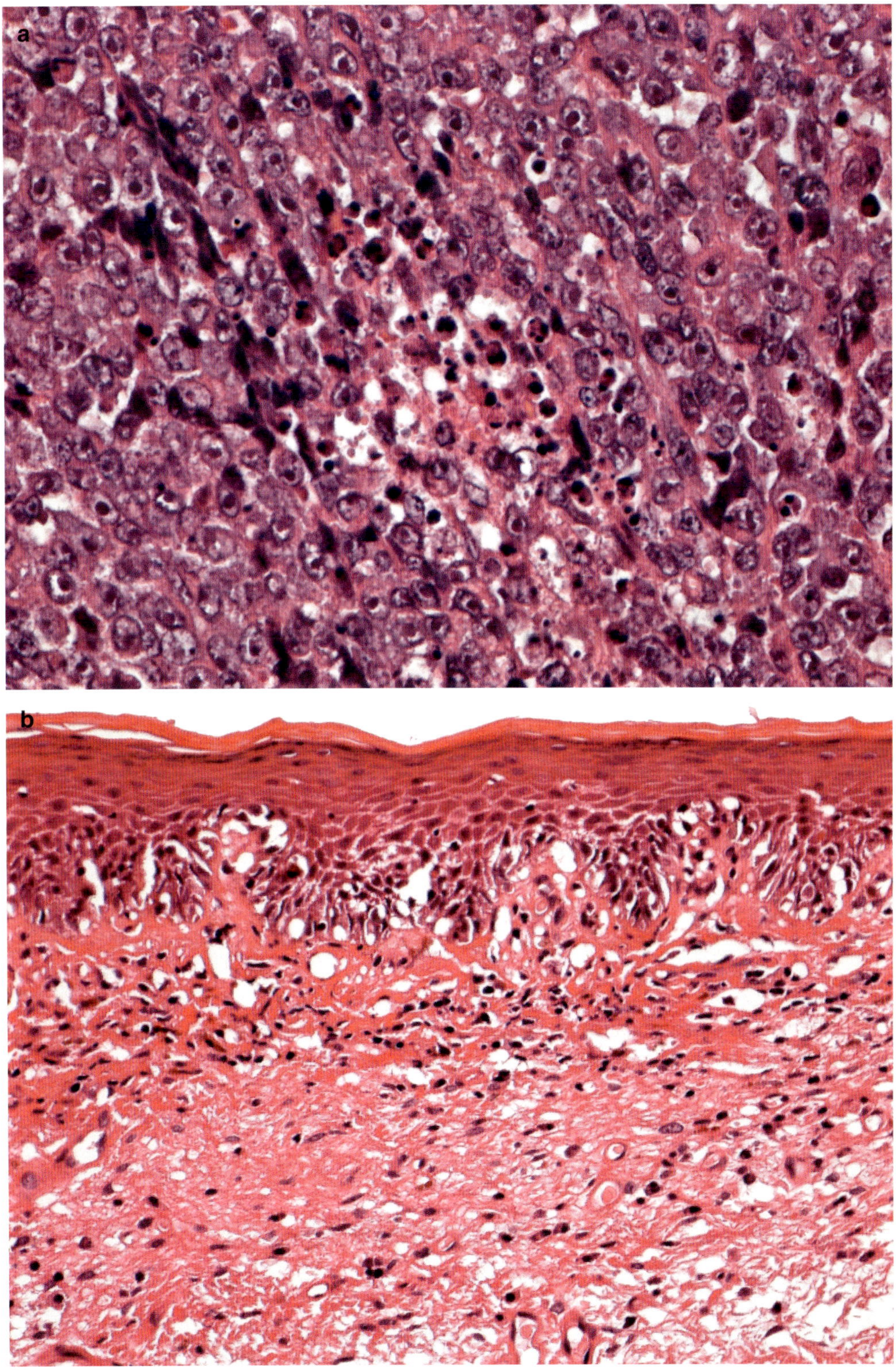

Fig. 5.17 (**a**) tumor necrosis may be identified. (**b**) Vulval lentiginous mucosal melanoma. An extensive and diffuse in situ melanoma is the characteristic finding in this subtype of melanoma. It is characterized by confluent and contiguous growth of single melanocytes in a lentiginous rather than nested arrangement. Cytological atypia may be subtle and pagetoid spread is rare

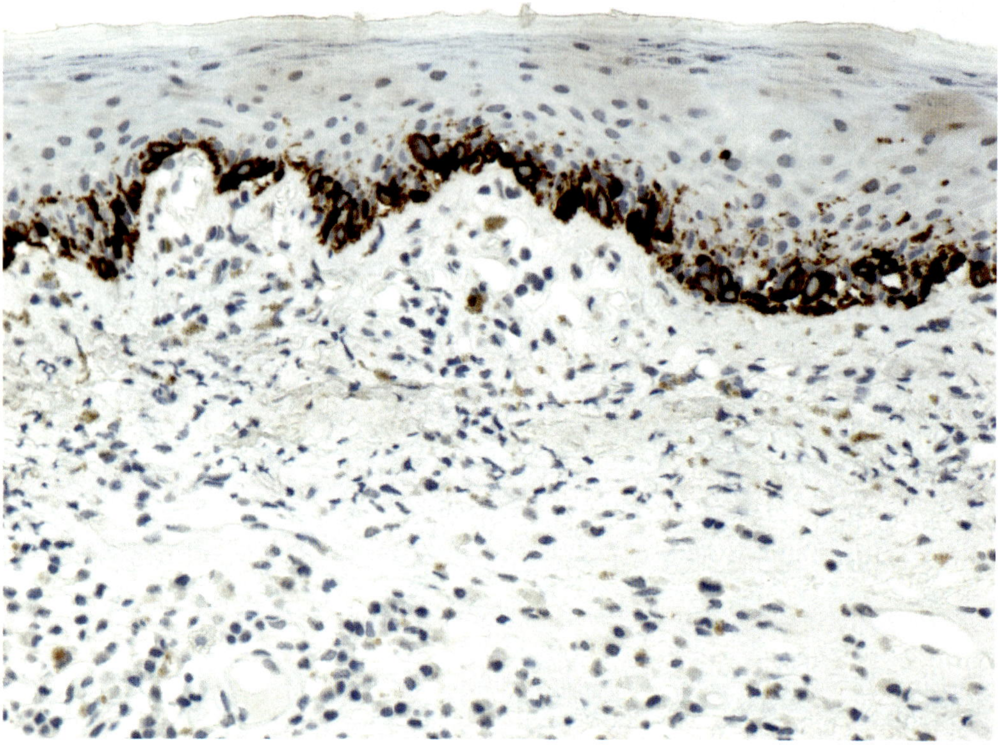

Fig. 5.18 Vulval lentiginous mucosal melanoma. Immunohistochemistry for Melan A highlights the confluent growth of melanocytes of the in situ component

Tumors frequently show extensive ulceration of the overlying epidermis (Fig. 5.13b). The invasive dermal component is cellular with expansile growth. It is composed of epithelioid or spindled melanocytes characteristically showing marked cytological atypia and nuclear pleomorphism (Fig. 5.14a). Intratumoral heterogeneity with mixed epithelioid and spindle cell differentiation may be identified especially in deeply invasive tumors (Fig. 5.14b). In addition, clear cell change, heavy melanin pigmentation, as well as rhabdoid features may be observed (Figs. 5.15a, b, 5.16a). The mitotic index is brisk including atypical forms, and tumor necrosis may be an additional finding (Figs. 5.16b, 5.17a). Lymphovascular invasion and microscopic satellites may also be noted in deeply invasive tumors. The mucosal lentiginous subtype is characterized by a broad and ill-defined junctional component extending far beyond the invasive aspect (Fig. 5.17b). The morphological features of the nodular and superficial spreading variants are identical to those seen at other anatomical locations. The melanocytic nature of the tumor can be confirmed by immunohistochemistry for S100 protein in addition to Melan A/Mart-1 and HMB-45. Melan A/Mart-1 immunohistochemistry is of particular diagnostic significance in the evaluation of peripheral margins and to highlight melanocyte density in small samples of lentiginous mucosal melanoma (Fig. 5.18).

Vaginal Melanoma

Vaginal melanoma is a rare disease with an estimated incidence of only 0.026/100,000, and it is significantly less common than vulval presentation [37]. Overall, melanoma represents about 4% of all vaginal malignancies [55].

Clinical Findings

The majority of tumors involve the distal third of the vaginal wall with nodular or polypoid appearances. The presenting sign is vaginal bleeding followed by detection of a mass [11, 56–58]. The mean age at presentation is 60 years and older and premenopausal manifestation is unusual [56, 57, 59]. The ethnic differences are less pronounced than in cutaneous or even vulval disease, and in a larger epidemiological study, no increased risk was identified for Caucasians [37]. Associated genital melanosis is very rare [10].

Staging, Prognosis, and Treatment

The overall prognosis for vaginal melanoma is poor with a median survival of 19 months and 5-year survival rates of only 13–20% and progression-free 5-year survival of 9.5% [37, 55, 56, 59, 60]. The AJCC criteria developed for cutaneous melanoma are also applied for the staging of vaginal tumors (Table 5.2). The disease course is characterized by local but more commonly distant recurrence, in particular with metastasis to lungs and liver [56]. The mainstay of treatment remains surgical excision, and wide local rather than aggressive surgery is currently advocated especially in the setting of adjuvant radiotherapy [50, 56].

Histological Findings

According to one more recent clinicopathological study, the majority of vaginal melanomas are nodular melanomas followed by mucosal lentiginous and unclassified subtypes [57]. Tumors are characteristically deeply invasive at presentation (Fig. 5.19a). The vertical growth phase is epithelioid, spindled, or mixed and composed of pleomorphic melanocytes showing brisk mitotic activity (Figs. 5.19b, 5.20a). Ulceration is present in the majority of tumors and tumor necrosis, lymphovascular invasions as well as microscopic satellites are detected in a significant subset of cases (Figs. 5.20b, 5.21a, b) [57]. While nodular tumors

Table 5.2 Melanoma staging and TNM classification of melanomas according to the 2002 AJCC staging criteria

Stage	TNM classification	Histological features
0	Tis N0 M0	Melanoma in situ
IA	T1a N0 M0	≤1 mm without ulceration and Clark level II/III
IB	T1b N0 M0	≤1 mm with ulceration or Clark level IV/V
	T2a N0 M0	1.01–2 mm without ulceration
IIA	T2b N0 M0	1.01–2 mm with ulceration
	T3a N0 M0	2.01–4 mm without ulceration
IIB	T3b N0 M0	2.01–4 mm with ulceration
	T4a N0 M0	>4 mm without ulceration
IIC	T4b N0 M0	>4 mm with ulceration
IIIA	T1–4a N1a M0	Single regional lymph node micrometastasis, non-ulcerated primary
	T1–4a N2a M0	2–3 regional lymph node micrometastasis, non-ulcerated primary
IIIB	T1–4b N1a M0	Single regional lymph node micrometastasis, ulcerated primary
	T1–4b N2a M0	2–3 regional lymph node micrometastasis, ulcerated primary
	T1–4a N1b M0	Single regional lymph node macrometastasis, non-ulcerated primary
	T1–4a N2b M0	2–3 regional lymph node macrometastasis, non-ulcerated primary
	T1–4a/b N2c M0	In transit/satellite metastasis without metastatic lymph node deposits
IIIC	T1–4b N1b M0	Single regional lymph node macrometastasis, ulcerated primary
	T1–4b N2b M0	2–3 regional lymph node macrometastasis, ulcerated primary
	Any T N3 M0	4 or more metastatic lymph nodes, matted nodes, gross extracapsular extension, or in transit/satellite metastasis and metastatic lymph node deposits
IV	Any T Any N M1a	Distant skin, subcutaneous, or nodal metastasis with normal LDH
	Any T Any N M1b	Lung metastasis with normal LDH
	Any T Any N M1c	All visceral metastasis with normal LDH or any distant metastasis with increased LDH

lack any significant adjacent in situ component (Fig. 5.22a), the mucosal lentiginous variant typically shows extensive spread of a predominantly lentiginous in situ melanoma (Fig. 5.22b). Immunohistochemistry, for S100 protein, Melan A/Mart-1, and HMB-45, is important to confirm the melanocytic nature, especially in nodular and ulcerated tumors and to assess margins of the mucosal lentiginous subtype (Fig. 5.23).

Pathogenesis

In keeping with their origin at sun-protected sites, mucosal melanomas show significant differences to their cutaneous counterparts and appear to be distinctive on a molecular level. As opposed to melanomas arising on intermittently sun-exposed skin, mucosal melanomas are characterized by a high degree of chromosomal aberrations and only rare BRAF mutations [61–63]. In contrast, mutations in the receptor tyrosine kinase c-kit are relatively commonly observed in mucosal melanomas [64, 65]. However, in a recent study, the incidence of c-kit mutations in vulval tumors was as high as 35%, while no c-kit mutations were detected in vaginal disease [66]. The identification of activating mutations in c-kit has implications for treatment with the successful use of imatinib for metastatic disease [67–69].

Differential Diagnosis

As discussed earlier, genital melanomas must be separated from genital melanosis and benign melanocytic nevi, in particular dysplastic and atypical genital nevi. Non-melanocytic tumors also enter the differential diagnosis. Most relevant is distinction from Paget's disease and poorly differentiated squamous cell carcinoma as there may be significant morphological overlap.

Paget's disease is characterized by an intraepidermal proliferation of epithelial cells. These cells are present as single cells or in small groups or nests. They are present at the level of the epidermal basal cell layer and show florid upward, so-called pagetoid spread. The morphological appearances are highly reminiscent of those seen in in situ melanoma. Occasionally, an invasive dermal component may also be present. Helpful histological clues to the correct diagnosis of Paget's disease include the presence of cytoplasmic mucin and glandular differentiation. The diagnosis can easily be confirmed by histochemistry with PAS/PAS-diastase-positive cells and immunohistochemistry with positivity for cytokeratins and CEA but negative staining for markers of melanocytic differentiation.

Helpful features in the distinction from poorly differentiated squamous cell carcinoma include the identification of better differentiated areas with evidence of keratinization and visualization of intercellular bridges in squamous cell carcinoma and the presence of an in situ component in melanoma. In difficult cases, the problem can usually be solved using immunohistochemistry for melanocytic markers such as S100 protein and Melan A in addition to cytokeratins.

Fig. 5.19 (**a**) Vaginal melanoma. Tumors are deeply invasive at presentation and often show extensive epidermal ulceration. (**b** and **5.20**). The invasive component shows significant cytological heterogeneity with areas of epithelioid cell change and brisk mitotic activity (**b**)

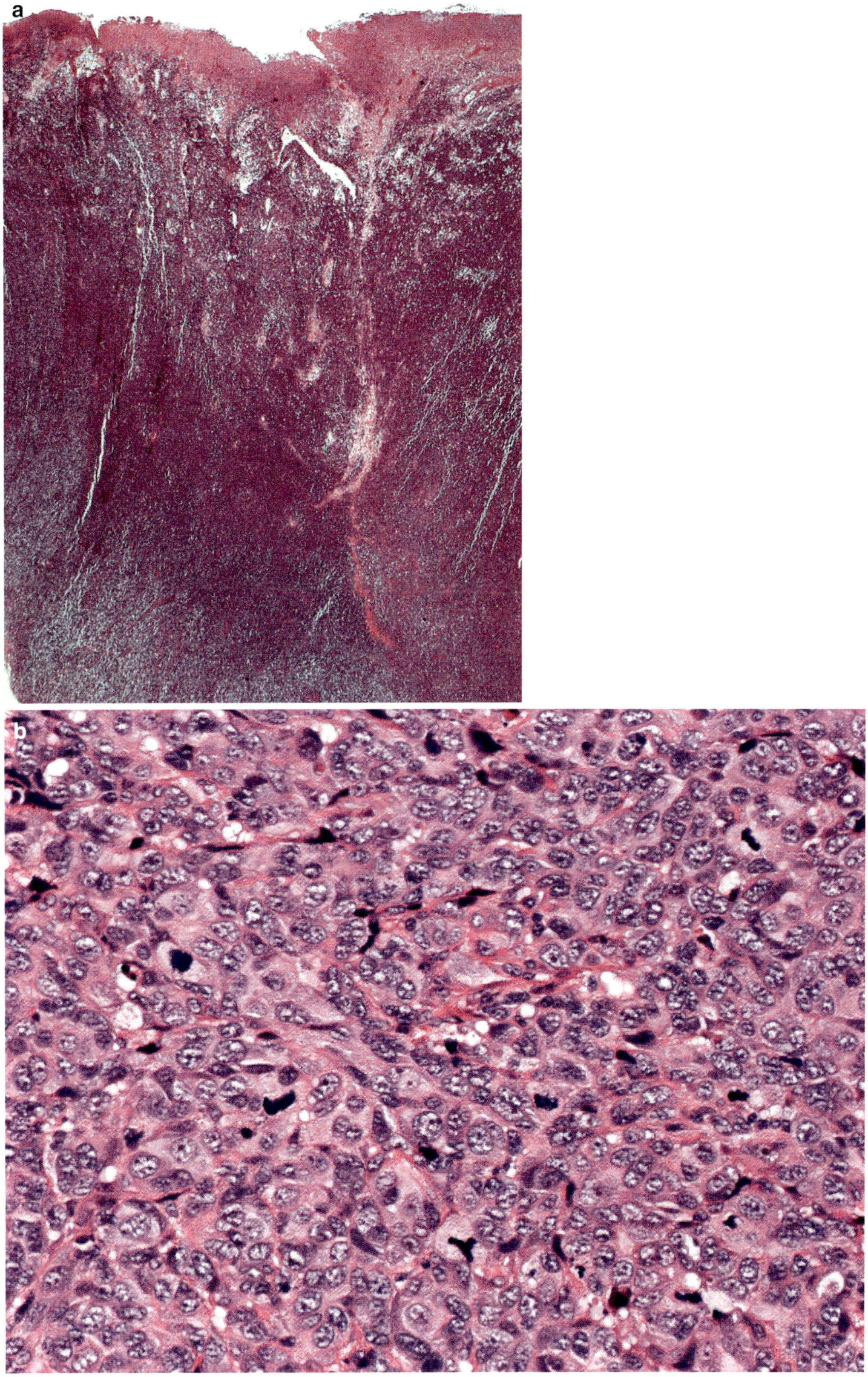
a
b

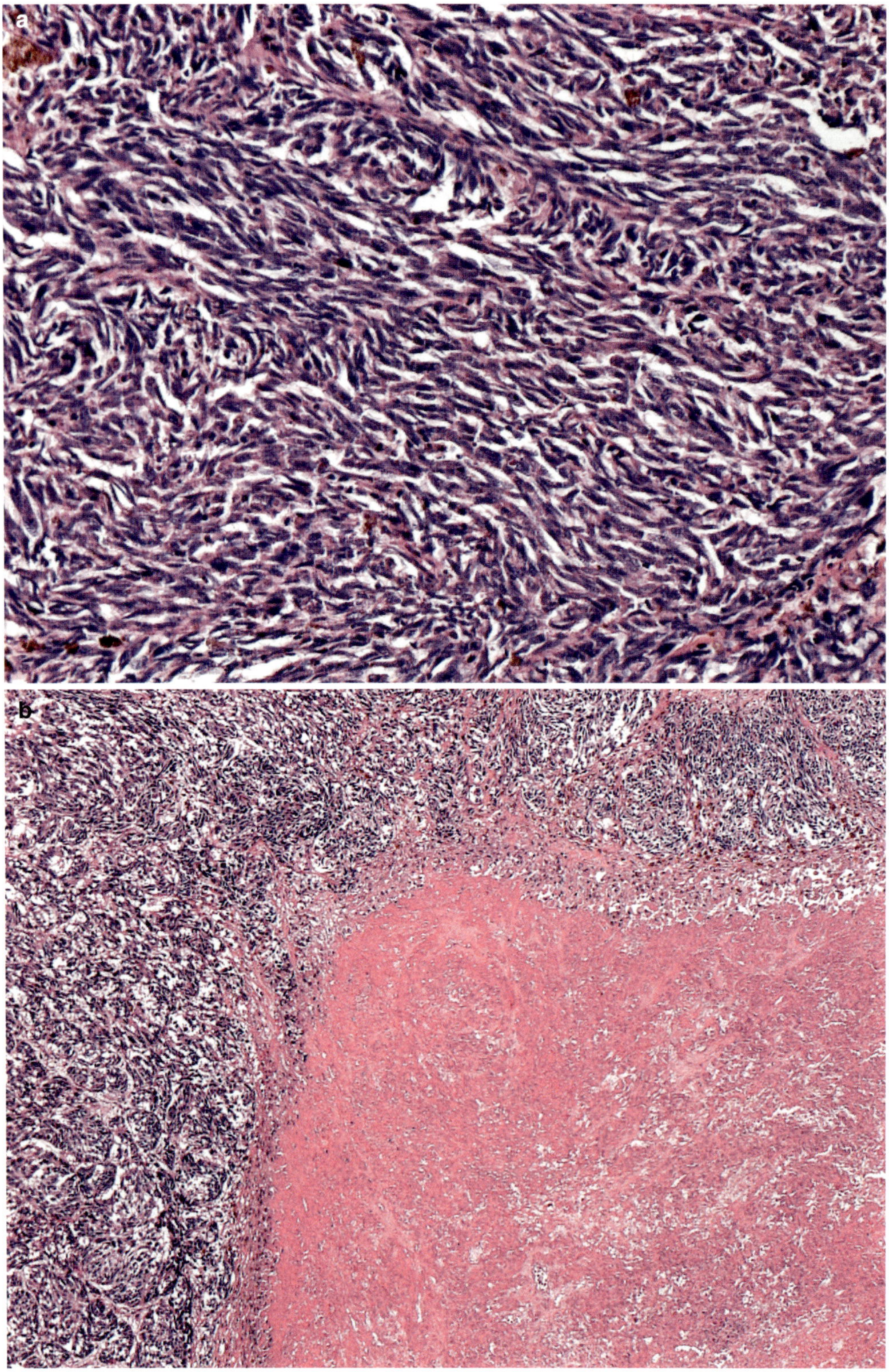

Fig. 5.20 Vaginal melanoma: spindle cell differentiation (**a**).Tumor necrosis (**b**)

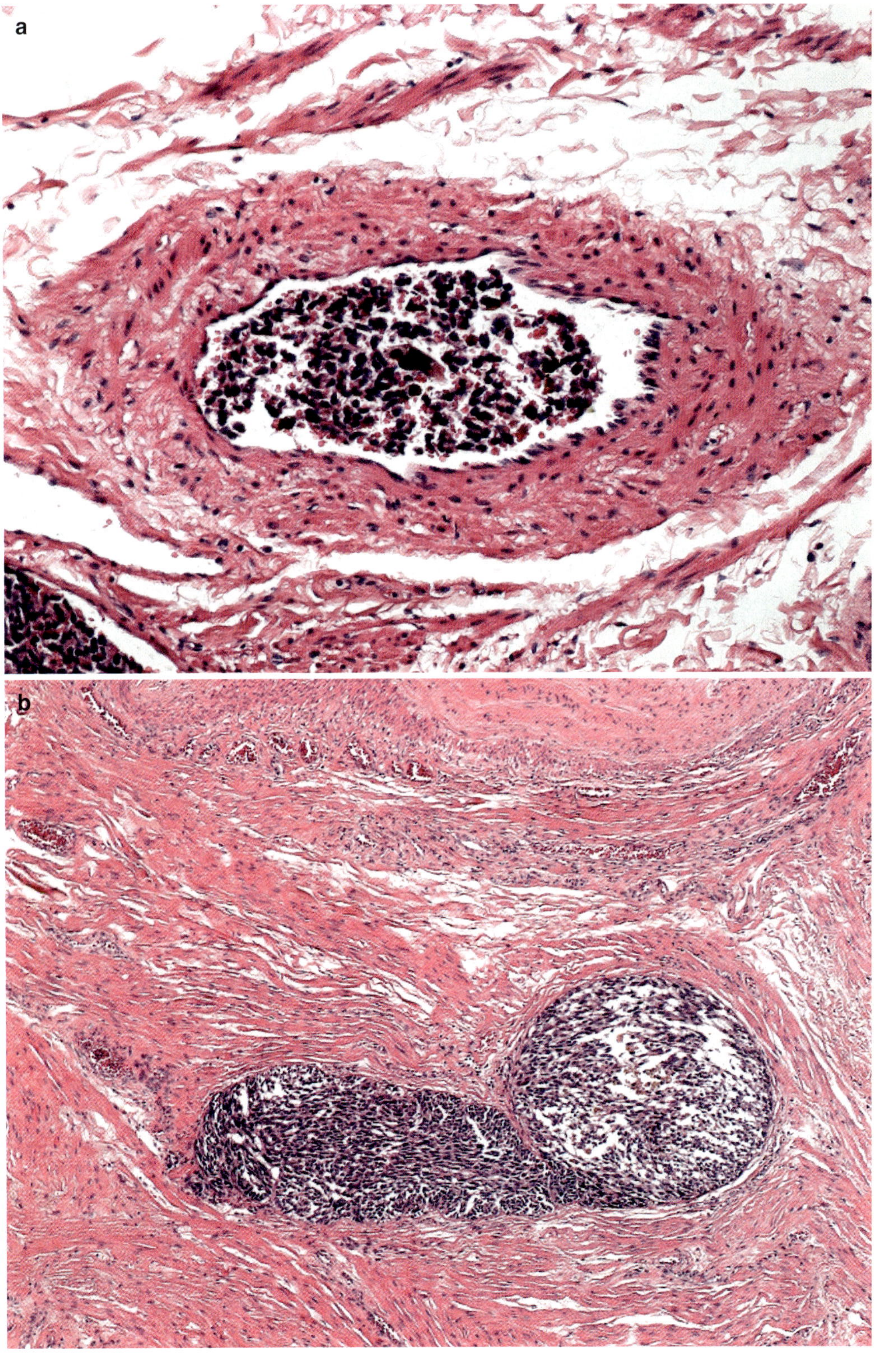

Fig. 5.21 (**a**) lymphovascular invasion and microscopic satellites (b) may be identified

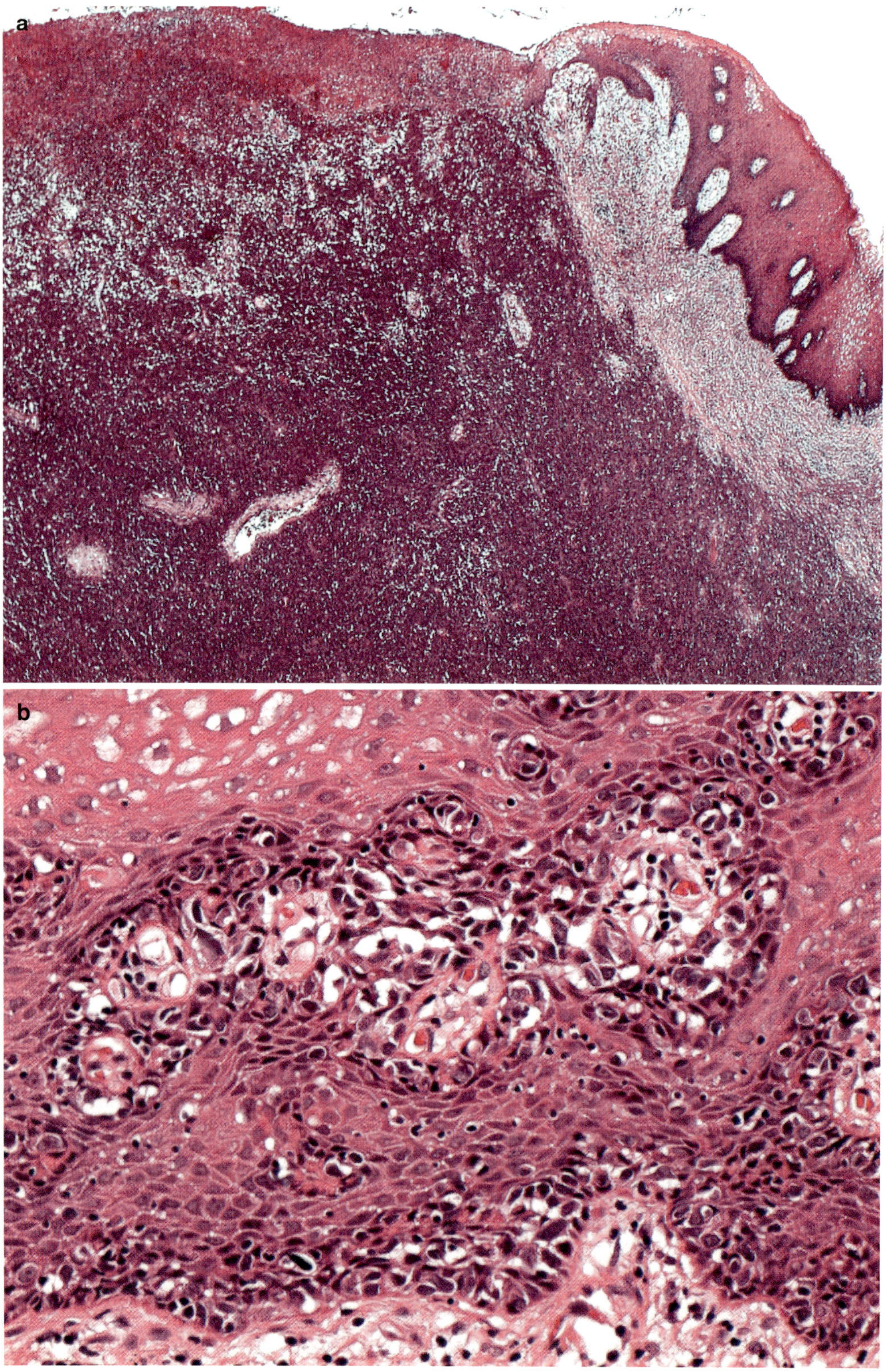

Fig. 5.22 (**a, b**) Vaginal melanoma. The nodular subtype is characterized by an invasive component without a significant radial growth phase. In contrast, an extensive adjacent in situ component composed of lentiginous melanocytes with contiguous growth is the hallmark of the lentiginous mucosal subtype

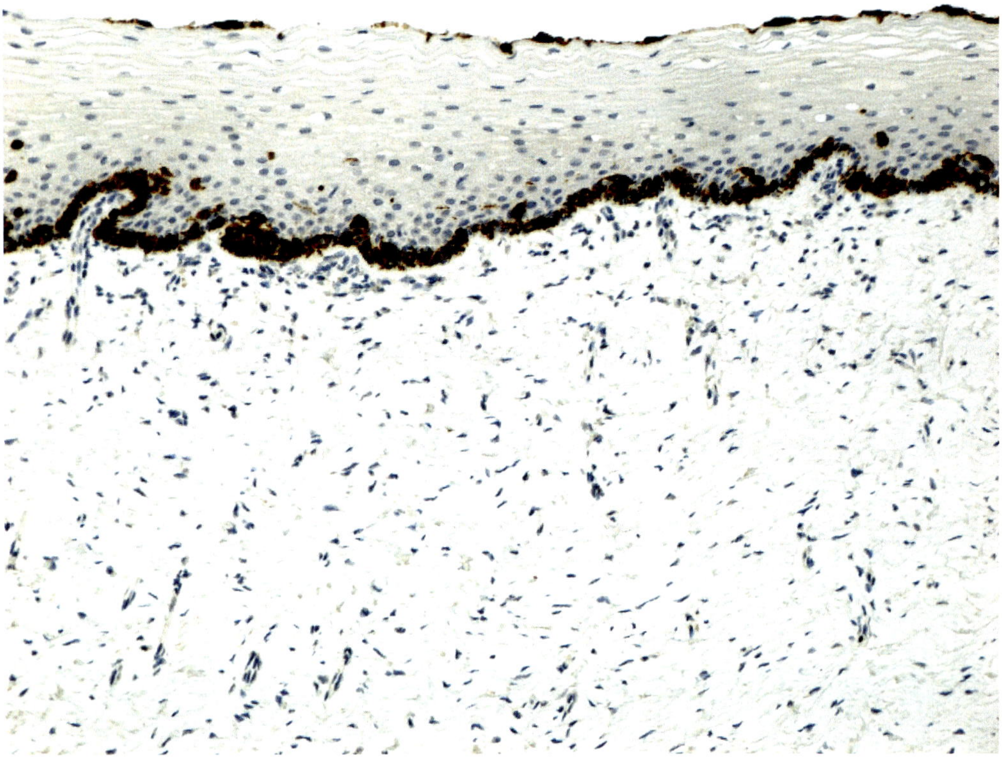

Fig. 5.23 Vaginal melanoma. Melan A immunohistochemistry highlights melanocyte density and the confluent melanocyte growth of the in situ component of the lentiginous mucosal melanoma

References

1. Mannone F, De Giorgi V, Cattaneo A, Massi D, De Magnis A, Carli P. Dermoscopic features of mucosal melanosis. Dermatol Surg. 2004;30(8):1118–23.
2. Rock B. Pigmented lesions of the vulva. Dermatol Clin. 1992;10(2):361–70.
3. Ferrari A, Buccini P, Covello R, et al. The ringlike pattern in vulvar melanosis: a new dermoscopic clue for diagnosis. Arch Dermatol. 2008;144(8):1030–4.
4. Ronger-Savle S, Julien V, Duru G, Raudrant D, Dalle S, Thomas L. Features of pigmented vulval lesions on dermoscopy. Br J Dermatol. 2011;164(1):54–61.
5. Jackson R. Melanosis of the vulva. J Dermatol Surg Oncol. 1984;10(2):119–21.
6. Lenane P, Keane CO, Connell BO, Loughlin SO, Powell FC. Genital melanotic macules: clinical, histologic, immunohistochemical, and ultrastructural features. J Am Acad Dermatol. 2000;42(4):640–4.
7. Barnhill RL, Albert LS, Shama SK, Goldenhersh MA, Rhodes AR, Sober AJ. Genital lentiginosis: a clinical and histopathologic study. J Am Acad Dermatol. 1990;22(3):453–60.
8. Sison-Torre EQ, Ackerman AB. Melanosis of the vulva. A clinical simulator of malignant melanoma. Am J Dermatopathol. 1985;7(Suppl):51–60.
9. Kerley SW, Blute ML, Keeney GL. Multifocal malignant melanoma arising in vesicovaginal melanosis. Arch Pathol Lab Med. 1991;115(9):950–2.
10. Lee RB, Buttoni Jr L, Dhru K, Tamimi H. Malignant melanoma of the vagina: a case report of progression from preexisting melanosis. Gynecol Oncol. 1984; 19(2):238–45.
11. Kemmett D, Ellis J, Spencer MJ, Hunter JA. The Laugier-Hunziker syndrome – a clinical review of six cases. Clin Exp Dermatol. 1990;15(2):111–4.
12. Veraldi S, Cavicchini S, Benelli C, Gasparini G. Laugier-Hunziker syndrome: a clinical, histopathologic, and ultrastructural study of four cases and review of the literature. J Am Acad Dermatol. 1991;25(4):632–6.
13. Lenane P, Sullivan DO, Keane CO, Loughlint SO. The Laugier-Hunziker syndrome. J Eur Acad Dermatol Venereol. 2001;15(6):574–7.
14. Lampe AK, Hampton PJ, Woodford-Richens K, Tomlinson I, Lawrence CM, Douglas FS. Laugier-Hunziker syndrome: an important differential diagnosis for Peutz-Jeghers syndrome. J Med Genet. 2003;40(6):e77.
15. Pandolfino TL, Cotell S, Katta R. Pigmented vulvar macules as a presenting feature of the Carney complex. Int J Dermatol. 2001;40(11):728–30.
16. Rudolph RI. Vulvar melanosis. J Am Acad Dermatol. 1990;23(5 Pt 2):982–4.

17. Estrada R, Kaufman R. Benign vulvar melanosis. J Reprod Med. 1993;38(1):5–8.
18. Al-Shraim MM. Angiomatoid giant cellular blue nevus of vaginal wall associated with pregnancy. Diagn Pathol. 2011;6:32.
19. Tobon H, Murphy AI. Benign blue nevus of the vagina. Cancer. 1977;40(6):3174–6.
20. Heim K, Hopfl R, Muller-Holzner E, Bergant A, Dapunt O. Multiple blue nevi of the vagina. A case report. J Reprod Med. 2000;45(1):42–4.
21. Ribe A. Melanocytic lesions of the genital area with attention given to atypical genital nevi. J Cutan Pathol. 2008;35 Suppl 2:24–7.
22. Polat M, Topcuoglu MA, Tahtaci Y, Hapa A, Yilmaz F. Spitz nevus of the genital mucosa. Indian J Dermatol Venereol Leprol. 2009;75(2):167–9.
23. Yamazhan M, Ertas IE, Kandiloglu G, Ozeren M. Cellular blue nevus of the vulva mimicking Bartholin's gland abscess in a 15-year-old girl: a case report. Arch Gynecol Obstet. 2012;285:1009–11.
24. Blickstein I, Feldberg E, Dgani R, Ben-Hur H, Czernobilsky B. Dysplastic vulvar nevi. Obstet Gynecol. 1991;78(5 Pt 2):968–70.
25. Elder DE. Precursors to melanoma and their mimics: nevi of special sites. Mod Pathol. 2006;19 Suppl 2:S4–20.
26. Tucker MA, Halpern A, Holly EA, et al. Clinically recognized dysplastic nevi. A central risk factor for cutaneous melanoma. JAMA. 1997;277(18): 1439–44.
27. Halpern AC, Guerry Dt, Elder DE, Trock B, Synnestvedt M, Humphreys T. Natural history of dysplastic nevi. J Am Acad Dermatol. 1993;29(1):51–7.
28. Friedman RJ, Ackerman AB. Difficulties in the histologic diagnosis of melanocytic nevi on the vulvae of premenopausal women. In: Ackerman AB, editor. Pathology of malignant melanoma. New York: Masson; 1981. p. 119.
29. Hosler GA, Moresi JM, Barrett TL. Nevi with site-related atypia: a review of melanocytic nevi with atypical histologic features based on anatomic site. J Cutan Pathol. 2008;35(10):889–98.
30. Christensen WN, Friedman KJ, Woodruff JD, Hood AF. Histologic characteristics of vulvar nevocellular nevi. J Cutan Pathol. 1987;14(2):87–91.
31. Brenn T. Atypical genital nevus. Arch Pathol Lab Med. 2011;135(3):317–20.
32. Gleason BC, Hirsch MS, Nucci MR, et al. Atypical genital nevi. A clinicopathologic analysis of 56 cases. Am J Surg Pathol. 2008;32(1):51–7.
33. Clark Jr WH, Hood AF, Tucker MA, Jampel RM. Atypical melanocytic nevi of the genital type with a discussion of reciprocal parenchymal-stromal interactions in the biology of neoplasia. Hum Pathol. 1998;29(1 Suppl 1):S1–24.
34. Carlson JA, Mu XC, Slominski A, et al. Melanocytic proliferations associated with lichen sclerosus. Arch Dermatol. 2002;138(1):77–87.
35. Nguyen LP, Emley A, Wajapeyee N, Green MR, Mahalingam M. BRAF V600E mutation and the tumour suppressor IGFBP7 in atypical genital naevi. Br J Dermatol. 2010;162(3):677–80.
36. Ragnarsson-Olding BK, Nilsson BR, Kanter-Lewensohn LR, Lagerlof B, Ringborg UK. Malignant melanoma of the vulva in a nationwide, 25-year study of 219 Swedish females: predictors of survival. Cancer. 1999;86(7):1285–93.
37. Weinstock MA. Malignant melanoma of the vulva and vagina in the United States: patterns of incidence and population-based estimates of survival. Am J Obstet Gynecol. 1994;171(5):1225–30.
38. Moxley KM, Fader AN, Rose PG, et al. Malignant melanoma of the vulva: an extension of cutaneous melanoma? Gynecol Oncol. 2011;122(3):612–7.
39. Stang A, Streller B, Eisinger B, Jockel KH. Population-based incidence rates of malignant melanoma of the vulva in Germany. Gynecol Oncol. 2005;96(1):216–21.
40. Raber G, Mempel V, Jackisch C, et al. Malignant melanoma of the vulva. Report of 89 patients. Cancer. 1996;78(11):2353–8.
41. Sugiyama VE, Chan JK, Shin JY, Berek JS, Osann K, Kapp DS. Vulvar melanoma: a multivariable analysis of 644 patients. Obstet Gynecol. 2007;110(2 Pt 1):296–301.
42. Egan CA, Bradley RR, Logsdon VK, Summers BK, Hunter GR, Vanderhooft SL. Vulvar melanoma in childhood. Arch Dermatol. 1997;133(3):345–8.
43. Hu DN, Yu GP, McCormick SA. Population-based incidence of vulvar and vaginal melanoma in various races and ethnic groups with comparisons to other site-specific melanomas. Melanoma Res. 2010;20(2): 153–8.
44. Moan J, Porojnicu AC, Dahlback A, Grant WB, Juzeniene A. Where the sun does not shine: is sunshine protective against melanoma of the vulva? J Photochem Photobiol B. 2010;101(2):179–83.
45. Wechter ME, Gruber SB, Haefner HK, et al. Vulvar melanoma: a report of 20 cases and review of the literature. J Am Acad Dermatol. 2004;50(4):554–62.
46. Ragnarsson-Olding BK, Kanter-Lewensohn LR, Lagerlof B, Nilsson BR, Ringborg UK. Malignant melanoma of the vulva in a nationwide, 25-year study of 219 Swedish females: clinical observations and histopathologic features. Cancer. 1999;86(7): 1273–84.
47. Verschraegen CF, Benjapibal M, Supakarapongkul W, et al. Vulvar melanoma at the M. D. Anderson Cancer Center: 25 years later. Int J Gynecol Cancer. 2001;11(5):359–64.
48. Raspagliesi F, Ditto A, Paladini D, et al. Prognostic indicators in melanoma of the vulva. Ann Surg Oncol. 2000;7(10):738–42.
49. Bradgate MG, Rollason TP, McConkey CC, Powell J. Malignant melanoma of the vulva: a clinicopathological study of 50 women. Br J Obstet Gynaecol. 1990;97(2):124–33.
50. Irvin Jr WP, Legallo RL, Stoler MH, Rice LW, Taylor Jr PT, Andersen WA. Vulvar melanoma: a retrospective analysis and literature review. Gynecol Oncol. 2001;83(3):457–65.

51. Suwandinata FS, Bohle RM, Omwandho CA, Tinneberg HR, Gruessner SE. Management of vulvar melanoma and review of the literature. Eur J Gynaecol Oncol. 2007;28(3):220–4.
52. Trimble EL, Lewis Jr JL, Williams LL, et al. Management of vulvar melanoma. Gynecol Oncol. 1992;45(3):254–8.
53. Trifiro G, Travaini LL, Sanvito F, et al. Sentinel node detection by lymphoscintigraphy and sentinel lymph node biopsy in vulvar melanoma. Eur J Nucl Med Mol Imaging. 2010;37(4):736–41.
54. Mulvany NJ, Sykes P. Desmoplastic melanoma of the vulva. Pathology. 1997;29(2):241–5.
55. Creasman WT, Phillips JL, Menck HR. A survey of hospital management practices for vulvar melanoma. J Am Coll Surg. 1999;188(6):670–5.
56. Frumovitz M, Etchepareborda M, Sun CC, et al. Primary malignant melanoma of the vagina. Obstet Gynecol. 2010;116(6):1358–65.
57. Gupta D, Malpica A, Deavers MT, Silva EG. Vaginal melanoma: a clinicopathologic and immunohistochemical study of 26 cases. Am J Surg Pathol. 2002;26(11):1450–7.
58. Borazjani G, Prem KA, Okagaki T, Twiggs LB, Adcock LL. Primary malignant melanoma of the vagina: a clinicopathological analysis of 10 cases. Gynecol Oncol. 1990;37(2):264–7.
59. Ragnarsson-Olding B, Johansson H, Rutqvist LE, Ringborg U. Malignant melanoma of the vulva and vagina. Trends in incidence, age distribution, and long-term survival among 245 consecutive cases in Sweden 1960–1984. Cancer. 1993;71(5):1893–7.
60. Cobellis L, Calabrese E, Stefanon B, Raspagliesi F. Malignant melanoma of the vagina. A report of 15 cases. Eur J Gynaecol Oncol. 2000;21(3):295–7.
61. Edwards RH, Ward MR, Wu H, et al. Absence of BRAF mutations in UV-protected mucosal melanomas. J Med Genet. 2004;41(4):270–2.
62. Curtin JA, Fridlyand J, Kageshita T, et al. Distinct sets of genetic alterations in melanoma. N Engl J Med. 2005;353(20):2135–47.
63. Bastian BC, Olshen AB, LeBoit PE, Pinkel D. Classifying melanocytic tumors based on DNA copy number changes. Am J Pathol. 2003;163(5):1765–70.
64. Yun J, Lee J, Jang J, et al. KIT amplification and gene mutations in acral/mucosal melanoma in Korea. APMIS. 2011;119(6):330–5.
65. Curtin JA, Busam K, Pinkel D, Bastian BC. Somatic activation of KIT in distinct subtypes of melanoma. J Clin Oncol. 2006;24(26):4340–6.
66. Omholt K, Grafstrom E, Kanter-Lewensohn L, Hansson J, Ragnarsson-Olding BK. KIT pathway alterations in mucosal melanomas of the vulva and other sites. Clin Cancer Res. 2011;17(12):3933–42.
67. Guo J, Si L, Kong Y, et al. Phase II, open-label, single-arm trial of imatinib mesylate in patients with metastatic melanoma harboring c-Kit mutation or amplification. J Clin Oncol. 2011;29(21):2904–9.
68. Carvajal RD, Antonescu CR, Wolchok JD, et al. KIT as a therapeutic target in metastatic melanoma. JAMA. 2011;305(22):2327–34.
69. Jiang X, Zhou J, Yuen NK, et al. Imatinib targeting of KIT-mutant oncoprotein in melanoma. Clin Cancer Res. 2008;14(23):7726–32.

Precursors of Vulvovaginal Squamous Cell Carcinoma

6

Richard Oparka and C. Simon Herrington

Abstract

The current classification of intraepithelial lesions of the vulva defines two distinct types of vulvar intraepithelial neoplasia (VIN), termed usual-type VIN (uVIN) and differentiated-type VIN (dVIN). uVIN occurs in younger women, is typically associated with high-risk HPV infection and hence with neoplasia at other anogenital sites. Vaginal intraepithelial neoplasia (VaIN) is also strongly related to HPV infection and is classified morphologically in a similar way to uVIN. Associated carcinomas are generally of warty or basaloid type. By contrast, dVIN occurs in older women, is not typically associated with HPV infection but rather shows a clinicopathological association with lichen sclerosus and HPV-negative keratinizing squamous cell carcinoma. This chapter describes these entities, highlighting the role played by HPV infection in the development of uVIN and VaIN, and discusses whether HPV-associated and non-HPV-associated VIN lesions equate to uVIN and dVIN, respectively.

Introduction

The Concept of Intraepithelial Neoplasia

There is good evidence that the majority of invasive carcinomas arise from noninvasive precursor lesions characterized by cytological and architectural features of malignancy but without either stromal invasion or metastasis. This principle applies to all carcinomas but is exemplified by, and was initially developed to describe, the precursors of squamous cell carcinoma. Historically, these lesions were termed "dysplasias" and "carcinoma in situ" (CIS), but in 1967, Richart described a new terminology, intraepithelial neoplasia, to describe noninvasive lesions of the cervical squamous epithelium (cervical intraepithelial neoplasia, CIN) [1]. This nomenclature is now in wide use, particularly in relation to cervical screening programs in the UK and the rest of Europe and has gradually been extended to other anatomical sites, initially in the anogenital region, for example, vulvar intraepithelial neoplasia (VIN) and vaginal

R. Oparka, BMSc, MBChB
Department of Pathology, Ninewells Hospital, Dundee DD1 9SY, UK

C.S. Herrington, MA., MBBS, DPhil, FRCP, FRCPath (✉)
Department of Pathology, Ninewells Hospital and Division of Cancer Research, Jacqui Wood Cancer Centre, University of Dundee, James Arrott Drive, DD1 9SY, UK
e-mail: s.herrington@dundee.ac.uk

L. Brown (ed.), *Pathology of the Vulva and Vagina*, Essentials of Diagnostic Gynecological Pathology, DOI 10.1007/978-0-85729-757-0_6, © Springer-Verlag London 2013 intraepithelial neoplasia (VaIN). Its use is no longer confined to squamous lesions, as demonstrated by its application to, for example, prostatic intraepithelial neoplasia (PIN) and (by some) endometrial intraepithelial neoplasia (EIN).

The concept of squamous intraepithelial neoplasia underpins the paradigm of squamous carcinogenesis, which holds that, as a lesion develops, the epithelium becomes progressively less well differentiated, with eventual basement membrane breach and consequent stromal invasion. The risk of stromal invasion increases as squamous differentiation is lost and therefore correlates with the proportion of the epithelium that is occupied by undifferentiated basaloid cells. This is expressed semiquantitatively by assessing the level of the epithelium at which maturation occurs and designating lesions that mature in the lower third as grade 1, the middle third as grade 2, and the upper third as grade 3 [2]. However, it is important to note that nuclear and cytoplasmic abnormalities are present at all levels of the epithelium in all grades, meaning that the concept of "partial dysplasia" developing into "full-thickness dysplasia" is not valid. This system has generally worked well, particularly for cervical disease, where it is used in the UK and Europe to direct patient management. The principles also work well for vaginal intraepithelial neoplasia (VaIN), which is generally associated with HPV infection and is strongly associated with a history of CIN [3]. However, there is increasing evidence that this approach does not accurately reflect the biology of these lesions which, for HPV-associated lesions, may be better represented by a two-tier system, such as the Bethesda system [4], which recognizes low-grade and high-grade squamous intraepithelial lesions: these correspond broadly to grade 1 and grade 2/3 intraepithelial neoplasia, respectively [5–7].

Vaginal Intraepithelial Neoplasia (VaIN)

VaIN is strongly associated with CIN and VIN, and is currently classified according to the principles outlined above using the system developed for CIN. HPV infection is the major etiological factor [8, 9], but VaIN is considerably less common than CIN, possibly due to the absence of a transformation zone in the vagina [3]. The mechanisms involved in the development of VaIN are similar to those for CIN and HPV-associated VIN and are therefore discussed below.

Vulvar Intraepithelial Neoplasia (VIN)

In view of the morphological similarity of intraepithelial lesions of the vulva to CIN, an analogous system was applied to the classification of VIN in the early 1980s [10–14]: this was adopted by the International Society for the Study of Vulvar Disease in 1986 [15, 16] and was incorporated into the World Health Organization classification in 1994 [17]. While this approach has a clear logic, and carried with it the added appeal of making terms such as erythroplasia of Queyrat and Bowen's disease obsolete, the analogy with cervical disease is not complete and translation of the CIN system to VIN is not entirely straightforward. The two main confounding issues are (1) the existence of two morphologically distinct forms of VIN—usual (also known as classic or undifferentiated) type and differentiated type—and (2) the overlapping but distinct morphological spectrum of usual-type VIN by comparison with CIN. This leads to imperfect translation between CIN and VIN, with a number of consequences.

First, when differentiated-type VIN lesions are correctly identified, VIN 1 (or low-grade VIN) is very uncommon, if it exists at all [18, 19]. This most likely relates to the differences between the biology of HPV infection in the cervix and vulva. CIN 1 is extremely common and is essentially a form of productive HPV infection (see below) of the metaplastic squamous epithelium of the transformation zone, which is biologically distinct from the squamous epithelium lining both the cutaneous and mucosal vulva. By contrast, productive HPV infection in the vulva is generally associated with low-risk HPV types and produces condylomata acuminata, which do not typically exhibit basal atypia. Indeed, in one

Table 6.1 International Society for the Study of Vulvar Disease 2004 classification of VIN

Type[a]	Associations and comments
Usual (uVIN)	Associated with high-risk HPV infection
1. Warty	Associated with HPV persistence factors such as cigarette smoking or immunocompromised states
2. Basaloid	Typically associated with warty/basaloid squamous cell carcinoma
3. Mixed (warty/basaloid)	
Differentiated (dVIN)	Associated with vulvar dermatoses, particularly lichen sclerosus
	Not associated with HPV infection
	Associated with a higher risk of invasive squamous cell carcinoma than uVIN
	Typically associated with keratinizing squamous cell carcinoma
Unclassified	Non-uVIN/dVIN (e.g., pagetoid type)

VIN vulvar intraepithelial neoplasia, *HPV* human papillomavirus
[a]Classification based on morphological criteria only, without considering the presence or absence of HPV

study, the majority of lesions initially considered to represent VIN 1 contained low-risk HPV types, suggesting overdiagnosis of VIN 1. This contrasted with a strong association between VaIN 1 and high-risk HPV types in the same study, underscoring the concept that VaIN is more closely related to CIN than to VIN [20]. Second, VIN 2 and VIN 3 very often coexist, and their morphological distinction is extremely subjective. This is to some extent also true for CIN and underpins the definition of high-grade SIL in the two-tier classification system.

These two factors, together with the identification of the differentiated form of VIN, led the International Society for the Study of Vulvar Disease to propose, in 2004, a modification to their classification such that (1) VIN 1 was no longer recognized, (2) all VIN lesions were regarded as high grade and hence the numerical grading system was dropped, and (3) two forms of VIN were recognized—usual type and differentiated type [19, 21] (see Table 6.1). Usual-type VIN was considered generally to be associated with HPV infection while differentiated-type VIN was not [22–26], but classification was based on morphological criteria only, without considering the presence or absence of HPV. A category of unclassified VIN was also included into which lesions that do not conform to the definitions of usual or differentiated type could be placed, for example, VIN of pagetoid type [21].

This classification has not been universally accepted for a number of reasons. First, there is not universal agreement that VIN 1 does not exist [8, 20, 27]. Second, the morphological recognition of differentiated-type VIN is challenging, particularly in the absence of an associated squamous cell carcinoma. And third, an absolute relationship between usual-type VIN and differentiated-type VIN, as defined morphologically, and the presence and absence of HPV infection, respectively, has not been convincingly demonstrated. However, for practical purposes, the recognition of differentiated-type VIN as an entity is important as it has modified thinking and to some extent clinical practice, particularly in patients with lichen sclerosus, as will be discussed below. Similarly, whatever one's views about the existence of VIN 1, it is undoubtedly rare [28], with most usual-type VIN lesions being unequivocally high grade: this is also useful pragmatically as the clear identification of lesions as high grade helps guide the treating clinician.

For practical purposes, the ISSVD classification is a useful approach to the morphological categorization of VIN lesions, but there may still be situations in which the term VIN 1 is appropriate. In addition, there is morphological overlap between VIN of usual and differentiated types, as will be discussed below. Nevertheless, the concept of differentiated-type VIN is helpful in the appropriate clinicopathological context.

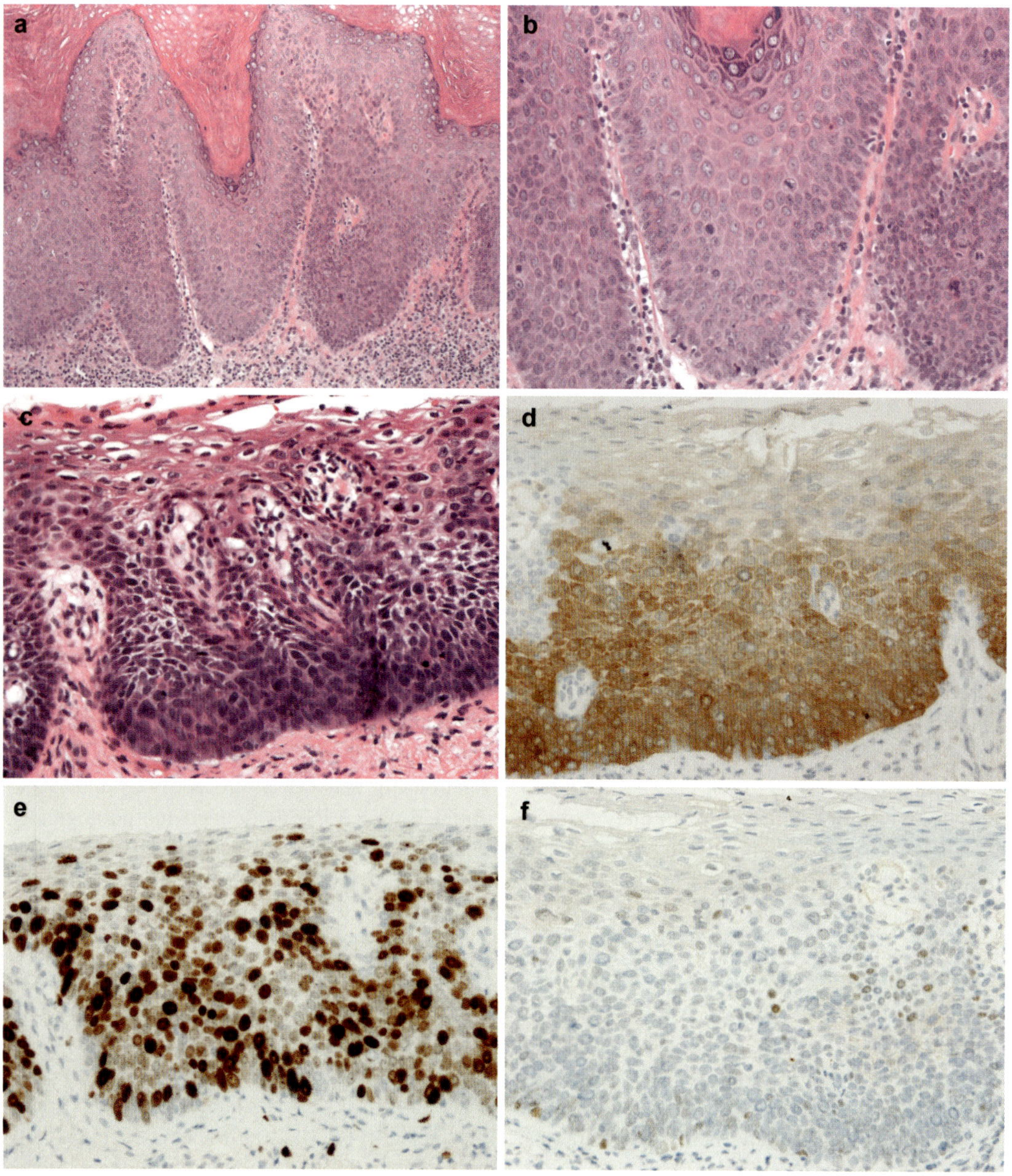

Fig. 6.1 Usual-type VIN may have a condylomatous architecture (**a**) and exhibit prominent keratinization, including the formation of a stratum granulosum (**b**). This is accompanied by proliferation of atypical basaloid cells, with abundant mitotic activity. The morphology may be more reminiscent of CIN, with more prominent HPV-associated changes including koilocytosis (**c**) indicating "warty" uVIN. The immunophenotype of this lesion is consistent with its association with HPV infection, with diffuse expression of p16 (**d**), extension of Ki67 expression into the upper layers of the epithelium (**e**), and only focal expression of p53, which is confined to the middle layers of the epithelium (**f**). Note that p16 expression does not extend into the upper epithelial layers, which is consistent with a switch to productive HPV infection (see text)

Usual-Type VIN

Usual-type VIN (uVIN) (Fig. 6.1) is associated with neoplastic lesions at other anogenital sites (including the vagina) and is subdivided into warty, basaloid, and mixed types [14, 21]. The warty form often has a condylomatous architecture and exhibits features associated with HPV infection such as koilocytosis, multinucleation, and dyskeratosis, which are seen in the upper layers of the epithelium. These features are accompanied by proliferation of atypical basaloid cells, with high nucleocytoplasmic ratio, nuclear hyperchromasia, and abundant mitotic figures throughout the epithelium. Abnormal mitotic figures are common, and apoptotic cells, which often possess densely eosinophilic cytoplasm, are frequent. Often, the appearances are reminiscent of CIN 2 and examples of CIN 3 in which there is noticeable HPV-associated change in the upper epithelium. Basaloid uVIN shows little or no maturation, and discernible HPV-associated changes are absent: this is analogous to CIN 3 with little or no maturation and corresponds to what was formerly termed carcinoma in situ. Mixed lesions, in which areas of both basaloid and warty uVIN are present, are common: this is not surprising, given that these are typically HPV-driven lesions. uVIN occurs preferentially in younger women, consistent with this association with HPV infection [14].

Differentiated-Type VIN

Differentiated-type VIN (dVIN) (Figs. 6.2 and 6.3) was first described as an "intraepithelial carcinoma of simplex type" in the 1960s by Abell and colleagues [29]. The term "differentiated" was introduced in 1977 by Hart as an alternative to "simplex" to emphasize the morphological appearance [14]. This entity is found in older women and is less common than uVIN, is frequently associated with invasive squamous cell carcinoma, which is often keratinizing in type, and is typically unassociated with HPV infection [26, 30]. It has a different morphological appearance from uVIN, the features being more subtle and easily confused with those of nonneoplastic epithelial disease, particularly squamous hyperplasia [14, 31]. This is compounded by the clinicopathological association of dVIN with lichen sclerosus and squamous hyperplasia, which are found in the majority of cases [26] and may be inflamed and therefore exhibit reactive changes. When seen adjacent to, or otherwise associated with, squamous cell carcinoma, the diagnosis of dVIN is easier to reach with certainty, but this diagnosis is a significantly greater challenge when there is no identifiable stromal invasion, particularly in small biopsies. Nevertheless, its recognition is important as, in the context of lichen sclerosus, dVIN is found more frequently in patients who subsequently develop invasive carcinoma [32].

The key histological features of dVIN are (1) basal keratinocyte atypia; (2) abnormal suprabasal keratinization, often accompanied by formation of whorls of differentiated cells, typically within rete pegs; (3) prominent nucleoli and intercellular bridges in suprabasal keratinocytes; (4) elongation and branching of rete pegs; and (5) epithelial acanthosis with prominent parakeratosis [14, 31]. Keratinocyte atypia is often present

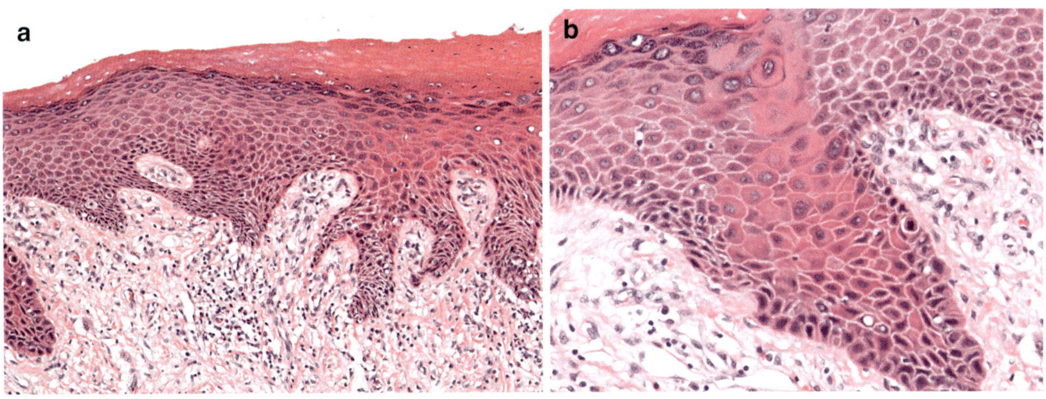

Fig. 6.2 Differentiated-type VIN is characterized by irregular elongation and fusion of rete pegs with basal keratinocyte atypia, separation of suprabasal keratinocytes with prominent intercellular bridges and nucleoli, and overlying parakeratosis (**a**). Higher power shows more clearly the abrupt suprabasal differentiation and the cytological features (**b**)

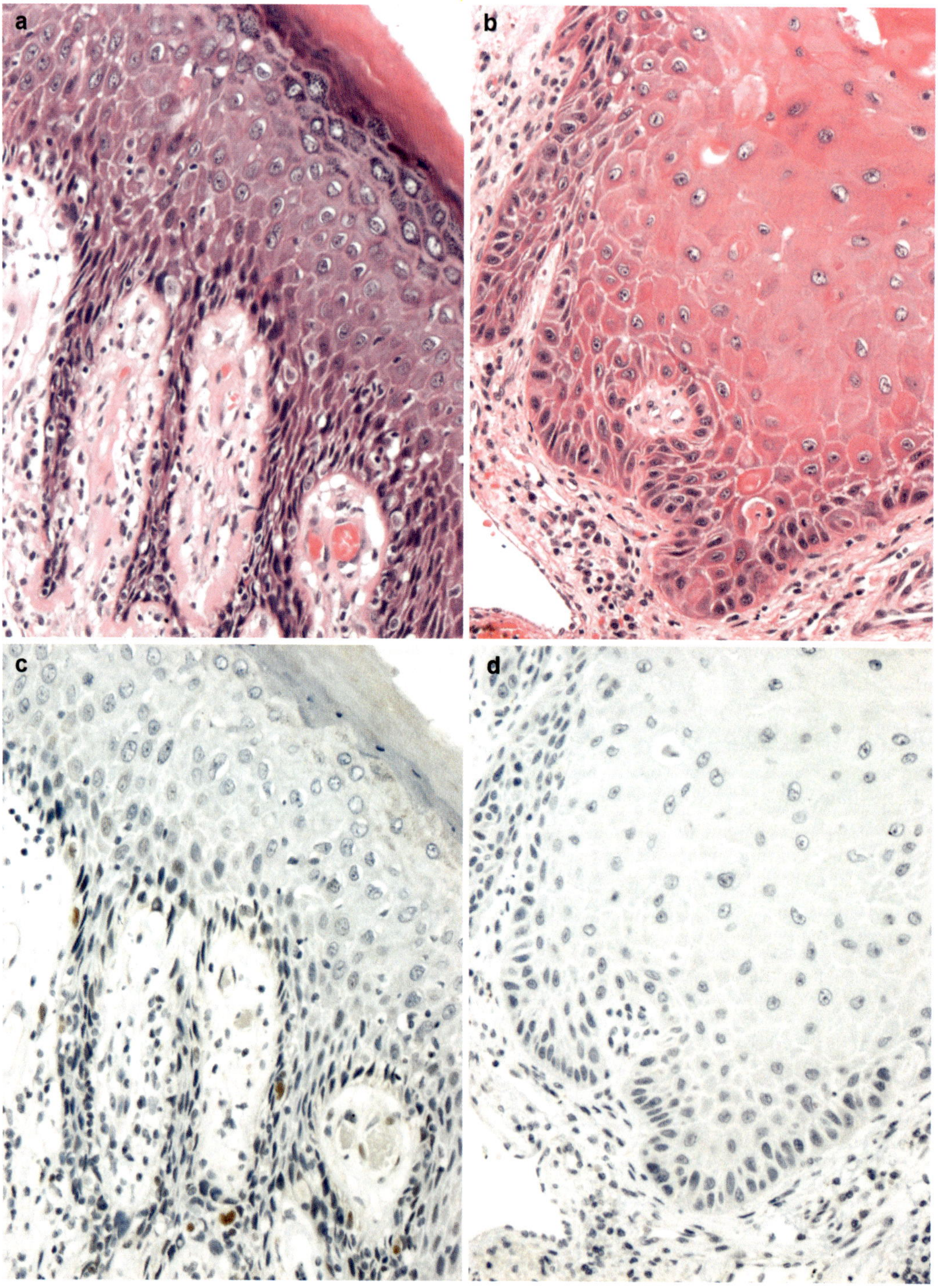

Fig. 6.3 Two areas showing features of differentiated VIN, taken from the same slide and adjacent to an invasive squamous cell carcinoma. Note the predominance of rete peg elongation and basal atypia, with less obvious suprabasal abnormality in (**a**), and more prominent suprabasal differentiation in (**b**). These regions show only focal, or no, p53 expression (**c** and **d**, respectively)

in inflammatory and other reactive nonneoplastic epithelial abnormalities, particularly squamous hyperplasia. The atypia of dVIN is generally more prominent, with notable mitotic activity including abnormal forms, the latter being a particularly useful feature in inflamed lesions. However, the degree of atypia is not as great as is seen in uVIN, being generally mild to moderate. Similarly, hyperplastic squamous epithelium may show spongiosis with associated separation of suprabasal keratinocytes and prominence of intercellular bridges, which may mimic dVIN. However, the presence of prominent nucleoli and an abnormal intraepithelial architecture, particularly the formation of intraepithelial whorls and keratin pearls, are helpful pointers to a diagnosis of dVIN. The lower power architecture of dVIN, with rete peg elongation and fusion together with thick parakeratosis, is typical and, when accompanied by the other features discussed above, helps to support the diagnosis. Finally, dVIN often occurs in the clinicopathological context of lichen sclerosus, and a clinical history, or the presence of histological features, of lichen sclerosus supports the diagnosis when the other morphological features are present.

Immunohistochemical Features of VIN

The concept that two pathways are involved in the development of VIN has led to the investigation of a variety of immunohistochemical markers both to support this hypothesis and to aid diagnosis. In particular, the expression of p16 has been used widely as a surrogate for high-risk HPV infection (see below and [33, 34]) and its expression supports a diagnosis of uVIN [34, 35]: this mirrors the use of p16 immunohistochemistry in the diagnosis of CIN. Other markers used in the diagnosis of CIN, such as Ki67, ProExC (topoisomerase II and MCM2), and HPV in situ hybridization [36, 37], have been less widely investigated in VIN, although it has been suggested that the pattern of Ki67 positivity may be of diagnostic help [38] and one report indicates that ProExC shows a similar staining pattern to CIN in uVIN [39]. dVIN is typically p16 negative, consistent with the concept that it is unassociated with HPV infection [35, 40]. The suggestion that p53 expression may be a marker of dVIN has not been substantiated, although the literature on this is conflicting [14, 35, 41]. Thus, there are, at the time of writing, no specific markers of dVIN. Nevertheless, where the differential diagnosis lies between uVIN and dVIN, it has been suggested that a panel of Ki67, p16, and p53 may be of value [35].

Is There an Overlap Between uVIN and dVIN?

The foregoing discussion implies that uVIN and dVIN, as defined morphologically, are essentially different disorders that arise via different mechanisms. However, a number of observations suggest that this is an oversimplification. First, features of uVIN and dVIN may coexist in the same lesion. It is not inconceivable that an epithelium prone to the development of dVIN, for example in a region of lichen sclerosus, may be infected by HPV and develop uVIN. However, a specific case illustrates a possible alternative explanation, namely that uVIN may on occasion show morphological features that mimic dVIN (Fig. 6.4): this is consistent with the observation by others that a minority of dVIN lesions contain HPV DNA [42]. Similarly, careful examination of lesions showing unequivocal features of dVIN not infrequently reveals regions with more marked epithelial atypia that mimics uVIN (Fig. 6.5). Indeed, a basaloid variant of dVIN has been proposed [43]. This morphological overlap suggests an alternative hypothesis, namely, that VIN may arise mechanistically via two pathways (HPV dependent and HPV independent) but that these two pathways may lead to similar morphological features. This does not negate the general association of HPV-associated disease with uVIN, and non-HPV-associated disease with dVIN, but calls into question the nonoverlapping morphological classification that equates uVIN with HPV-associated disease and dVIN with non-HPV-associated disease.

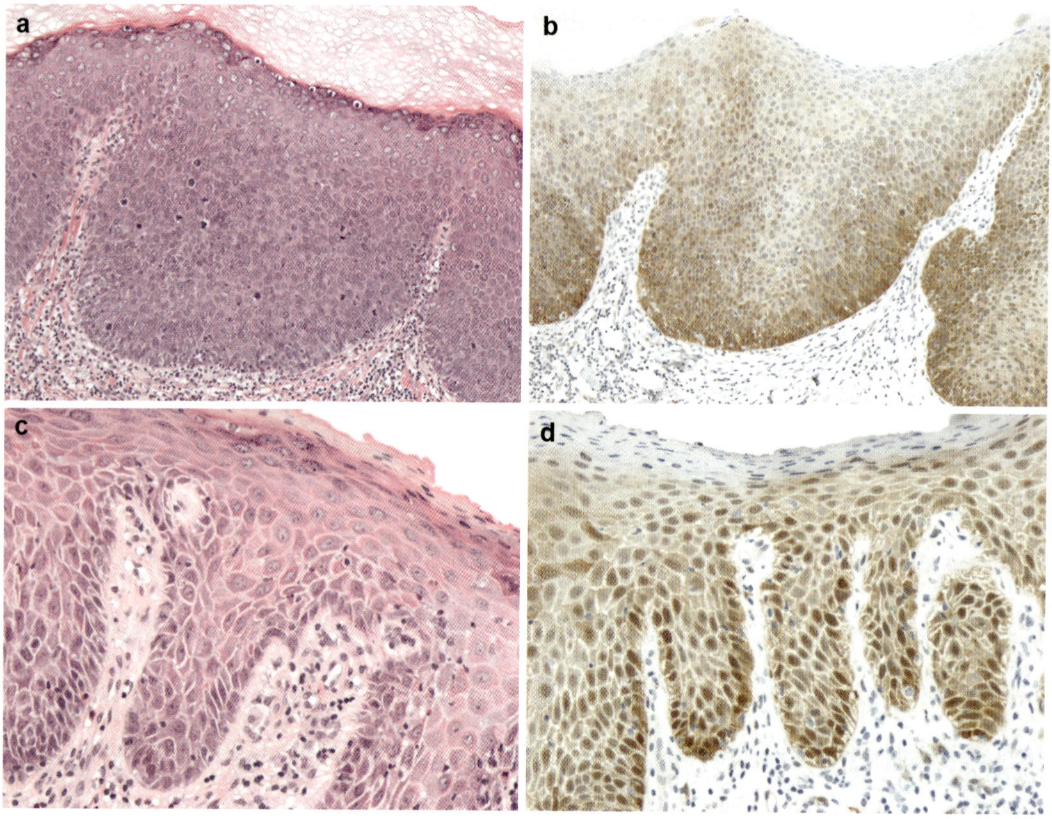

Fig. 6.4 In this case, a region of basaloid VIN of usual type (**a**) was flanked by abnormal epithelium showing features suggestive of differentiated-type VIN (**c**). However, p16 immunostaining shows strong expression in both regions (**b** and **d** respectively) suggesting that they both represent HPV-associated abnormalities

In the following sections, the mechanisms involved in the development of HPV-associated and non-HPV-associated squamous intraepithelial neoplasia are reviewed and the evidence supporting this hypothesis discussed.

HPV Infection and HPV-Associated VaIN and VIN

Although the link between sexual activity and lower genital tract neoplasia, particularly cervical carcinoma, had been well known since the nineteenth century [44], the involvement of HPV infection did not achieve widespread acceptance until the late 1990s. zur Hausen first postulated that HPV infection was important in lower genital tract neoplasia in the 1970s [45, 46], at a time when herpes simplex virus was thought to be the most likely etiological agent for cervical carcinoma [45]. However, despite the isolation of HPV 16 from a cervical carcinoma in 1983 [47], there remained doubt about the involvement of HPV, which was considered by some to be a passenger infection rather than one of pathogenetic importance. This view was reinforced by the apparent demonstration, using at that time newly developed PCR-based techniques, that HPV infection was ubiquitous. However, the recognition that the high sensitivity of PCR made it susceptible to sample contamination [48] led to methodological refinement and the eventual demonstration that HPV infection did indeed associate strongly with neoplasia, with almost 100% of cervical carcinomas containing HPV DNA in a carefully controlled multinational study published in 1999 [49]. Since then, the development of prophylactic HPV vaccines has reinforced the

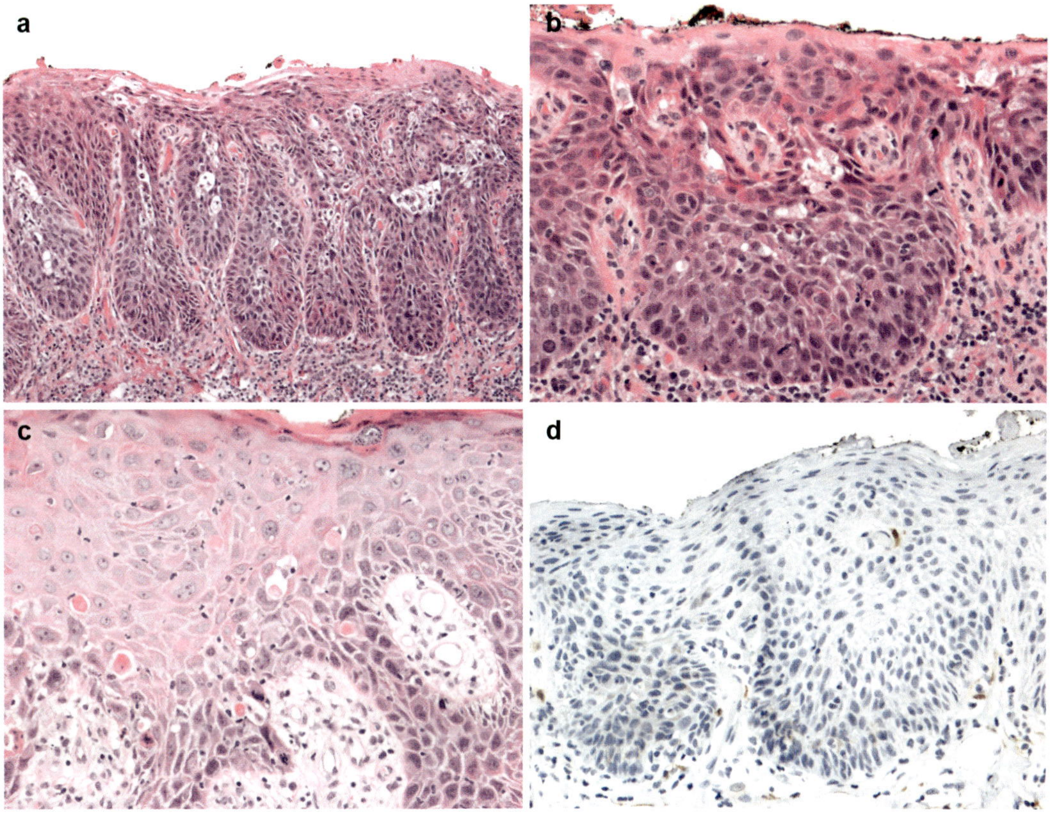

Fig. 6.5 In this case, areas showing atypia extending into the suprabasal epithelium (**a**, **b**) were present adjacent to epithelium showing more typical appearances of differentiated-type VIN (**c**): widespread lichen sclerosus was also present. p16 immunostaining was negative (**d**). Taken in isolation, the abnormalities in panels (**a**) and (**b**) show features suggestive of VIN of usual type but, on the basis of the associated morphological features (**c**) and p16 negativity (**d**), are more likely to indicate dVIN

role of HPV infection with the demonstration that prevention of HPV infection prevents HPV-associated intraepithelial neoplasia, including that in the vagina and vulva [50, 51].

Over 120 HPV types have been identified, all of which have a strong propensity to infect squamous epithelium [52, 53]. Anogenital infection is caused by HPVs of the alpha genus, which contains approximately 30 HPV types. These types vary in their association with neoplastic disease and hence have been divided into low-risk types, which are associated with benign warts/condylomata, and high-risk types, which are associated with neoplastic disease. VaIN and uVIN, but not dVIN, are typically associated with infection with similar high-risk mucosal HPV types to those found in CIN [9, 54].

HPV Infection

HPVs belong to the *Papillomaviridae* family and have a small circular double-stranded DNA genome that is approximately 8,000 bp in length [55] (Fig. 6.6a). Viral replication is tightly associated with squamous differentiation (Fig. 6.6b), which explains the relationship between HPV infection and squamous epithelial disorders. The viral genome contains eight open reading frames (ORFs), which encode proteins that direct viral DNA replication and virion production. The genome is divided into early (E) and late (L) regions, based on the relationship between viral gene expression and the viral life cycle, separated by a long control region (LCR), also known as the upstream regulatory region (URR), which

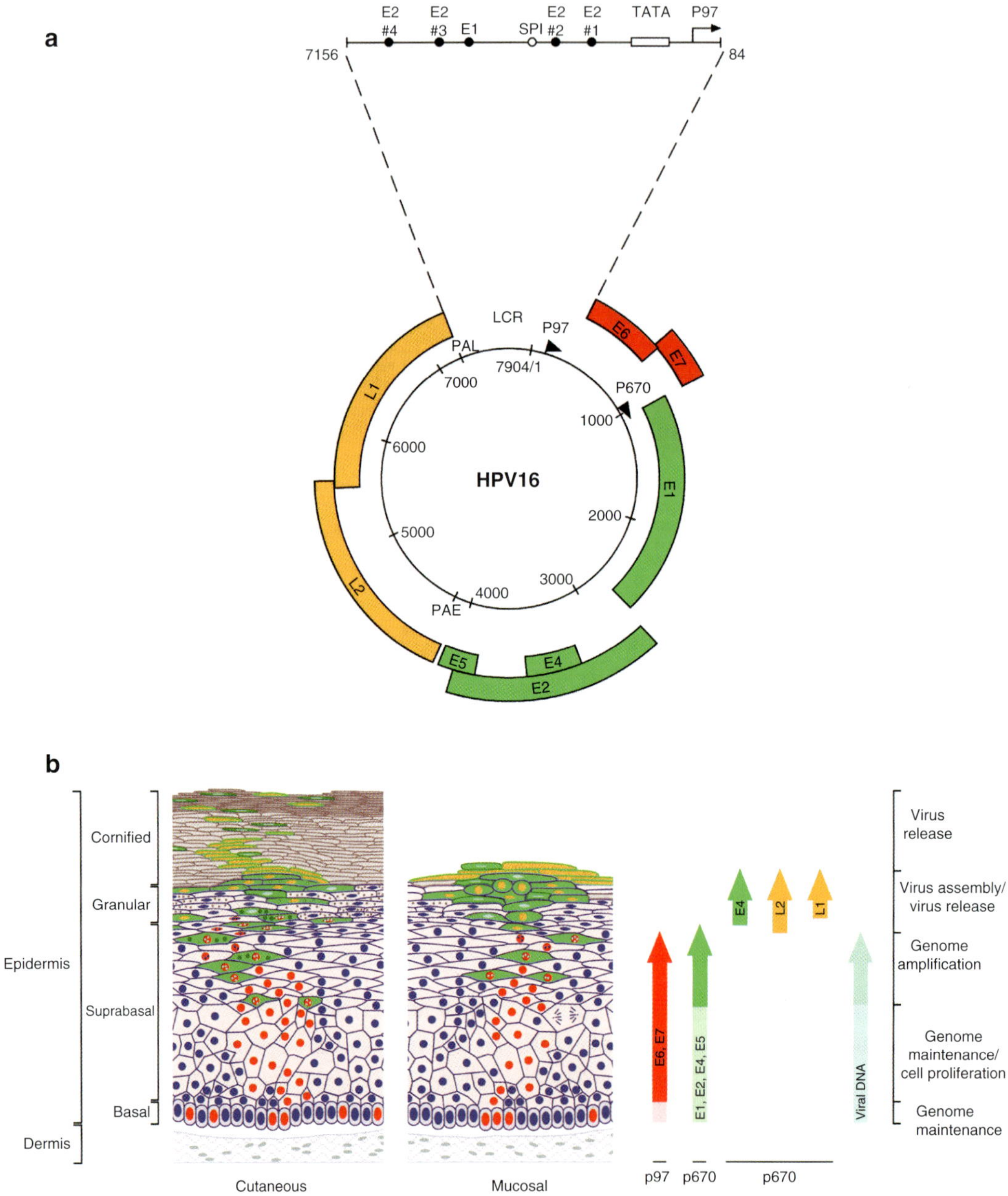

Fig. 6.6 (**a**) Pictorial representation of the human papillomavirus genome. (**b**) The relationship between viral gene expression and squamous differentiation (Reproduced with permission from [56])

contains enhancer and promoter elements, glucocorticoid response elements, and the origin of DNA replication [57].

The E1 protein is involved in viral DNA replication and is the only viral gene product to possess enzyme activity. It acts as a helicase but also forms a heterodimer with the E2 protein [58, 59]. The E2 protein regulates the expression of viral early genes, particularly E6 and E7, through E2 binding sites in the URR. It also plays a role in viral DNA replication, through its binding to E1, and is important for genome maintenance through its ability to tether the HPV genome to host cell chromatin [56, 58, 60]. The E4 ORF contributes to the E1^E4 protein

[61–63]. This fusion protein is involved late in the viral life cycle and is thought to play a role in collapse of the cytoskeleton, perhaps in preparation for viral exit. The E5 protein has proved difficult to study, partly as a result of its hydrophobicity, and little is known of its function [64]. However, it does cooperate with the HPV E6 oncoprotein to induce koilocytosis in human cervical cells and keratinocytes in vitro [65], and downregulates the expression of surface HLA molecules thereby aiding evasion of the immune response [66].

The E6 and E7 ORFs encode the main transforming proteins. These are capable of immortalization and neoplastic transformation under appropriate conditions. They are discussed further below.

The L1 and L2 ORFs encode the major and minor capsid proteins, respectively. These proteins form the icosahedral capsid coat of the virus [67] and have been used to produce the virus-like particles that constitute the prophylactic vaccines developed for immunization against HPV infection [68].

The Early Events in HPV Infection

The viral life cycle begins with infection of dividing basal squamous epithelial cells [56]. Metaplastic epithelium between squamous and glandular epithelia, particularly the cervical transformation zone, is a particular target for viral infection as the replicating cells are easily accessible [56]. Both capsid proteins (L1 and L2) are involved in the initial binding of the virus to basal keratinocytes. For the majority of HPV types, this involves interaction with heparan sulfate proteoglycans expressed on the keratinocyte cell surface [69], although secondary receptors, for example, integrins, are likely to be involved [70]. The virus then enters the cell by slow endocytosis and disassembles in late endosomes and/or lysosomes, following which viral DNA is released.

The E2 protein is involved in the transport of viral DNA to the host nucleus and promotes its binding to host DNA [71]. In basal epithelial cells, the viral genome is maintained in an extrachromosomal form (episome) and low-level replication occurs in parallel with the host cell cycle. Only the early promoter (e.g., p97 in HPV 16, see Fig. 6.6a) is active in basal cells [72]. The E6 and E7 proteins are expressed at this stage and promote expansion of the infected cell population, allowing suprabasal cells to continue to express S-phase-associated proteins in the presence of squamous epithelial differentiation [73].

The most important function of the E6 protein is to counteract the effects of p53 [74]. The E6-associated protein (E6-AP) binds to E6, and this complex can then bind to p53 with subsequent ubiquitination and degradation by proteolysis. E6-driven ubiquitination of p53 can also occur in the absence of E6AP as demonstrated by its occurrence in E6AP null mice [75]. Loss of p53 leads to loss of cell cycle inhibition by the cyclin-dependent kinase inhibitor (CDKI) p21 and potentiation of the effects of the various cyclin/cyclin-dependent kinase (CDK) complexes, promoting cell cycle progression [73]. Abrogation of p53 function by E6 results in the failure of G1/S arrest and predisposes the cell to accumulating DNA damage and developing a transformed phenotype [76]: variation in this property between HPV types is likely to explain in part their different associations with neoplastic disease. E6 also activates telomerase reverse transcriptase (hTERT) [77], which can cooperate with the abrogation of pRb function to immortalize keratinocytes [78]. Furthermore, E7 appears to act synergistically with E6 in activating hTERT but is unable to do so in isolation [79].

The E7 protein is structurally and functionally similar to proteins produced by other human DNA viruses, for example the E1A protein and large T antigen of adenoviruses and Simian virus 40, respectively [80]. E7 binds to a variety of endogenous "pocket proteins," the most important of which is the retinoblastoma protein (pRb), which plays a central regulatory role at the G1/S boundary of the cell cycle. By binding to pRb, E7 removes the inhibitory effect of hypophosphorylated pRb on E2F. This leads to transcription of a number of cell cycle mediators including cyclins E and A. E7 also binds to the pocket proteins p107 and p130 [81], which have similar effects to pRb on other members of the E2F family (E2F4 and E2F5, respectively). p130 is expressed in differentiated cells within higher levels of the epithelium, whereas p107 levels are increased when quiescent cells begin to divide [82]. The E7 protein therefore has multiple target binding sites throughout the epithelium as cells progress through the maturation process. E7 can also activate E2F-related transcription, hence promoting synthesis of S-phase components, without binding to pRb [83], and has also been shown to interact with other cellular complexes, including the TATA box binding proteins (TBP), which may have wider-ranging effects on transcription [84].

E7 has been shown to abrogate the inhibitory role of CDKIs, particularly p16, p21, and p27, thereby promoting cell cycle progression [85, 86]. At first sight, this appears inconsistent with the marked upregulation of p16 expression seen in lesions associated with high-risk HPV infection. However, as E7 abrogates the function of pRb and therefore substitutes functionally for the phosphorylation of pRb by CDK4, the CDK4 inhibitor p16 no longer has an effect at the G1/S checkpoint. Therefore, although p16 expression is upregulated by the loss of pRb [87], it is functionally ineffective. Nevertheless, this increase in p16 expression is useful as a surrogate marker for E7-expressing high-risk HPV infection [33, 88]. It is of note that low-risk HPV infection is not associated with elevated p16 expression as the E7 proteins of these HPV types do not efficiently abrogate pRb function (see below).

In addition to their cell cycle effects, HPVs have also evolved mechanisms to interfere with apoptotic signals. In the early phases of viral infection, inhibition of the apoptotic response is essential for viral survival and genome maintenance. In the late phases of infection, however, the initiation of apoptosis helps virion release. It is not surprising therefore that HPV proteins are capable of exerting both pro- and anti-apoptotic effects.

The E6 and E7 proteins play important roles in the evasion of apoptosis during the early phases of HPV infection. One of the many roles of p53 is to stimulate pro-apoptotic molecules in response to cellular damage. Clearly, the E6-mediated degradation of p53 leads to loss of p53 function and hence loss of this apoptotic response. E6 also has p53-independent anti-apoptotic effects, for example, by inducing the ubiquitination of Bak [89]. It can also bind to the cytoplasmic death domain of the TNF receptor, inhibiting the downstream activation of caspase-8 [90].

E7 has similar anti-apoptotic effects, many of which counteract the functions of E2, which is pro-apoptotic (see below). For example, E7 decreases the activation of the caspase cascade initiator pro-caspase-8 [91]. In experimental models, E7 immortalized cells appear almost completely resistant to cell death via the extrinsic pathway. However, treatment with the nuclear export inhibitor leptomycin B induces rapid apoptosis of primary keratinocytes expressing HPV 16 E7, indicating that the anti-apoptotic effects of E7 can be overcome: this has potential therapeutic implications [92, 93].

The Late Events in HPV Infection

The differentiation-dependent promoter, for example, p670 in HPV 16 (see Fig. 6.6a), is located within the E7 ORF in many HPV types. This promoter is only activated in suprabasal "differentiated" cells, leading to increased expression of E1, E2, E4, and E5. This produces a switch to productive infection, with consequent viral genome amplification, disruption of the cellular scaffold through the effects of the E1^E4 protein, packaging of viral DNA in an icosahedral capsid composed of the L1 and L2 proteins, and release of mature virions [63, 94, 95].

The pro-apoptotic effects of the HPV proteins are important in late viral infection. E6 undergoes posttranslational splicing to form truncated proteins termed E6*I and E6**I, which counteract the effect of E6 on p53 [90]. It is also postulated that E6*I can directly induce apoptosis [96].

As well as being a trans-repressor of E6 and E7 expression, and a viral replication protein, E2 has strong pro-apoptotic effects [97] through induction of the caspase cascade by direct caspase-8 activation [98]. This combination of functions makes intuitive sense as the net effect of E2 expression is to inhibit E6 and E7 while inducing both viral DNA replication and host cell apoptosis.

The HPV E1^E4 protein also plays an important part in disruption of the host cell to enable viral release after replication. It binds to and degrades intermediate filaments, disrupting the keratin network, and has also been shown to bind to mitochondria, altering the mitochondrial membrane potential and inducing apoptosis [95].

High-Risk Versus Low-Risk HPV Types

All HPV types have a similar genome capable of expressing similar proteins, and it is therefore not immediately clear why certain HPV types have a far greater propensity for malignant transformation than others (Table 6.2). One important difference is that the viral DNA in low-risk HPV infection remains in an extrachromosomal episomal form, whereas the DNA from the high-risk types often integrates into the host DNA and this integration is associated with neoplastic transformation [99, 100]. Furthermore, the circular viral genome breaks relatively constantly in the E1/E2 region during integration. This leads to loss of viral DNA replication coupled with upregulation of E6 and E7 expression and hence enhanced disruption of cell cycle checkpoints in cells in which productive HPV infection can no longer occur. Moreover, the upregulation of E6 and E7 expression leads to inhibition of apoptosis, while the loss of E2 expression removes its pro-apoptotic effect.

The E6 and E7 proteins of high- and low-risk HPVs also differ in their ability to interact with cellular proteins. For example, high-risk HPV E6 proteins degrade p53 much more effectively than low-risk HPV E6 proteins [101]. Similarly, high-risk HPV E7 proteins bind to pRb with greater affinity than low-risk HPV E7 [102]. In addition, the E6 proteins of low-risk HPV types lack the PDZ-binding domains that allow the virus to interact with many host proteins (e.g., MAGUK) promoting transformation [103]. Finally, high-risk (HPV 16), but not low-risk (HPV 6) E6 and E7 proteins can cooperate to induce mitotic defects and genomic instability [104].

These differences between low- and high-risk HPVs explain in part the differences in the squamous epithelial abnormalities associated with these HPV types. Low-risk HPVs interfere with cell cycle control to induce viral DNA replication in postmitotic suprabasal squamous epithelial cells. Expression of viral proteins is coordinated with squamous differentiation, leading to production of virions in concert with desquamation of surface epithelial cells. It is important to appreciate that high-risk HPVs can produce a similar outcome and would not survive if they were unable to complete a productive life cycle. However, the disruption of coordinated expression of high-risk HPV genes, for example, by HPV integration, leads to inappropriate high-level expression, particularly of E6 and E7, in dividing cells with consequent genetic instability with accumulation of secondary genetic changes and inhibition of apoptosis, resulting eventually in neoplastic transformation.

Table 6.2 The classification of common HPV types by their association with anogenital neoplasia

Low-risk HPV types	*Common* HPV 6, 11 *Less common* HPV 42, 44, 53, 54, 62, and 66
High-risk HPV types	*Common* HPV 16, 18 *Less common* HPV 31, 33, 35, 39, 45, 51, 52, 56, 58, 59, and 68

HPV Infection and Intraepithelial Neoplasia

From a morphological point of view, productive HPV infection produces a characteristic cytopathic effect, namely koilocytosis, in which nuclear enlargement is accompanied by the formation of a perinuclear halo. This indicates vegetative viral replication and is seen typically in viral warts and low-grade intraepithelial lesions, particularly of the cervix and vagina, in which the viral life cycle proceeds relatively normally. It may also be seen in some high-grade lesions of the cervix (CIN 2 and 3), vagina (VaIN 2 and 3), and vulva (particularly uVIN of warty type). This implies that productive HPV infection can still occur in high-grade intraepithelial lesions, which at first seems inconsistent with the arguments presented above. However, there is evidence that episomal and integrated HPV sequences can coexist in HPV-infected cells [100], and hence it is possible that lesions in which HPV infection is driving expansion of basaloid cells through the expression of E6 and E7 may retain the ability to undergo a switch to productive HPV infection. Increasing morphological abnormality, with a more prominent basaloid phenotype, is associated with increasing dysregulation of E6 and E7 gene expression and loss of this switch.

Non-HPV-Associated VIN

The Lichen Sclerosus-Differentiated VIN Concept

Clinicopathological studies indicate that there is an association between lichen sclerosus and an elevated risk of the development of squamous cell carcinoma [105]. However, the nature of this elevated risk, and whether it is mediated through a noninvasive precursor lesion, is less well established. Lichen sclerosus is typically associated with squamous epithelial atrophy, but epithelial hyperplasia is often also present, particularly where there is a local clinical abnormality. This hyperplastic epithelium is often inflamed and therefore shows reactive changes, which complicate further the definition and recognition of dVIN. However, it is unlikely that squamous hyperplasia is a direct precursor of invasive squamous cell carcinoma [106].

As described above, dVIN was first described in the 1960s [29]. The morphological criteria for its diagnosis are subtle and to some extent subjective. However, there is increasing recognition that this entity exists and that it is associated with both lichen sclerosus [105] and vulvar squamous cell carcinoma [106], which is often keratinizing in type [14]. This association with squamous cell carcinoma is stronger than for uVIN [106], and the carcinomas that arise in the context of dVIN are more likely to recur [107]. Moreover, the strong association between dVIN and invasive squamous cell carcinoma [106], the existence of dVIN in the absence of invasive squamous cell carcinoma [41, 106], and the demonstration that dVIN can progress to invasive carcinoma [108] provide compelling evidence that it is a true precursor lesion.

The acceptance of dVIN as an entity has been hampered by the lack of specific markers. Unlike uVIN, where there is consistent expression of markers associated with HPV infection such as p16 (Fig. 6.4), no equivalent markers exist for dVIN. Moreover, lesions that mimic dVIN can be seen in association with uVIN and vice versa (see above). There is, however, general acceptance that dVIN is not associated with HPV infection [109]. An alternative approach would be to define dVIN on the basis of a combination of the presence of the appropriate morphological features coupled with absence of HPV infection, perhaps as defined by p16 negativity (Fig. 6.5). This certainly has the appeal of greater objectivity, but the issue of morphological subjectivity remains. It has been suggested that basal keratinocyte Ki67 expression might be used as a "positive" marker of dVIN, but again, this is not entirely straightforward [38].

Early reports suggested that increased p53 expression, as identified by immunohistochemistry, could be used as a marker for dVIN [14, 26]. However, this has not stood the test of time and it is likely that p53 expression in this context reflects upregulation of wild-type p53, which is related more to inflammatory and reactive mechanisms than to the presence of dVIN [41]. Thus, p53 expression is variable and of little help diagnostically (Fig. 6.3) [41]. There is a single report of p53 mutation in dVIN [110]. This carefully controlled study identified consistent p53 mutations in microdissected dVIN lesions, but at the time of writing, the findings have not been confirmed.

Thus, the molecular pathology of dVIN and its associated squamous cell carcinomas remains unclear. There is a need for a "positive" marker of this entity, but identification of such a marker is currently hampered by the imperfect definition and identification of these lesions. Based on current evidence, perhaps the most appropriate approach would be to define dVIN on the basis of p16 negativity, with or without the absence of HPV, coupled with the appropriate morphological features. Careful analysis of series of uVIN and dVIN lesions defined in this way is likely to improve understanding of their molecular pathogenesis.

Conclusion

The current classification of intraepithelial lesions of the vulva defines two distinct types of VIN, termed usual-type VIN (uVIN) and differentiated-type VIN (dVIN). uVIN occurs in younger women, is typically associated with high-risk HPV infection and hence with neoplasia at other anogenital sites. VaIN is also strongly related to HPV infection and is classified morphologically in a similar way. Associated carcinomas are generally of warty or basaloid type. By contrast, dVIN occurs in older women, is not typically associated with HPV infection but rather shows a clinicopathological association with lichen sclerosus and HPV-negative keratinizing squamous cell carcinoma. There is, however, evidence of a degree of morphological overlap between uVIN and dVIN, and it may be more appropriate to consider HPV-associated and non-HPV-associated pathways to the development of VIN. Further studies are needed to explore the precise relationship between these pathways and lesion morphology.

References

1. Richart RM. Natural history of cervical intraepithelial neoplasia. Clin Obstet Gynecol. 1967;10(4):748–84.
2. Herrington CS, Wells M. Premalignant and malignant squamous lesions of the cervix. In: Fox H, Wells M, editors. Haines and Taylor obstetrical and gynaecological pathology. 4th ed. Edinburgh: Churchill Livingstone; 2002.
3. Tavassoli F, Devilee P, editors. Pathology and genetics of tumours of the breast and female genital organs. Lyon: IARC Press; 2003.
4. Henry MR. The Bethesda system 2001: an update of new terminology for gynecologic cytology. Clin Lab Med. 2003;23(3):585–603.
5. Wilson G. The classification of cervical intraepithelial neoplasia. Histopathology. 2002;40(4):380–5.
6. Ismail S, Fiander A. Grading cervical intraepithelial neoplasia. Histopathology. 2002;40(4):385–90.
7. Heatley MK. How should we grade CIN? Histopathology. 2002;40(4):377–80.
8. Srodon M, Stoler MH, Baber GB, Kurman RJ. The distribution of low and high-risk HPV types in vulvar and vaginal intraepithelial neoplasia (VIN and VaIN). Am J Surg Pathol. 2006;30(12):1513–8.
9. De Vuyst H, Clifford GM, Nascimento MC, Madeleine MM, Franceschi S. Prevalence and type distribution of human papillomavirus in carcinoma and intraepithelial neoplasia of the vulva, vagina and anus: a meta-analysis. Int J Cancer. 2009;124(7):1626–36.
10. Crum CP, Fu YS, Levine RU, Richart RM, Townsend DE, Fenoglio CM. Intraepithelial squamous lesions of the vulva: biologic and histologic criteria for the distinction of condylomas from vulvar intraepithelial neoplasia. Am J Obstet Gynecol. 1982;144(1):77–83.
11. Crum CP, Braun LA, Shah KV, Fu YS, Levine RU, Fenoglio CM, et al. Vulvar intraepithelial neoplasia: correlation of nuclear DNA content and the presence of a human papilloma virus (HPV) structural antigen. Cancer. 1982;49(3):468–71.
12. Crum CP. Vulvar intraepithelial neoplasia: the concept and its application. Hum Pathol. 1982;13(3):187–9.
13. Crum CP, Liskow A, Petras P, Keng WC, Frick HC. Vulvar intraepithelial neoplasia (severe atypia and carcinoma in situ). A clinicopathologic analysis of 41 cases. Cancer. 1984;54(7):1429–34.
14. Hart WR. Vulvar intraepithelial neoplasia: historical aspects and current status. Int J Gynecol Pathol. 2001;20(1):16–30.
15. Wilkinson E, Kneale B, Lunch P. Report of the ISSVD terminology committee. J Reprod Med. 1986;31(10):973–4.
16. Wilkinson EJ. Normal histology and nomenclature of the vulva, and malignant neoplasms, including VIN. Dermatol Clin. 1992;10(2):283–96.
17. Scully R, Bonfiglio T, Kurman R, Silverberg S, Wilkinsonm E. Histologic typing of female genital tract tumours. In: Scully R, Poulsen H, Sobin L, editors. World health organisation international histological classification of tumours. Berlin: Springer; 2004.
18. Scurry J, Campion M, Scurry B, Kim SN, Hacker N. Pathologic audit of 164 consecutive cases of vulvar intraepithelial neoplasia. Int J Gynecol Pathol. 2006;25(2):176–81.
19. Scurry J, Wilkinson EJ. Review of terminology of precursors of vulvar squamous cell carcinoma. J Low Genit Tract Dis. 2006;10(3):161–9.
20. Logani S, Lu D, Quint WGV, Ellenson LH, Pirog EC. Low-grade vulvar and vaginal intraepithelial neoplasia: correlation of histologic features with human papillomavirus DNA detection and MIB-1 immunostaining. Mod Pathol. 2003;16(8):735–41.
21. Sideri M, Jones RW, Wilkinson EJ, Preti M, Heller DS, Scurry J, et al. Squamous vulvar intraepithelial neoplasia: 2004 modified terminology, ISSVD Vulvar Oncology Subcommittee. J Reprod Med. 2005;50(11):807–10.
22. Park JS, Jones RW, McLean MR, Currie JL, Woodruff JD, Shah KV, et al. Possible etiologic heterogeneity of

vulvar intraepithelial neoplasia. A correlation of pathologic characteristics with human papillomavirus detection by in situ hybridization and polymerase chain reaction. Cancer. 1991;67(6):1599–607.
23. Haefner HK, Tate JE, McLachlin CM, Crum CP. Vulvar intraepithelial neoplasia: age, morphological phenotype, papillomavirus DNA, and coexisting invasive carcinoma. Hum Pathol. 1995;26(2):147–54.
24. Hørding U, Junge J, Poulsen H, Lundvall F. Vulvar intraepithelial neoplasia III: a viral disease of undetermined progressive potential. Gynecol Oncol. 1995; 56(2):276–9.
25. van Beurden M, ten Kate FJ, Smits HL, Berkhout RJ, de Craen AJ, van der Vange N, et al. Multifocal vulvar intraepithelial neoplasia grade III and multicentric lower genital tract neoplasia is associated with transcriptionally active human papillomavirus. Cancer. 1995;75(12):2879–84.
26. Yang B, Hart WR. Vulvar intraepithelial neoplasia of the simplex (differentiated) type: a clinicopathologic study including analysis of HPV and p53 expression. Am J Surg Pathol. 2000;24(3):429–41.
27. Medeiros F, Nascimento AF, Crum CP. Early vulvar squamous neoplasia: advances in classification, diagnosis, and differential diagnosis. Adv Anat Pathol. 2005;12(1):20–6.
28. Micheletti L, Barbero M, Preti M, Zanotto Valentino MC, Chiringhello B, Pippione M. Vulvar intraepithelial neoplasia of low grade: a challenging diagnosis. Eur J Gynaecol Oncol. 1994;15(1):70–4.
29. Abell MR. Intraepithelial carcinomas of epidermis and squamous mucosa of vulva and perineum. Surg Clin North Am. 1965;45(5):1179–98.
30. Kruse A-J, Bottenberg MJH, Tosserams J, Slangen B, van Marion AMW, van Trappen PO. The absence of high-risk HPV combined with specific p53 and p16INK4a expression patterns points to the HPV-independent pathway as the causative agent for vulvar squamous cell carcinoma and its precursor simplex VIN in a young patient. Int J Gynecol Pathol. 2008;27(4):591–5.
31. van de Nieuwenhof HP, van der Avoort IAM, de Hullu JA. Review of squamous premalignant vulvar lesions. Crit Rev Oncol Hematol. 2008;68(2):131–56.
32. van de Nieuwenhof HP, Bulten J, Hollema H, Dommerholt RG, Massuger LFAG, van der Zee AGJ, et al. Differentiated vulvar intraepithelial neoplasia is often found in lesions, previously diagnosed as lichen sclerosus, which have progressed to vulvar squamous cell carcinoma. Mod Pathol. 2011;24(2):297–305.
33. Klaes R, Benner A, Friedrich T, Ridder R, Herrington S, Jenkins D, et al. p16INK4a immunohistochemistry improves interobserver agreement in the diagnosis of cervical intraepithelial neoplasia. Am J Surg Pathol. 2002;26(11):1389–99.
34. Riethdorf S, Neffen EF, Cviko A, Löning T, Crum CP, Riethdorf L. p16INK4A expression as biomarker for HPV 16-related vulvar neoplasias. Hum Pathol. 2004;35(12):1477–83.
35. Hoevenaars BM, van der Avoort IAM, de Wilde PCM, Massuger LFAG, Melchers WJG, de Hullu JA, et al. A panel of p16(INK4A), MIB1 and p53 proteins can distinguish between the 2 pathways leading to vulvar squamous cell carcinoma. Int J Cancer. 2008;123(12): 2767–73.
36. Kong C, Balzer B, Troxell M, Patterson B, Longacre T. p16INK4A immunohistochemistry is superior to HPV in situ hybridization for the detection of high-risk HPV in atypical squamous metaplasia. Am J Surg Pathol. 2007;31(1):33–43.
37. Kong CS, Beck AH, Longacre TA. A panel of 3 markers including p16, ProExC, or HPV ISH is optimal for distinguishing between primary endometrial and endocervical adenocarcinomas. Am J Surg Pathol. 2010;34(7):915–26.
38. van der Avoort IAM, van der Laak JAWM, Paffen A, Grefte JMM, Massuger LFAG, de Wilde PCM, et al. MIB1 expression in basal cell layer: a diagnostic tool to identify premalignancies of the vulva. Mod Pathol. 2007;20(7):770–8.
39. Chen H, Gonzalez JL, Brennick JB, Liu M, Yan S. Immunohistochemical patterns of ProEx C in vulvar squamous lesions: detection of overexpression of MCM2 and TOP2A. Am J Surg Pathol. 2010;34(9): 1250–7.
40. Ruhul Quddus M, Xu C, Steinhoff MM, Zhang C, Lawrence WD, Sung CJ. Simplex (differentiated) type VIN: absence of p16INK4 supports its weak association with HPV and its probable precursor role in non-HPV related vulvar squamous cancers. Histopathology. 2005;46(6):718–20.
41. Liegl B, Regauer S. p53 immunostaining in lichen sclerosus is related to ischaemic stress and is not a marker of differentiated vulvar intraepithelial neoplasia (d-VIN). Histopathology. 2006;48(3):268–74.
42. Skapa P, Zamecnik J, Hamsikova E, Salakova M, Smahelova J, Jandova K, et al. Human papillomavirus (HPV) profiles of vulvar lesions: possible implications for the classification of vulvar squamous cell carcinoma precursors and for the efficacy of prophylactic HPV vaccination. Am J Surg Pathol. 2007; 31(12):1834–43.
43. Ordi J, Alejo M, Fusté V, Lloveras B, del Pino M, Alonso I, et al. HPV-negative vulvar intraepithelial neoplasia (VIN) with basaloid histologic pattern: an unrecognized variant of simplex (differentiated) VIN. Am J Surg Pathol. 2009;33(11):1659–65.
44. Rigoni-Stern D. Fatti statistica relativi alle malattie cancerose. Giornale per servire ai progressi della Paologica e della Terapoa. 1842;2:507–17.
45. Hausen zur H. Condylomata acuminata and human genital cancer. Cancer Res. 1976;36:794.
46. Hausen zur H. Human papillomaviruses and their possible role in squamous cell carcinomas. Curr Top Microbiol Immunol. 1977;78:1–30.
47. Dürst M, Gissmann L, Ikenberg H, Hausen zur H. A papillomavirus DNA from a cervical carcinoma and its prevalence in cancer biopsy samples from different geographic regions. Proc Natl Acad Sci USA. 1983;80(12):3812–5.
48. Zitz JC, McLachlin CM, Tate JE, Mutter GL, Crum CP. Restriction fragment length polymorphism

analysis of isotype-labeled polymerase chain reaction-amplified human papillomavirus DNA combines sensitivity with built-in contaminant detection. Mod Pathol. 1994;7(3):407–11.
49. Walboomers J, Jacobs M, Manos M, Bosch F, Kummer J, Shah K, et al. Human papillomavirus is a necessary cause of invasive cervical cancer worldwide. J Pathol. 1999;189(1):12–9.
50. Joura E, Leodolter S, Hernandez-Avila M, Wheeler C, Perez G, Koutsky L, et al. Efficacy of a quadrivalent prophylactic human papillomavirus (types 6, 11, 16, and 18) L1 virus-like-particle vaccine against high-grade vulval and vaginal lesions: a combined analysis of three randomised clinical trials. Lancet. 2007; 369(9574):1693–702.
51. Medeiros LR, Rosa DD, Da Rosa MI, Bozzetti MC, Zanini RR. Efficacy of human papillomavirus vaccines: a systematic quantitative review. Int J Gynecol Cancer. 2009;19(7):1166–76.
52. de Villiers E-M, Fauquet C, Broker TR, Bernard H-U, Hausen zur H. Classification of papillomaviruses. Virology. 2004;324(1):17–27.
53. Bernard H-U, Burk RD, Chen Z, van Doorslaer K, Hausen zur H, de Villiers E-M. Classification of papillomaviruses (PVs) based on 189 PV types and proposal of taxonomic amendments. Virology. 2010;40(1):70–9.
54. de Koning MNC, Quint WGV, Pirog EC. Prevalence of mucosal and cutaneous human papillomaviruses in different histologic subtypes of vulvar carcinoma. Mod Pathol. 2008;21(3):334–44.
55. Hebner CM, Laimins LA. Human papillomaviruses: basic mechanisms of pathogenesis and oncogenicity. Rev Med Virol. 2006;16(2):83–97.
56. Doorbar J. Molecular biology of human papillomavirus infection and cervical cancer. Clin Sci. 2006;110(5):525–41.
57. Moodley M, Sewart S, Herrington CS, Chetty R, Pegoraro R, Moodley J. The interaction between steroid hormones, human papillomavirus type 16, E6 oncogene expression, and cervical cancer. Int J Gynecol Cancer. 2003;13(6):834–42.
58. Chiang CM, Ustav M, Stenlund A, Ho TF, Broker TR, Chow LT. Viral E1 and E2 proteins support replication of homologous and heterologous papillomaviral origins. Proc Natl Acad Sci USA. 1992;89(13): 5799–803.
59. Wilson VG, West M, Woytek K, Rangasamy D. Papillomavirus E1 proteins: form, function, and features. Virus Genes. 2002;24(3):275–90.
60. Longworth MS, Laimins LA. Pathogenesis of human papillomaviruses in differentiating epithelia. Microbiol Mol Biol Rev. 2004;68(2):362–72.
61. Fang L, Budgeon LR, Doorbar J, Briggs ER, Howett MK. The human papillomavirus type 11 E1^E4 protein is not essential for viral genome amplification. Virology. 2006;351(2):271–9.
62. Wilson R, Ryan GB, Knight GL, Laimins LA, Roberts S. The full-length E1E4 protein of human papillomavirus type 18 modulates differentiation-dependent viral DNA amplification and late gene expression. Virology. 2007;362(2):453–60.
63. Khan J, Davy CE, McIntosh PB, Jackson DJ, Hinz S, Wang Q, et al. Role of calpain in the formation of human papillomavirus type 16 e1^e4 amyloid fibers and reorganization of the keratin network. J Virol. 2011;85(19):9984–97.
64. DiMaio D, Mattoon D. Mechanisms of cell transformation by papillomavirus E5 proteins. Oncogene. 2001;20(54):7866–73.
65. Krawczyk E, Suprynowicz FA, Hebert JD, Kamonjoh CM, Schlegel R. The HPV-16 E5 oncoprotein translocates calpactin I to the perinuclear region. J Virol. 2011;85:10968–75.
66. Campo MS, Graham SV, Cortese MS, Ashrafi GH, Araibi EH, Dornan ES, et al. HPV-16 E5 down-regulates expression of surface HLA class I and reduces recognition by CD8 T cells. Virology. 2010;407(1):137–42.
67. Zhou J, Frazer I. Papovaviridae: capsid structure and capsid protein function. In: Lacey C, editor. Papillomavirus reviews: current research on papillomaviruses. Leeds: Leeds University Press; 1996. p. 93–100.
68. Cutts F, Franceschi S, Goldie S, Castellsague X, de Sanjose S, Garnett G, et al. Human papillomavirus and HPV vaccines: a review. Bull World Health Organ. 2007;85(9):719–26.
69. Schiller JT, Day PM, Kines RC. Current understanding of the mechanism of HPV infection. Gynecol Oncol. 2010;118:S12–7.
70. McMillan NA, Payne E, Frazer IH, Evander M. Expression of the alpha6 integrin confers papillomavirus binding upon receptor-negative B-cells. Virology. 1999;261(2):271–9.
71. Oliveira JG, Colf LA, McBride AA. Variations in the association of papillomavirus E2 proteins with mitotic chromosomes. Proc Natl Acad Sci USA. 2006;103(4): 1047–52.
72. Conway MJ, Meyers C. Replication and assembly of human papillomaviruses. J Dent Res. 2009;88(4): 307–17.
73. Southern S, Herrington CS. Disruption of cell cycle control by human papillomaviruses with special reference to cervical carcinoma. Int J Gynecol Cancer. 2000;10(4):263–74.
74. Werness BA, Levine AJ, Howley PM. Association of human papillomavirus types 16 and 18 E6 proteins with p53. Science. 1990;248(4951):76–9.
75. Massimi P, Shai A, Lambert P, Banks L. HPV E6 degradation of p53 and PDZ containing substrates in an E6AP null background. Oncogene. 2008;27(12): 1800–4.
76. Thomas J, Laimins L, Ruesch M. Perturbation of cell cycle control by E6 and E7 oncoproteins of human papillomaviruses. Papillomavirus Rep. 1998;9:59–64.
77. Klingelhutz AJ, Foster SA, McDougall JK. Telomerase activation by the E6 gene product of human papillomavirus type 16. Nature. 1996;380(6569):79–82.
78. Kiyono T, Foster SA, Koop JI, McDougall JK, Galloway DA, Klingelhutz AJ. Both Rb/p16INK4a inactivation and telomerase activity are required to immortalize human epithelial cells. Nature. 1998; 396(6706):84–8.

79. Liu X, Roberts J, Dakic A, Zhang Y, Schlegel R. HPV E7 contributes to the telomerase activity of immortalized and tumorigenic cells and augments E6-induced hTERT promoter function. Virology. 2008;375(2):611–23.
80. Munger K, Basile J, Duensing S, Eichten A, Gonzalez S, Grace M, et al. Biological activities and molecular targets of the human papillomavirus E7 oncoprotein. Oncogene. 2001;20(54):7888–98.
81. Helt A-M, Galloway DA. Mechanisms by which DNA tumor virus oncoproteins target the Rb family of pocket proteins. Carcinogenesis. 2003;24(2):159–69.
82. Classon M, Dyson N. p107 and p130: versatile proteins with interesting pockets. Exp Cell Res. 2001;264(1):135–47.
83. Hwang SG, Lee D, Kim J, Seo T, Choe J. Human papillomavirus type 16 E7 binds to E2F1 and activates E2F1-driven transcription in a retinoblastoma protein-independent manner. J Biol Chem. 2002;277(4):2923–30.
84. Massimi P, Pim D, Banks L. Human papillomavirus type 16 E7 binds to the conserved carboxy-terminal region of the TATA box binding protein and this contributes to E7 transforming activity. J Gen Virol. 1997;78(10):2607–13.
85. Zerfass-Thome K, Zwerschke W, Mannhardt B, Tindle R, Botz JW, Jansen-Dürr P. Inactivation of the cdk inhibitor p27KIP1 by the human papillomavirus type 16 E7 oncoprotein. Oncogene. 1996;13(11):2323–30.
86. Jones DL, Alani RM, Münger K. The human papillomavirus E7 oncoprotein can uncouple cellular differentiation and proliferation in human keratinocytes by abrogating p21Cip1-mediated inhibition of cdk2. Genes Dev. 1997;11(16):2101–11.
87. Li Y, Nichols MA, Shay JW, Xiong Y. Transcriptional repression of the D-type cyclin-dependent kinase inhibitor p16 by the retinoblastoma susceptibility gene product pRb. Cancer Res. 1994;54(23):6078–82.
88. Klaes R, Friedrich T, Spitkovsky D, Ridder R, Rudy W, Petry U, et al. Overexpression of p16(INK4A) as a specific marker for dysplastic and neoplastic epithelial cells of the cervix uteri. Int J Cancer. 2001;92(2):276–84.
89. Jackson S, Harwood C, Thomas M, Banks L, Storey A. Role of Bak in UV-induced apoptosis in skin cancer and abrogation by HPV E6 proteins. Genes Dev. 2000;14(23):3065–73.
90. Filippova M, Parkhurst L, Duerksen-Hughes PJ. The human papillomavirus 16 E6 protein binds to Fas-associated death domain and protects cells from Fas-triggered apoptosis. J Biol Chem. 2004;279(24):25729–44.
91. Duensing S, Münger K. Mechanisms of genomic instability in human cancer: insights from studies with human papillomavirus oncoproteins. Int J Cancer. 2004;109(2):157–62.
92. Gray LJ, Bjelogrlic P, Appleyard VCL, Thompson AM, Jolly CE, Lain S, et al. Selective induction of apoptosis by leptomycin B in keratinocytes expressing HPV oncogenes. Int J Cancer. 2007;120(11):2317–24.
93. Jolly CE, Gray LJ, Parish JL, Lain S, Herrington CS. Leptomycin B induces apoptosis in cells containing the whole HPV 16 genome. Int J Oncol. 2009;35(3):649–56.
94. Bryan JT, Brown DR. Association of the human papillomavirus type 11 E1^E4 protein with cornified cell envelopes derived from infected genital epithelium. Virology. 2000;277(2):262–9.
95. Raj K, Berguerand S, Southern S, Doorbar J, Beard P. E1^E4 Protein of human papillomavirus type 16 associates with mitochondria. J Virol. 2004;78(13):7199–207.
96. Pim D, Banks L. HPV-18 E6*I protein modulates the E6-directed degradation of p53 by binding to full-length HPV-18 E6. Oncogene. 1999;18(52):7403–8.
97. Webster K, Parish J, Pandya M, Stern PL, Clarke AR, Gaston K. The human papillomavirus (HPV) 16 E2 protein induces apoptosis in the absence of other HPV proteins and via a p53-dependent pathway. J Biol Chem. 2000;275(1):87–94.
98. Demeret C, Garcia-Carranca A, Thierry F. Transcription-independent triggering of the extrinsic pathway of apoptosis by human papillomavirus 18 E2 protein. Oncogene. 2003;22(2):168–75.
99. Winder D, Pett M, Foster N, Shivji M, Herdman M, Stanley M, et al. An increase in DNA double-strand breaks, induced by Ku70 depletion, is associated with human papillomavirus 16 episome loss and de novo viral integration events. J Pathol. 2007;213(1):27–34.
100. Pett M, Coleman N. Integration of high-risk human papillomavirus: a key event in cervical carcinogenesis? J Pathol. 2007;212(4):356–67.
101. Hiller T, Poppelreuther S, Stubenrauch F, Iftner T. Comparative analysis of 19 genital human papillomavirus types with regard to p53 degradation, immortalization, phylogeny, and epidemiologic risk classification. Cancer Epidemiol Biomarkers Prev. 2006;15(7):1262–7.
102. Münger K, Werness BA, Dyson N, Phelps WC, Harlow E, Howley PM. Complex formation of human papillomavirus E7 proteins with the retinoblastoma tumor suppressor gene product. EMBO J. 1989;8(13):4099–105.
103. Watson RA, Thomas M, Banks L, Roberts S. Activity of the human papillomavirus E6 PDZ-binding motif correlates with an enhanced morphological transformation of immortalized human keratinocytes. J Cell Sci. 2003;116(24):4925–34.
104. Duensing S, Lee LY, Duensing A, Basile J, Piboonniyom S, Gonzalez S, et al. The human papillomavirus type 16 E6 and E7 oncoproteins cooperate to induce mitotic defects and genomic instability by uncoupling centrosome duplication from the cell division cycle. Proc Natl Acad Sci USA. 2000;97(18):10002–7.

105. Scurry J. Does lichen sclerosus play a central role in the pathogenesis of human papillomavirus negative vulvar squamous cell carcinoma? The itch-scratch-lichen sclerosus hypothesis. Int J Gynecol Cancer. 1999;9(2):89–97.
106. Eva LJ, Ganesan R, Chan KK, Honest H, Luesley DM. Differentiated-type vulval intraepithelial neoplasia has a high-risk association with vulval squamous cell carcinoma. Int J Gynecol Cancer. 2009;19(4):741–4.
107. Eva LJ, Ganesan R, Chan KK, Honest H, Malik S, Luesley DM. Vulval squamous cell carcinoma occurring on a background of differentiated vulval intraepithelial neoplasia is more likely to recur: a review of 154 cases. J Reprod Med. 2008;53(6): 397–401.
108. Roma AA, Hart WR. Progression of simplex (differentiated) vulvar intraepithelial neoplasia to invasive squamous cell carcinoma: a prospective case study confirming its precursor role in the pathogenesis of vulvar cancer. Int J Gynecol Pathol. 2007;26(3):248–53.
109. van de Nieuwenhof HP, van Kempen LCLT, de Hullu JA, Bekkers RLM, Bulten J, Melchers WJG, et al. The etiologic role of HPV in vulvar squamous cell carcinoma fine tuned. Cancer Epidemiol Biomarkers Prev. 2009;18(7):2061–7.
110. Pinto AP, Miron A, Yassin Y, Monte N, Woo TYC, Mehra KK, et al. Differentiated vulvar intraepithelial neoplasia contains TP53 mutations and is genetically linked to vulvar squamous cell carcinoma. Mod Pathol. 2010;23(3):404–12.

7 Squamous Cell Carcinoma and Basal Cell Carcinoma of the Vulva and Squamous Cell Carcinoma of the Vagina

Laurence Brown

Abstract

Squamous carcinoma of the vulva and vagina is increasing in incidence and appears to be related to HPV infection in younger women and chronic irritation in older women. Individualized treatment aims to prevent unnecessary surgery by recognizing early stage disease amenable to simple excision and is focusing on sentinel node analysis for vulval cancer. Care must be taken to distinguish squamous carcinoma from benign mimics such as wart, verruca vulgaris, herpes simplex, hyperplasia, keratoacanthoma, verruciform xanthoma, papillomatosis, and polyps. Basal cell carcinoma of the vulva is a rare disease that must be separated from squamous carcinoma in order to prevent overtreatment.

Vulva

Squamous Carcinoma

This malignant tumor of vulval stratified squamous epithelium grows as a nodule, elevated plaque, ulcer, or larger papillary excrescence. Any part of the vulva may be involved, but most occur on the labia majora or labia minora with a significant minority on the clitoris, clitoral hood, interlabial sulcae, fourchette, or margins of the introitus [1, 2]. Opposing vulval lips may support "kissing" tumors (Fig. 7.1a, b). The WHO classifies these tumors by histology into keratinizing, non-keratinizing, basaloid, and warty subtypes [3].

Keratinizing Squamous Carcinoma

Keratinizing squamous carcinoma is the subtype that is most commonly preceded or associated with differentiated VIN [4] and can be graded on the basis of the degree of keratinization. Subsequent improvements to this system use a combination of histological and cytological scoring [5, 6].

In practice, squamous carcinoma is graded by a modified 3-grade Broders system [7], but this is of limited prognostic utility (see below).

Well-differentiated tumors show infiltrating tongues and nests of cells with smooth, rounded contours. The infiltrative foci are more than

L. Brown, B.Sc., MBBS, FRCPath
Department of Histopathology,
Leicester Royal Infirmary,
Infirmary Square, Leicester LE1 5WW, UK
e-mail: laurence.brown@uhl-tr.nhs.uk

L. Brown (ed.), *Pathology of the Vulva and Vagina*, Essentials of Diagnostic Gynecological Pathology,
DOI 10.1007/978-0-85729-757-0_7, © Springer-Verlag London 2013

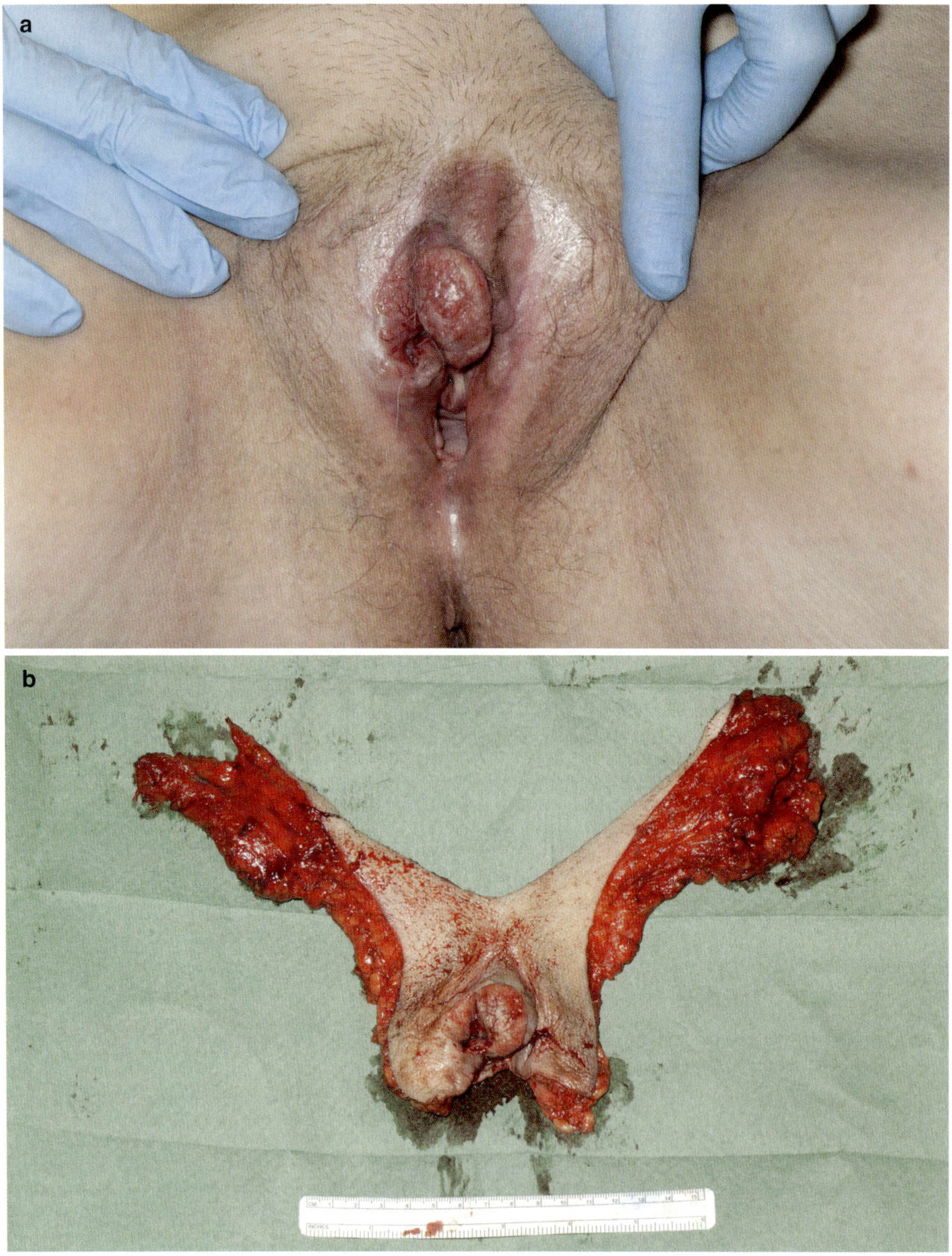

Fig. 7.1 (**a**) Clinically advanced squamous carcinoma of the right labium minus and major, extending onto the clitoral hood. (**b**) Vulvectomy specimen—"butterfly" excision of advanced carcinoma seen in (**a**) sparing the posterior vulva and fourchette, but including bilateral inguinal lymph node dissections (Courtesy of Dr. Sophia Julian)

two-thirds keratinized with central foci of keratin that can occupy most of the nest forming a squamous pearl. Nuclei show minimal pleomorphism, with atypia tending to be limited to the periphery of the epithelial nests. Mitoses are scarce (Fig. 7.2a)

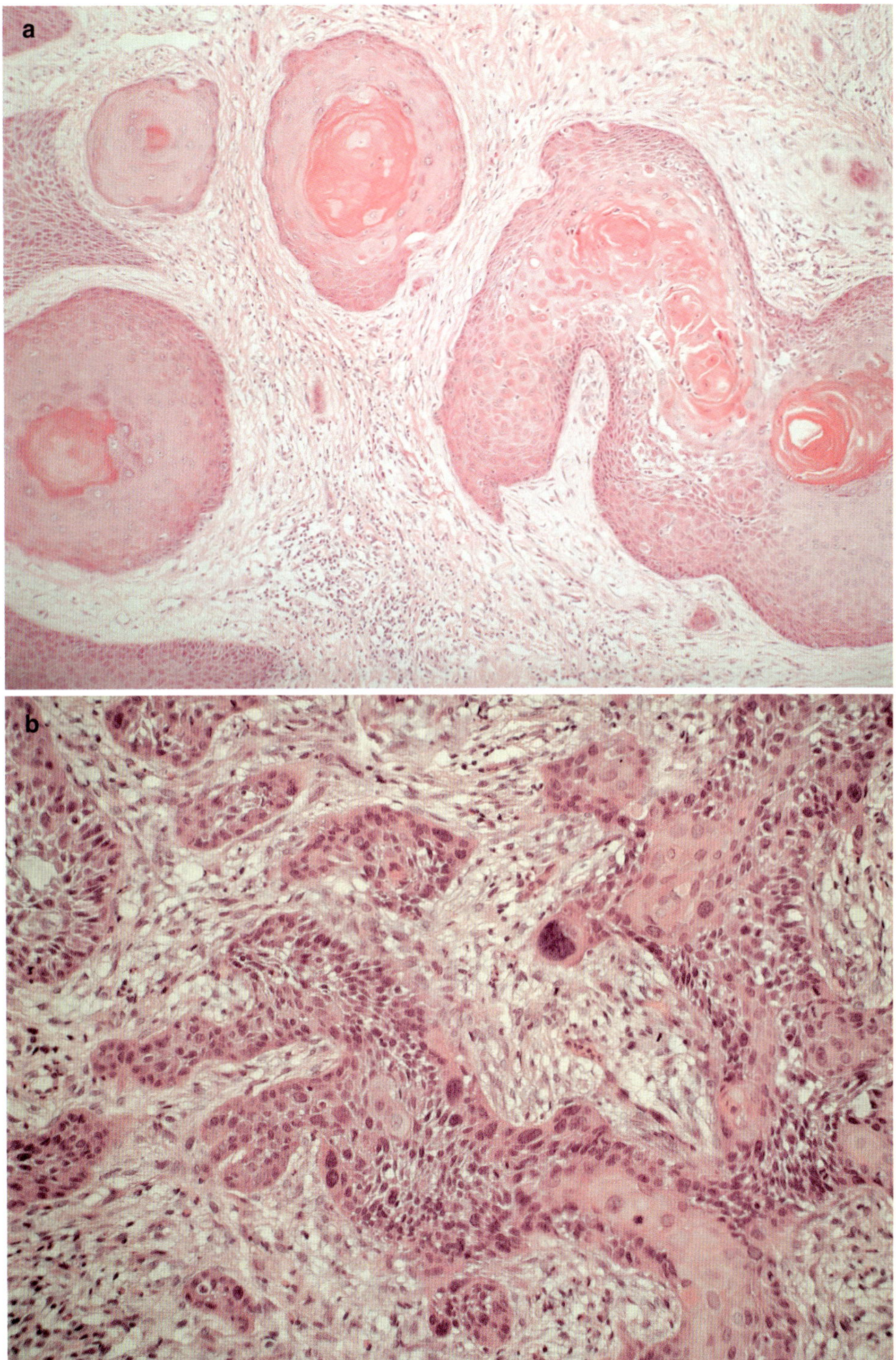

Fig. 7.2 (**a**) Well-differentiated squamous cell carcinoma showing more than 70% keratinization. (**b**) Moderately differentiated squamous carcinoma showing 50% keratinization

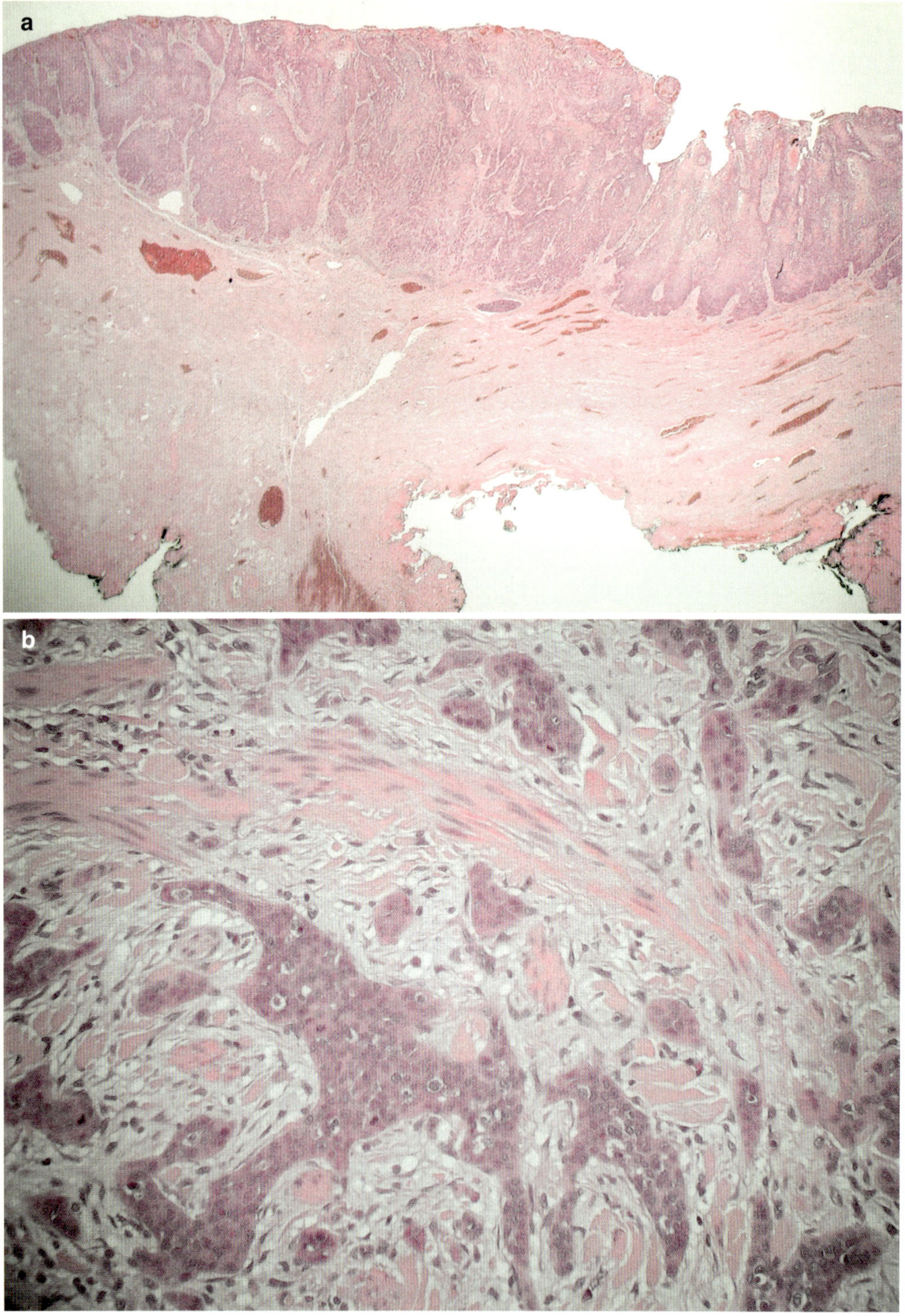

Fig. 7.3 (**a**) Poorly differentiated squamous carcinoma showing very little keratinization. (d) Poorly differentiated squamous carcinoma with a few individually keratinized cells

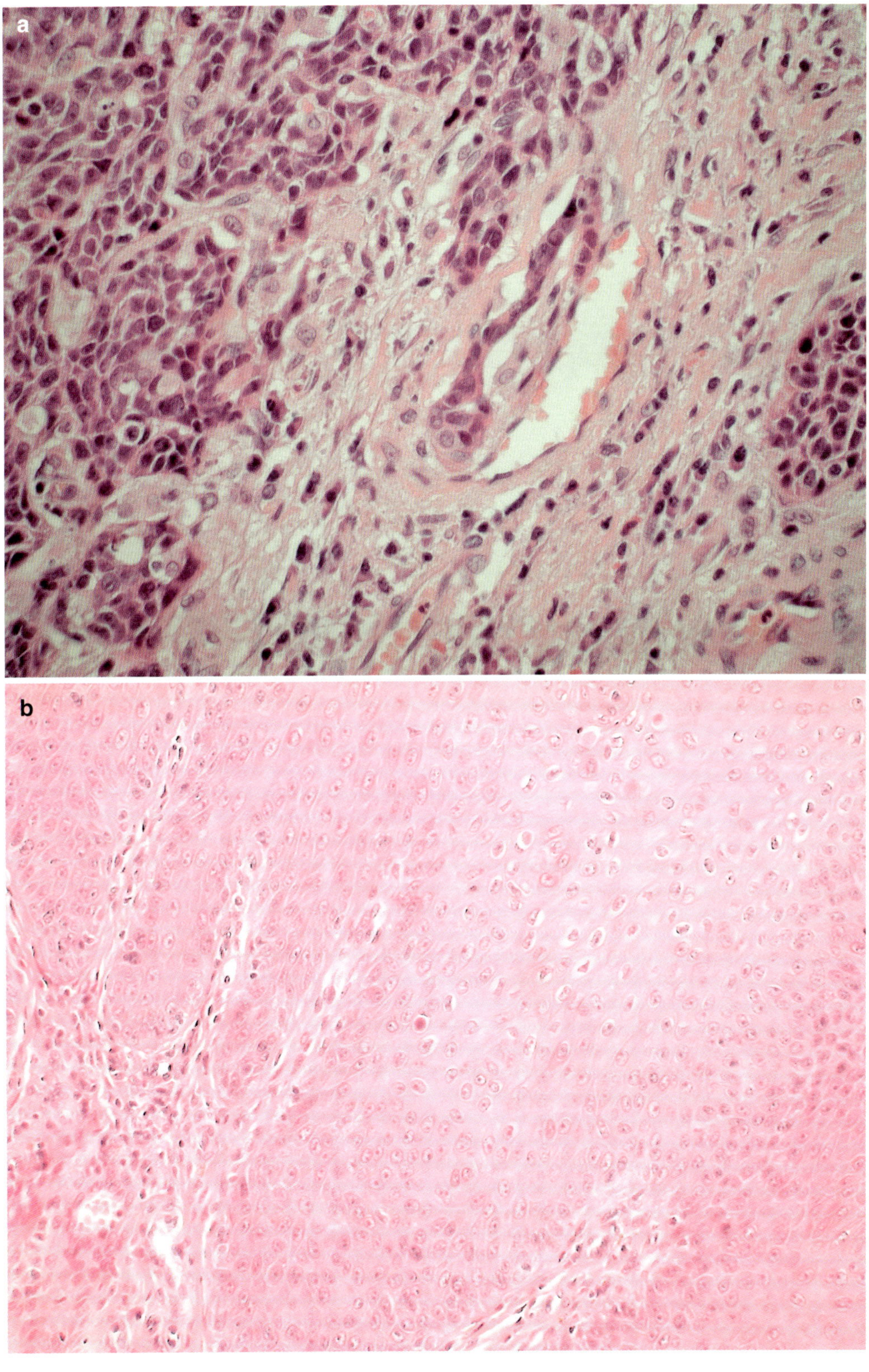

Fig. 7.4 (**a**) Basaloid squamous carcinoma with no keratinization. (**b**) Warty squamous carcinoma. Note the variable chromatin of the atypical koilocytes

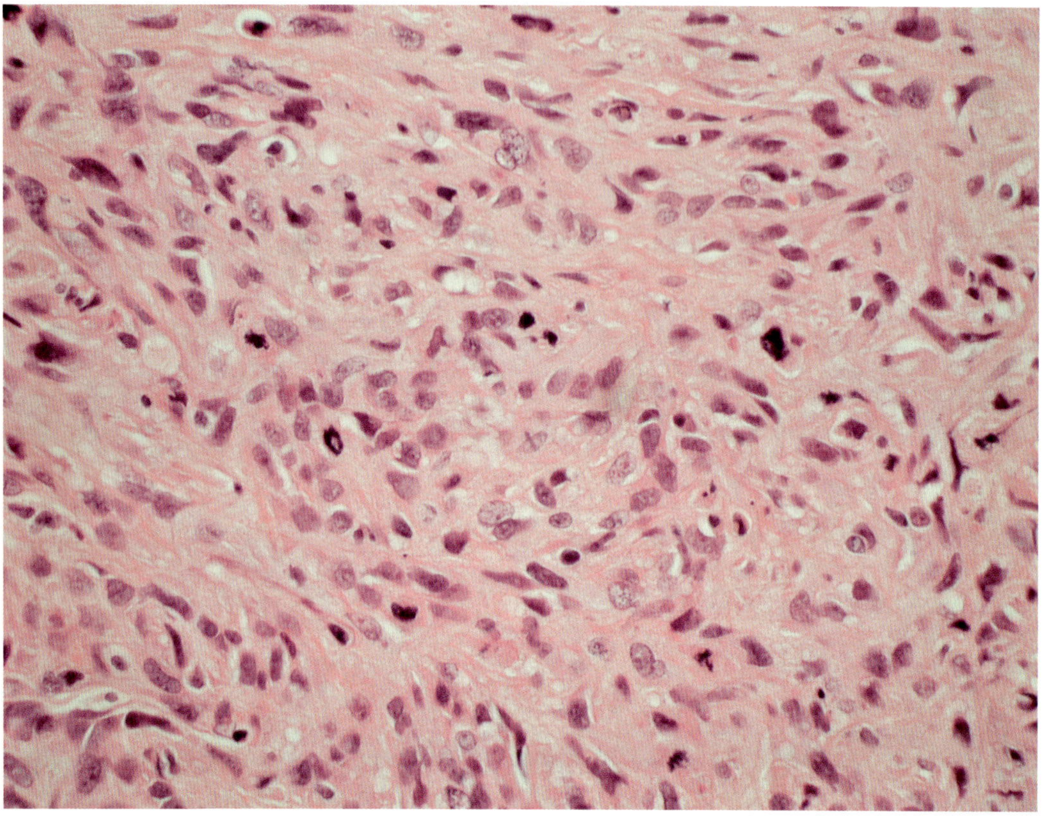

Fig. 7.5 Spindle and epithelioid cells in a sarcomatoid squamous carcinoma

Moderately differentiated tumors have more sharply angulated outlines to the invasive foci, and between one-third and two-thirds of the cell nests are keratinized. There is more nuclear pleomorphism with nuclei occupying up to one-third of the cell diameter. Mitotic figures and less well-differentiated cells are scattered through the cell nests (Fig. 7.2b).

Poorly differentiated tumors feature infiltrating cells, perhaps individually poorly keratinized, arranged more randomly in sheets, cords, or small nests without central keratinization. In the absence of obvious nesting, the tumor/stromal border can be very irregular. Mitoses may be numerous, atypical, and scattered through the tumor islands (Fig. 7.3a, b).

Keratinizing squamous carcinoma is generally negative for p16 and positive for p53, mirroring the reactivity of d-VIN and providing further proof of d-VIN as a precursor lesion and the lack of HPV as a cause [8]. To be considered positive, p53 reaction should be strongly nuclear [9].

Non-keratinizing Squamous Carcinoma

These are tumors in which there is no obvious cytoplasmic keratinization. Tumors with a spindle cell stroma can cause confusion with sarcomas or carcinosarcomas [10] (see section "Sarcomatoid squamous carcinoma").

Basaloid Squamous Carcinoma

This is a tumor composed more predominantly of small, non-keratinizing cells and tends to occur in women under 50, with a high incidence of association with high-grade VIN and HPV infection, particularly in women under 40 [11, 12]

(Fig. 7.4a). The tumors show p16 reactivity and tend to be p53 negative, contrasting with the etiology of keratinizing tumors [9]. Younger women seem particularly at risk if immunosuppressed [13], and there have been several reports such tumors developing in young women with Fanconi's syndrome [12, 14], Hodgkin's disease [12], renal allograft [15–17], HIV seropositivity [18], chemotherapy [13], and liver disease [13].

Warty Squamous Carcinoma

These tumors show the more recognizable features of HPV infection, appearing as keratinized, warty, often grossly exophytic masses on the vulva. The tumors account for 7–10% of vulvar carcinomas and show marked epithelial acanthosis with koilocytosis, dyskeratosis, multinucleation, and wrinkled irregular nuclei (Fig. 7.4b). The adjacent epithelium can also show similar changes of HPV infection or gross warty change, with or without VIN [19]. Most are associated with u-VIN and are p16 positive and p53 negative, indicating the HPV etiology [8, 9].

Sarcomatoid Squamous Carcinoma

A poorly differentiated, aggressive variant features a spindle cell, sarcomatoid morphology [10, 20] (Fig. 7.5). By light microscopy, mucin stains are negative and electron microscopy shows tonofilaments and desmosomes [10]. Immunohistochemistry of the spindle cell component demonstrates cytokeratins, indicating metaplastic derivation from epithelial cells [21]. The tumor can metastasize as either keratinizing squamous carcinoma or as a sarcomatoid version.

Incidence/Epidemiology

Carcinoma of the vulva is rare, representing less than 1% of all cancers and 3–6% of all gynecological cancers. Most patients are aged between 50 and 80 [22]. The risk of metastasis and death from squamous carcinoma of the vulva is far higher than squamous carcinoma elsewhere on the skin, with a 5-year survival of 58% for vulval cancer comparing to essentially 100% 5-year survival for non-melanoma skin cancer [23]. The incidence is increasing, probably due to a combination of rising rates of HPV infection secondary to more liberal sexual standards, smoking and increased detection [24, 25], particularly in western societies. The worldwide incidence was estimated to be 27,000 in 2006 [26]. The highest rates in 2002 were in the USA and northern and eastern Europe of 1.5/100,000, with slightly lower rates of 1.3/100,000 in western Europe with the lowest 0.25/100,000 in eastern Asia.

In the UK, in 2007, there were 1,120 new cases, equating to a rate of 3.6/100,000. In the years 2004–2008, there were, on average, 373 deaths a year in the UK.

As might be anticipated, the risk of death from vulval carcinoma rises sharply with age, with death rates of 0.1/100,000 under 44 years, 0.5/100,000 for age range 45–64 years, 6/100,000 for women over 65 years, and 12/100,000 for those over 80 years. The death rate from vulval cancer has been dropping steadily over the past 40 years, falling by 62% for those aged 45–64 and 29% for those over 65. The statistical research team of the CRUK calculated that the lifetime risk of developing vulval cancer for women in the UK is 1 in 316 [24].

Of all the common gynecological cancers, some work from Israel [27] and Denmark [28] indicates that the diagnosis of vulval carcinoma can be the most delayed: nearly twice that of cervical carcinoma, about two and a half times that of endometrial cancer and slightly more than three times that for ovarian carcinoma. This is mainly accounted for by the patients' reluctance to seek medical advice, presumably because the symptoms are not as troubling as for these other three malignancies. Overall, there appears to be no grounds for the perception that significant delay is caused by the GPs' reluctance to examine [29, 30].

There are two different types of squamous carcinoma of the vulva in women: those occurring in younger patients, associated with u-VIN and

HPV infection [11], and those of older women linked to chronic irritation, d-VIN, lichen sclerosus, and squamous hyperplasia. It is possible that a small number of cases may arise from an intraepithelial squamous carcinoma that has morphological similarities to Paget's disease—the so-called Pagetoid squamous carcinoma in situ [31]. Immunosuppression and pregnancy are associated with more rapidly progressing lesions at an earlier age [32–34].

Prognostic Factors for Squamous Carcinoma Vulva

The prognosis of squamous carcinoma depends primarily on stage, and this is determined by the size of the lesion, the depth of invasion, spread beyond the vulva, the presence and number of involved lymph nodes, the size of metastasis in the nodes and the presence of extranodal spread [35, 36]. Overall, the 1-year survival is now 96.4–100% for stage I, 87.6–100% for stage II, 75–86% for stage III and 29–35% for stage IV [22, 35, 36]. The 5-year survival stages I–IV is 78.5%, 58.8%, 43.2%, 13%, respectively [22]. Survival is inversely proportional to age: 100% of those under 30 will be alive at 5 years; this drops to 65–54% for those aged 60–80 and 32% for those over 80 [22, 37].

The grade of differentiation can influence the progression of some cases [38], and this is most marked for poor differentiation [39, 40], but compared to stage, degree of differentiation has very little impact on survival [6, 41, 42].

The FIGO staging system was revised in 2009 [43], to clarify the impact of the number and size of lymph node metastasis (Table 7.1). Invasion equal to or less than 1 mm predicts a negligible risk of lymph node metastasis [44] and overall, positive lymph nodes reduce the 10-year survival by approximately two-thirds to a half, being 90–76% for negative nodes and 32–39.5% for node positive cases [14–16]. Extranodal extension in one or more nodes reduces 5-year survival from 80–51% to 30–15% [14, 17] (Fig. 7.6a). Overall survival can be linked to the number of involved nodes [45], extracapsular spread and how many of the nodes are more than 50% replaced by metastasis [46], but involvement of only one or two nodes has a risk of recurrence similar to node-negative patients [35]. In support of the FIGO staging system, bilateral node involvement was no more important than the number of nodes involved [47]. A study that did not confirm the relationship of multiple node involvement, by itself, to poor prognosis found that other parameters of poor prognosis such as size of metastasis and extranodal extension were linked to number of involved nodes [48].

Table 7.1 FIGO 2009 staging for carcinoma of the vulva [43]

Stage I: Tumor confined to the vulva
Stage I A: Tumor confined to the vulva or perineum, ≤2 cm in size with stromal invasion ≤1 mm[a], negative nodes
Stage I B: Tumor confined to the vulva or perineum, > 2 cm in size or with stromal invasion >1 mm[a], negative nodes
Stage II: Tumor of any size with extension to adjacent perineal structures (1/3 lower urethra, 1/3 lower vagina, anus), negative nodes
Stage III: Tumor of any size with or without extension to adjacent perineal structures (1/3 lower urethra, 1/3 lower vagina, anus) with positive inguinofemoral lymph nodes
Stage III A: (i) One lymph node metastasis (≥5 mm) or (ii) One to two lymph node metastasis(es) (<5 mm)
Stage III B (i) Two or more lymph nodes metastases (≥5 mm) or (ii) Three or more lymph nodes metastases (<5 mm)
Stage III C: Positive nodes with extracapsular spread
Stage IV: Tumor invades other regional structures (2/3 upper urethra, 2/3 upper vagina) or distant structures
Stage IV A: Tumor invades any of the following:
(i) Upper urethra and/or vaginal mucosa, bladder mucosa, rectal mucosa, or fixed to pelvic bone
(ii) Fixed or ulcerated inguinofemoral lymph nodes
Stage IV B: Any distant metastasis including pelvic lymph nodes

NB: Vascular space involvement, either venous or lymphatic, does not alter the staging

[a]The depth of invasion is defined as the measurement of the tumor from the epithelial-stromal junction of the adjacent most superficial epithelial papilla to the deepest point of invasion

Lymphovascular space involvement (Fig. 7.6b) does not alter the stage, but has been shown to be an independent prognostic variable [48], relating

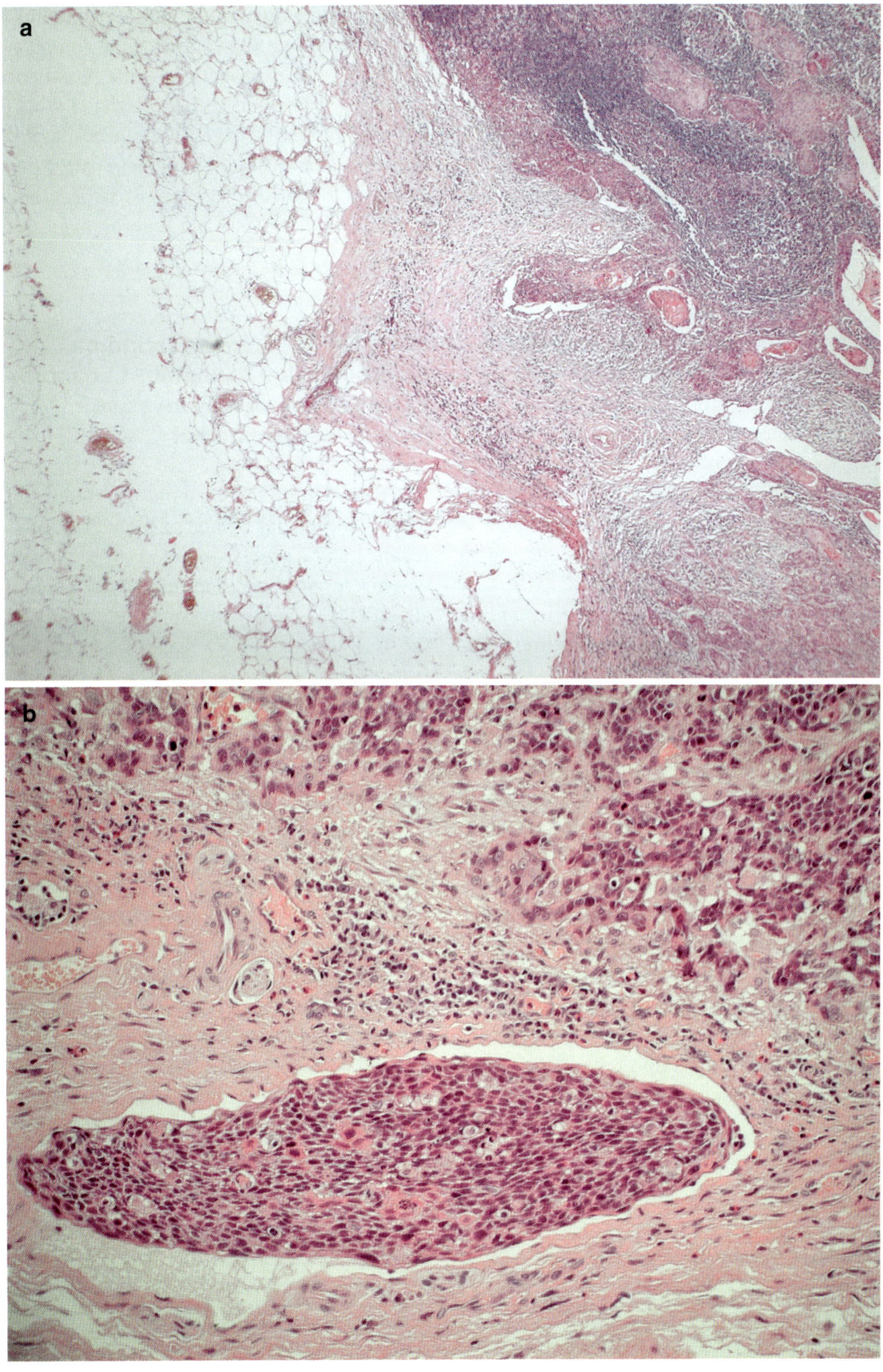

Fig. 7.6 (**a**) Metastatic squamous carcinoma in a lymph node extending into the extranodal tissue. Note the desmoplastic stromal reaction. (**b**) Lymphovascular involvement by poorly differentiated squamous carcinoma

both to recurrence and metastasis. Excision with pathological margins (after fixation) of less than 8 mm has been shown by some to be associated with local recurrence [10, 18, 39], but not by all.

In a series of 145 women with stage 1 or 2 tumors, neither Ag NOR counts nor proliferation as measured by Ki67 had any bearing on lymph node metastasis or prognosis [49].

Lymph node metastasis has been linked to S phase fraction and Her2 status [50]. Retinoblastoma protein (pRp) expression is not linked to outcome, but there is reduced expression with advancing stage [21, 51]. Neither p53 mutations [15, 20] nor DNA ploidy appear to influence outcome but aneuploidy has been linked to poor prognosis in some studies [12, 18, 20]. HPV infection is linked to p16 and p14 expression and is inversely proportional to p53 expression. High p14 correlates with longer survival [21].

In a study where a third of the series of 101 squamous carcinomas developed recurrent disease, recurrence was associated with stage, lymph node involvement, size of the lesion (>2.5 cm), positive margins and accompanying VIN 2/3 [52]. Hence, the removal of all the carcinoma is important to prevent recurrent disease. Groin recurrence has a bleak prognosis [53]. The accuracy of surgery can be improved by per-operative frozen section of the margins including skin, urethral and the Cloquet node [54], using parallel, tangential cuts to the margin. This reduces sampling artifact, but compromises an assessment of the tumor-free distance to the resection margin. The authors attained 100% diagnostic accuracy for the node by frozen section with 98.6% accuracy for the margins, but this took up to 44 min (mean 24.4 min) and could have huge resource implications.

Increased numbers of tissue eosinophils are said to be an indication of invasion and may correlate to a better prognosis, while blood eosinophilia has been said to be associated with poor outcome [25, 26]. However, tissue eosinophilia is also caused by arthropod bite and parasite infestation as shown by a report of two cases with squamous hyperplasia and Enterobious vermicularis infestation [55].

Stage 1A Squamous Carcinoma (Microinvasive Squamous Carcinoma, Early or Superficially Invasive Squamous Carcinoma)

The terminology for squamous carcinoma invading the superficial stroma of the vulva is so confusing and poorly defined [56] that the classifications of microinvasive carcinoma, superficial and early invasion are abandoned for the well-defined FIGO stage 1A: less than or equal to 1 mm invasion in a lesion less than 2 cm in diameter with no nodal metastasis [43]. The importance of recognizing this stage is that, if completely excised, there is a negligible risk of metastasis [57].

Clinically, these carcinomas appear no different to VIN. Histologically, invasion takes the form of small buds, single cells, fine cords, or thin tongues of cells invading the stroma through the epithelial basement membrane (Fig. 7.7a). It can be difficult to distinguish invasion from tangential cuts through irregular epithelial down growths, so multiple levels are usually necessary to establish the morphology. The outline of invasive foci is often less well delineated from the stroma and can be sharply pointed, branching, or irregular (Fig. 7.7b). This contrasts with the more

Fig. 7.7 (**a**) Squamous carcinoma stage 1a invading the superficial stroma. Note the desmoplastic stromal reaction. (**b**) This is almost the smallest discernable example of stromal invasion. The infiltrating epithelium is more eosinophilic than the basal epithelium from which it arose and has an irregular, sharply pointed contour

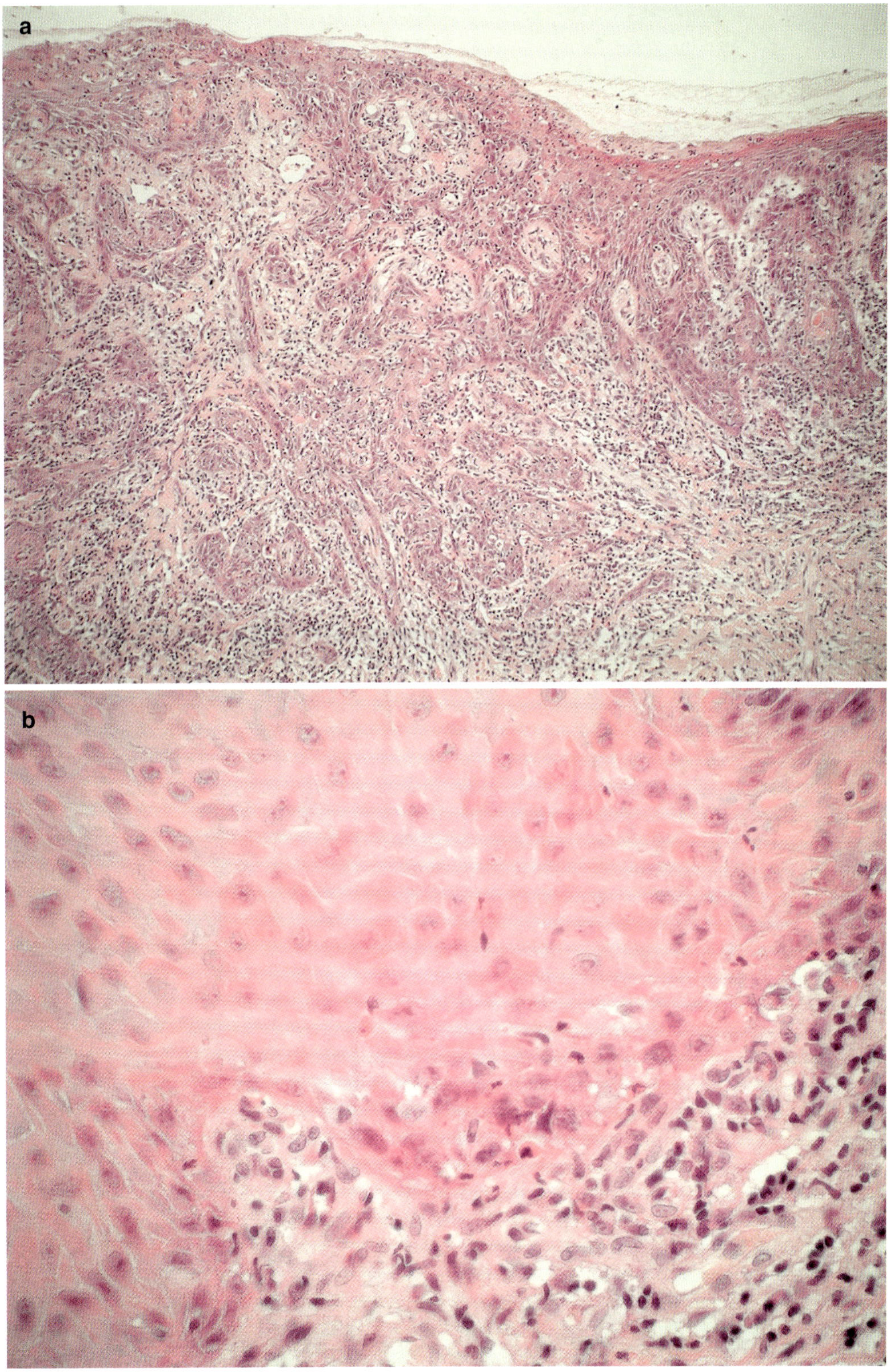

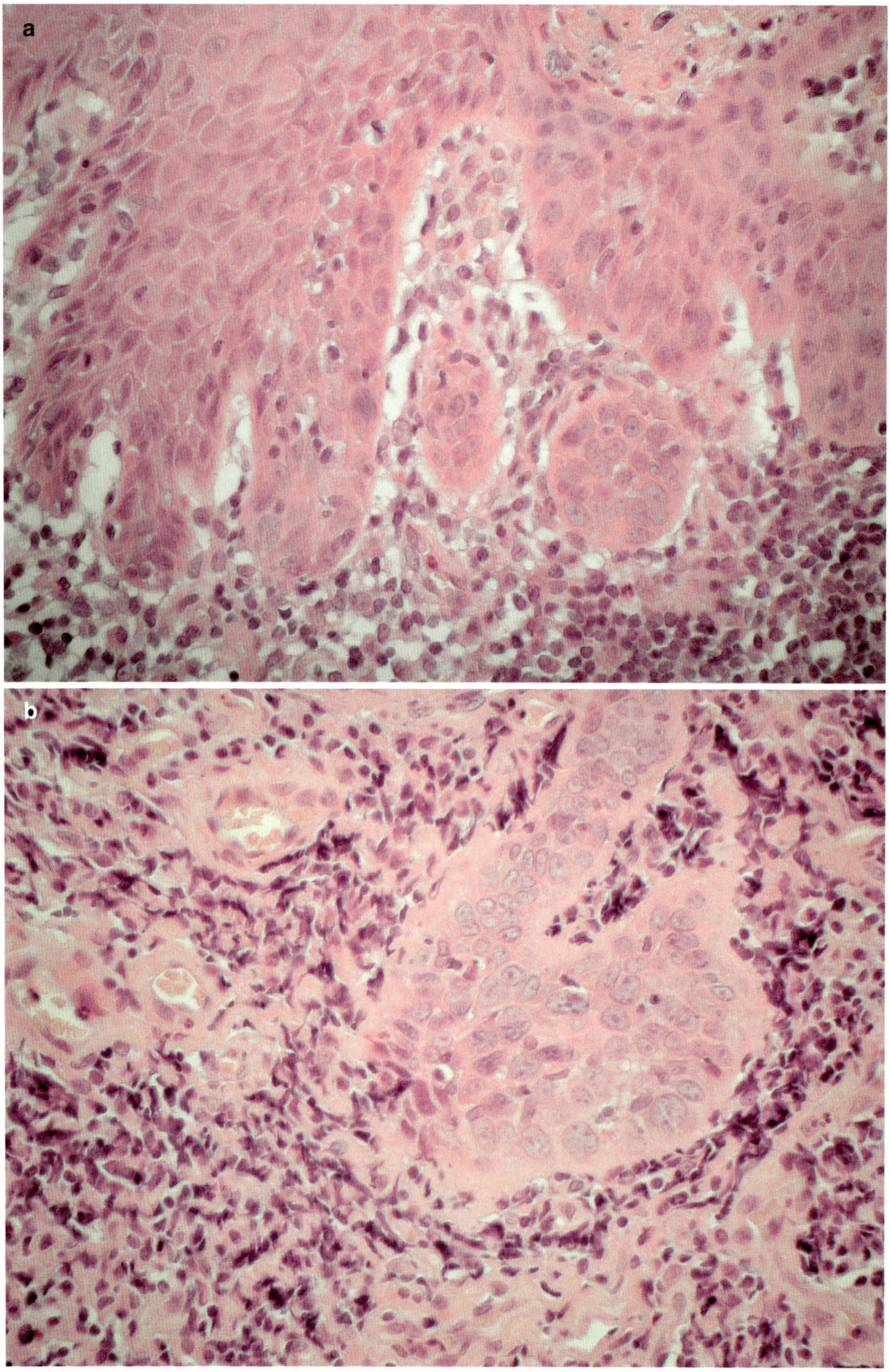

Fig. 7.8 (**a**) This is noninvasive: note the preserved basement membrane and rounded contour to the epithelial downgrowth. (**b**) Higher power view to show the rounded profile of noninvasive buds of epithelium

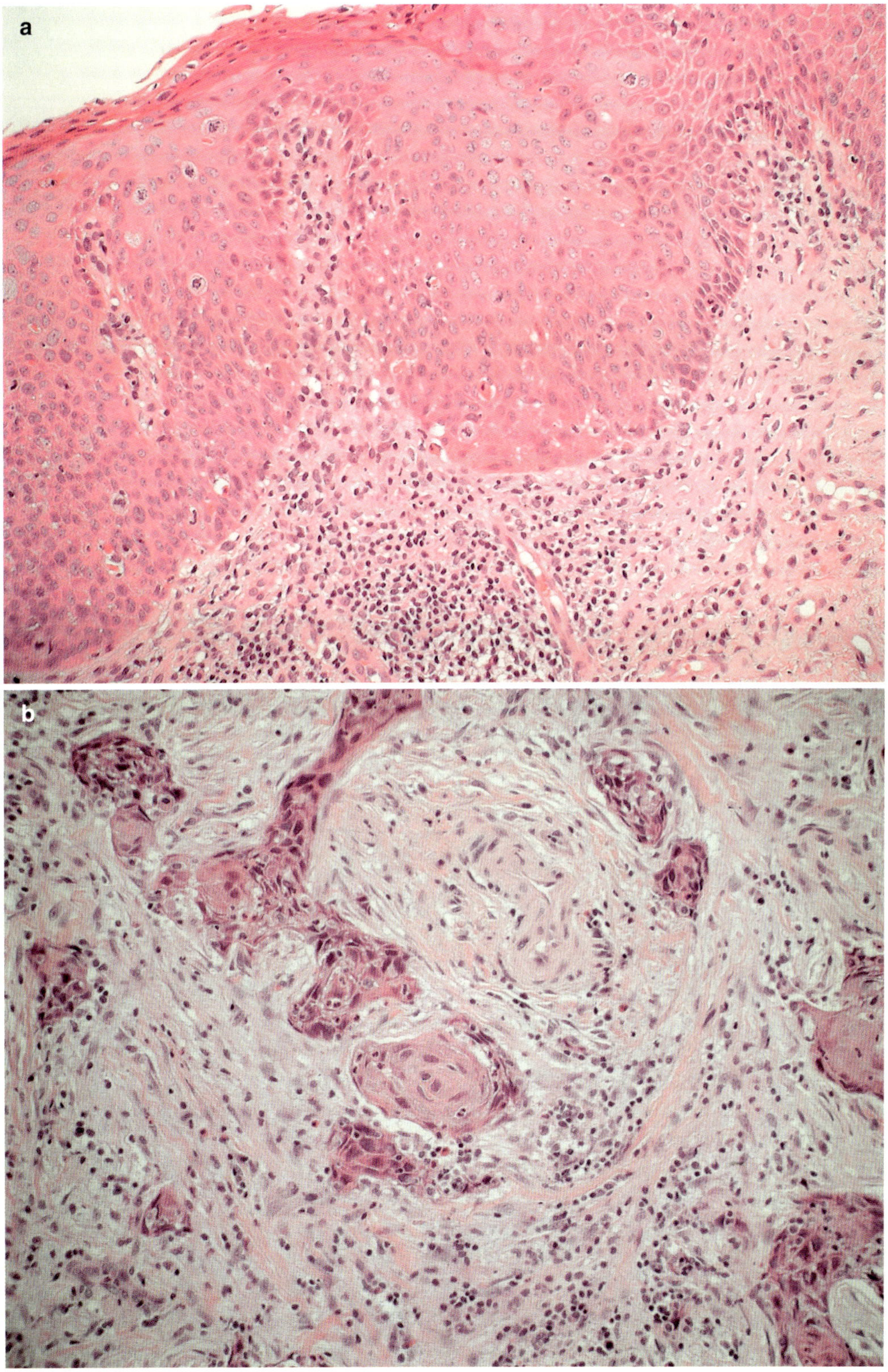

Fig. 7.9 (**a**) More obvious keratinization in a superficially invasive stage 1a squamous carcinoma. (**b**) Prominent stromal desmoplastic reaction to islands of moderately differentiated squamous carcinoma infiltrating around a small arteriole

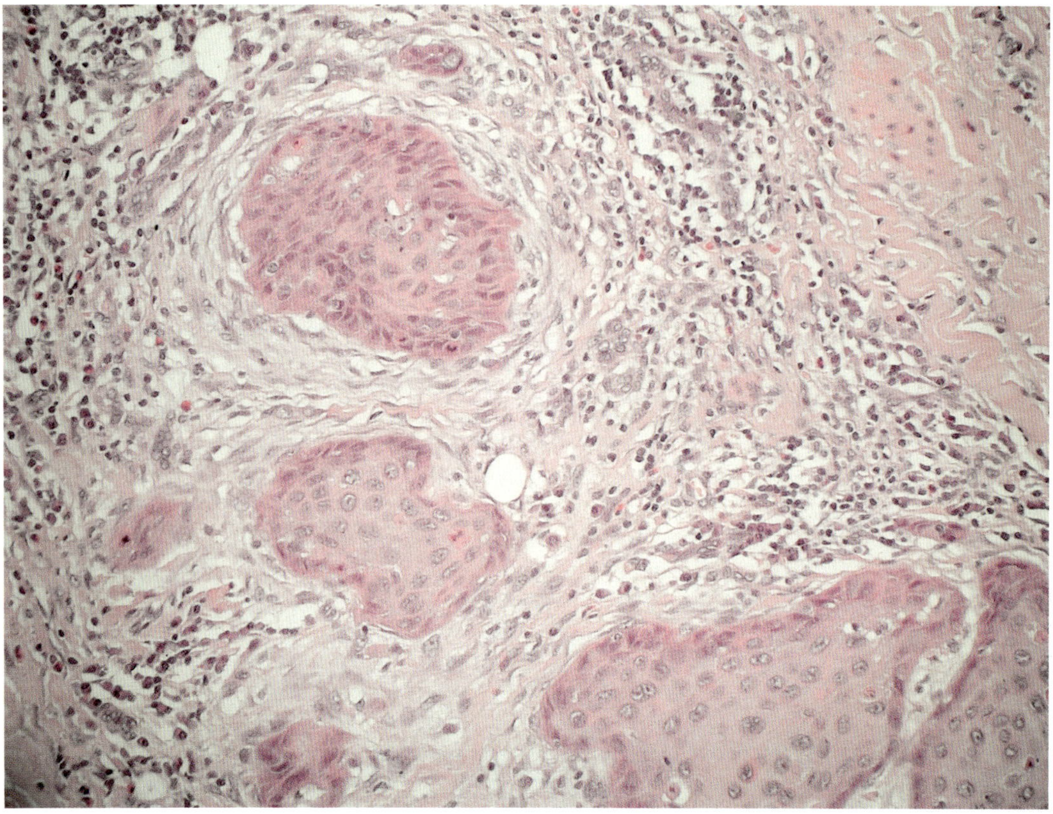

Fig. 7.10 Stromal desmoplasia around moderately differentiated squamous carcinoma

rounded outline of noninvasive epithelial pegs (Fig. 7.8a, b). The invasive cells may exhibit paradoxical differentiation and appear more eosinophilic or keratinized than the basal layer from which they arise (Fig. 7.9a). Other features that help the diagnosis of invasion include a desmoplastic stromal response and irregularity of contour of the invasive tongues (Fig. 7.9b, 7.10).

The method for measuring invasion is critical and is different to the measurement of depth of invasion in the cervix. Conceptually, invasion could be measured from the surface of the tumor or the granular cell layer to the deepest point of invasion, from the deepest rete ridge to the deepest point of invasion [57], or from the epithelial basement membrane from which the tumor appears to arise [58]. However, these may not be reproducible because the granular cell layer may be absent, there may be surface ulceration, or dysplastic basement epithelial layers can be difficult to distinguish from the invasive cells. Measurement of tumor volume (approximated to a truncated cone) is difficult, requires a complex formula and has not been shown to correlate with behavior [56, 57]. Consequently, studies have shown that the most reproducible method to establish those lesions which have the least risk of metastasis is to *measure invasion to the deepest point of the invasive focus from the dermoepidermal junction of the next most superficial dermal papilla* [43, 57]. Hence, a few buds of cells arising from the tip of an epithelial downgrowth acquire more depth than might be initially appreciated and thus more significance with regard to potential metastasis. The lateral extent of the tumor must also be assessed in the third dimension by correlating the position of the tumor in several blocks. If tumor involves more than seven adjacent blocks which are 3 mm or more in thickness, then the tumor maximum dimension is greater than 20 mm and is too large to be included in stage 1a.

Vascular space involvement has not been shown to influence the incidence of metastasis and so does not affect the stage [43, 56].

The risk of lymph mode metastasis with invasion equal to or less than 1 mm is very low, but is not zero. By 2007 [59], nine instances of metastasis from validated cases of stage 1a squamous carcinoma had been reported. Lymph node recurrences have occurred at 3–36 months [59–64]. There is a greater risk of rapid metastasis in immunosuppressed women [15]. The risk of metastasis is not thought to be sufficient to warrant lymphadenectomy for stage 1a cases, but sentinel node biopsy could play an important role in individualizing treatment for these women [60].

Risk of Metastasis

The pattern of lymph node spread is well documented and predictable [65]. Unilateral tumors spread to the ipsilateral nodes; midline tumors can spread bilaterally. This might require only ipsilateral node surgery [66] and clearly supports the role of sentinel node assessment (see below). Up to 20–30% of stage 1 or stage 2 vulval carcinomas will have lymph node metastasis. But groin node dissection comes with high morbidity. The challenge is to identify those tumors that pose a lower risk of metastasis, independent of stage. Epidermal growth factor receptor is overexpressed in squamous carcinoma of the vulva, as with similar tumors of the cervix and vagina [67]. A study [68] designed to determine whether those squamous carcinomas of the vulva which did not express EGRF presented a lower risk of metastasis confirmed EGFR expression in 68% of tumors. There was insufficient correlation between EGFR expression and nodal metastasis to allow prediction of metastasis. Even after the inclusion of other risk parameters, the prediction would give a false-negative rate of 6%.

One small study of 51 cases of squamous carcinoma showed that when a prominent fibromyxoid stromal response developed instead of the more usual desmoplastic reaction to invasion, there was an association with age, worse survival and more extensive lymph node metastasis [69]. The authors postulated that the collagen laid down in a desmoplastic response might offer some protection not provided by the immature collagen in the loose myxoid stroma that they felt typified the fibromyxoid stromal response. The hyaluronic acid of the myxoid component of the stroma might allow tumor cell mobility and also contribute to a more aggressive behavior. Further work is needed in a larger series to categorize these stromal reactions more fully.

Inguinal Node Dissection for Squamous Carcinoma

The classical treatment of carcinoma of the vulva is radical dissection and removal of most of the vulva including each set of labia, the clitoris and fourchette in continuity with the groin nodes (inguinofemoral lymphadenectomy) on both sides in a butterfly incision. This is a drastic operation that leads to significant local morbidity with risks of wound infection, lymphedema of the legs, lymphocyst, thromboembolism and extended hospital admission. Modern surgical techniques have sought to limit morbidity by reducing the extent of the vulval surgery to the lesion and surrounding tissues (simple vulvectomy, hemi-vulvectomy, or wide local excision) and removing the regional groin nodes in separate parts, giving a three block removal. Unilateral dissections are employed if the primary lesion is well localized to one side. Midline lesions require bilateral groin node dissections. This has been shown to have led to an increase in local recurrences but no reduction in survival [70]. Groin recurrence is recognized to have a very poor prognosis [65].

Latterly, sentinel node dissection has been introduced in some centers in an attempt to reduce the problems of lymphedema and lymphocyst associated with full node dissection [71]. Theoretically, if the first node draining an anatomical area (the sentinel node) is tumor-free, then the nodes receiving subsequent drainage should not contain metastases [30, 32]. Detailed examination of the sentinel node is employed to detect any metastastic disease. If the node is shown to be tumor-free, then a full nodal dissection on that side should not be necessary and morbidity can be lessened.

The sentinel node is identified clinically by a ^{99m}Technetium-nanocolloid (^{99m}Tc)-labeled injection into the vulval lymphatic drainage [72], usually by injecting around the lesion. Per-operatively, identification of the sentinel node is further assisted by blue dye that is injected in the same way. Following work on breast, skin, and gastric cancer, initial studies indicate that it might be possible to replace this 2-stage technique with a 1-stage fluorescent imaging system [33]. There is less likelihood of missing the sentinel node if the primary lesion has not been locally resected before definitive surgery. It might be that surgery alters lymphatic drainage around the tumor, compromising the investigation [73].

A review of 15 studies [74] showed a detection rate of 82–100% for the sentinel node, with false-negative results most often occurring for those women with midline tumors, where the lymph drainage is not as predictable.

Usually one or two, but occasionally up to four sentinel lymph nodes are identified. These can be evaluated by frozen section per-operatively or by conventional histology or by serial sectioning with immunohistochemistry [75]. The recommendation is for blocking the node at one block for every 5 mm of node diameter. Negative nodes are subjected to 200-μm serial sectioning with immunohistochemistry for pancytokeratins [74]. Conventional histopathology of sentinel nodes is accepted in some major centers [73].

A micrometastasis, drawing on studies of breast cancer, is defined as one less than 2 mm in diameter [76]. Micrometastasis in a sentinel node, identified after the initial dissection by serial sectioning, was shown to be associated with groin recurrence in one case [77], but it is possible that this was as part of a more extensive node dissection [78]. The detection of squamous cell micrometastases is made easier by immunohistochemistry for cytokeratins [79]. But serial sectioning has been shown by some to be as effective as immunohistochemistry in identifying metastases [76] and in a series of 110 nodes that were negative by conventional histology [80] immunohistochemistry picked up no metastases that had been missed. Conversely, ultrastaging identified micrometastases in two nodes previously judged negative by conventional sectioning [72]. A small study showed that 6/13 patients with micrometastases, identified by serial sectioning and cytokeratin immunohistochemistry, died compared to four who died in the group without micrometastases [81]. A 1-mm micrometastasis in a sentinel node biopsy was followed by a groin scar recurrence [82]. As yet, the pathological significance of micrometastases has to be established.

Immunohistochemistry and conventional histology sometimes identify aneucleate cellular fragments. These do not behave as metastases and a node containing such deposits should be regarded as negative [83].

The Groningen International Study on Sentinel Nodes in Vulval Cancer (GROINSS-V) [43] has been set up to examine prospectively the safety and use of sentinel node biopsy in this site. Their protocol for lymph node examination requires all of the nodes to be embedded in blocks taken at 2–3 mm. One H&E and two unstained sections are taken from each block and, then, if negative 500 μm step sections are taken. Immuno for AE1/3, spare, and H&E are taken of each. The number of involved nodes, size of the metastasis and any extranodal spread is reported. The therapeutic objective is for complete absence of groin recurrence following identification of sentinel nodes. For early stage (T1, T2), this has been achieved in a series of 34 patients [84], but GROINSS-V showed 6 recurrences in 403 patients (2%) [85].

The clinical significance of micrometastases has been controversial, with the implication for recurrent or distant metastatic disease not established.

In an attempt to clarify whether nodes identified as positive by ultrastaging alone had the same prognostic implications as metastasis identified by conventional histology, the GROINSS study used two histopathologists to review those 307 of their 403 patients where there were suitable samples [43]. In 164 groin dissections, one or two positive nodes had been identified. Immunohistochemistry identified micrometastases in 36/304 (12%) of patients with previously negative nodes. The risk of spread to the non-sentinel nodes was not found to be increased with the number of positive sentinel nodes per groin but was related to the size of the sentinel node metastasis. The risk of metastasis to the non-sentinel nodes was 4.2% for isolated tumor cells, 10% for ≤1 mm, 11.1% for >1–2 mm, 13.3% for >2–5 mm, 38.5% for >5–10 mm and 62.5% for ≥10 mm.

Increasing size of sentinel node metastasis reduced survival at 5 years: a few small scattered cells gave 97% survival, 2 mm gave 88% survival. 2–5 mm gave 70%, and >5 mm gave 69%. The authors therefore concluded that they could not establish a minimum size below which there was negligible risk of spread, yet they conceded that they could not say whether this alone influenced survival because all their patients with positive nodes (with any size of metastasis) received lymph node clearance. Yet the risk of groin recurrence is unrelated to the size of sentinel node metastasis and groin recurrence with uninvolved sentinel nodes was found to be 2.9% [46]. This could equally well be used as an argument *against* ultrastaging as with the Breast Screening Programme [86] where sentinel nodes are not ultrastaged. Clearly, more work is required to establish the relevance of micrometastases in lymph nodes in vulval cancer.

It has been suggested that at least ten lymph nodes represents an adequate inguinal dissection [87], but the removal of more than seven lymph nodes has a higher association with local complications such as lymphedema [88].

Adenoid Squamous Carcinoma (Pseudoangiosarcomatous Squamous Cell Carcinoma, Pseudovascular Squamous Carcinoma, Pseudoglandular Squamous Carcinoma)

Rarely, acantholysis in squamous carcinoma (Fig. 7.11) results in multiple anastomosing cords of squamous cells and the spaces between these

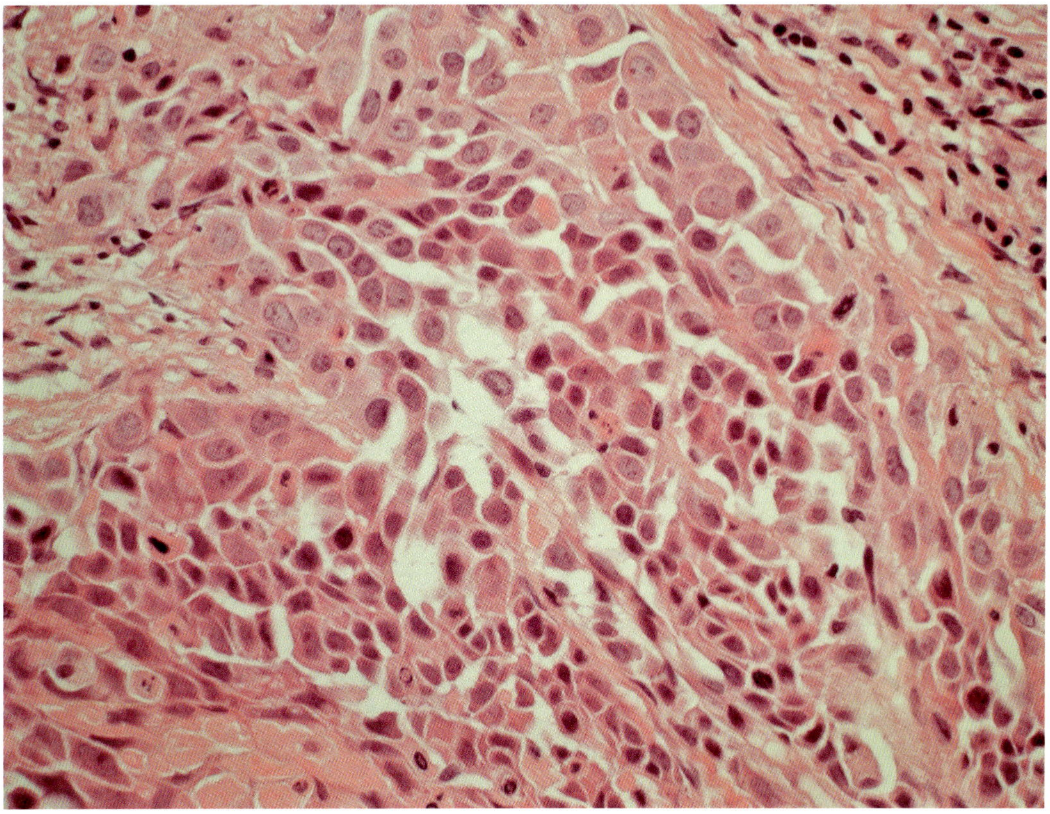

Fig. 7.11 Acantholytic squamous carcinoma. The cellular discohesion gives rise to intercellular clefts and gland-like spaces

cells looking like vascular channels with peripherally placed atypical nuclei [89]. Adenoid variants [90] of squamous carcinoma show larger intercellular spaces where connections between cells have broken down to give pseudoglandular spaces. A distinction must be made between true acantholysis and mucin production in an adenosquamous carcinoma. The series reported by Underwood shows a good example of pseudoangiosarcomatous growth in an acantholytic squamous carcinoma but also includes tumors that represent true mixtures of squamous and glandular cells where there is mucin production [91], at variance with the original description of adenoid squamous carcinomas at this site where the absence of mucin is emphasized [90].

Vascular markers are negative, but note that some true angiosarcomas can produce cytokeratins. Consequently, a mixture of cytokeratin markers, such as EA1/3, MNF116, and EMA, and endothelial markers such as CD31, CD34, and factor VIII is necessary to confirm the diagnosis [47, 50]. Horn et al [89]. prefer the term pseudoangiosarcomatous squamous cell carcinoma (PSCC) as it presents a spurious resemblance to angiosarcoma, but the entity encompasses adenoid squamous carcinoma and pseudoglandular squamous carcinoma.

Most cases are HPV negative [92], although some of Carson's series were probably true adenosquamous carcinomas with mucin production. One case, in a woman of 69, contained HPV DNA by pcr and showed strong $p16^{INK4a}$ positivity [93] It is more common to find associated lichen sclerosus and chronic irritation, mainly in older women (age range 57–84), although one case was in a woman of 44 [89].

This type of squamous carcinoma is more common on the head and neck where it was postulated that the breakdown of intercellular connections was caused by sunlight damage. However, in the vulva, lungs [94], breast [95], mouth [96], and cervix [97], it is clear that ultraviolet radiation cannot be the cause.

These tumors tend to have an aggressive behavior [93] with a higher rate of lymph node metastasis [45, 48]. In one series, survival for adenoid squamous carcinoma was only 58% at 3 years compared to 96.5% for squamous carcinoma [92].

Verrucous Carcinoma

This appears as a large, often very large, papillary, warty, or fungating lesion that can extend over the labia majora to involve the majority of the vulva [98, 99]. The tumor more commonly occurs in the skin, larynx, and mouth, rarely in the vagina and cervix [100] with case reports in the endometrium [101] and ovary [102].

Essentially a well-differentiated type of vulval squamous carcinoma of middle-aged to elderly women [103, 104], this variant differs from the usual types of squamous carcinoma by its pushing, apparently non-infiltrative growth pattern, characterized by bulbous, florid epithelial pegs [98] (Fig. 7.12). The epithelium is arranged in acanthotic papillary folds, often hyperkeratotic or extremely hyperkeratotic to give an appearance at low and medium magnification that is similar to a condyloma. This has lead to much confusion historically with the so-called Giant Condyloma of Buschke Lowenstein. However, it

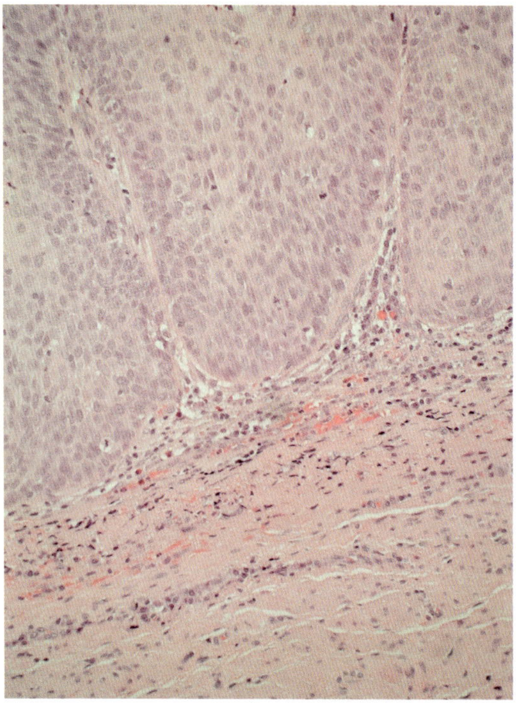

Fig. 7.12 Verrucous carcinoma. The epithelial downgrowths have rounded profiles that burrow deeply into the stroma. The epithelium is mildly dysplastic

is now thought that this does not represent a separate entity and that all such lesions represent verrucous squamous carcinoma.

The epithelium usually shows little atypia with few mitoses, no atypical mitoses, and basaloid cells limited to the lowest 1–3 layers, supported by the finding of Mib1 limited to the basal layers [104]. The uniform production of keratin filaments, shown by AE1/3 reactivity throughout the whole thickness of the epithelium except the basal layer, contrasts with the scattered reactivity of the usual types of squamous carcinoma and with the basal–only reactivity of normal epithelium [99, 104]. Not all authors accept koilocytosis as part of the pattern [103], but some do [98, 99]. There are reports of HPV 6/11 [105] but not all studies have shown HPV presence [103, 104]. There is no association with u-VIN, but it is possible that this tumor may arise in the vulva from a thickening of the epithelium that shows some similarities to differentiated VIN but differs in possessing papillomatosis and parakeratosis and loss of the granular cell layer. This has been called vulvar acanthosis with altered differentiation (VAAD) [103].

The epithelium grows down into the dermis in smoothly contoured protrusions that seem to maintain a defined boundary from the stroma. The difficulty in diagnosis comes from appreciating that these blunt contoured, bulbous epithelial downgrowths are invasive and that deep invasion and recurrence are typical of the natural history of the disease.

Although metastasis is rare [98], it is reported to the regional, but not distant lymph nodes [106]. Treatment is by surgical excision. Radiotherapy has been associated with transformation to more aggressive behavior [107].

In contrast to HPV-related usual type of squamous carcinoma, verrucous carcinoma was found not to exhibit ploidy abnormalities [51] and to be negative for p16 in two cases [9]. Some cases are negative for retinoblastoma protein (pRp) [51]. Accumulated evidence is allowing recognition that this is a subset of the HPV-negative squamous carcinoma group occurring in older women [103].

There has been a single case report of the tumor in a 41-year-old who also had Turner's syndrome [108].

Plasmacytoid Carcinoma

This is a rare and aggressive variant of squamous carcinoma that has been reported in an elderly woman [109]. The tumor consists of plasmacytoid- and spindle-shaped cells but distinction from lymphoid or sarcomatoid tumors can be made using markers more specific for squamous carcinoma such as AE2, CK5/6, and p63.

Differential Diagnosis of Squamous Carcinoma

Pseudocarcinomatous Hyperplasia (PCH) Associated with Granular Cell Tumors

The marked epithelial hyperplasias that can overlay granular cell tumors of the vulva can be a significant cause of confusion with squamous carcinoma [110]. The granular cell tumor can be overshadowed by the irregular downgrowths of squamous epithelium that can have sufficient architectural abnormalities including keratin horn cysts to raise the suspicion of carcinoma. Strands of epithelium with single groups of cell can infiltrate the stroma, but a desmoplastic reaction is not seen. Vulvar granular cell tumor is only rarely correctly diagnosed clinically and the separation of PCH from squamous carcinoma can be extremely difficult. The most helpful features are recognition of the underlying granular cell tumor and the absence of severe atypia. Restriction of the downgrowths to the papillary dermis, absence of large nucleoli, few mitoses, and rarity of horn cysts are less helpful in identifying a benign proliferation.

Pseudocarcinomatous Hyperplasia (PCH) Associated with Granuloma Inguinale

Squamous cell carcinoma may coexist with granuloma inguinale rarely, but a diagnostic problem is distinguishing the pseudocarcinomatous hyperplasia that overlies and borders the lesions of granuloma inguinale. Recognizing the typical inflammatory reaction of granuloma inguinale and Donovan bodies, as well as the absence of nuclear atypia and abnormal mitoses, aids the diagnosis. See Chap. 2.

Amyloid

Marked squamous hyperplasia overlying deposits of amyloid in systemic amyloidosis can mimic squamous carcinoma clinically. The presence of Congo Red-positive collections in the stroma confirms the diagnosis of amyloid [111].

Vulval Warts, Genital Warts

Condyloma Acuminatum

Vulval warts (pl: Condylomata acuminata) are HPV-associated squamous papillomas that may be single, multiple, or so numerous that they can cover large areas of the vulva. They can be situated on the skin or mucosa of the vulva and may extend on to the perineum and perianal areas. Caused by viral infection with HPV 6 and 11 typically [112], they are usually transmitted by sexual contact and occur more often in the immunocompromised [113], presenting occasionally as overgrown, large, often recurrent masses [114]. Genital warts occur in children and have been cited as a marker for childhood sexual abuse, but HPV DNA is carried on the fingers of genital wart sufferers, and it has been suggested that genital contact is not always necessary for transmission [115]. It is also possible that infection has occurred during birth by direct transmission from the mother and that the infection has remained latent until the development of the condyloma. Another potential for the misdiagnosis of childhood sexual abuse comes from confusion of vulvar verruca vulgaris (see below) with condyloma. A series of young girls aged 2–5 years were shown to have HPV 2-related verrucae vulgares. These lesions are similar to those found elsewhere on the body and show marked hyperkeratosis and acanthosis and differ in showing less hyperkeratosis than condylomata. However, the authors stress that a firm distinction from condyloma acuminatum can only be made by DNA studies [116].

Grossly each lesion appears as single, or more commonly multiple papillary fronds covered by skin or mucosa. Large, irregular, or heavily keratinized lesions can be confused clinically with squamous carcinoma. They are much larger than the small, fine lesions of vulvar papillomatosis, which are not associated with HPV infection [117].

Histologically, fibrovascular cores are covered by acanthotic stratified squamous epithelium that in at least some areas show the cytopathic effects of HPV infection (Fig. 7.13a). This may result in koilocytosis (scooped out cells) where there is a degree of cytoplasmic clearing around a slightly hyperchromatic nucleus that possesses a wrinkled nuclear membrane. These cells should not be confused with the glycogen-containing “cellules claires” that also show cytoplasmic clearing, but without nuclear abnormalities. Koilocytes are also frequently seen in usual type of VIN [118].

The epithelium can be parakeratotic, hyperkeratotic, or non-keratinized. Typically, there may be large, irregular keratohyaline granules in the stratum granulosum, associated with regular maturation upwards from the basal layers. Mitoses should be limited to the basal layers of the epithelium, but the epithelium should not show deeply hyperchromatic nuclei or abnormal, variable chromatin patterns with atypical mitoses (Fig. 7.13b), the presence of which raise the possibility of usual or d-VIN in a squamous papilloma [118].

It has long been recognized that podophyllin treatment for vulval warts may cause apoptosis, nuclear enlargement and hyperchromasia where the history of podophyllin application assists the diagnosis. More recently, a report details five cases of condylomas in young women where nuclear changes in the superficial epithelial layers, in the absence of such treatment, resembled some of the features of podophyllin effect. The authors have called this pseudobowenoid change in a condyloma [119]. The lack of basal cell atypia helps to exclude intraepithelial neoplasia.

The warty surface of lymphangioma circumscriptum can also be confused with carcinoma or condylomata [120], but in this condition there is a proliferation of thin-walled lymphatics in the superficial stroma, and there are no features of

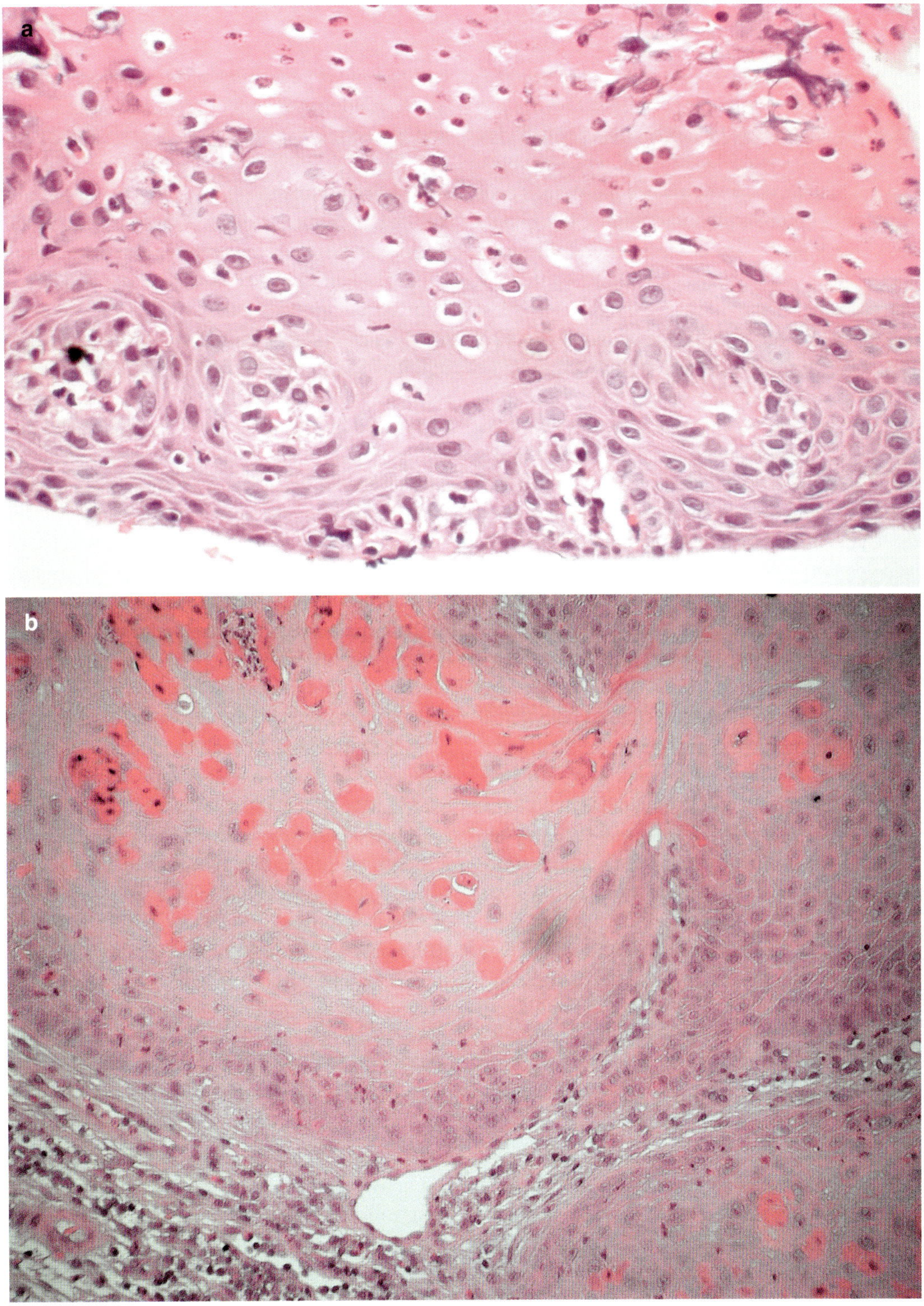

Fig. 7.13 (**a**) Epithelium from a condyloma acuminatum to show koilocytes. The nuclear profile is irregular and wrinkled, but there is little variation in chromatin pattern, and there are no atypical mitoses. (**b**) The epithelial cells in this condyloma show dyskeratosis, but little atypia and no mitotic activity

HPV infection in the epithelium. Paget's disease may result in marked squamous hyperplasia of the epithelium that is permeated by the Paget's cells, and this may cause clinical confusion with neoplasia. Paget's cells may be numerous; in which case the diagnosis should be obvious, but squamous hyperplasia can occur even when the Paget's cells are scanty. Immunostaining with CK7 should reveal the Paget's cells and prevent misdiagnosis [121]. In systemic amyloidosis, the epithelium can become hyperplastic overlying amyloid deposits in the vulva, mimicking condyloma [122, 123]. Granulomatous disease of the vulva can be associated with overlying squamous proliferations that can look like condylomas clinically. This can be caused by schistosomiasis [124] where warts may occur in contrast to the more usual ulcer [125]. The diagnosis can be made by identifying the characteristic ova with terminal spines (*S. hematobium*) related to the granulomata.

Verruca Vulgaris

Verruca vulgaris [116] appears to be more common in children than in adults. Verrucae tend not to exhibit florid papillary growth, but both verrucae and condylomas can show papillomatosis, koilocytosis, and prominent keratohyaline layers, although verrucae tend to show more hyperkeratosis. HPV 2 is present in verrucae in contrast to the HPV 6/11 of condyloma acuminatum, probably due to auto-transmission from skin lesions [126]. Because the histological features of each overlap, HPV genotyping is a more reliable way of making the diagnosis. This is particularly important in childhood warts as condyloma can be sexually transmitted but verrucae are not.

Herpes Simplex

In patients with AIDS, there can be such profound hyperplasia of the vulvar epithelium infected by herpes simplex [127, 128] to cause confusion with squamous carcinoma. Grossly exophytic squamous areas can form that show irregular downgrowths, mitotic activity, and nuclear atypia. A dense inflammatory response, including abundant plasma cells can underlie the lesion. Classical herpetic inclusions aid the diagnosis, but immunohistochemistry might be necessary to confirm the presence of the virus. Hypertrophic vulvar herpes infection should be considered in any immunosuppressed patient where epithelial hyperplasia raises a suspicion of malignancy.

Keratoacanthoma

Keratoacanthoma [129–131] forms a keratotic nodule or papule, often with a prominent central crater growing on the labia majora of middle-aged to elderly women. It usually occurs on sun-damaged skin, so is rare on the vulva with only four reported cases. The history is of rapid enlargement, up to 2 cm in diameter, with one documented to increase from pea-sized to 1.5 cm diameter in a few weeks [131]. Those reported on the vulva have all been excised, although subsequent involution elsewhere on the body is not unusual.

Histologically, the acanthotic epidermis forms a cup around a central accumulation of keratin. This cup is characteristically buttressed by well-formed epidermal shoulders and the base of the invagination is made up of irregular sheets of glassy, eosinophilic keratinocytes. The epidermal downgrowths are delineated by a sharp margin from the dermis. Early lesions may show mitotic activity in the base, but this progressively lessens, contributing to regression.

A biopsy from the base of the lesion poses real difficulty in differentiating from squamous carcinoma, but the most helpful features include fewer mitoses, lack of accompanying VIN, absence of HPV and a well-formed central keratin mass. The single cell infiltration seen in a squamous cell carcinoma is not a feature of a keratoacanthoma. Some of the features that have been said to be characteristic such as intraepithelial neutrophils and intraepithelial elastic fibers, wider lateral than deep extension, parakeratosis, and dyskeratosis are not always discriminatory [74, 75], and there is a belief among some dermatopathologists that even with excisional biopsy [129] a distinction cannot be made, resulting in these being called keratoacanthoma-like squamous carcinomas.

Outside the vulva, this is a largely academic argument as for most lesions, whether SCC or keratoacanthoma, excision is curative. However, on the vulva, where metastasis from squamous carcinoma is more common, this distinction is important to ensure that further surgery or adjuvant therapy is not given inappropriately for a benign self-limiting lesion.

It might be anticipated that squamous carcinoma proliferates more rapidly and undergoes apoptosis less often than a keratoacanthoma [132], but there are no biomarkers that distinguish the two reliably [133]. A tissue marker array study has shown statistically significant higher expression of an apoptosis inhibitor, Bcl-xL in squamous carcinoma [134], but there are no practical applications of this reported so far.

This differential is not easily resolved, but given the rarity of keratoacanthoma on this site, it is probably not a significant issue. The most prudent approach would seem to be wide consultation with dermatopathologists who accept keratoacanthoma as a diagnostic entity [135].

Verruciform Xanthoma

This is a very rare lesion representing less than 1% of all benign vulval tumors [136]. Only 19 cases have been reported to date and most are seen in women with another vulvar condition such as lichen sclerosus, lichen planus, Paget's disease, or prior irradiation [77, 78]. A common feature appears to be damaged to the epithelium and dermis [137]. This condition presents as a nodule or papillary, wart-like plaque. Histologically, there is a dermal accumulation of non-Langerhans foamy histiocytes that contain lipid and diastase resistant PAS-positive material associated with an overlying exophytic, papillary epithelium (Fig. 7.14). The histiocytes are CD68-postive and are sited between the acanthotic epidermal ridges and may be accompanied by lymphocytes, plasma cells, neutrophils, and eosinophils. Although recurrence has been recorded [136], these are benign conditions that can be distinguished from verrucous carcinoma by the histiocyte population and lack of invasion into the stroma.

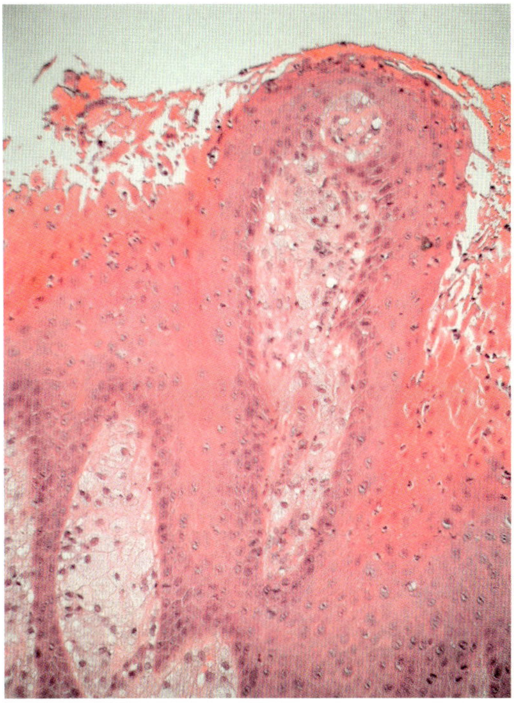

Fig. 7.14 Verruciform xanthoma to show acanthotic papillary epithelium over stroma containing foam cells

Vestibular Papillomatosis (Micropapillomatosis Labialis)

A condition of multiple or single small vestibular papillomas, often distributed symmetrically around the introitus on the hymenal ring, sometimes extending into the vagina, formed by fine fibrovascular cores covered by thin, normal, or mildly acanthotic squamous epithelium (Fig. 7.15). They are usually smaller than 6 mm and tend to be solitary in older women. These lesions have been found in one-third of one series of 40 asymptomatic women [138] and to be asymptomatic in 50% of 18 women [139]. The papillomas tend to be much smaller [117] than condyloma acuminatum, and there are no cytopathic changes of HPV infection such as koilocytosis, dyskeratosis, multinucleation, or irregularity of nuclear outline. Most regress spontaneously [140]. Earlier studies suggested that vulvar papillomatosis is caused by HPV [139], but that may have been related to HPV infections elsewhere on the vulva and other work suggests that viral DNA can be detected no more frequently than in controls [79, 80].

Fibroepithelial Polyp

Vulvovaginal fibroepithelial polyps (also see section "Vagina" and Chap. 8) are single or multiple

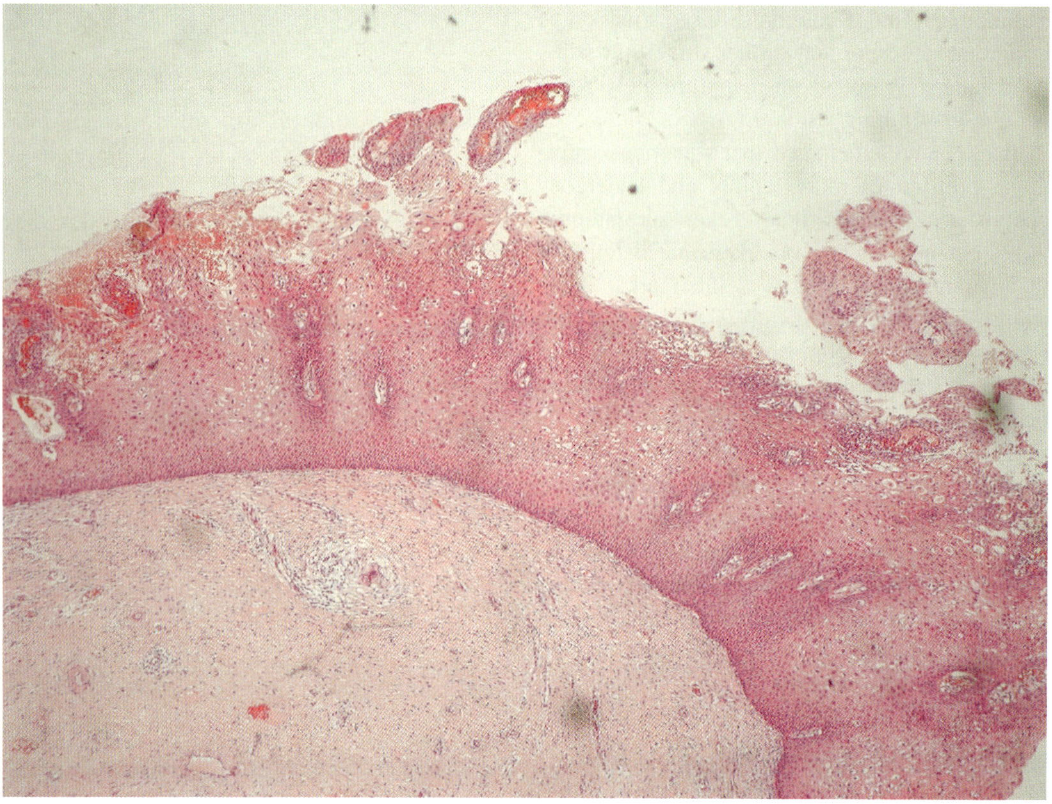

Fig. 7.15 Micropapillomatosis showing the very fine fibrovascular cores covered by focally inflamed squamous epithelium

lesions composed of a mainly fibrous, fibrovascular core covered by stratified squamous epithelium that exhibits varying degrees of glycogenation and keratinization (Fig. 7.16a). They are usually small to moderate sized 1 mm–2 cm, but can grow much larger if edematous [141]. The stroma may be loose or dense and contain the specialized atypical stellate or swallow-tailed fibroblasts characteristic of the vulval subepithelial layer (Fig. 7.16b). The covering epithelium may contain glycogenated epithelial cells that can be distinguished from koilocytes by their smooth nuclear contour in contrast to the enlarged, wrinkled, or irregular nuclei of koilocytes. Nevertheless, a small proportion of cases appear to be related to low-risk HPV infection [142].

Moderate or marked epithelial hyperplasia and acanthosis are not usually seen in these polyps and, if present, should suggest a vulvar wart (condyloma acuminatum). Intraepithelial neoplasia and Paget's disease can involve the surface epithelium. It is possible that the polyps grow as a result of the effect of estrogen on the subepithelial stroma, and this has been proposed as a cause of hypertrophy of the labia minora [143]. Estrogen receptors have been identified in the vulval stroma of infants illustrated by a rapidly growing vulvar fibroepithelial polyp that was reported in a 7-month-old that was resected at age 14 months and which recurred when the girl was 3 years old [144].

Seborrheic Keratosis (Basal Cell Papilloma)

Seborrheic keratoses (SKs) are common benign lesions of the skin of the mons pubis or labia majora, presenting as elsewhere on the body as keratotic or greasy raised plaques with variable degrees of papillomatosis. As there is often variable melanin pigment in the keratinocytes, they

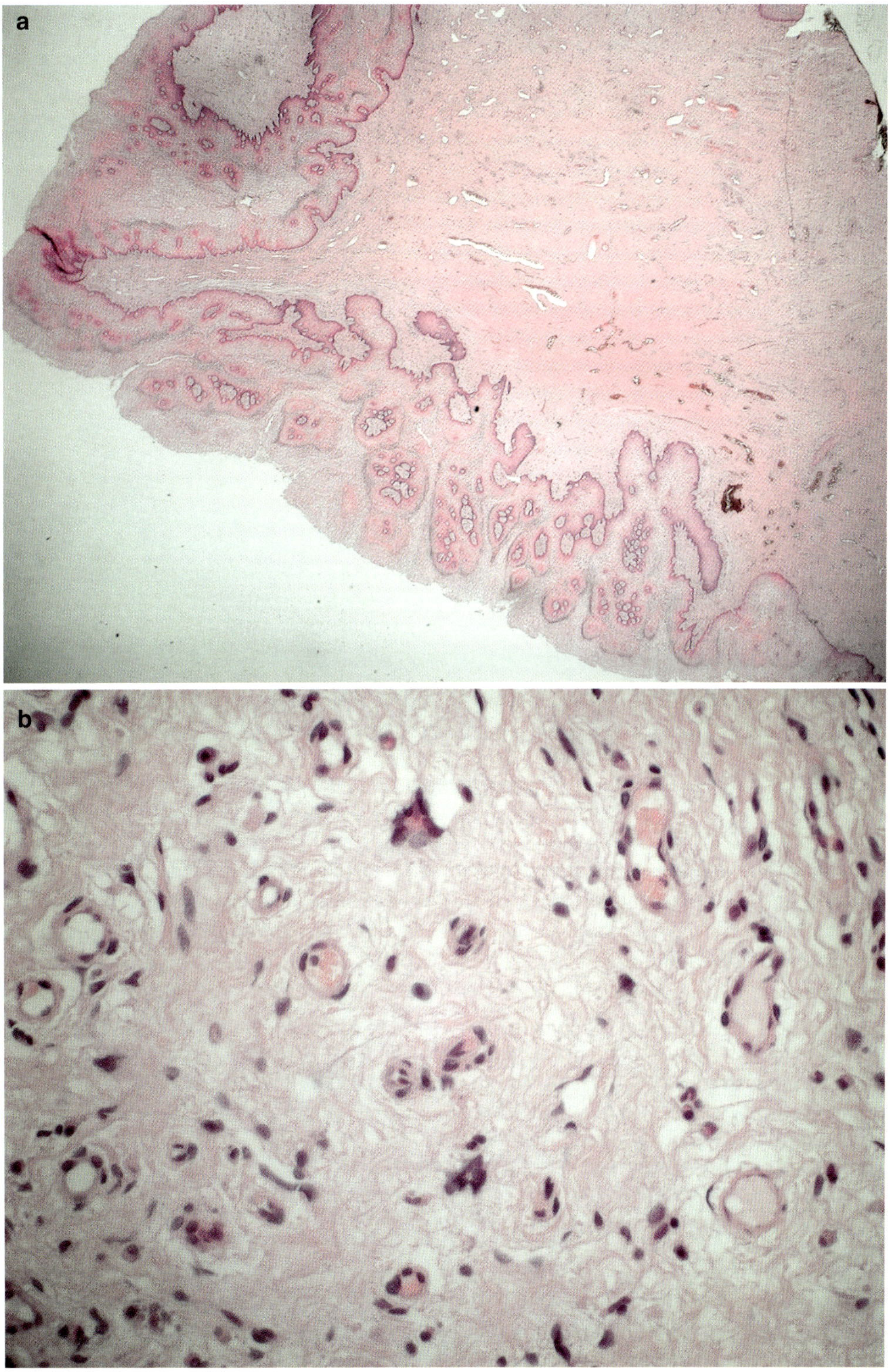

Fig. 7.16 (**a**) Vulvovaginal fibroepithelial polyp showing a fibrovascular core covered by slightly hyperplastic stratified squamous epithelium. (**b**) High-power view of the stroma of a vulvovaginal polyp to show the atypical swallow-tailed and floret-like fibroblasts

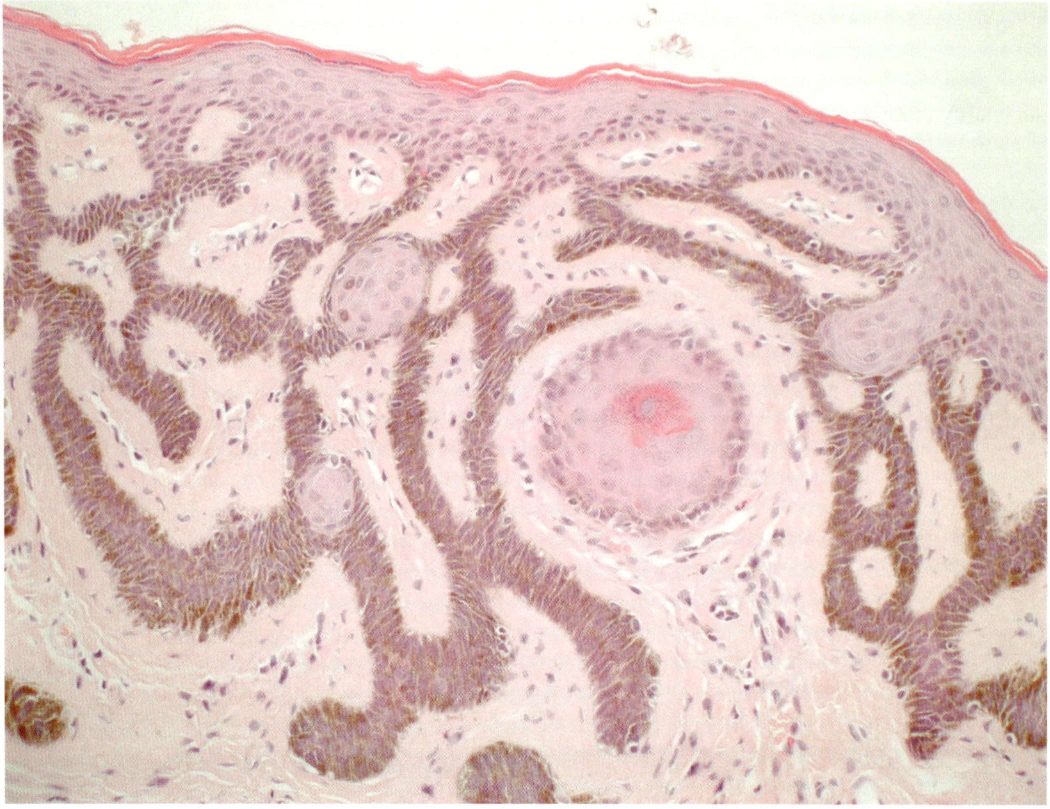

Fig. 7.17 Reticulate (adenoid) form of seborrheic keratosis showing bands of pigmented epithelium anastomosing in the dermis and incorporating squamoid areas

can raise a clinical concern of malignant melanoma [145, 146]. Dermoscopy can be used to examine the lesions clinically for the characteristic pores which are openings of the horn cysts [145].

Histologically, there is an exophytic proliferation of regular basaloid cells showing no atypia or abnormal mitoses forming sheets, bands, or anastomosing strands (Fig. 7.17). Keratin inclusions form horn cysts. Histological confusion with squamous carcinoma can arise when mechanical trauma or other chronic irritation leads to the development of more eosinophilic epithelioid cell groups—so-called squamous eddies. This may be accompanied by mild cytological atypia and some mitotic activity, but the absence of invasion or abnormal mitoses distinguishes seborrheic keratosis from squamous carcinoma. One study found 72% of vulvar seborrheic keratoses contained HPV 6, in contrast to 2% of nongenital seborrheic keratoses [142], building on a previous report suggesting that SKs in the anogenital region were variants of condylomata acuminata [147]. However, Mib1 reactivity was the same in genital and nongenital SKs, suggesting either superinfection with HPV on vulvar SKs derived from other etiologies or unrecognized HPV in cutaneous SK.

Inverted Follicular Keratosis

Inverted follicular keratosis shows similarities to irritated seborrheic keratosis with the development of squamous eddies in a proliferation of basaloid cells forming an invagination of epithelium into the dermis [148]. Seborrheic keratoses of the vulva are common: it is thought that inverted follicular keratosis is akin to seborrheic keratosis involving a pilosebaceous unit, possibly caused by regular genital shaving.

The endophytic growth of basaloid cells with squamous differentiation in this lesion can cause confusion with squamous carcinoma as the cells can show nuclear atypia and mitotic activity in the squamous eddies. However, distinguishing features include the symmetry of the lesion, absence of a desmoplastic stromal reaction, low nuclear/cytoplasmic ratio, smooth nuclear outline, and absence of abnormal mitoses.

Vulval Angiokeratoma

Angiokeratomas are benign and usually arise as asymptomatic gray, dark blue, red, purple, warty, smooth, or raised papules on the skin of the labia majora, or more rarely the clitoris [149–151], in women under 50. Most are unilateral and multiple, usually under 1 cm in size. Histologically, the small veins, venules, and capillaries of the papillary dermis are dilated and may be thrombosed. Overlying and partially enclosing these vessels, the epidermis exhibits papillomatosis, hyperkeratosis and irregular acanthosis, often with a collarette around the superficial dermal vessels. It is likely that loss of support for the vasculature associated with hydrostatic effects leads to vascular dilatation and secondary effects in the overlying epithelium. This effect can be exaggerated in pregnancy when there can be marked growth of the lesion [151].

Warty Dyskeratoma

More commonly seen on the head and neck of elderly patients, this has been reported on the vulva, where it can be confused with squamous carcinoma. Warty dyskeratoma appears as a papule or nodule with a keratinized surface or central plug [90, 91]. Supra-basal acantholysis of the squamous epithelium around a central keratotic plug is a typical diagnostic feature. Acantholytic squamous carcinoma is rare on the vulva, being more typically seen on sun-exposed sites, but the small regular lesions that are likely to cause diagnostic difficulty can be distinguished from warty dyskeratoma by more widespread acantholysis, abnormal nuclear morphology, and atypical mitoses.

Basal Cell Carcinoma

Basal cell carcinoma is the most commonly occurring skin malignancy, with approximately 2% of these occurring on the vulva [152], representing 2–5% [153] of all primary malignant tumors at this site. This is a disease of old age, with most detected between 65 and 90 years old [152–154].

6/10 cases of basal cell carcinoma of the vulva were positive for p16 and p53 [9] in contrast to the HPV-associated basaloid squamous carcinomas. These tumors are not thought to be caused by HPV, which seems only to be present as the epidermodysplasia verruciformis-linked subtypes 8, 15, and 36 in sunlight-associated BCCs [155].

This tumor usually presents as a nodule, "wart," "papilloma," pigmented area, or larger fungating mass, most often grown to 2 cm in diameter by time of treatment, but can be up to 6.5 cm in size [152, 153], although very large tumors, 10 cm in diameter, have been recorded [156, 157]. Around 1 in 4 is ulcerated [152]. The lesion can cause itching [153, 158, 159] and may mislead the clinicians to treat as an inflammatory of allergic condition, especially when the lesion causes non-localized symptoms. Local recurrence is reported following incomplete excision and in metastasizing tumors [153].

There are very rare reports of metastasis with a rate of 0.0028–0.55% from all sites with only eight reported from the vulva [153, 157, 160–165]. Spread is related to delay in diagnosis, depth of invasion—greater than 10 mm [157], morphic growth pattern [153], bleeding at presentation and may be associated with atypia in the squamous component [166]. As anticipated, metastasis is to the regional nodes where death can be due to local complications [153], and there has been a report of spread to the head of femur in an elderly woman [167].

Histologically, vulvar basal cell carcinomas resemble extra-genital forms and have the typical peripheral palisade of more regular cells around sheets, nests, cords and adenoid proliferations [168]. There is potential for confusion of adenoid forms with adenoid cystic carcinoma arising from Bartholin's glands, but in contrast adenoid basal cell carcinomas show far less nuclear pleomorphism and do not possess the PAS-positive basophilic intraluminal product or insidiously infiltrative growth pattern, often along perineural lymphatics of adenoid cystic carcinomas [165, 168]. Adenoid basal cell carcinomas can usually be seen to be originating from the epidermis, in contrast to adenoid cystic carcinomas, which are usually deeply situated and related to Bartholin's gland remnants [168]. The tumor cells are small and round or elongated with little or moderate cytoplasm. Mitoses, usually non-atypical, recorded as up to 66/10 hpf (area 0.152 mm^2) with a mean of 17/10 hpf [153]. There may be pillar-type keratinization (without a granular cell layer). Larger tumors tend to have more infiltrating growth patterns although purely morpheic types are rare at this site [153].

Unlike most cases of extra-genital basal cell carcinoma, the lesion is clearly unlikely to be associated with sunlight exposure in this site and associated solar damage to the tissues has not been reported [153], but there are reports of occurrence in Gorlin's (nevoid basal cell carcinoma) syndrome [169] and occurring in areas of Paget's disease [170]. There is no association with HPV, but six out of ten vulvar basal cell carcinomas were found to be positive with p16 [9]. Lichen sclerosus is not thought to play a role [153], but chronic irritation, infection, irradiation, and arsenic have been cited.

Basal Cell Carcinomas with a Malignant Squamous Component (Basosquamous Carcinoma, Metatypical Basal Cell Carcinoma)

Tumors that show features intermediate between basal cell carcinomas and squamous carcinomas have been termed metatypical basal cell carcinomas or basosquamous carcinomas and are rare, even more so on the vulva [119, 120]. Clinically, the lesions may appear less well defined than a typical basal cell carcinoma, appearing as a plaque or a flat-edged ulcer and may be associated with multiple similar extra-genital carcinomas. The tumors show a malignant squamous component, often representing squamous carcinoma extending out and infiltrating from more typical basal cell carcinoma. The more usual arrangement of basaloid cells encompassing central squamous areas without atypia should be termed a basal cell carcinoma with squamous areas or a keratotic basal cell carcinoma [171]. The presence of banal squamous keratinizing elements in a BCC has no effect on behavior or prognosis, but it is possible that a malignant squamous element can behave like squamous carcinoma, especially as recurrence appears more common than BCC. There is little documented evidence of behavior in this site, with no agreed basis for more aggressive therapy [154]. Nevertheless, the infiltrating cells react strongly for membranous and cytoplasmic BerEP4, confirming a basal cell carcinoma and allowing a distinction from collision tumors [172].

Vagina

Squamous Cell Carcinoma

Squamous carcinoma of the vagina is a rare disease most often seen in women over 50 [173], with a mean age of around 66 years [174]. There is a peak incidence in women aged 70–79, representing about 2% of genital neoplasias [175]. However, as with the vulva, there is a bimodal age distribution with around 30–40% occurring in the under 50s. In these younger women, squamous carcinoma in this site is associated with intraepithelial neoplasia of the cervix (and hence the probability of prior hysterectomy or cervical surgery) and to a lesser extent, vulva [176]. Most tumors present as bleeding, with a mass detectable clinically; around a quarter of cases are asymptomatic or detected by cytology [177, 178].

Grossly, the tumors may present as a white patch or aceto-white area in the vagina with underlying microscopic foci of invasion, as a papule, larger nodule, papillary mass, fungating lesion, encircling or constricting tumor, or ulcer. Histologically, keratinizing or non-keratinizing tongues of squamous carcinoma invade the stroma and in younger women there may be koilocytic change [179]. There are no significant morphological differences to squamous carcinomas of the vulva or cervix (Fig. 7.18).

By convention, squamous carcinoma of the upper third of the vagina arising less than 5 years

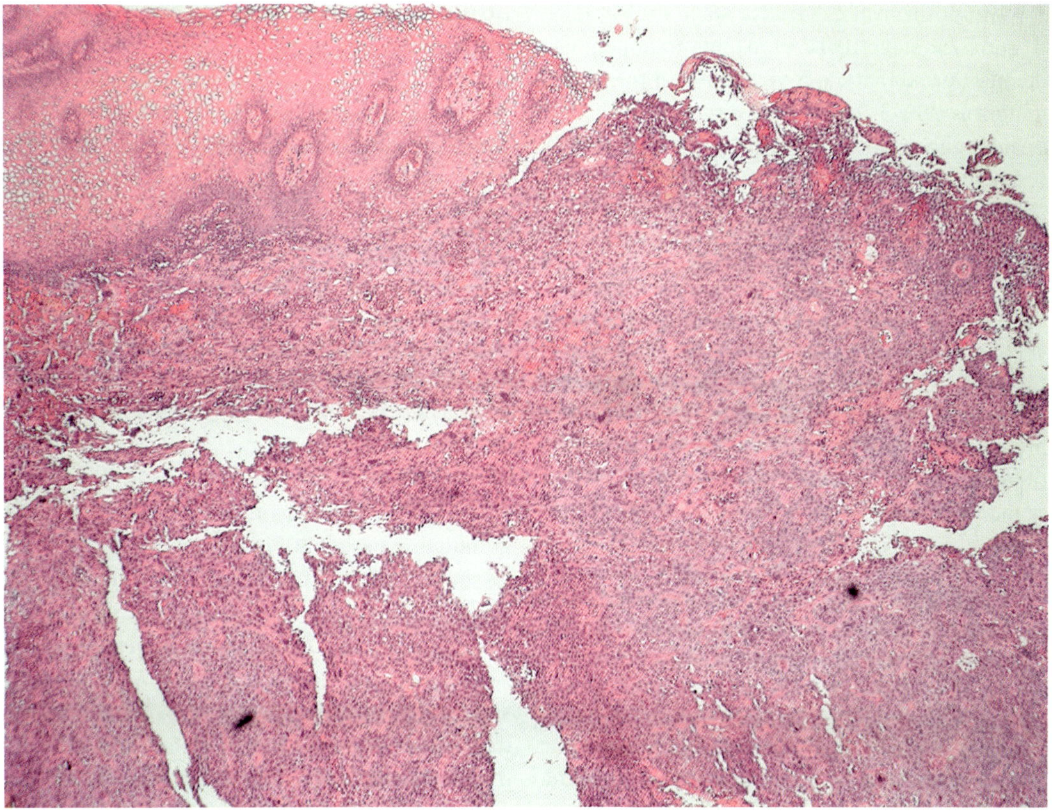

Fig. 7.18 Poorly differentiated squamous carcinoma of the vagina invading beneath glycogenated vaginal epithelium

after treatment for carcinoma of the cervix is regarded to be recurrent cervical tumor [176, 180]. Radiotherapy for carcinoma of cervix poses an additional predisposing risk [176]. There is a higher incidence of other genital infections in this younger age group, probably relating to numbers of sexual partners [176]. Risk factors for older women appear to be late menarche [176] and earlier menopause, suggesting hormonal factors such as the lack of the protective effect of estrogen on the vaginal epithelium [181]. There are case reports of squamous carcinoma developing in chronic prolapse [182, 183], so trauma and chronic irritation may also play a role.

Although there is a weak association with tumor grade (where poorly differentiated lesions behave more aggressively [184]), the prognosis is most closely associated with stage (Table 7.2) at diagnosis [184, 186, 187]. Advanced age has been identified as an adverse prognostic indicator [187, 188], but other studies have not confirmed this [174, 184]. Immunosuppression and coinfection with HIV or HTLV1 may result in a more aggressive course [189, 190]. In common with squamous carcinoma of the vulva in young women and the cervix, other risk factors include multiple sexual partners, smoking, and early age at first intercourse [191].

Table 7.2 FIGO 2006 staging for carcinoma of vagina [173]

Stage I: limited to vaginal wall
Stage II: Into para-vaginal tissue
Stage III: Extension to pelvic side wall
Stage IVA: Mucosa of bladder/rectum (+ urethra proposed 2009 [185]), beyond pelvis
Stage IVB: Distant metastasis

Overall survival is 84% for stage I, 75% stage II, and 57% stage III/IV [174], but treatment can modify this so that the 5-year survival for stage I tumors is 90% if treated by surgery and 63% if treated with radiotherapy alone, for stage II 70% if amenable to surgery and 57% after radiotherapy. Stage III and IV survival figures are 47% for surgery, 45% for radiotherapy, 60% for combined surgery and radiotherapy and 71% for those few patients who received surgery, radiotherapy and chemotherapy [175]. Tumor size has been poorly recorded in the past, but there is an indication that a diameter >4 cm is associated with a poorer prognosis [172, 178, 180, 187]. Individualization of treatment may involve sentinel node dissection in the future [192], but the drainage is not as predictable as in the vulva, necessitating detailed node mapping before dissection [193].

Verrucous Carcinoma

Verrucous carcinoma of the vagina appears to be very rare, not least because the diagnostic criteria have been contradictory [194–196]. The distinction must be made between those lesions with a similar appearance to verrucous carcinoma of the vulva and extensive HPV-associated warty squamous carcinoma [197]or condylomas [198]. Verrucous carcinoma will exhibit the typical exophytic growth pattern with a burrowing invasive base. It should be HPV-negative and may be associated with verrucous carcinoma of the vulva [103]. The tumors have a grossly exophytic growth pattern with marked acanthosis, papillomatosis, and hyperkeratosis. The epithelial downgrowths have a pushing advancing edge with rounded or smooth-contoured epithelial downgrowths. The epithelial cells lack atypia and proliferation in basaloid cells will be limited to the basal layers [194]. Infiltration by single cells or narrow strands of cells is not typical of verrucous carcinoma and should suggest a diagnosis of more typical squamous carcinoma. As with verrucous carcinoma of the vulva, this lesion can invade deeply into the wall of the vagina and beyond, but distant metastasis is rare [194, 196]. Similarly, radiotherapy may result in a more aggressive behavior [196].

Squamous Carcinoma Following Surgery

An artificial vagina can be constructed for congenital absence or malformation, gender reassignment and following ablative surgery. The lining of the newly constructed vagina is usually made from an autologous graft, either split skin, myocutaneous grafts, or by refashioning of the penile or scrotal skin. There have been many reports of squamous carcinoma [199–203] including verrucous subtypes [204] in this context. The artificial vagina may be subject to long-term irritation from intercourse or a prosthetic phallus designed to maintain patency of the new organ. This may cause inflammation, irritation, and the growth of granulation tissue [205], suggesting carcinogenesis in the context of chronic cell turnover and healing. Squamous carcinoma can even develop in this site when a space has been created by dissection between the bladder and the vagina and no skin has been used. In this case, the tumor has developed in metaplastic squamous epithelium that has grown around the prosthetic phallus and can be disguised by granulation tissue [206]. Human papilloma virus may also be implicated, especially when the skin of the donor site was normal before transplantation and when the recipient has been sexually active [199] or there are other HPV-associated lesions such as genital warts [200]. It is entirely understandable that there could be a higher risk of squamous carcinoma developing in a neovagina following surgery for vaginal intraepithelial neoplasia (VAIN) [201].

To date, only one case of squamous carcinoma arising in residual vaginal in a female to male transsexual has been reported [207].

Squamous carcinoma has been reported developing in episiotomy scars [202].

Squamotransitional Carcinoma of the Vagina

This is a very rare lesion with only six recorded cases that shows a mixture of squamous and transitional epithelial components [203, 208]. Positive reactions for CK7 and p16 and the presence of HPV 16 with negative reaction for CK20 distinguish this lesion from transitional carcinoma arising in the urinary tract (CK7-positive, CK20-positive, HPV-negative) and show a link to squamous carcinoma. A similar subtype is recorded in the cervix [209].

Lymphoepithelial-Like Carcinoma of the Vagina

This is an extremely rare lesion with only two cases reported to date [207, 210]. These tumors are similar to those of the nasopharynx and show infiltrating syncytial sheets of epithelioid cells lacking squamous or glandular features mixed with a dense inflammatory infiltrate of lymphocytes, plasma cells, and eosinophils. The epithelioid cells display obviously malignant features with high-grade nuclei, prominent nucleoli, and abundant eosinophilic cytoplasm.

The lymphoid population is predominantly T cell with a smaller B cell component. Unlike these carcinomas of the head and neck, Epstein-Barr virus was not identified in either of the two cases reported.

Differential Diagnosis of Squamous Carcinoma

Fibroepithelial Polyp of the Vagina

These vaginal lesions present as single or multiply fronded mucosal—covered polyps. The subject is covered more fully in Chap. 8. Morphologically similar to polyps of the vulva and cervix, they are composed of an often richly vascularized stromal core in which there are abundant atypical myofibroblasts, covered by stratified squamous epithelium [191, 192]. These polyps are derived from the hormonally reactive subepithelial layer that extends from the vulva to the endocervix which provides a loose layer on which the epithelium can move during intercourse and which might have some expansive and contractile role in parturition [211]. The atypical myofibroblasts have multipointed, stellate, or swallow-tailed outlines and may possess multiple nuclei, often arranged in wreath to form a floret-like cell.

Mitoses are usually rare, but hypercellular, mitotically active pseudosarcomatous variants can be confused with malignant proliferations [212], particularly if the mitoses are atypical. Pointers to the benign nature of these lesions are the absence of a collagenous band separating the atypical myofibroblasts from the epidermis (cambium layer), diffuse distribution of individual multinucleate cells and a common association with pregnancy or other hormonal alterations such as Tamoxifen treatment [211–213]. The stroma does not contain bone, cartilage, or striated muscle cells [211]. The stromal cells react with most commonly with desmin, vimentin, estrogen, and progesterone receptors [214] and to a lesser extent with smooth muscle actin [211]. Electron microscopy shows collagen production and contractile microfilaments, confirming myofibroblastic cells [211].

The major differential diagnosis is with cervicovaginal myofibroblastoma. Fibroepithelial polyp possesses similar atypical stromal myofibroblasts, but lacks the high cellularity with myxoid and edematous areas that characterize the myofibroblastoma [215, 216], although it is possible that these two entities form part of the same spectrum of changes.

Tubulo-Squamous Polyp of the Vagina

A series of ten cases reported in 2007 [217] characterized a fibroepithelial polyp of the upper vagina occurring at ages 39–78 ranging in size from 1 to 3 cm containing squamous and glandular stromal elements. The epithelium is arranged as stromal cysts and nests lined by focally glycogenated or basaloid [218] squamous epithelium. Within the squamous nests are tubules are lined by low cuboidal epithelium that reacts for prostatic acid phosphatase and/or prostate specific antigen. Occasional tubules may be lined solely by cuboidal epithelium. The epithelial cells possess bland nuclei with no mitotic activity and often with grooved chromatin. Complex arrangements of tubules may give a cribriform arrangement. These epithelial elements bear similarities to prostate ducts and may have arisen as examples of ectopic prostate-like tissue, prostatic metaplasia or be related to the Skene glands [217]. The epithelium is supported by a loose fibrous or edematous stroma containing thin-walled blood vessels. It is likely that previously reported examples of Brenner tumor of the vagina were tubulo-squamous polyps.

Sebaceous glands [219], mucinous differentiation with goblet cells [220], and necrotic, focally calcified or keratinous cyst contents [217, 219] have been described.

The squamous elements react focally for CD10 and more diffusely for AE1/3, CK7, LP34, 34betaE12 and CK5/6. The cuboidal glandular cells react for EA1/3, CK7, and luminally for CD10. The stroma is negative for cytokeratins and CD10. ER is positive in the squamous and stromal cells. PR reacts for the stromal but not the epithelial cells [217]. Basaloid cells are positive for p63 [218]. Hardly any cells react for Mib1.

An awareness of this benign entity should prevent confusion with mixed tumors of the vagina which usually occur at the hymenal ring and which show a more prominent spindle cell stroma that is unreactive for cytokeratins. Fibroepithelial polyps do not contain epithelial elements within the stroma. The absence of nuclear atypia and an infiltrative growth pattern combined with low proliferative index help to separate tubulo-squamous polyps from adenoid basal cell carcinoma, basaloid squamous carcinoma and small cell neuroendocrine carcinoma.

References

1. Japaze H, Garcia-Bunuel R, Woodruff JD. Primary vulvar neoplasia: a review of in situ and invasive carcinoma, 1935–1972. Obstet Gynecol. 1977;49(4):404–11.
2. Herod JJ, Shafi MI, Rollason TP, Jordan JA, Luesley DM. Vulvar intraepithelial neoplasia: long term follow up of treated and untreated women. Br J Obstet Gynaecol. 1996;103(5):446–52.
3. Tavassoli FA, Devilee P. Pathology and genetics of tumours of the breast and female genital organs. WHO Classification of tumours. Lyon: IARC Press; 2003.
4. Chiesa-Vottero A, Dvoretsky PM, Hart WR. Histopathologic study of thin vulvar squamous cell carcinomas and associated cutaneous lesions: a correlative study of 48 tumors in 44 patients with analysis of adjacent vulvar intraepithelial neoplasia types and lichen sclerosus. Am J Surg Pathol. 2006;30(3):310–8.
5. Husseinzadeh N, Wesseler T, Schneider D, Schellhas H, Nahhas W. Prognostic factors and the significance of cytologic grading in invasive squamous cell carcinoma of the vulva: a clinicopathologic study. Gynecol Oncol. 1990;36(2):192–9.
6. Andreasson B, Nyboe J. Value of prognostic parameters in squamous cell carcinoma of the vulva. Gynecol Oncol. 1985;22(3):341–51.
7. Broders A. Squamous cell epithelioma of the skin. A study of 256 cases. Ann Surg. 1921;73:141–60.
8. Trimble CL, Hildesheim A, Brinton LA, Shah KV, Kurman RJ. Heterogeneous etiology of squamous carcinoma of the vulva. Obstet Gynecol. 1996;87(1):59–64.
9. Santos M, Montagut C, Mellado B, Garcia A, Ramon y Cajal S, Cardesa A, et al. Immunohistochemical staining for p16 and p53 in premalignant and malignant epithelial lesions of the vulva. Int J Gynecol Pathol. 2004;23(3):206–14.
10. Steeper TA, Piscioli F, Rosai J. Squamous cell carcinoma with sarcoma-like stroma of the female genital tract. Clinicopathologic study of four cases. Cancer. 1983;52(5):890–8.
11. Al-Ghamdi A, Freedman D, Miller D, Poh C, Rosin M, Zhang L, et al. Vulvar squamous cell carcinoma in young women: a clinicopathologic study of 21 cases. Gynecol Oncol. 2002;84(1):94–101.
12. Choo YC. Invasive squamous carcinoma of the vulva in young patients. Gynecol Oncol. 1982;13(2):158–64.
13. Carter J, Carlson J, Fowler J, Hartenbach E, Adcock L, Carson L, et al. Invasive vulvar tumors in young women – a disease of the immunosuppressed? Gynecol Oncol. 1993;51(3):307–10.
14. Mousavi A, Abbasi F, Abadi AG, Hashemi FA. Vulvar squamous cell carcinoma associated with Fanconi's anemia. Int J Hematol. 2010;91(3):498–500.
15. Volgger B, Marth C, Zeimet A, Muller-Holzner E, Ruth N, Dapunt O. Fulminant course of a microinvasive vulvar carcinoma in an immunosuppressed woman. Gynecol Oncol. 1997;65(1):177–9.
16. Caterson RJ, Furber J, Murray J, McCarthy W, Mahony JF, Sheil AG. Carcinoma of the vulva in two young renal allograft recipients. Transplant Proc. 1984;16(2):559–61.
17. Leckie GB, Cotton RE. Simultaneous in situ carcinoma of the cervix, vulva and perineum after immunosuppressive therapy for renal transplantation. Br J Obstet Gynaecol. 1977;84(2):143–8.
18. Brown JE, Sunborg MJ, Kost E, Cosin JA, Winter 3rd WE. Vulvar cancer in human immunodeficiency virus-seropositive premenopausal women: a case series and review of the literature. J Low Genit Tract Dis. 2005;9(1):7–10.
19. Preston M. Squamous cell carcinoma of the vulva presenting amongst gigantic vulval warts. J Obstet Gynaecol. 2005;25(3):316.
20. Choi DS, Lee JW, Lee SJ, Choi CH, Kim TJ, Lee JH, et al. Squamous cell carcinoma with sarcomatoid features of the vulva: a case report and review of literature. Gynecol Oncol. 2006;103(1):363–7.
21. Santeusanio G, Schiaroli S, Anemona L, Sesti F, Valli E, Piccione E, et al. Carcinoma of the vulva with sarcomatoid features: a case report with immunohistochemical study. Gynecol Oncol. 1991;40(2):160–3.

22. Beller U, Quinn MA, Benedet JL, Creasman WT, Ngan HY, Maisonneuve P, et al. Carcinoma of the vulva. FIGO 26th Annual Report on the Results of Treatment in Gynecological Cancer. Int J Gynaecol Obstet. 2006;95 Suppl 1:S7–27.
23. CRUK. Vulval cancer – UK incidence statistics. 2010. http://info.cancerresearchuk.org/cancerstats/types/vulva/incidence/#Worldwide. Accessed in 2011.
24. CRUK. Vulval cancer – UK incidence statistics. 2010. http://info.cancerresearchuk.org/cancerstats/types/vulva/incidence/#Worldwide. Accessed in 2011.
25. Joura EA, Losch A, Haider-Angeler MG, Breitenecker G, Leodolter S. Trends in vulvar neoplasia. Increasing incidence of vulvar intraepithelial neoplasia and squamous cell carcinoma of the vulva in young women. J Reprod Med. 2000;45(8):613–5.
26. Sankaranarayanan R, Ferlay J. Worldwide burden of gynaecological cancer: the size of the problem. Best Pract Res Clin Obstet Gynaecol. 2006;20(2):207–25.
27. Piura B, Rabinovich A, Cohen Y, Friger M, Glezerman M. Squamous cell carcinoma of the vulva in the south of Israel: a study of 50 cases. J Surg Oncol. 1998;67(3): 174–81.
28. Vandborg MP, Christensen RD, Kragstrup J, Edwards K, Vedsted P, Hansen DG, et al. Reasons for diagnostic delay in gynecological malignancies. Int J Gynecol Cancer. 2011;21(6):967–74.
29. Ansink A. Vulvar squamous cell carcinoma. Semin Dermatol. 1996;15(1):51–9.
30. Coleman RL, Santoso JT. Vulvar carcinoma. Curr Treat Options Oncol. 2000;1(2):177–90.
31. Armes JE, Lourie R, Bowlay G, Tabrizi S. Pagetoid squamous cell carcinoma in situ of the vulva: comparison with extramammary paget disease and nonpagetoid squamous cell neoplasia. Int J Gynecol Pathol. 2008;27(1):118–24.
32. Bakour SH, Jaleel H, Weaver JB, Kehoe S, Radcliffe KW. Vulvar carcinoma presenting during pregnancy, associated with recurrent bone marrow hypoplasia: a case report and literature review. Gynecol Oncol. 2002;87(2):207–9.
33. Heller DS, Cracchiolo B, Hameed M, May T. Pregnancy-associated invasive squamous cell carcinoma of the vulva in a 28-year-old. HIV-negative woman. A case report. J Reprod Med. 2000;45(8): 659–61.
34. Regan MA, Rosenzweig BA. Vulvar carcinoma in pregnancy: a case report and literature review. Am J Perinatol. 1993;10(4):334–5.
35. Chan JK, Sugiyama V, Pham H, Gu M, Rutgers J, Osann K, et al. Margin distance and other clinico-pathologic prognostic factors in vulvar carcinoma: a multivariate analysis. Gynecol Oncol. 2007;104(3):636–41.
36. Tantipalakorn C, Robertson G, Marsden DE, Gebski V, Hacker NF. Outcome and patterns of recurrence for International Federation of Gynecology and Obstetrics (FIGO) stages I and II squamous cell vulvar cancer. Obstet Gynecol. 2009;113(4):895–901.
37. Kumar S, Shah JP, Bryant CS, Imudia AN, Morris RT, Malone Jr JM. A comparison of younger vs older women with vulvar cancer in the United States. Am J Obstet Gynecol. 2009;200(5):e52–5.
38. Nicoletto MO, Parenti A, Del Bianco P, Lombardi G, Pedrini L, Pizzi S, et al. Vulvar cancer: prognostic factors. Anticancer Res. 2010;30(6):2311–7.
39. Rhodes CA, Cummins C, Shafi MI. The management of squamous cell vulval cancer: a population based retrospective study of 411 cases. Br J Obstet Gynaecol. 1998;105(2):200–5.
40. Husseinzadeh N, Zaino R, Nahhas WA, Mortel R. The significance of histologic findings in predicting nodal metastases in invasive squamous cell carcinoma of the vulva. Gynecol Oncol. 1983;16(1):105–11.
41. Drew PA, al-Abbadi MA, Orlando CA, Hendricks JB, Kubilis PS, Wilkinson EJ. Prognostic factors in carcinoma of the vulva: a clinicopathologic and DNA flow cytometric study. Int J Gynecol Pathol. 1996;15(3): 235–41.
42. Ansink A, Mooi WJ, van Doornewaard G, van Tinteren H, Heintz AP, Ivanyi D. Cytokeratin subtypes and involucrin in squamous cell carcinoma of the vulva. An immunohistochemical study of 41 cases. Cancer. 1995;76(4):638–43.
43. Pecorelli S. Revised FIGO staging for carcinoma of the vulva, cervix, and endometrium. Int J Gynaecol Obstet. 2009;105(2):103–4.
44. Oonk MH, Hollema H, de Hullu JA, van der Zee AG. Prediction of lymph node metastases in vulvar cancer: a review. Int J Gynecol Cancer. 2006;16(3):963–71.
45. Ndubisi B, Kaminski PF, Olt G, Sorosky J, Singapuri K, Hackett T, et al. Staging and recurrence of disease in squamous cell carcinoma of the vulva. Gynecol Oncol. 1995;59(1):34–7.
46. van der Velden J, van Lindert AC, Lammes FB, ten Kate FJ, Sie-Go DM, Oosting H, et al. Extracapsular growth of lymph node metastases in squamous cell carcinoma of the vulva. The impact on recurrence and survival. Cancer. 1995;75(12):2885–90.
47. Fons G, Hyde SE, Buist MR, Schilthuis MS, Grant P, Burger MP, et al. Prognostic value of bilateral positive nodes in squamous cell cancer of the vulva. Int J Gynecol Cancer. 2009;19(7):1276–80.
48. Raspagliesi F, Hanozet F, Ditto A, Solima E, Zanaboni F, Vecchione F, et al. Clinical and pathological prognostic factors in squamous cell carcinoma of the vulva. Gynecol Oncol. 2006;102(2):333–7.
49. Emanuels AG, Burger MP, Hollema H, Koudstaal J. Quantitation of proliferation-associated markers Ag-NOR and Ki-67 does not contribute to the prediction of lymph node metastases in squamous cell carcinoma of the vulva. Hum Pathol. 1996;27(8):807–11.
50. Gordinier ME, Steinhoff MM, Hogan JW, Peipert JF, Gajewski WH, Falkenberry SS, et al. S-Phase fraction, p53, and HER-2/neu status as predictors of nodal metastasis in early vulvar cancer. Gynecol Oncol. 1997;67(2):200–2.
51. Lerma E, Matias-Guiu X, Lee SJ, Prat J. Squamous cell carcinoma of the vulva: study of ploidy, HPV, p53, and pRb. Int J Gynecol Pathol. 1999;18(3): 191–7.

52. Preti M, Ronco G, Ghiringhello B, Micheletti L. Recurrent squamous cell carcinoma of the vulva: clinicopathologic determinants identifying low risk patients. Cancer. 2000;88(8):1869–76.
53. Gonzalez Bosquet J, Magrina JF, Gaffey TA, Hernandez JL, Webb MJ, Cliby WA, et al. Long-term survival and disease recurrence in patients with primary squamous cell carcinoma of the vulva. Gynecol Oncol. 2005;97(3):828–33.
54. Horn LC, Wagner S. Frozen section analysis of vulvectomy specimens: results of a 5-year study period. Int J Gynecol Pathol. 2010;29(2):165–72.
55. Konanahalli P, Menon P, Walsh MY, McCluggage WG. Enterobious vermicularis (pinworm) infestation of the vulva: report of 2 cases of a pseudoneoplastic lesion mimicking squamous carcinoma. Int J Gynecol Pathol. 2010;29(5):490–3.
56. Buckley CH, Butler EB, Fox H. Vulvar intraepithelial neoplasia and microinvasive carcinoma of the vulva. J Clin Pathol. 1984;37(11):1201–11.
57. Wilkinson EJ, Rico MJ, Pierson KK. Microinvasive carcinoma of the vulva. Int J Gynecol Pathol. 1982; 1(1):29–39.
58. Wells M, Jenkins M. Selected topics in the histopathology of the vulva. Curr Diagn Pathol. 1994;1:41–7.
59. Vernooij F, Sie-Go DM, Heintz AP. Lymph node recurrence following stage IA vulvar carcinoma: two cases and a short overview of literature. Int J Gynecol Cancer. 2007;17(2):517–20.
60. Sidor J, Diallo-Danebrock R, Eltze E, Lelle RJ. Challenging the concept of microinvasive carcinoma of the vulva: report of a case with regional lymph node recurrence and review of the literature. BMC Cancer. 2006;6:157.
61. Van Der Velden J, Kooyman CD, Van Lindert AC, Heintz AP. A stage Ia vulvar carcinoma with an inguinal lymph node recurrence after local excision. A case report and literature review. Int J Gynecol Cancer. 1992;2(3):157–9.
62. Atamdede F, Hoogerland D. Regional lymph node recurrence following local excision for microinvasive vulvar carcinoma. Gynecol Oncol. 1989;34(1):125–8.
63. Hicks ML, Hempling RE, Piver MS. Vulvar carcinoma with 0.5 mm of invasion and associated inguinal lymph node metastasis. J Surg Oncol. 1993;54(4):271–3.
64. Schausberger C, Six L, Horvat R, Joura EA. Groin metastasis after extensive microinvasive vulvar cancer. A case report. J Reprod Med. 2007;52(2):78–80.
65. Figge DC, Tamimi HK, Greer BE. Lymphatic spread in carcinoma of the vulva. Am J Obstet Gynecol. 1985;152(4):387–94.
66. Gonzalez Bosquet J, Magrina JF, Magtibay PM, Gaffey TA, Cha SS, Jones MB, et al. Patterns of inguinal groin metastases in squamous cell carcinoma of the vulva. Gynecol Oncol. 2007;105(3):742–6.
67. Berchuck A, Rodriguez G, Kamel A, Soper JT, Clarke-Pearson DL, Bast Jr RC. Expression of epidermal growth factor receptor and HER-2/neu in normal and neoplastic cervix, vulva, and vagina. Obstet Gynecol. 1990;76(3 Pt 1):381–7.
68. Oonk MH, de Bock GH, van der Veen DJ, Ten Hoor KA, de Hullu JA, Hollema H, et al. EGFR expression is associated with groin node metastases in vulvar cancer, but does not improve their prediction. Gynecol Oncol. 2007;104(1):109–13.
69. Ambros RA, Malfetano JH, Mihm Jr MC. Clinicopathologic features of vulvar squamous cell carcinomas exhibiting prominent fibromyxoid stromal response. Int J Gynecol Pathol. 1996;15(2):137–45.
70. de Hullu JA, Oonk MH, van der Zee AG. Modern management of vulvar cancer. Curr Opin Obstet Gynecol. 2004;16(1):65–72.
71. Crosbie EJ, Slade RJ, Ahmed AS. The management of vulval cancer. Cancer Treat Rev. 2009;35(7):533–9.
72. de Hullu JA, Doting E, Piers DA, Hollema H, Aalders JG, Koops HS, et al. Sentinel lymph node identification with technetium-99m-labeled nanocolloid in squamous cell cancer of the vulva. J Nucl Med. 1998;39(8):1381–5.
73. Crosbie EJ, Winter-Roach B, Sengupta P, Sikand KA, Carrington B, Murby B, et al. The accuracy of the sentinel node procedure after excision biopsy in squamous cell carcinoma of the vulva. Surg Oncol. 2010;19(4): e150–4.
74. Hampl M, Hantschmann P, Michels W, Hillemanns P. Validation of the accuracy of the sentinel lymph node procedure in patients with vulvar cancer: results of a multicenter study in Germany. Gynecol Oncol. 2008;111(2):282–8.
75. Puig-Tintore LM, Ordi J, Vidal-Sicart S, Lejarcegui JA, Torne A, Pahisa J, et al. Further data on the usefulness of sentinel lymph node identification and ultrastaging in vulvar squamous cell carcinoma. Gynecol Oncol. 2003;88(1):29–34.
76. Moore RG, Granai CO, Gajewski W, Gordinier M, Steinhoff MM. Pathologic evaluation of inguinal sentinel lymph nodes in vulvar cancer patients: a comparison of immunohistochemical staining versus ultrastaging with hematoxylin and eosin staining. Gynecol Oncol. 2003;91(2):378–82.
77. Tamussino KF, Bader AA, Lax SF, Aigner RM, Winter R. Groin recurrence after micrometastasis in a sentinel lymph node in a patient with vulvar cancer. Gynecol Oncol. 2002;86(1):99–101.
78. de Hullu JA, van der Zee AG. Tammussino et al.: groin recurrence after micrometastasis in a sentinel lymph node in a patient with vulvar cancer. Gynecol Oncol. 2003;89(1):189–90; author reply 191.
79. Knopp S, Holm R, Trope C, Nesland JM. Occult lymph node metastases in early stage vulvar carcinoma patients. Gynecol Oncol. 2005;99(2):383–7.
80. Leys CM, Hartenbach EM, Hafez GR, Mahvi DM. Screening for occult nodal metastasis in squamous cell carcinoma of the vulva. Int J Gynecol Pathol. 2000;19(3):243–7.
81. Narayansingh GV, Miller ID, Sharma M, Welch CJ, Sharp L, Parkin DE, et al. The prognostic significance of micrometastases in node-negative squamous cell carcinoma of the vulva. Br J Cancer. 2005;92(2): 222–4.

82. Moss EL, Hirschowitz L, Luesley DM. Skin scar recurrence following removal of a sentinel lymph node containing a solitary micrometastasis of squamous cell vulval cancer. Gynecol Oncol. 2011; 121(1):239–40.
83. TjinAsjoe FM, van Bekkum E, Ewing P, Burger CW, Ansink AC. Sentinel node procedure in vulvar squamous cell carcinoma: a histomorphologic review of 32 cases. The significance of anucleate structures on immunohistochemistry. Int J Gynecol Cancer. 2008;18(5):1032–6.
84. Johann S, Klaeser B, Krause T, Mueller MD. Comparison of outcome and recurrence-free survival after sentinel lymph node biopsy and lymphadenectomy in vulvar cancer. Gynecol Oncol. 2008;110(3):324–8.
85. Van der Zee AG, Oonk MH, De Hullu JA, Ansink AC, Vergote I, Verheijen RH, et al. Sentinel node dissection is safe in the treatment of early-stage vulvar cancer. J Clin Oncol. 2008;26(6):884–9.
86. Programme NBS. Pathology reporting of breast disease. NHS Breast Screening Programme publication; 2005. p. 58.
87. Le T, Elsugi R, Hopkins L, Faught W, Fung-Kee-Fung M. The definition of optimal inguinal femoral nodal dissection in the management of vulva squamous cell carcinoma. Ann Surg Oncol. 2007;14(7):2128–32.
88. Walker KF, Day H, Abu J, Nunns D, Williamson K, Duncan T. Do surgical techniques used in groin lymphadenectomy for vulval cancer affect morbidity rates? Int J Gynecol Cancer. 2011;21(8):1495–9.
89. Horn LC, Liebert UG, Edelmann J, Hockel M, Einenkel J. Adenoid squamous carcinoma (pseudoangiosarcomatous carcinoma) of the vulva: a rare but highly aggressive variant of squamous cell carcinoma-report of a case and review of the literature. Int J Gynecol Pathol. 2008;27(2):288–91.
90. Lasser A, Cornog JL, Morris JM. Adenoid squamous cell carcinoma of the vulva. Cancer. 1974;33(1):224–7.
91. Underwood JW, Adcock LL, Okagaki T. Adenosquamous carcinoma of skin appendages (adenoid squamous cell carcinoma, pseudoglandular squamous cell carcinoma, adenocanthoma of sweat gland of Lever) of the vulva: a clinical and ultrastructural study. Cancer. 1978;42(4):1851–8.
92. Carson LF, Twiggs LB, Okagaki T, Clark BA, Ostrow RS, Faras AJ. Human papillomavirus DNA in adenosquamous carcinoma and squamous cell carcinoma of the vulva. Obstet Gynecol. 1988;72(1):63–7.
93. Giordano G, D'Adda T, Merisio C, Gnetti L. Vulvar acantholytic squamous carcinoma: a case report with immunohistochemical and molecular study. Int J Gynecol Pathol. 2005;24(3):303–6.
94. Nappi O, Swanson PE, Wick MR. Pseudovascular adenoid squamous cell carcinoma of the lung: clinicopathologic study of three cases and comparison with true pleuropulmonary angiosarcoma. Hum Pathol. 1994;25(4):373–8.
95. Parramore B, Hanly M, Yeh KA, McNeely T. Acantholytic variant of squamous cell carcinoma of the breast: a case report. Am Surg. 1999;65(5):467–9.
96. Papadopoulou E, Tosios KI, Nikitakis N, Papadogeorgakis N, Sklavounou-Andrikopoulou A. Acantholytic squamous cell carcinoma of the gingiva: report of a case and review of the literature. Oral Surg Oral Med Oral Pathol Oral Radiol Endod. 2010;109(6):e67–71.
97. Horie Y, Kato M. Pseudovascular squamous cell carcinoma of the uterine cervix: a lesion that may simulate an angiosarcoma. Pathol Int. 1999;49(2):170–4.
98. Japaze H, Van Dinh T, Woodruff JD. Verrucous carcinoma of the vulva: study of 24 cases. Obstet Gynecol. 1982;60(4):462–6.
99. Brisigotti M, Moreno A, Murcia C, Matias-Guiu X, Prat J. Verrucous carcinoma of the vulva. A clinicopathologic and immunohistochemical study of five cases. Int J Gynecol Pathol. 1989;8(1):1–7.
100. Degefu S, O'Quinn AG, Lacey CG, Merkel M, Barnard DE. Verrucous carcinoma of the cervix: a report of two cases and literature review. Gynecol Oncol. 1986;25(1):37–47.
101. Illanes D, Broman J, Meyer B, Kredentser D, McElrath T, Timmins 3rd P. Verrucous carcinoma of the endometrium: case history, pathologic findings, brief review of literature and discussion. Gynecol Oncol. 2006;102(2):375–7.
102. Fancher TT, Hamzi MH, Macaron SH, Magno WB, Dudrick SJ, Palesty JA. Hybrid verrucous-squamous cell carcinoma of the ovary with synchronous squamous cell carcinoma of the endometrium. Int J Surg Pathol. 2008;16(1):91–5.
103. Nascimento AF, Granter SR, Cviko A, Yuan L, Hecht JL, Crum CP. Vulvar acanthosis with altered differentiation: a precursor to verrucous carcinoma? Am J Surg Pathol. 2004;28(5):638–43.
104. Gualco M, Bonin S, Foglia G, Fulcheri E, Odicino F, Prefumo F, et al. Morphologic and biologic studies on ten cases of verrucous carcinoma of the vulva supporting the theory of a discrete clinico-pathologic entity. Int J Gynecol Cancer. 2003;13(3):317–24.
105. Kondi-Paphitis A, Deligeorgi-Politi H, Liapis A, Plemenou-Frangou M. Human papilloma virus in verrucus carcinoma of the vulva: an immunopathological study of three cases. Eur J Gynaecol Oncol. 1998;19(3):319–20.
106. Levitan Z, Kaplan AL, Kaufman RH. Advanced squamous cell carcinoma of the vulva after treatment for verrucous carcinoma. A case report. J Reprod Med. 1992;37(10):889–92.
107. Gadducci A, De Punzio C, Facchini V, Rispoli G, Fioretti P. The therapy of verrucous carcinoma of the vulva. Observations on three cases. Eur J Gynaecol Oncol. 1989;10(4):284–7.
108. Iwamoto I, Kijima Y, Fujino T, Yoshinaga M, Douchi T. Verrucous carcinoma of the vulva in Turner syndrome. Gynecol Oncol. 2004;92(1):380–3.
109. Tran TA, Carlson JA. Plasmacytoid squamous cell carcinoma of the vulva. Int J Gynecol Pathol. 2008;27(4):601–5.
110. Wolber RA, Talerman A, Wilkinson EJ, Clement PB. Vulvar granular cell tumors with pseudocarcinomatous

hyperplasia: a comparative analysis with well-differentiated squamous carcinoma. Int J Gynecol Pathol. 1991;10(1):59–66.
111. Persoons JH, Sutorius FJ, Koopman RJ, Schaafsma MR, van Doorn GA. Vulvar paraneoplastic amyloidosis with the appearance of a vulvar carcinoma. Am J Obstet Gynecol. 1999;180(4):1041–4.
112. Nuovo GJ, Friedman D, Richart RM. In situ hybridization analysis of human papillomavirus DNA segregation patterns in lesions of the female genital tract. Gynecol Oncol. 1990;36(2):256–62.
113. Chiasson MA, Ellerbrock TV, Bush TJ, Sun XW, Wright Jr TC. Increased prevalence of vulvovaginal condyloma and vulvar intraepithelial neoplasia in women infected with the human immunodeficiency virus. Obstet Gynecol. 1997;89(5 Pt 1):690–4.
114. Marshburn PB, Trofatter Jr KF. Recurrent condyloma acuminatum in women over age 40: association with immunosuppression and malignant disease. Am J Obstet Gynecol. 1988;159(2):429–33.
115. Sonnex C, Strauss S, Gray JJ. Detection of human papillomavirus DNA on the fingers of patients with genital warts. Sex Transm Infect. 1999;75(5):317–9.
116. Aguilera-Barrantes I, Magro C, Nuovo GJ. Verruca vulgaris of the vulva in children and adults: a nonvenereal type of vulvar wart. Am J Surg Pathol. 2007;31(4):529–35.
117. Moyal-Barracco M, Leibowitch M, Orth G. Vestibular papillae of the vulva. Lack of evidence for human papillomavirus etiology. Arch Dermatol. 1990;126(12):1594–8.
118. Crum CP, Fu YS, Levine RU, Richart RM, Townsend DE, Fenoglio CM. Intraepithelial squamous lesions of the vulva: biologic and histologic criteria for the distinction of condylomas from vulvar intraepithelial neoplasia. Am J Obstet Gynecol. 1982;144(1):77–83.
119. Nucci MR, Genest DR, Tate JE, Sparks CK, Crum CP. Pseudobowenoid change of the vulva: a histologic variant of untreated condylata acuminatum. Mod Pathol. 1996;9(4):375–9.
120. Harwood CA, Mortimer PS. Acquired vulval lymphangiomata mimicking genital warts. Br J Dermatol. 1993;129(3):334–6.
121. Brainard JA, Hart WR. Proliferative epidermal lesions associated with anogenital Paget's disease. Am J Surg Pathol. 2000;24(4):543–52.
122. Konig A, Wennemuth G, Soyer HP, Hoffmann R, Happle R, Krause W. Vulvar amyloidosis mimicking giant condylomata acuminata in a patient with multiple myeloma. Eur J Dermatol. 1999;9(1):29–31.
123. Schiera A, Pini M, Pioltelli P, Rossi E, Valente MG, Crippa D. Perianal condyloma-like lesions in multiple myeloma associated amyloidosis. Eur J Dermatol. 2004;14(3):193–5.
124. Goldsmith PC, Leslie TA, Sams V, Bryceson AD, Allason-Jones E, Dowd PM. Lesions of schistosomiasis mimicking warts on the vulva. BMJ. 1993; 307(6903):556–7.
125. Poggensee G, Kiwelu I, Weger V, Goppner D, Diedrich T, Krantz I, et al. Female genital schistosomiasis of the lower genital tract: prevalence and disease-associated morbidity in northern Tanzania. J Infect Dis. 2000; 181(3):1210–3.
126. Handley J, Hanks E, Armstrong K, Bingham A, Dinsmore W, Swann A, et al. Common association of HPV 2 with anogenital warts in prepubertal children. Pediatr Dermatol. 1997;14(5):339–43.
127. Domfeh B, Silasi DA, Lindo F, Parkash V. Chronic hypertrophic vulvar herpes simulating neoplasia. Int J Gynecol Pathol. 2012;31(1):33–7.
128. Mosunjac M, Park J, Wang W, Tadros T, Siddiqui M, Bagirov M, et al. Genital and perianal herpes simplex simulating neoplasia in patients with AIDS. AIDS Patient Care STDS. 2009;23(3):153–8.
129. Chen W, Koenig C. Vulvar keratoacanthoma: a report of two cases. Int J Gynecol Pathol. 2004;23(3): 284–6.
130. Gilbey S, Moore DH, Look KY, Sutton GP. Vulvar keratoacanthoma. Obstet Gynecol. 1997;89(5 Pt 2):848–50.
131. Rhatigan RM, Nuss RC. Keratoacanthoma of the vulva. Gynecol Oncol. 1985;21(1):118–23.
132. Connolly M, Narayan S, Oxley J, de Berker DA. Immunohistochemical staining for the differentiation of subungual keratoacanthoma from subungual squamous cell carcinoma. Clin Exp Dermatol. 2008;33(5):625–8.
133. Kaabipour E, Haupt HM, Stern JB, Kanetsky PA, Podolski VF, Martin AM. p16 expression in keratoacanthomas and squamous cell carcinomas of the skin: an immunohistochemical study. Arch Pathol Lab Med. 2006;130(1):69–73.
134. Vasiljevic N, Andersson K, Bjelkenkrantz K, Kjellstrom C, Mansson H, Nilsson E, et al. The Bcl-xL inhibitor of apoptosis is preferentially expressed in cutaneous squamous cell carcinoma compared with that in keratoacanthoma. Int J Cancer. 2009;124(10):2361–6.
135. Mandrell JC, Santa Cruz D. Keratoacanthoma: hyperplasia, benign neoplasm, or a type of squamous cell carcinoma? Semin Diagn Pathol. 2009;26(3):150–63.
136. Reich O, Regauer S. Recurrent verruciform xanthoma of the vulva. Int J Gynecol Pathol. 2004; 23(1):75–7.
137. Cumberland L, Dana A, Resh B, Fitzpatrick J, Goldenberg G. Verruciform xanthoma in the setting of cutaneous trauma and chronic inflammation: report of a patient and a brief review of the literature. J Cutan Pathol. 2010;37(8):895–900.
138. van Beurden M, van der Vange N, de Craen AJ, Tjong AHSP, ten Kate FJ, ter Schegget J, et al. Normal findings in vulvar examination and vulvoscopy. Br J Obstet Gynaecol. 1997;104(3):320–4.
139. Welch JM, Nayagam M, Parry G, Das R, Campbell M, Whatley J, et al. What is vestibular papillomatosis? A study of its prevalence, aetiology and natural history. Br J Obstet Gynaecol. 1993;100(10): 939–42.
140. Bergeron C, Ferenczy A, Richart RM, Guralnick M. Micropapillomatosis labialis appears unrelated to

human papillomavirus. Obstet Gynecol. 1990;76(2): 281–6.
141. Orosz Z, Lehoczky O, Szoke J, Pulay T. Recurrent giant fibroepithelial stromal polyp of the vulva associated with congenital lymphedema. Gynecol Oncol. 2005;98(1):168–71.
142. Bai H, Cviko A, Granter S, Yuan L, Betensky RA, Crum CP. Immunophenotypic and viral (human papillomavirus) correlates of vulvar seborrheic keratosis. Hum Pathol. 2003;34(6):559–64.
143. Heller DS, Kuye OO. Recurrent hypertrophy of the labia minora: a hormonally related lesion possibly related to fibroepithelial stromal polyps of the vulva. J Low Genit Tract Dis. 2011;15(1):69–70.
144. Wani Y, Fujioka Y. A vulvar fibroepithelial stromal polyp appearing in infancy. Am J Dermatopathol. 2009;31(5):465–7.
145. de Giorgi V, Massi D, Salvini C, Mannone F, Carli P. Pigmented seborrheic keratoses of the vulva clinically mimicking a malignant melanoma: a clinical, dermoscopic-pathologic case study. Clin Exp Dermatol. 2005;30(1):17–9.
146. Venkatesan A. Pigmented lesions of the vulva. Dermatol Clin. 2010;28(4):795–805.
147. Li J, Ackerman AB. "Seborrheic keratoses" that contain human papillomavirus are condylomata acuminata. Am J Dermatopathol. 1994;16(4):398–405; discussion 406–8.
148. Roth LM, Look KY. Inverted follicular keratosis of the vulvar skin: a lesion that can be confused with squamous cell carcinoma. Int J Gynecol Pathol. 2000;19(4):369–73.
149. Cohen PR, Young Jr AW, Tovell HM. Angiokeratoma of the vulva: diagnosis and review of the literature. Obstet Gynecol Surv. 1989;44(5):339–46.
150. McNeely TB. Angiokeratoma of the clitoris. Arch Pathol Lab Med. 1992;116(8):880–1.
151. Yamazaki M, Hiruma M, Irie H, Ishibashi A. Angiokeratoma of the clitoris: a subtype of angiokeratoma vulvae. J Dermatol. 1992;19(9):553–5.
152. de Giorgi V, Salvini C, Massi D, Raspollini MR, Carli P. Vulvar basal cell carcinoma: retrospective study and review of literature. Gynecol Oncol. 2005;97(1):192–4.
153. Feakins RM, Lowe DG. Basal cell carcinoma of the vulva: a clinicopathologic study of 45 cases. Int J Gynecol Pathol. 1997;16(4):319–24.
154. Palladino VS, Duffy JL, Bures GJ. Basal cell carcinoma of the vulva. Cancer. 1969;24(3):460–70.
155. Wieland U, Ritzkowsky A, Stoltidis M, Weissenborn S, Stark S, Ploner M, et al. Communication: papillomavirus DNA in basal cell carcinomas of immunocompetent patients: an accidental association?TITLE. J Invest Dermatol. 2000;115(1):124–8.
156. Dudzinski MR, Askin FB, Fowler Jr WC. Giant basal cell carcinoma of the vulva. Obstet Gynecol. 1984;63(3 Suppl):57S–60.
157. Sworn MJ, Hammond GT, Buchanan R. Metastatic basal cell carcinoma of the vulva. Case report. Br J Obstet Gynaecol. 1979;86(4):332–4.
158. Kanitakis J, Arbona-Vidal E, Faure M. Extensive pigmented vulvar basal-cell carcinoma presenting as pruritus in an elderly woman. Dermatol Online J. 2011;17(1):8.
159. Saini R, Sarnoff DS. Basal cell carcinoma of the vulva presenting as unilateral pruritus. J Drugs Dermatol. 2008;7(3):288–90.
160. Perrone T, Twiggs LB, Adcock LL, Dehner LP. Vulvar basal cell carcinoma: an infrequently metastasizing neoplasm. Int J Gynecol Pathol. 1987;6(2):152–65.
161. Mizushima J, Ohara K. Basal cell carcinoma of the vulva with lymph node and skin metastasis – report of a case and review of 20 Japanese cases. J Dermatol. 1995;22(1):36–42.
162. Gleeson NC, Ruffolo EH, Hoffman MS, Cavanagh D. Basal cell carcinoma of the vulva with groin node metastasis. Gynecol Oncol. 1994;53(3):366–8.
163. Winkelmann SE, Llorens AS. Metastatic basal cell carcinoma of the vulva. Gynecol Oncol. 1990;38(1): 138–40.
164. Hoffman MS, Roberts WS, Ruffolo EH. Basal cell carcinoma of the vulva with inguinal lymph node metastases. Gynecol Oncol. 1988;29(1):113–9.
165. Cruz-Jimenez PR, Abell MR. Cutaneous basal cell carcinoma of vulva. Cancer. 1975;36(5):1860–8.
166. Farmer ER, Helwig EB. Metastatic basal cell carcinoma: a clinicopathologic study of seventeen cases. Cancer. 1980;46(4):748–57.
167. Mulayim N, Foster Silver D, Tolgay Ocal I, Babalola E. Vulvar basal cell carcinoma: two unusual presentations and review of the literature. Gynecol Oncol. 2002;85(3):532–7.
168. Merino MJ, LiVolsi VA, Schwartz PE, Rudnicki J. Adenoid basal cell carcinoma of the vulva. Int J Gynecol Pathol. 1982;1(3):299–306.
169. Giuliani M, Di Stefano L, Zoccali G, Angelone E, Leocata P, Mascaretti G. Gorlin syndrome associated with basal cell carcinoma of the vulva: a case report. Eur J Gynaecol Oncol. 2006;27(5):519–22.
170. Ishizawa T, Mitsuhashi Y, Sugiki H, Hashimoto H, Kondo S. Basal cell carcinoma within vulvar Paget's disease. Dermatology. 1998;197(4):388–90.
171. Carr RA, Taibjee S, Sanders DSA. Basaloid skin tumours: basal cell carcinoma. Curr Diagn Pathol. 2007;13:252–72.
172. Beer TW, Shepherd P, Theaker JM. Ber EP4 and epithelial membrane antigen aid distinction of basal cell, squamous cell and basosquamous carcinomas of the skin. Histopathology. 2000;37(3):218–23.
173. Beller U, Benedet JL, Creasman WT, Ngan HY, Quinn MA, Maisonneuve P, et al. Carcinoma of the vagina. FIGO 26th annual report on the results of treatment in gynecological cancer. Int J Gynaecol Obstet. 2006;95 Suppl 1:S29–42.
174. Shah CA, Goff BA, Lowe K, Peters 3rd WA, Li CI. Factors affecting risk of mortality in women with vaginal cancer. Obstet Gynecol. 2009;113(5):1038–45.
175. Creasman WT, Phillips JL, Menck HR. The National Cancer Data Base report on cancer of the vagina. Cancer. 1998;83(5):1033–40.

176. Hellman K, Silfversward C, Nilsson B, Hellstrom AC, Frankendal B, Pettersson F. Primary carcinoma of the vagina: factors influencing the age at diagnosis. The Radiumhemmet series 1956–96. Int J Gynecol Cancer. 2004;14(3):491–501.
177. Eddy GL, Marks Jr RD, Miller 3rd MC, Underwood Jr PB. Primary invasive vaginal carcinoma. Am J Obstet Gynecol. 1991;165(2):292–6; discussion 296–8.
178. Andersen ES. Primary carcinoma of the vagina: a study of 29 cases. Gynecol Oncol. 1989;33(3):317–20.
179. Pride GL, Schultz AE, Chuprevich TW, Buchler DA. Primary invasive squamous carcinoma of the vagina. Obstet Gynecol. 1979;53(2):218–25.
180. Eddy GL, Singh KP, Gansler TS. Superficially invasive carcinoma of the vagina following treatment for cervical cancer: a report of six cases. Gynecol Oncol. 1990;36(3):376–9.
181. Brinton LA, Nasca PC, Mallin K, Schairer C, Rosenthal J, Rothenberg R, et al. Case–control study of in situ and invasive carcinoma of the vagina. Gynecol Oncol. 1990;38(1):49–54.
182. Iavazzo C, Vorgias G, Vecchini G, Katsoulis M, Akrivos T. Vaginal carcinoma in a completely prolapsed uterus. A case report. Arch Gynecol Obstet. 2007;275(6):503–5.
183. Batista TP, Morais JA, Reis TJ, Macedo FI. A rare case of invasive vaginal carcinoma associated with vaginal prolapse. Arch Gynecol Obstet. 2009;280(5): 845–8.
184. Otton GR, Nicklin JL, Dickie GJ, Niedetzky P, Tripcony L, Perrin LC, et al. Early-stage vaginal carcinoma – an analysis of 70 patients. Int J Gynecol Cancer. 2004;14(2):304–10.
185. Petru E, Luck HJ, Stuart G, Gaffney D, Millan D, Vergote I. Gynecologic Cancer Intergroup (GCIG) proposals for changes of the current FIGO staging system. Eur J Obstet Gynecol Reprod Biol. 2009; 143(2):69–74.
186. Davis KP, Stanhope CR, Garton GR, Atkinson EJ, O'Brien PC. Invasive vaginal carcinoma: analysis of early-stage disease. Gynecol Oncol. 1991;42(2):131–6.
187. Tjalma WA, Monaghan JM, de Barros Lopes A, Naik R, Nordin AJ, Weyler JJ. The role of surgery in invasive squamous carcinoma of the vagina. Gynecol Oncol. 2001;81(3):360–5.
188. Hellman K, Lundell M, Silfversward C, Nilsson B, Hellstrom AC, Frankendal B. Clinical and histopathologic factors related to prognosis in primary squamous cell carcinoma of the vagina. Int J Gynecol Cancer. 2006;16(3):1201–11.
189. Lee YC, Holcomb K, Buhl A, Holden J, Abulafia O. Rapid progression of primary vaginal squamous cell carcinoma in a young HIV-infected woman. Gynecol Oncol. 2000;78(3 Pt 1):380–2.
190. Miyazaki K, Yamaguchi K, Tohya T, Ohba T, Takatsuki K, Okamura H. Human T-cell leukemia virus type I infection as an oncogenic and prognostic risk factor in cervical and vaginal carcinoma. Obstet Gynecol. 1991;77(1):107–10.
191. Daling JR, Madeleine MM, Schwartz SM, Shera KA, Carter JJ, McKnight B, et al. A population-based study of squamous cell vaginal cancer: HPV and cofactors. Gynecol Oncol. 2002;84(2):263–70.
192. van Dam P, Sonnemans H, van Dam PJ, Verkinderen L, Dirix LY. Sentinel node detection in patients with vaginal carcinoma. Gynecol Oncol. 2004;92(1): 89–92.
193. Frumovitz M, Gayed IW, Jhingran A, Euscher ED, Coleman RL, Ramirez PT, et al. Lymphatic mapping and sentinel lymph node detection in women with vaginal cancer. Gynecol Oncol. 2008;108(3):478–81.
194. Ramzy I, Smout MS, Collins JA. Verrucous carcinoma of the vagina. Am J Clin Pathol. 1976;65(5): 644–53.
195. Jones MJ, Levin HS, Ballard Jr LA. Verrucous squamous cell carcinoma of the vagina; case report. Report of a case and review of the literature. Cleve Clin Q. 1981;48(2):305–13.
196. Wood WG, Giustini FG, Sohn S, Aranda RR. Verrucous carcinoma of the vagina. South Med J. 1978;71(4):368–71.
197. Okagaki T, Clark BA, Zachow KR, Twiggs LB, Ostrow RS, Pass F, et al. Presence of human papillomavirus in verrucous carcinoma (Ackerman) of the vagina Immunocytochemical, ultrastructural, and DNA hybridization studies. Arch Pathol Lab Med. 1984;108(7):567–70.
198. Robertson DI, Maung R, Duggan MA. Verrucous carcinoma of the genital tract: is it a distinct entity? Can J Surg. 1993;36(2):147–51.
199. Baltzer J, Zander J. Primary squamous cell carcinoma of the neovagina. Gynecol Oncol. 1989;35(1): 99–103.
200. Harder Y, Erni D, Banic A. Squamous cell carcinoma of the penile skin in a neovagina 20 years after male-to-female reassignment. Br J Plast Surg. 2002;55(5):449–51.
201. Gallup DG, Castle CA, Stock RJ. Recurrent carcinoma in situ of the vagina following split-thickness skin graft vaginoplasty. Gynecol Oncol. 1987;26(1): 98–102.
202. Van Dam PA, Irvine L, Lowe DG, Fisher C, Barton DP, Shepherd JH. Carcinoma in episiotomy scars. Gynecol Oncol. 1992;44(1):96–100.
203. Rose PG, Stoler MH, Abdul-Karim FW. Papillary squamotransitional cell carcinoma of the vagina. Int J Gynecol Pathol. 1998;17(4):372–5.
204. Abrenio JK, Chung HI, Pomante R. Verrucous carcinoma arising from an artificial vagina. Obstet Gynecol. 1977;50(1 Suppl):18s–21.
205. Steiner E, Woernle F, Kuhn W, Beckmann K, Schmidt M, Pilch H, et al. Carcinoma of the neovagina: case report and review of the literature. Gynecol Oncol. 2002;84(1):171–5.
206. Bobin JY, Zinzindohoue C, Naba T, Isaac S, Mage G. Primary squamous cell carcinoma in a patient with vaginal agenesis. Gynecol Oncol. 1999;74(2):293–7.
207. Dietl J, Horny HP, Kaiserling E. Lymphoepithelioma-like carcinoma of the vagina: a case report with

special reference to the immunophenotype of the tumor cells and tumor-infiltrating lymphoreticular cells. Int J Gynecol Pathol. 1994;13(2):186–9.
208. Patrelli TS, Silini EM, Berretta R, Thai E, Gizzo S, Bacchi Modena A, et al. Squamotransitional cell carcinoma of the vagina: diagnosis and clinical management: a literature review starting from a rare case report. Pathol Oncol Res. 2011;17(1):149–53.
209. Koenig C, Turnicky RP, Kankam CF, Tavassoli FA. Papillary squamotransitional cell carcinoma of the cervix: a report of 32 cases. Am J Surg Pathol. 1997;21(8):915–21.
210. McCluggage WG. Lymphoepithelioma-like carcinoma of the vagina. J Clin Pathol. 2001;54(12):964–5.
211. Mucitelli DR, Charles EZ, Kraus FT. Vulvovaginal polyps. Histologic appearance, ultrastructure, immunocytochemical characteristics, and clinicopathologic correlations. Int J Gynecol Pathol. 1990;9(1):20–40.
212. Nucci MR, Young RH, Fletcher CD. Cellular pseudosarcomatous fibroepithelial stromal polyps of the lower female genital tract: an underrecognized lesion often misdiagnosed as sarcoma. Am J Surg Pathol. 2000;24(2):231–40.
213. Maenpaa J, Soderstrom KO, Salmi T, Ekblad U. Large atypical polyps of the vagina during pregnancy with concomitant human papilloma virus infection. Eur J Obstet Gynecol Reprod Biol. 1988;27(1):65–9.
214. Hartmann CA, Sperling M, Stein H. So-called fibroepithelial polyps of the vagina exhibiting an unusual but uniform antigen profile characterized by expression of desmin and steroid hormone receptors but no muscle-specific actin or macrophage markers. Am J Clin Pathol. 1990;93(5):604–8.
215. Stewart CJ, Amanuel B, Brennan BA, Jain S, Rajakaruna R, Wallace S. Superficial cervico-vaginal myofibroblastoma: a report of five cases. Pathology. 2005;37(2):144–8.
216. Laskin WB, Fetsch JF, Tavassoli FA. Superficial cervicovaginal myofibroblastoma: fourteen cases of a distinctive mesenchymal tumor arising from the specialized subepithelial stroma of the lower female genital tract. Hum Pathol. 2001;32(7):715–25.
217. McCluggage WG, Young RH. Tubulo-squamous polyp: a report of ten cases of a distinctive hitherto uncharacterized vaginal polyp. Am J Surg Pathol. 2007;31(7):1013–9.
218. Stewart CJ. Tubulo-squamous vaginal polyp with basaloid epithelial differentiation. Int J Gynecol Pathol. 2009;28(6):563–6.
219. Chaturvedi A, Padel A. Tubulo-squamous polyp of the vagina with sebaceous glands: novel features in an uncommon recently described entity. Int J Gynecol Pathol. 2010;29(5):494–6.
220. Tong B, Clarke BA, Ghazarian D. Tubulo-squamous polyp with mucinous differentiation: a unique morphological variant. Int J Gynecol Pathol. 2011;30(5):518–9.

Vulvovaginal Mesenchymal Lesions

8

W. Glenn McCluggage

Abstract

The wide variety of mesenchymal lesions that involve the vulvovaginal region can result in diagnostic difficulties for pathologists, in part because of their relative rarity but also because of overlapping morphological features. They can be divided into those lesions which are specific to or characteristic of this site and those which can occur at any site with no predilection for the vulvovaginal region. Many of the site-specific or characteristic lesions are thought to arise from the specialized subepithelial stroma of the lower female genital tract that extends from the cervix to the vulva; the stromal cells of this region are hormone responsive and exhibit positive immunohistochemical staining with estrogen receptor (ER) and progesterone receptor (PR). As a consequence, most of the site-specific mesenchymal lesions are positive with ER and PR. Immunoreactivity with both desmin and CD34 is also common; this constitutes an unusual immunophenotype since mesenchymal lesions at other sites are uncommonly positive with both markers. The best known of the site-specific lesions is aggressive angiomyxoma, an infiltrative neoplasm with a marked propensity for local recurrence following excision. Recent developments with regard to aggressive angiomyxoma include the description of occasional metastasizing cases, the potential value of gonadotropin-releasing hormone agonists in management and the emergence of HMGA2 as a valuable diagnostic marker. Most of the other site-specific mesenchymal lesions are well circumscribed and exhibit little tendency for local recurrence. These include angiomyofibroblastoma, fibroepithelial stromal polyp, superficial myofibroblastoma of the lower female genital tract, and cellular angiofibroma. Smooth muscle tumors also occur in this region and

W.G. McCluggage, FRCPath
Department of Pathology,
Royal Group of Hospitals,
Grosvenor Road, Belfast BT 12 6BA,
Northern Ireland
e-mail: glenn.mccluggage@belfasttrust.hscni.net

L. Brown (ed.), *Pathology of the Vulva and Vagina*, Essentials of Diagnostic Gynecological Pathology,
DOI 10.1007/978-0-85729-757-0_8, © Springer-Verlag London 2013

are more likely than their uterine counterparts to have an epithelioid or myxoid appearance. Vulvovaginal smooth muscle neoplasms exhibit a propensity for local recurrence and the morphological features which predict malignant behavior differ from uterine smooth muscle neoplasms. Relatively, recently described mesenchymal lesions in the vulvovaginal region include massive vulval edema, prepubertal vulval fibroma, and reactive fibroblastic and myofibroblastic proliferation of the vulva (cyclist's nodule). Gastrointestinal stromal tumors have been described as primary neoplasms in the rectovaginal septum and vagina (termed extragastrointestinal stromal tumors). A wide range of other mesenchymal lesions potentially occur in this region, and it is stressed that when dealing with a vulvovaginal mesenchymal lesion, as well as considering the site-specific lesions, pathologists should consider a wide range of diagnoses since many mesenchymal lesions potentially occur in this region.

Introduction

A wide variety of mesenchymal lesions, neoplastic and nonneoplastic and benign and malignant, can involve the vulvovaginal region. These lesions not uncommonly result in diagnostic problems for pathologists, in part because of their relative rarity but also because of overlapping morphological features [1–4]. Some of the lesions are relatively specific to or are characteristic of the vulvovaginal region while others may occur at any site with no predeliction for this area. Table 8.1 lists the site-specific or characteristic mesenchymal lesions in this region. When faced with a vulvovaginal mesenchymal lesion, pathologists often consider the site-specific or characteristic entities but fail to think of other lesions which have no predeliction for this area but which may potentially occur here. Morphologically bland mesenchymal lesions are a particular problem [1–4], and it is important to distinguish between the various entities since their behavior may differ markedly. For example, aggressive angiomyxoma is a locally infiltrative neoplasm with a marked tendency to local recurrence following excision whereas other lesions such as angiomyofibroblastoma, cellular angiofibroma, and superficial myofibroblastoma of the lower female genital tract are well circumscribed with limited tendency to local recurrence. Many of the site-specific vulvovaginal mesenchymal lesions are thought to arise from the specialized subepithelial stroma of the lower female genital tract which is vascular, often has a somewhat myxoid appearance and may contain atypical fibroblast-like cells, including multinucleate forms (Fig. 8.1a). This zone extends from the cervix to the vulva; the stromal cells of this region are hormone responsive and exhibit positive immunohistochemical staining with estrogen receptor (ER) (Fig. 8.1b) and progesterone receptor (PR). As a consequence, most of the mesenchymal lesions specific to this site are positive with ER and PR. This zone is also positive with desmin and CD34 and, probably as a direct consequence, immunoreactivity with both desmin (Fig. 8.1c) and CD34 (Fig. 8.1d) is common in vulvovaginal mesenchymal lesions; this constitutes an unusual immunophenotype since mesenchymal lesions at other sites are uncommonly positive with both markers.

Table 8.1 Site-specific or characteristic vulvovaginal mesenchymal lesions

Aggressive (deep) angiomyxoma
Angiomyofibroblastoma
Superficial myofibroblastoma of the lower female genital tract
Cellular angiofibroma
Fibroepithelial stromal polyp
Smooth muscle neoplasms
Prepubertal vulval fibroma
Massive vulval edema
Reactive fibroblastic and myofibroblastic proliferation of the vulva ("cyclists nodule")

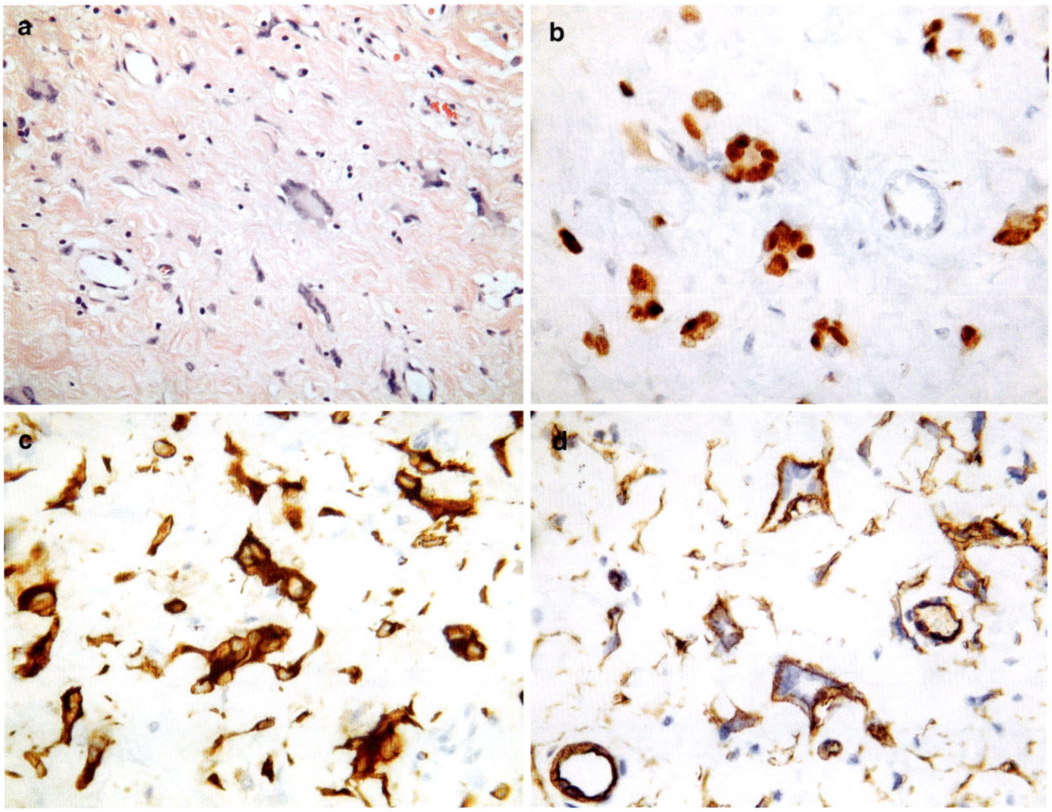

Fig. 8.1 Atypical fibroblasts, including multinucleate forms, are a normal feature in the vulvovaginal subepithelial stroma (**a**). This zone is often positive with ER (**b**), desmin (**c**), and CD34 (**d**)

In distinguishing the various mesenchymal lesions, immunohistochemistry plays a relatively minor role because of immunophenotypic overlap, although there are some important exceptions.

Given the overlapping morphology and immunophenotype and the relative rarity of the various mesenchymal lesions at this site, such that an individual pathologist is unlikely to see more than an occasional case in his or her practice, a specialist opinion should be considered; this has the added advantage of facilitating accrual of series of significant numbers of thesc uncommon lesions.

Aggressive (Deep) Angiomyxoma

Aggressive angiomyxoma, synonymously referred to as deep angiomyxoma by the World Health Organization [5], was first described in 1983 as "aggressive angiomyxoma of the female pelvis and perineum" [6]. It is an uncommon infiltrative but morphologically bland mesenchymal neoplasm with a propensity for local recurrence following excision.

Clinical Features

Aggressive angiomyxoma usually involves the deep soft tissues of the vulvovaginal region, pelvis, and perineum of females in the reproductive age group [7–9]. Similar neoplasms have been described in the inguinoscrotal region of males [10]. At presentation, aggressive angiomyxoma is often a large lesion which fills much of the pelvis, displacing rather than directly invading the pelvic structures. Occasional examples form a polypoid mass, although this is relatively uncommon. Aggressive angiomyxoma, like many other vulvovaginal mesenchymal lesions, is clinically often thought to

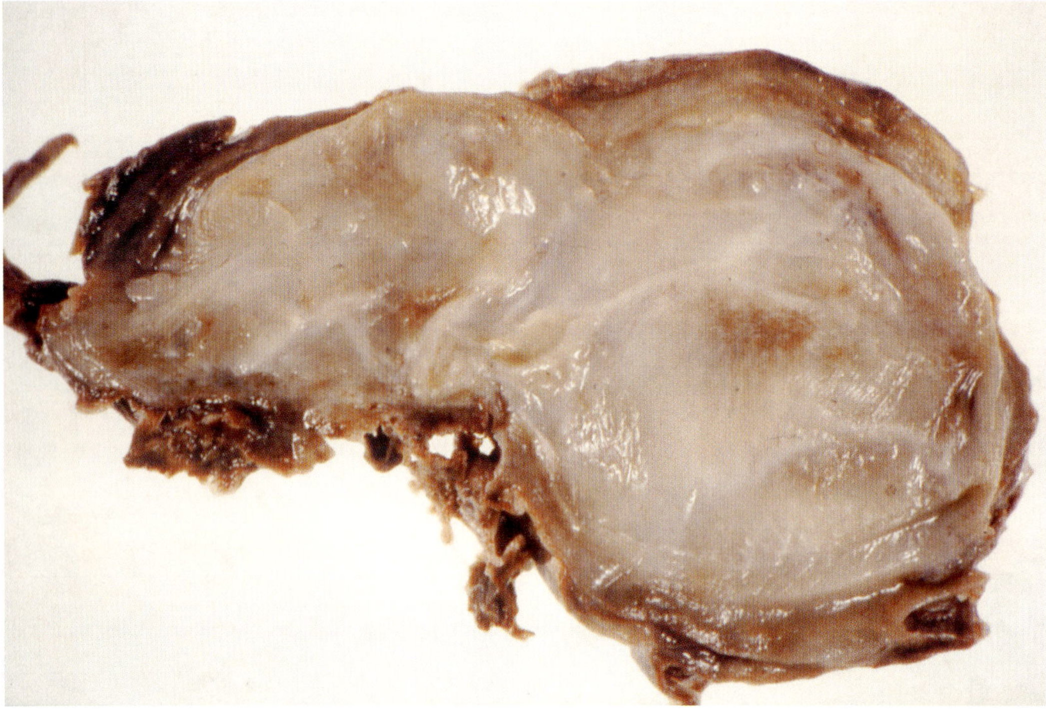

Fig. 8.2 Gross photomicrograph of aggressive angiomyoma showing a large mass with a gelatinous or myxoid cut surface

represent a cystic lesion, such as a Bartholin's gland cyst. It is a locally infiltrative neoplasm with a distinct propensity for local recurrence following excision, especially in lesions that are not adequately excised and extend to the resection margins. Often, there is deeper extension than is appreciated on clinical examination and total excision with a rim of surrounding normal tissue may be difficult. Tumor recurrence may be delayed, and there may be multiple local recurrences. A case of metastasizing aggressive angiomyxoma was described in the older literature [11] and more recently a seemingly bona fide example of an aggressive angiomyxoma that metastasized to the lungs following multiple local recurrences and resulted in the patient's death has been reported [12]; however, the development of metastatic disease is an extremely rare phenomenon. As discussed later, almost all aggressive angiomyxomas are hormone receptor (ER and PR) positive. This, together with the observation that occasional cases exhibit rapid growth during pregnancy, suggests that aggressive angiomyxoma is a hormone-responsive neoplasm that could respond to hormonal manipulation. There have been a few reports of aggressive angiomyxoma which have demonstrated a dramatic response to gonadotrophin-releasing hormone agonists (GnRH agonists) with marked diminution in size [13, 14]. These agents can be considered following excision if the lesion extends to or close to the resection margins or in a recurrent lesion where further excision is not feasible. They may also be useful in reducing the size of recurrent neoplasms, thus potentially allowing less radical surgery. Management of aggressive angiomyxoma with GnRH agonists has a similar rationale to the use of these agents in the treatment of uterine leiomyomas [15].

Gross Features

Grossly, aggressive angiomyxoma is typically large and poorly circumscribed with a gelatinous or myxoid consistency (Fig. 8.2). Often on slicing the specimen, the tumor tenaciously sticks to the knife. Some areas may have a more fibrous consistency.

Microscopic Features

Aggressive angiomyxoma is a uniform low cellularity neoplasm, the constituent cells having small bland ovoid to short spindle-shaped nuclei and indiscernible cytoplasm. Occasional cells with stellate-shaped nuclei may be present and the neoplastic cells are embedded in an abundant myxoid stroma (Fig. 8.3a). Mitotic activity and nuclear atypia are virtually absent. Stromal mast cells and extravasated erythrocytes are common. Numerous stromal blood vessels of varying caliber, ranging from thin-walled, capillary-like vessels to large vessels with thick muscular walls, are present. Perivascular smooth muscle fibers radiating from thick-walled blood vessels are a characteristic feature (Fig. 8.3b), and bundles of smooth muscle may be present in the stroma remote from blood vessels. Relatively unusual features include small foci of increased cellularity and a more fibrous stroma; the latter is especially a feature of recurrent tumors. Aggressive angiomyxomas have an infiltrative edge, often with entrapment of adipose tissue and skeletal muscle at the periphery. In occasional cases, foci resembling angiomyofibroblastoma are present, as discussed later.

Ancillary Techniques

The myxoid stroma is Alcian blue positive. The immunophenotype of aggressive angiomyxoma overlaps considerably with many of the other site-specific vulvovaginal mesenchymal lesions. The cells are invariably positive for vimentin and, in some cases, smooth muscle actin (SMA) and CD34. Most cases are desmin, ER (Fig. 8.4a), and PR positive [16, 17]; androgen receptor positivity has been described in cases in males. The architectural transcription factor HMGA2 (formerly known as HMGIC), located on chromosome 12q15, is often rearranged in aggressive angiomyxoma, resulting in aberrant HMGA2 protein expression (Fig. 8.4b), and this is emerging as a useful marker of aggressive angiomyxoma [18–24]. In one study, HMGA2 nuclear immunoreactivity, usually diffuse, was found in 10 of 12 aggressive angiomyxomas [24]. Most, but not all, of the other vulvovaginal mesenchymal lesions studied were negative, except for leiomyomas where a significant number were positive [24]. Blood vessels and native vulvovaginal connective tissues are HMGA2 negative [24]. In a patient with a history of aggressive angiomyxoma, it may be extremely difficult in a re-excision specimen to distinguish between residual or recurrent tumor and native vulvovaginal connective tissue for a number of reasons. Recurrent neoplasms may have a more fibrous appearance, and native vulvovaginal connective tissue has a somewhat myxoid consistency and contains numerous vascular channels. HMGA2 may be useful both in the evaluation of surgical margins and in the assessment of the presence or absence of residual disease in re-excision specimens. There is not a perfect correlation between HMGA2 gene rearrangement, as demonstrated by molecular techniques, and protein expression; in other words, in some cases, there is HMGA2 rearrangement without protein expression and vice versa [21, 22]. The HMGA2 gene has also been shown to be rearranged in cases of uterine leiomyoma, intravenous leiomyomatosis, endometrial polyps and nongynecological mesenchymal neoplasms, including lipomas, leiomyomas, chondroid tumors, and pulmonary hamartomas [23, 25]; in some of these, nuclear HMGA2 expression can be demonstrated.

Differential Diagnosis and Pitfalls

The differential diagnosis chiefly includes the other mesenchymal lesions discussed in this chapter. Aggressive angiomyxoma is the most important of the site-specific vulvovaginal mesenchymal lesions because of its marked propensity for local recurrence, and so it is important to accurately establish this diagnosis. Most of the other lesions are well circumscribed while aggressive angiomyxoma almost invariably has an infiltrative margin. It tends to be more overtly myxoid, both on gross and microscopic evaluation, and less cellular than the other mesenchymal lesions. HMGA2 may be useful in the distinction from other lesions with the exception of leiomyomatous neoplasms.

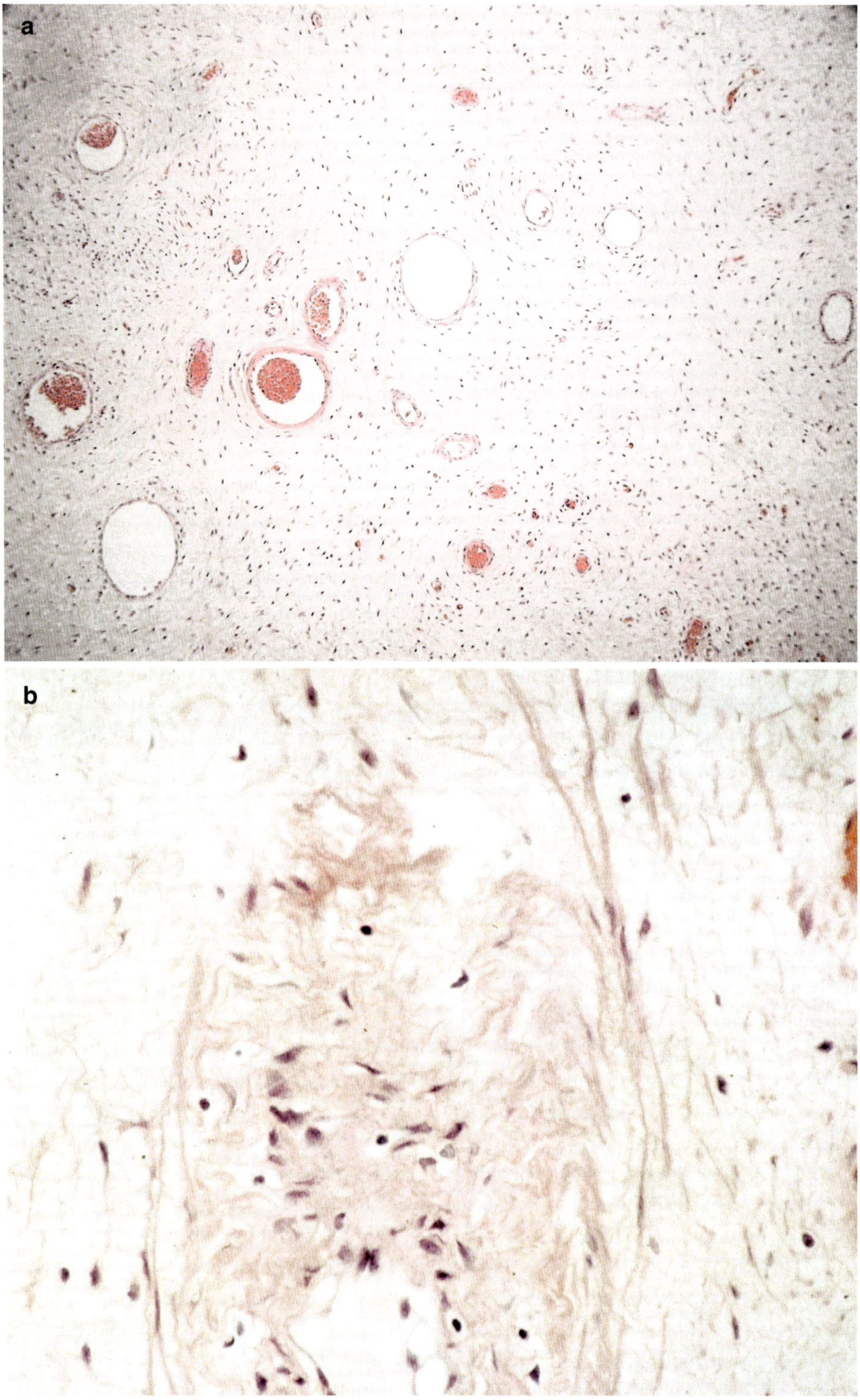

Fig. 8.3 Typical morphology of aggressive angiomyxoma with uniform appearance of bland spindle-shaped cells in a hypocellular myxoid stroma containing many blood vessels (**a**). Smooth muscle fibers sometimes radiate from the muscle coat of thick-walled blood vessels (**b**)

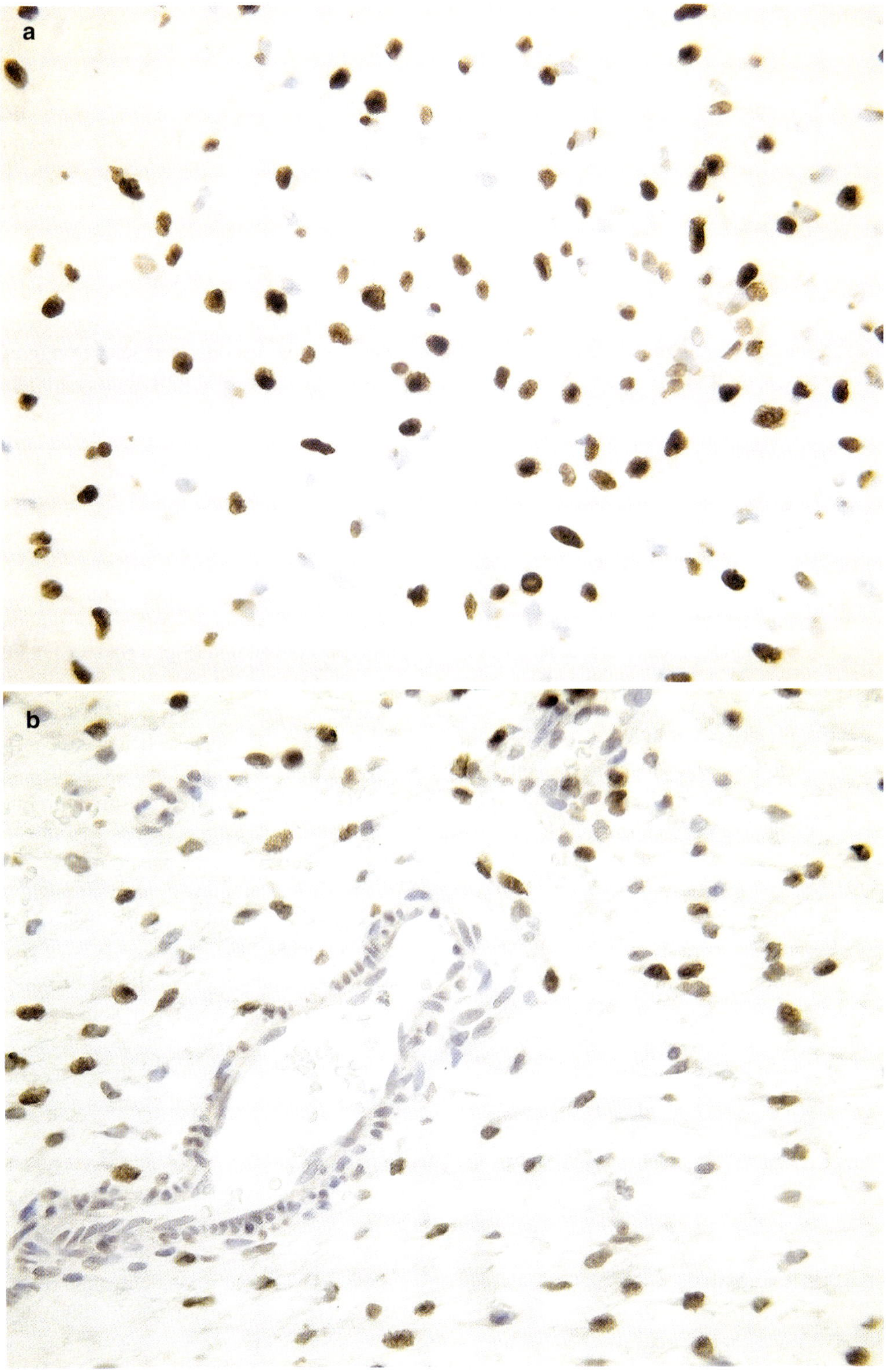

Fig. 8.4 Aggressive angiomyxoma exhibiting positive nuclear staining with ER (**a**) and HMGA2 (**b**); the nuclei of the blood vessels are negative with the latter

Angiomyofibroblastoma

Angiomyofibroblastoma was first described in 1992 as a benign vulval mesenchymal neoplasm distinct from aggressive angiomyxoma [26].

Clinical Features

Angiomyofibroblastoma typically occurs on the vulva, and more uncommonly in the vagina, of women in the reproductive and early postmenopausal years [27–32]. It is typically clinically thought to represent a cyst, although occasionally it presents as a polypoid lesion. A purported example has been reported in the fallopian tube [33]. Angiomyofibroblastoma almost always exhibits a benign behavior. Occasional cases recur locally following excision, especially those that have been "shelled-out." In contrast to aggressive angiomyxoma, when angiomyofibroblastoma recurs, the recurrence is nondestructive in that it can usually be easily removed. However, there have been occasional reports of sarcomatous transformation in angiomyofibroblastoma (see later), and it is probable that this has a small risk of malignant change, although further studies of well characterized cases are required to confirm this.

Gross Features

Angiomyofibroblastoma, in contrast to aggressive angiomyxoma, is a grossly well-circumscribed lesion and is typically less than 5 cm in diameter, although occasionally larger than this. The cut surface is usually pale or tan in color. Although the consistency may be slightly myxoid, there is not the obvious myxoid quality of aggressive angiomyxoma.

Microscopic Features

Histology shows a well-circumscribed but unencapsulated lesion. Although some lesions have a uniform cellularity throughout, characteristically there are alternating hypocellular and hypercellular areas (Fig. 8.5a). Many, usually thin-walled, capillary-like vascular channels are present. The nuclei may be ovoid to spindle-shaped, but there are typically foci, especially in the more cellular areas, where cells with an epithelioid appearance and abundant eosinophilic cytoplasm are present (Fig. 8.5b). Plasmacytoid cells may occur where the epithelioid nuclei have an eccentric location. Occasional multinucleate cells may be present. In the cellular foci, the epithelioid and plasmacytoid cells may be arranged in small groups or cords and tend to aggregate around blood vessels. Mitotic figures are rare or absent. The stroma is usually fibrous but focally may be edematous or myxoid. Scattered stromal mast cells and lymphocytes are common. Adipose tissue may be present, especially around the periphery, and a lipomatous variant containing abundant adipose tissue has been described [34, 35]; away from the lipomatous areas, the morphological features are otherwise typical of angiomyofibroblastoma (Fig. 8.6).

Rare neoplasms at this site contain areas resembling both angiomyofibroblastoma and aggressive angiomyxoma, and it has been suggested that these are related neoplasms in a spectrum of tumors exhibiting myofibroblastic differentiation [36]. These "hybrid" tumors are usually large infiltrative neoplasms mostly resembling aggressive angiomyxoma with small foci reminiscent of angiomyofibroblastoma. It is recommended that these be regarded as having potential for locally aggressive behavior and, as such, akin to aggressive angiomyxoma.

In one report of a recurrent tumor, the original neoplasm contained areas of typical angiomyofibroblastoma and sarcomatous areas resembling malignant fibrous histiocytoma [37]; the recurrent neoplasm was purely sarcomatous. A series of angiomyofibroblastomas with sarcomatous areas has been reported in abstract form [38]. The sarcomatous elements were of two types, one that morphologically resembled angiomyofibroblastoma and the other consisting of poorly differentiated sarcoma resembling leiomyosarcoma or undifferentiated sarcoma. The two types were termed malignant angiomyofibroblastoma and dedifferentiated angiomyofibroblastoma respectively [38].

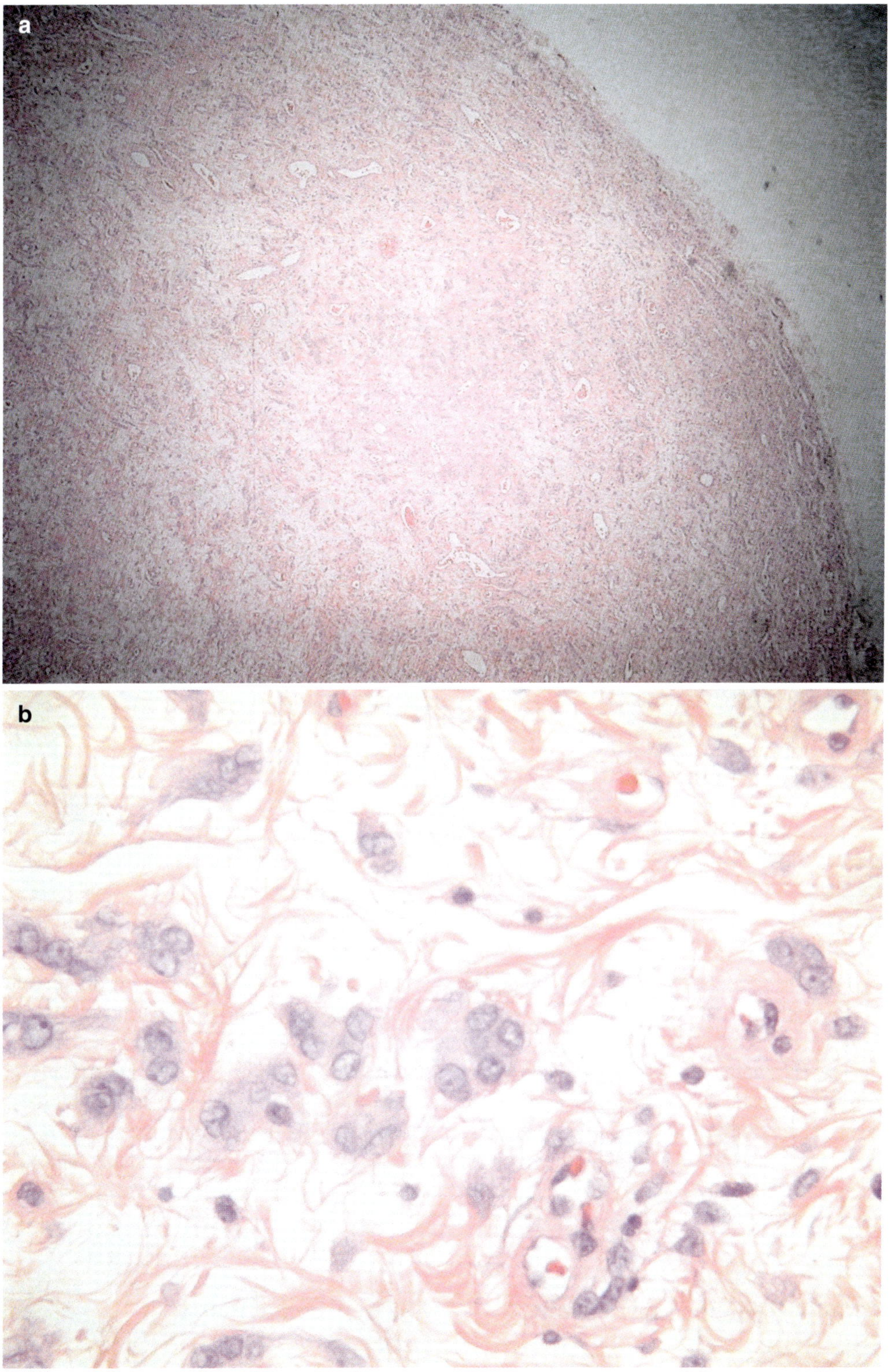

Fig. 8.5 Angiomyofibroblastoma with well-circumscribed edge and areas of varying cellularity (**a**). Groups of cells with an epithelioid appearance are a characteristic feature (**b**)

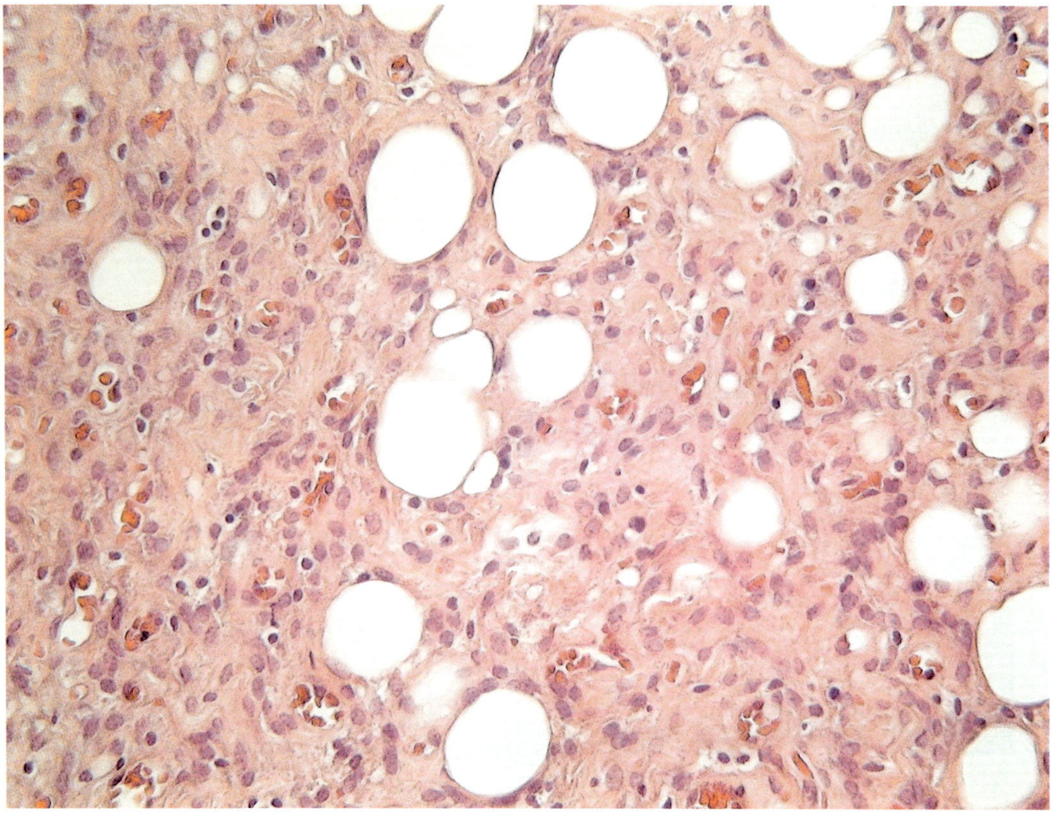

Fig. 8.6 Lipomatous variant of angiomyofibroblastoma containing abundant adipose tissue

Ancillary Techniques

The tumor cells are invariably immunoreactive with vimentin and are often desmin positive (Fig. 8.7). SMA may be positive but less commonly than desmin. There is typically nuclear staining with ER and PR and some cases are positive with CD34. There is much immunophenotypic overlap between angiomyofibroblastoma and aggressive angiomyxoma. In a single case of angiomyofibroblastoma, HMGA2 transcripts were identified using molecular techniques [39], although HMGA2 immunohistochemistry is negative [24].

Differential Diagnosis and Pitfalls

The differential diagnosis includes the other site-specific vulvovaginal mesenchymal lesions and other morphologically bland mesenchymal lesions which are not specific to this site. In contrast to aggressive angiomyxoma, angiomyofibroblastoma is well circumscribed, has a less myxoid and more fibrous stroma, is more cellular, and typically contains a population of epithelioid or plasmacytoid tumor cells. Blood vessels are usually thin-walled, in contrast to aggressive angiomyxoma which generally has a component of thick-walled vessels. While there is considerable immunophenotypic overlap with regard to ER, PR, desmin, SMA, and CD34, HMGA2 nuclear positivity favors aggressive angiomyxoma.

Fibroepithelial Polyp

Fibroepithelial polyp (fibroepithelial stromal polyp) is a relatively common polypoid lesion occurring on the vulva and vagina.

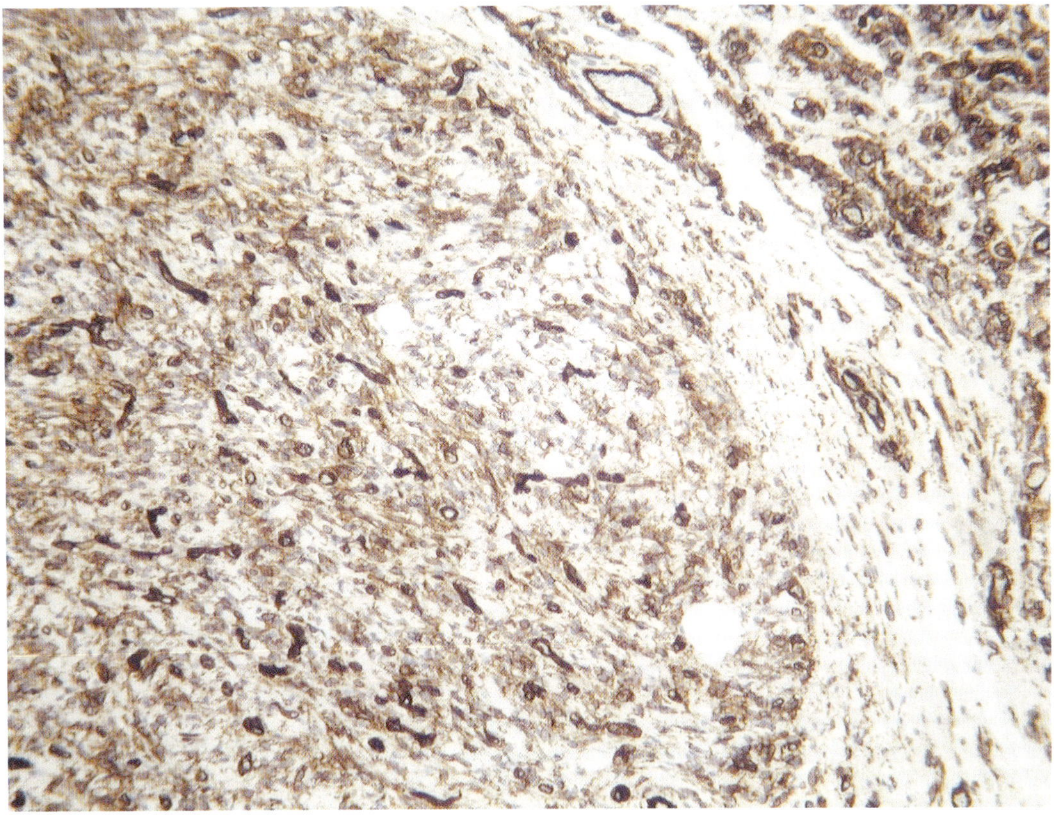

Fig. 8.7 Angiomyofibroblastoma exhibiting diffuse desmin positivity

Clinical Features

This polyp is the most common of the vulvovaginal mesenchymal lesions and may occur on the vulva or in the vagina, usually in women of reproductive age [40–42]. There may be a hormonal association since some patients are pregnant at diagnosis or there may be a history of hormonal usage or tamoxifen therapy [40–43]. However, the propensity for detection in pregnancy may simply be due to these lesions being discovered at antenatal examination; occasionally, the polyps regress in the puerperium. Sometimes, fibroepithelial polyps are multiple. These are benign lesions and local excision is usually curative. Rare cases recur locally, but the recurrence is nondestructive and re-excision can be undertaken. Sometimes, these polypoid lesions tort and undergo hemorrhagic necrosis.

Gross Features

On gross examination, these are polypoid lesions of varying size which are usually round but occasionally have a villiform appearance. They may be broad-based or sessile.

Microscopic Features

Fibroepithelial polyps are covered by squamous epithelium that is unremarkable or mildly thickened. Deep to the surface, within the core of the polyp, cells with spindle- and stellate-shaped nuclei are present (Fig. 8.8a). The cells are usually widely separated (Fig. 8.8b). Multinucleate cells or cells with multilobed nuclei are commonly present, sometimes with a wreath-like appearance (Fig. 8.9). The stromal cells, which are modified fibroblasts, usually extend right

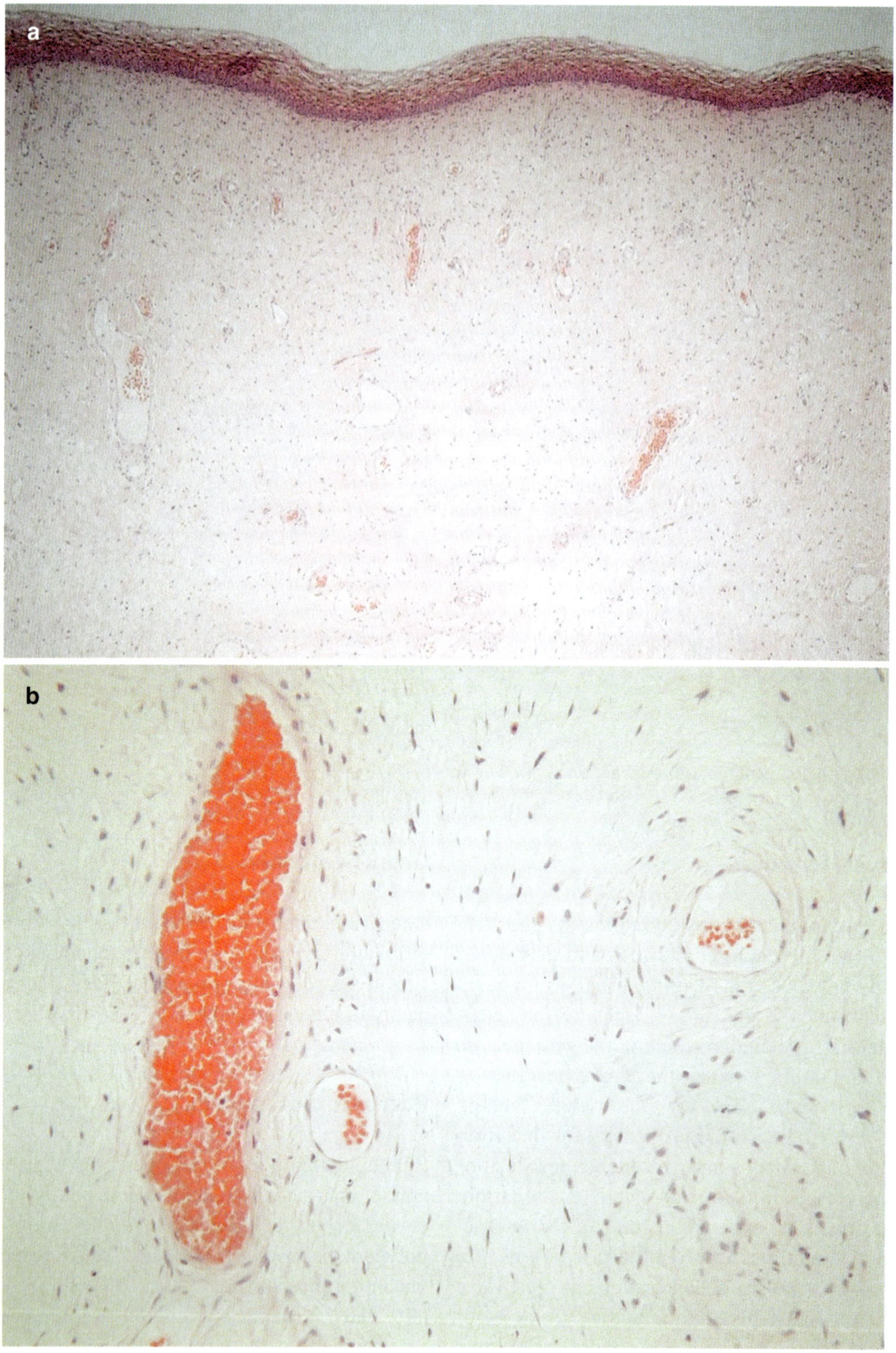

Fig. 8.8 Fibroepithelial polyp covered by unremarkable squamous epithelium with an underlying edematous and vascular stroma (**a**). Out of context, the edematous and vascular stroma could be mistaken for aggressive angiomyoma (**b**)

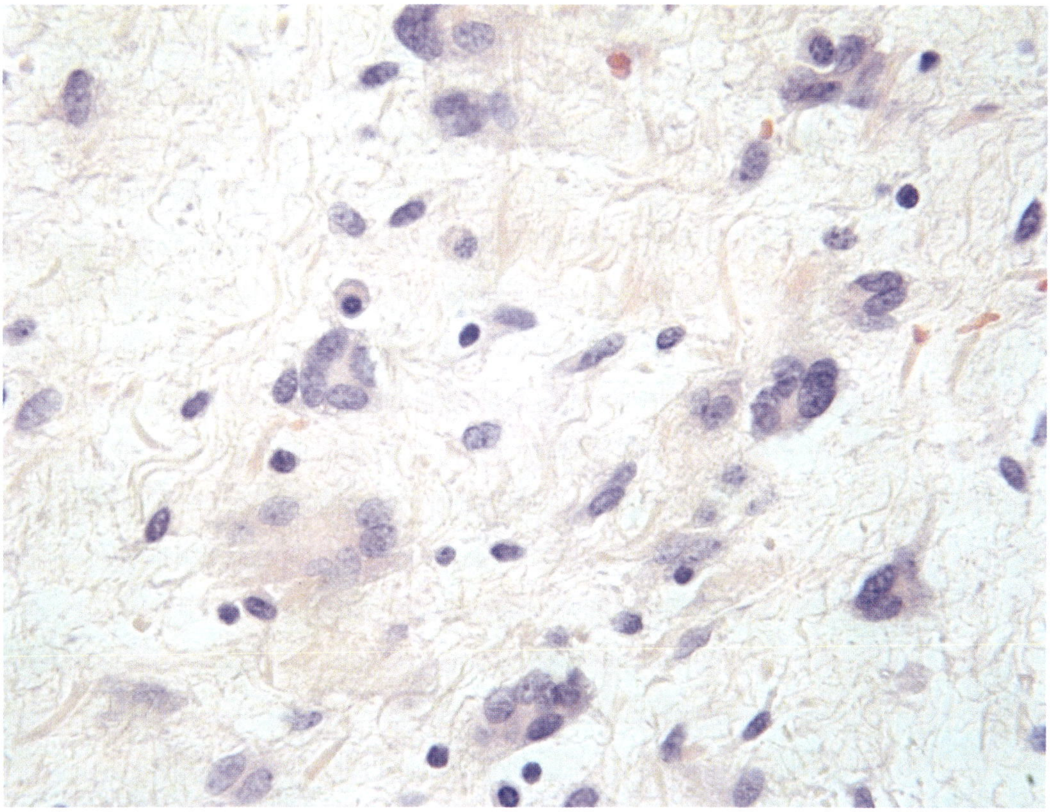

Fig. 8.9 Multinucleate stromal cells are common in fibroepithelial polyps

up to the epithelial-stromal junction without an uninvolved Grenz zone, and this is a useful diagnostic feature since most of the other vulvovaginal mesenchymal lesions are separated from the overlying surface epithelium by a Grenz zone. The stroma may be fibrous, edematous or somewhat myxoid (Fig. 8.8b). Stromal edema and myxoid change are especially common in larger lesions. The stroma often contains many vascular channels, especially thin-walled blood vessels, which are usually most prominent towards the center of the lesion. Occasionally, especially in cases which have undergone torsion, the endothelial cells may exhibit a degree of nuclear atypia (Fig. 8.10a). Torsion may also result in surface ulceration and extensive hemorrhagic necrosis. Sometimes, the lesion is more cellular and the stromal cells have a somewhat epithelioid appearance with round nuclei (Fig. 8.10b). Entrapped squamous or glandular epithelium is sometimes present within the stromal core, the glands representing skin appendage structures. Collections of inflammatory cells may be present.

Rarely, especially but not exclusively in pregnancy, a variety of features can be present that result in consideration of a sarcoma [44–50]. These features, which may be present singly or in combination, include marked stromal hypercellularity, bizarre nuclear features, numerous mitotic figures (occasionally >10 per 10 high-power fields), and atypical mitoses (Fig. 8.11) [50]. The terms cellular pseudosarcomatous fibroepithelial polyp and pseudosarcoma botryoides have both been used for lesions that exhibit these histological features [44–50], but it is recommended that such cases be reported as fibroepithelial polyp with the atypical features being described and stated to be of no clinical significance.

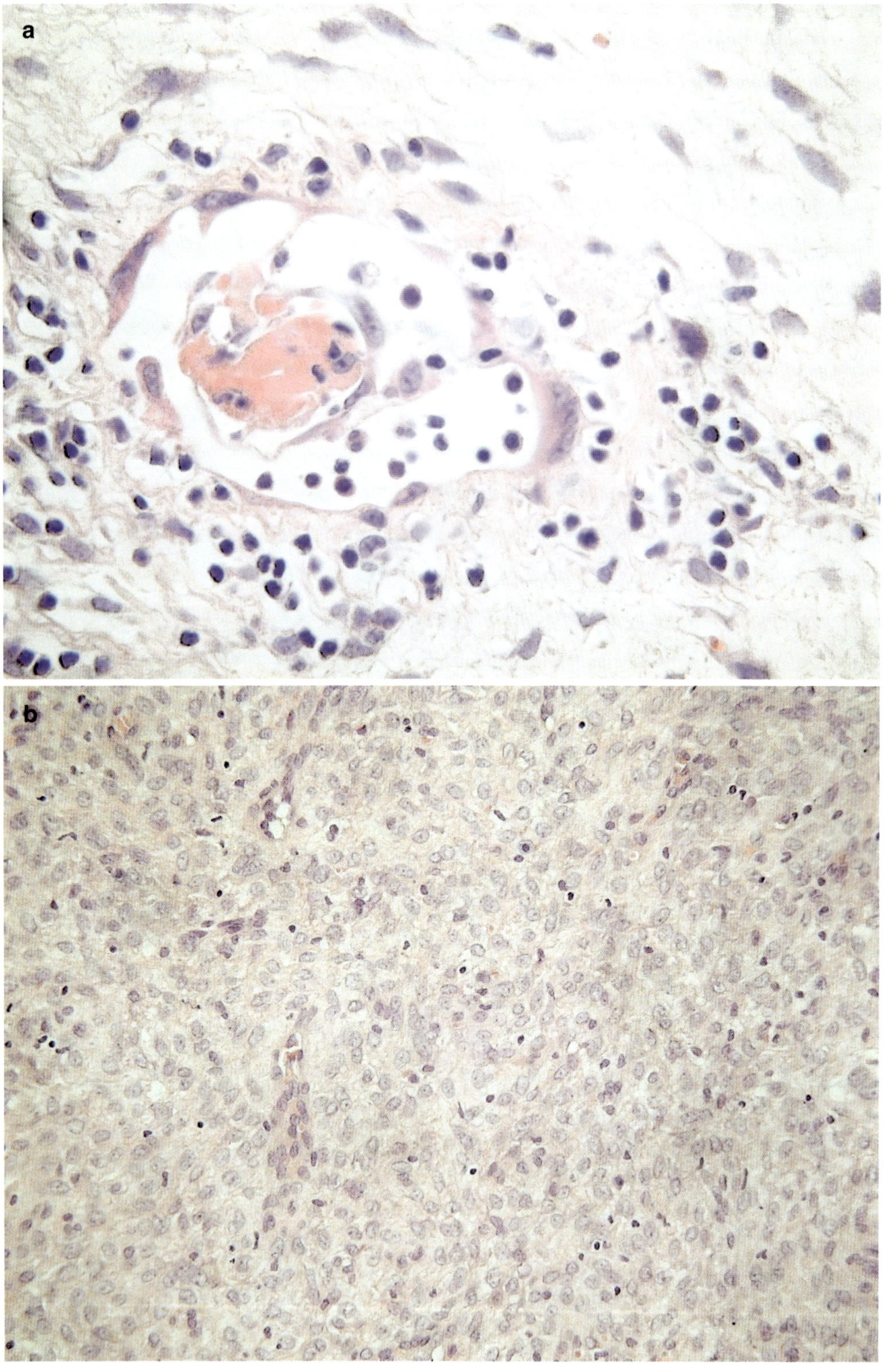

Fig. 8.10 Unusual features in some fibroepithelial polyps include atypical endothelial cells (**a**), an epithelioid appearance to the stroma (**b**)

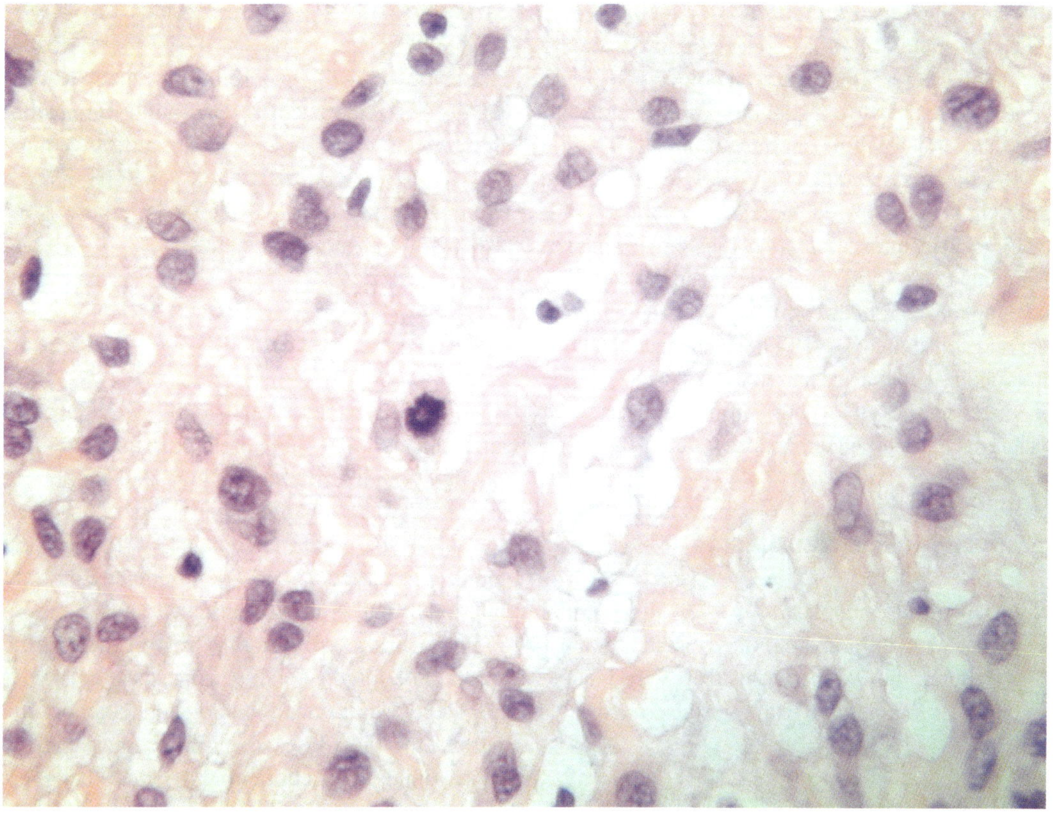

Fig. 8.11 Fibroepithelial polyp: stromal mitotic figures which are most commonly seen in pregnancy

Ancillary Techniques

The lesional cells are typically immunoreactive with vimentin, desmin, ER, and PR and less commonly with CD34 and SMA [40–42]. They are negative with S100 and cytokeratins. HMGA2 is usually negative, although in the only study to examine this, occasional cases were positive [24].

Differential Diagnosis and Pitfalls

The diagnosis is usually straightforward. However, difficulties may occur with large lesions, especially those that exhibit stromal edema or myxoid change; the latter can result in consideration of aggressive angiomyxoma, and taken out of context, areas within some fibroepithelial polyps could be compatible with a diagnosis of aggressive angiomyxoma. Appreciation of the polypoid nature of the lesion assists in establishing a diagnosis (aggressive angiomyxoma is only rarely polypoid), and the presence of multinucleate stromal cells is much more typical of fibroepithelial polyp than aggressive angiomyxoma. HMGA2 positivity favors the latter. A useful diagnostic feature in fibroepithelial polyp is that the stromal cells extend up to the epithelial-stromal junction without an uninvolved Grenz zone. This feature may be useful in the distinction from angiomyofibroblastoma, cellular angiofibroma, and superficial myofibroblastoma of the lower female genital tract which are usually separated from the overlying epithelium by a zone of uninvolved tissue; in fact, these lesions are often "shelled-out" with no overlying epithelium present in the specimen. Angiomyofibroblastoma and cellular angiofibroma usually present as "cysts" rather than polyps. Myofibroblastoma of the lower female genital tract (discussed later) presents as a polypoid lesion and may exhibit overlapping morphological features with fibroepithelial polyp. However, in myofibroblastoma of the lower female genital tract, there is typically an uninvolved Grenz zone deep to the surface squamous epithelium, and there are often multiple architectural patterns.

A variety of sarcomas may rarely enter into the differential diagnosis in those cases with atypical cytological features. Embryonal rhabdomyosarcoma (sarcoma botyroides) usually occurs in the vagina in a younger age group, a cambium layer is often present and cells with cross striations are seen. Positive immunohistochemical staining with skeletal muscle markers, such as myogenin and myoD1, assists in diagnosis of embryonal rhabdomyosarcoma.

Smooth Muscle Neoplasms

Smooth muscle neoplasms in the vulvovaginal region are uncommon, but not rare, and are much less frequent than in the uterus. Most are located in the vulva but vaginal examples also occur.

Clinical Features

Vulvovaginal smooth muscle neoplasms occur over a wide age range and clinically are often thought to be a cystic lesion, such as a Bartholin's cyst. They are usually well circumscribed and most are less than 5 cm [51–53]. There are few studies of vulvovaginal smooth muscle neoplasms with long-term follow-up, and so the features which predict recurrent or metastatic potential (discussed later) are not well established. However, vulvovaginal smooth muscle neoplasms have a potential for local recurrence, especially when "shelled-out." Some tumors recur many years after local excision and recurrences often exhibit more worrisome histological features, such as increased cellularity and mitotic activity, than in the primary neoplasm. Vulvar leiomyomatosis is a rare condition characterized by a multinodular proliferation of smooth muscle [54–57]. Rarely, patients with vulvar leiomyomatosis also have smooth muscle tumors in the esophagus, and there may be an association with Alport's syndrome [54–57].

Gross Features

These are typically well-circumscribed lesions, usually less than 5 cm in maximum dimension, although larger examples with an infiltrative margin occur uncommonly. They generally have a white whorled cut surface and are similar in consistency to uterine leiomyomas.

Microscopic Features

Histologically, these are usually well circumscribed, and there are three principal patterns, namely, spindled, myxohyaline, and epithelioid (Fig. 8.12). These patterns may be pure or mixed within an individual neoplasm. Although the spindle cell type is most common, epithelioid and, in particular, myxohyaline variants are more common in the vulvovaginal region than in the uterus. The spindle cell type consists of cells with elongated blunt-ended nuclei and eosinophilic cytoplasm (Fig. 8.12a), similar to most uterine leiomyomas. The epithelioid type is characterized by the presence of cells with round nuclei and abundant cytoplasm which may be eosinophilic or clear (Fig. 8.12b). In the myxohyaline variant, spindle-shaped or epithelioid cells are set in a myxohyaline stroma (Fig. 8.13), sometimes resulting in a nested, lacy, or plexiform appearance. Mucin pools may be present. The myxohyaline and epithelioid patterns may result in diagnostic problems but a clue to diagnosis is that there is often merging of these foci with areas of more usual smooth muscle differentiation.

The criteria that predict malignant behavior in uterine smooth muscle neoplasms cannot be extrapolated to vulvovaginal smooth muscle tumors. Features which predict recurrent potential in vulvovaginal smooth muscle neoplasms include any degree of mitotic activity or nuclear pleomorphism or an infiltrative growth pattern [1–4, 52, 53]. In the presence of any of these features, the possibility of local recurrence (which may be late) should be stated in the pathology report and even neoplasms not exhibiting these features may recur. It is useful to state in the pathology report that even when the morphology is bland and of a benign

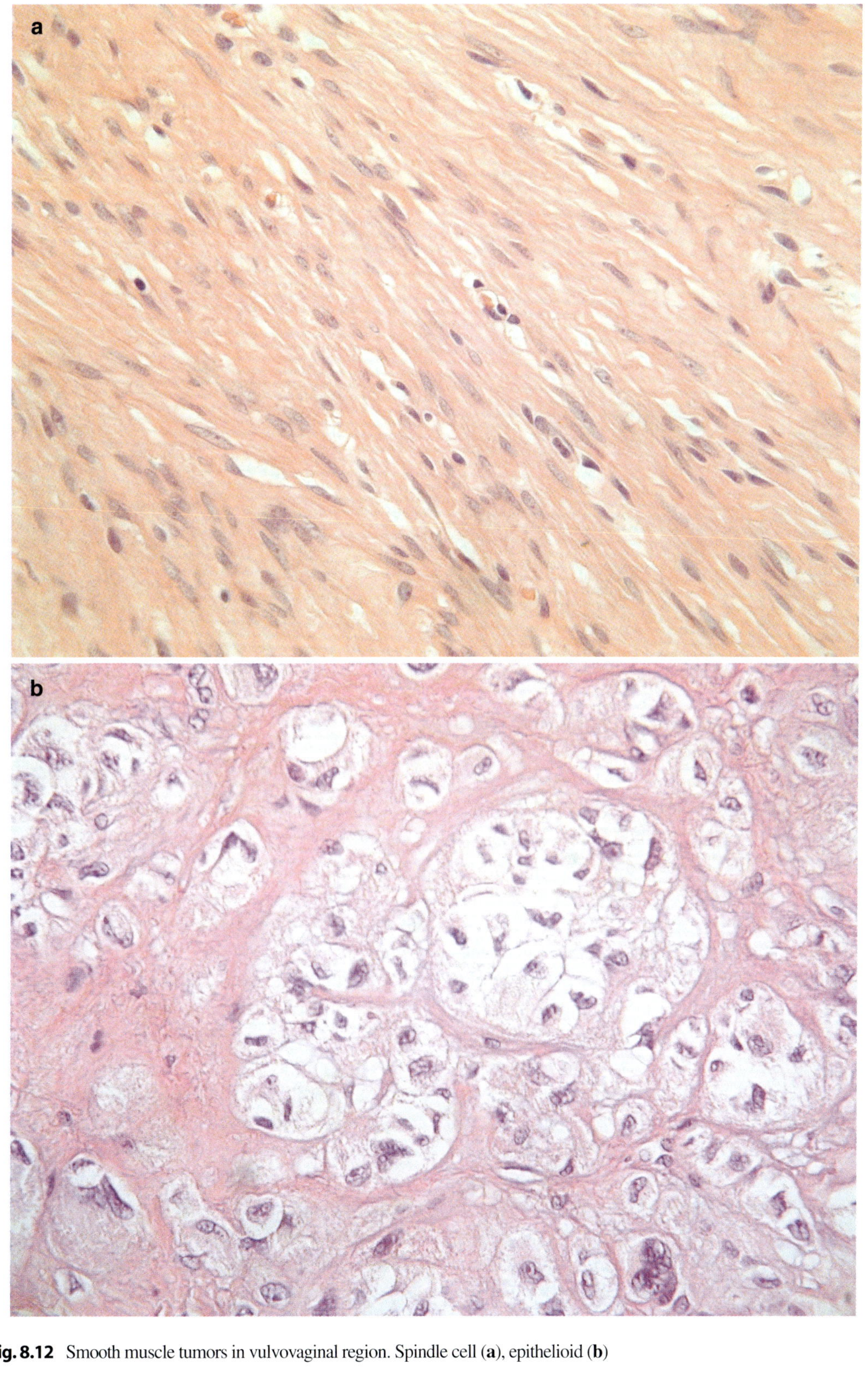

Fig. 8.12 Smooth muscle tumors in vulvovaginal region. Spindle cell (**a**), epithelioid (**b**)

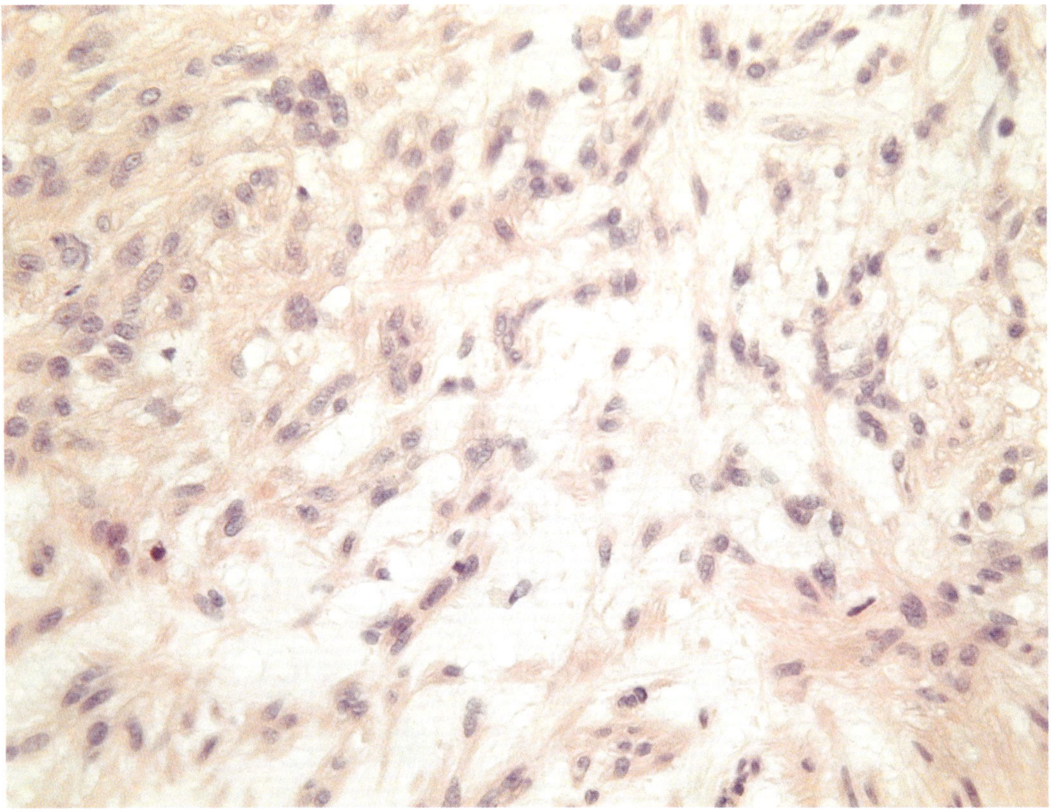

Fig. 8.13 Smooth muscle tumours: myxohyaline variants occur

leiomyoma, there is a possibility of local recurrence. The term "atypical smooth muscle tumor" has been proposed for lesions which do not fulfill the criteria for a diagnosis of leiomyosarcoma (see below) but which have any of the adverse features listed above [1]. In such cases, wide local excision is recommended whenever possible. However, the lesions are often initially "shelled-out" and the clinician may be reluctant to undertake further surgery given that the site of excision may not be grossly apparent and the problems associated with radical excision in this area.

The most commonly used criteria to predict metastatic potential in vulvovaginal smooth muscle neoplasms are those proposed by Tavassoli and Norris [53]. Tumors exhibiting three or more of the following features are classified as leiomyosarcoma: >5 cm in size, infiltrative margin, >5 mitotic figures per 10 high-power fields and moderate to severe cytological atypia. Coagulative tumor cell necrosis is also a worrying feature. Most leiomyosarcomas at this site exhibit obvious malignant morphological features.

Ancillary Techniques

The tumor cells are typically positive for the smooth muscle markers SMA, desmin, and h-caldesmon. ER and PR are also generally positive. A significant percentage exhibits nuclear positivity with HMGA2 [24]. Some of these neoplasms exhibit nuclear positivity with WT1, and it has been suggested that there are two broad groups of inguinal smooth muscle neoplasm, namely, an ER- and WT1-positive group of Mullerian-type smooth muscle tumors which are usually morphologically benign and associated with a good prognosis, and an ER and WT1 negative group which morphologically often comprise leiomyosarcoma and which have a guarded prognosis [58].

Differential Diagnosis and Pitfalls

The differential diagnosis can be wide and includes many of the other lesions discussed in this chapter. The histological features described and diffuse immunoreactivity with smooth muscle markers (especially h-caldesmon) assists in establishing a diagnosis. It is stressed that many other vulvovaginal mesenchymal lesions are positive with smooth muscle markers, especially desmin, although it is helpful that cellular angiofibroma, one of the main lesions in the differential diagnosis, is usually negative or at the most focally positive.

Cellular Angiofibroma

Cellular angiofibroma is an uncommon mesenchymal neoplasm that usually occurs on the vulva. Since the original description in 1997 [59], there have been several further reports [60–66] and these neoplasms may occur in females and males [66].

Clinical Features

Cellular angiofibroma usually arises in middle aged females and is clinically often thought to represent a cyst. Unlike most of the other site-specific vulvovaginal mesenchymal lesions, cellular angiofibroma has a marked predilection for the vulva with only occasional examples reported in the vagina [59–66]. Occasional cases have exhibited local recurrence following excision [60]. One study reported 13 cases of cellular angiofibroma (12 in females, 1 in a male) with morphological evidence of atypia or sarcomatous transformation [67]. Follow-up in these cases revealed no evidence of an adverse outcome.

Gross Features

These are usually well-circumscribed lesions with a firm gray-white cut surface and most are less than 5 cm in dimension.

Microscopic Features

The classical morphology is of a well-circumscribed but unencapsulated lesion, often with entrapped adipose tissue at the periphery. The lesion is usually moderately cellular and composed of a uniform population of bland spindle-shaped cells in a fibrous stroma with bundles of wispy collagen. Occasionally, there is vague nuclear palisading. Mitotic figures, although generally sparse, may be easily identified in some cases. Numerous blood vessels are typically present which are of small to medium size, often with thick hyalinized walls (Fig. 8.14), this being one of the characteristic histological features of cellular angiofibroma; however, vessels with think hyalinized walls are not always present. Stromal mast cells may be present.

One report focused on lesions which deviated from the typical morphological picture and expanded on the histological spectrum of cellular angiofibroma [65]. In some cases, there were vessels without thick hyalinized walls and in others hypocellular hyalinized areas were present. Other unusual features included a hemangiopericytomatous vascular pattern, stromal lymphoid aggregates, myxoid areas, and focal marked nuclear pleomorphism (Fig. 8.15), reminiscent of symplastic change within a uterine leiomyoma; the latter usually occurred in association with adipocytes [65].

In the previously referred to series of cases which exhibited atypia or sarcomatous transformation [67], in some cases, there were scattered foci of atypical cells without mitotic activity. In the cases which exhibited sarcomatous transformation, there was an abrupt transition between benign and malignant areas. The sarcomatous component either consisted of pleomorphic liposarcoma, atypical lipomatous tumor, or undifferentiated sarcoma [67].

Ancillary Techniques

Cellular angiofibroma is positive with vimentin and usually, although not always, negative with SMA, desmin, and h-caldesmon [59–66]. Occasional cases are focally positive with these

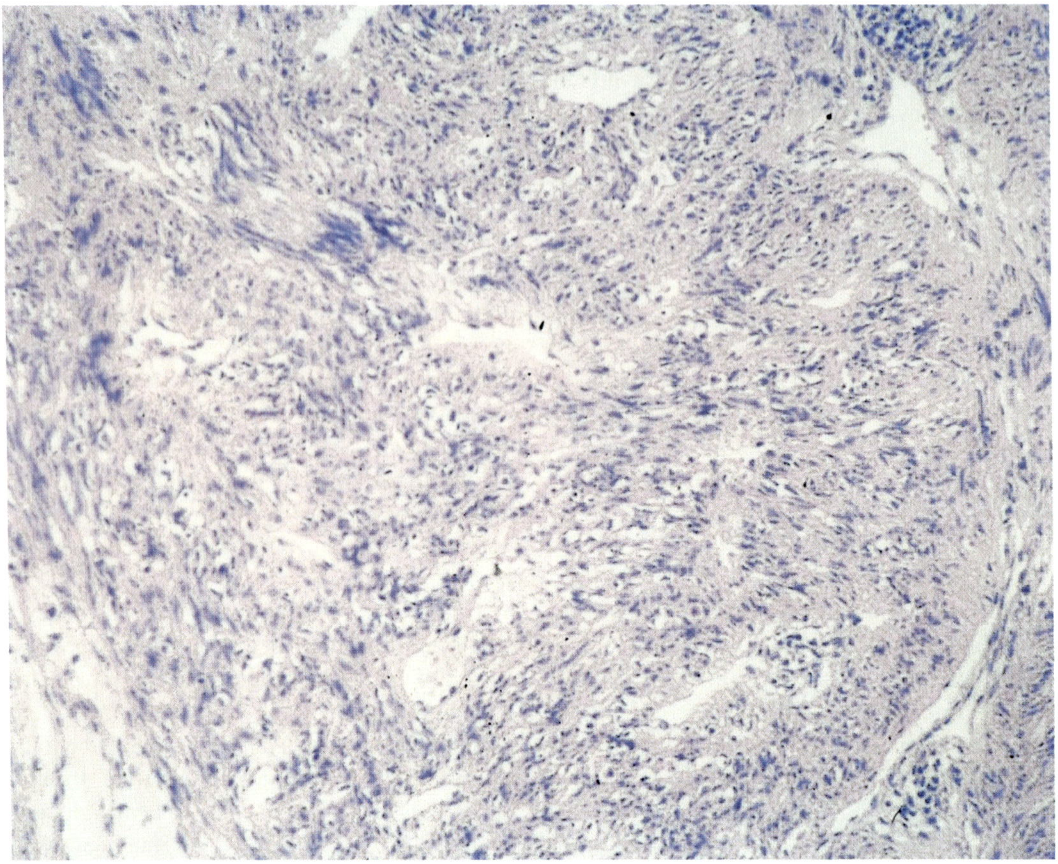

Fig. 8.14 Typical appearance of cellular angiofibroma with bland spindle-shaped cells and blood vessels with thick hyalinized walls

smooth muscle markers. An absence of staining with smooth muscle markers may be useful in diagnosis since most of the other site-specific vulvovaginal mesenchymal lesions are at least focally positive, especially with desmin. CD34 is not uncommonly positive with 60% of cases being immunoreactive in one series [66]. Most examples exhibit positive nuclear staining with ER and PR [59–66]. Some cases are CD10 positive. EMA positivity has been reported in a single case and S100 is negative [65]. On the basis of negative staining with smooth muscle markers and ultrastructural examination of a single case [60], it is suggested that cellular angiofibroma exhibits fibroblastic rather than myofibroblastic differentiation, the latter being a feature of many of the other site-specific vulvovaginal mesenchymal lesions. Overexpression of p16 in the atypical cells and in the sarcomatous components suggests that this may be implicated in malignant transformation of cellular angiofibroma [67].

Abnormalities of chromosome 13q14, including deletions and monoallelic loss, have been reported in cellular angiofibroma [68]. Spindle cell lipoma and extramammary myofibroblastoma have also been shown to exhibit 13q loss; this suggests a genetic relationship between these three lesions which exhibit overlapping morphological and immunophenotypic features, including CD34 expression, and it may be that they form part of a morphological spectrum.

Differential Diagnosis and Pitfalls

Distinction from aggressive angiomyxoma is based on the circumscription of cellular

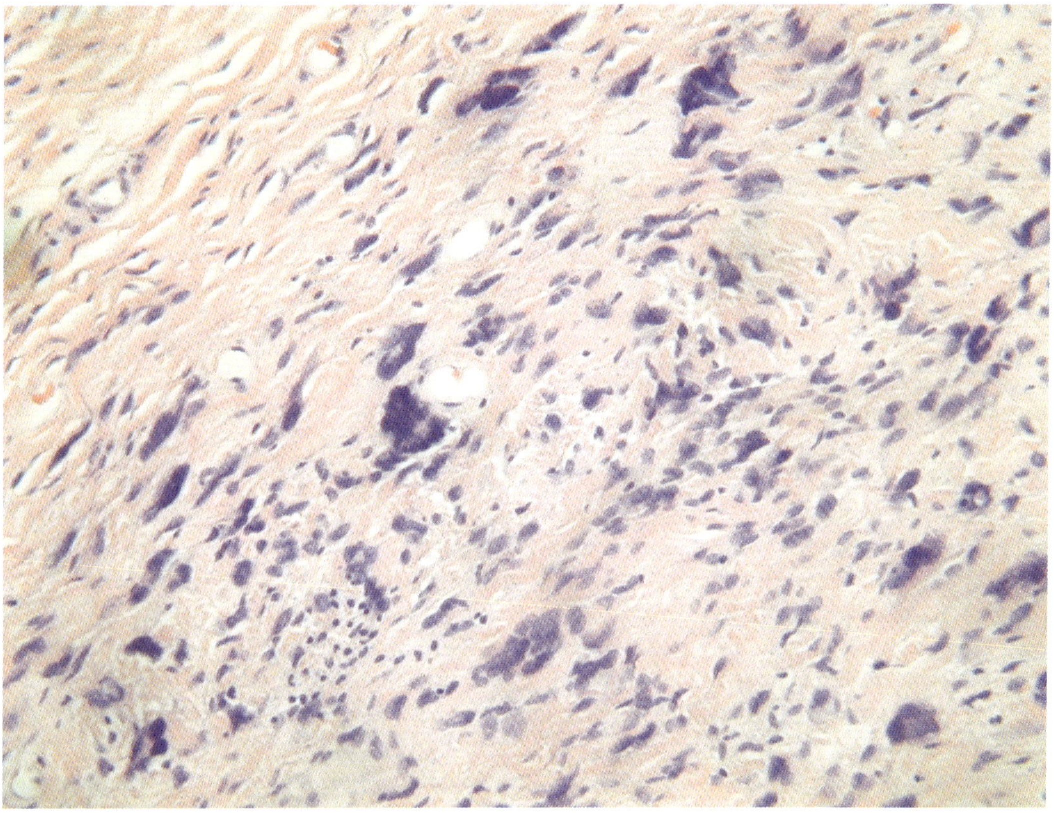

Fig. 8.15 Unusual morphologic features in cellular angiofibroma include foci of markedly atypical nuclei with a symplastic-like appearance; these are usually seen in relation to adipose tissue

angiofibroma, its higher cellularity, a more fibrous and less myxoid stroma, and a greater tendency for hyalinization of vessel walls. HMGA2 is negative. In comparison to angiomyofibroblastoma, cellular angiofibroma is more monomorphic without epithelioid or plasmacytoid cells and without a perivascular increase in cellularity. The vessels in angiomyofibroblastoma are generally thin-walled in contrast to the thick hyalinized vessels found, at least focally, in most cellular angiofibromas. The presence of adipose tissue within cellular angiofibroma and the character of the cells may result in consideration of a spindle cell lipoma, and as discussed it may be that these lesions are part of a morphological spectrum. However, vessels with hyalinized walls are not a feature of spindle cell lipoma, which usually contains more adipose tissue and is more consistently positive for CD34 than cellular angiofibroma.

Often, the main differential diagnosis considered on the morphology is a smooth muscle neoplasm. This is an important distinction to make since mitotic figures are not uncommon in cellular angiofibroma, but any mitotic activity in a vulvovaginal smooth muscle neoplasm is worrisome and indicates a potential for local recurrence. In this distinction, positive staining, especially when diffuse, with one or more of the smooth muscle markers desmin, SMA, and h-caldesmon is supportive of a smooth muscle neoplasm since cellular angiofibroma is usually negative.

Superficial Myofibroblastoma of the Lower Female Genital Tract (Superficial Cervicovaginal Myofibroblastoma)

In 2001, Laskin et al. described a distinctive mesenchymal tumor arising in the superficial lamina propria of the cervix and vagina [69]. The term superficial cervicovaginal myofibroblastoma was proposed to encompass the superficial location in the cervix or vagina and presumed myofibroblastic differentiation. A subsequent series of cases involved the vagina and the vulva, and the term superficial myofibroblastoma of the lower female genital tract was proposed since some neoplasms have a vulval location [70].

Clinical Features

These occur in premenopausal or postmenopausal patients and usually present as polypoid lesions most commonly involving the vagina and less often the cervix or vulva. Some patients have been taking tamoxifen, raising the possibility of an association with this medication [69–71]. Based on the reported cases, superficial myofibroblastoma of the lower female genital tract is a benign lesion, although there is uncommonly local recurrence following excision [69–71]. Metastasis or malignant transformation has not been reported.

Gross Features

Grossly these are well circumscribed. They are often, but not always, polypoid in appearance.

Microscopic Features

Histological examination shows a well-circumscribed but unencapsulated lesion covered by unremarkable or thickened squamous epithelium. Deep to the surface epithelium, there is usually an uninvolved Grenz zone, although rarely the lesion extends up to the epithelial-stromal junction. There are typically areas of varying cellularity with cells with bland ovoid, spindle-, or stellate-shaped nuclei, often with a somewhat wavy appearance, embedded in a finely collagenous stroma, sometimes with thicker collagen bundles. Multiple patterns, including lacelike, sieve-like and fascicular, and resulting in a heterogeneous appearance, are a characteristic feature, as are myxoid or edematous foci (Fig. 8.16a). Few or no mitoses are present.

Ancillary Techniques

The cells are positive with vimentin and usually with desmin [69–71]. CD34 and SMA are positive in some cases and most neoplasms are ER and PR positive. S100, EMA, and cytokeratins are negative. Desmin staining typically highlights the ramifying dendritic processes of many of the tumor cells (Fig. 8.16b). The immunophenotype is nonspecific and identical to many of the other site-specific vulvovaginal mesenchymal lesions.

Differential Diagnosis and Pitfalls

Perhaps the main differential diagnosis is a cellular fibroepithelial polyp since both lesions typically have a polypoid gross appearance. The Grenz zone which is typical of superficial myofibroblastoma of the lower female genital tract is not a feature of fibroepithelial polyp and the former is characterized by a more heterogenous appearance with a variety of architectural patterns. This lesion is distinguished from aggressive angiomyxoma by its circumscription, more heterogenous appearance and negative staining with HMGA2. Angiomyofibroblastoma often contains a population of epithelioid or plasmacytoid cells and is more vascular than superficial myofibroblastoma of the lower female genital tract. Negative staining with S100 helps to exclude a neural lesion since some of the morphological features, such as the presence of wavy nuclei, may raise this possibility.

Prepubertal Vulval Fibroma

This lesion was initially described by two different groups in 2004 and 2005 [72, 73]. In the first publication, the lesion was designated "prepubertal vulval fibroma" [72] and in the second "childhood asymmetric labium majus enlargement"

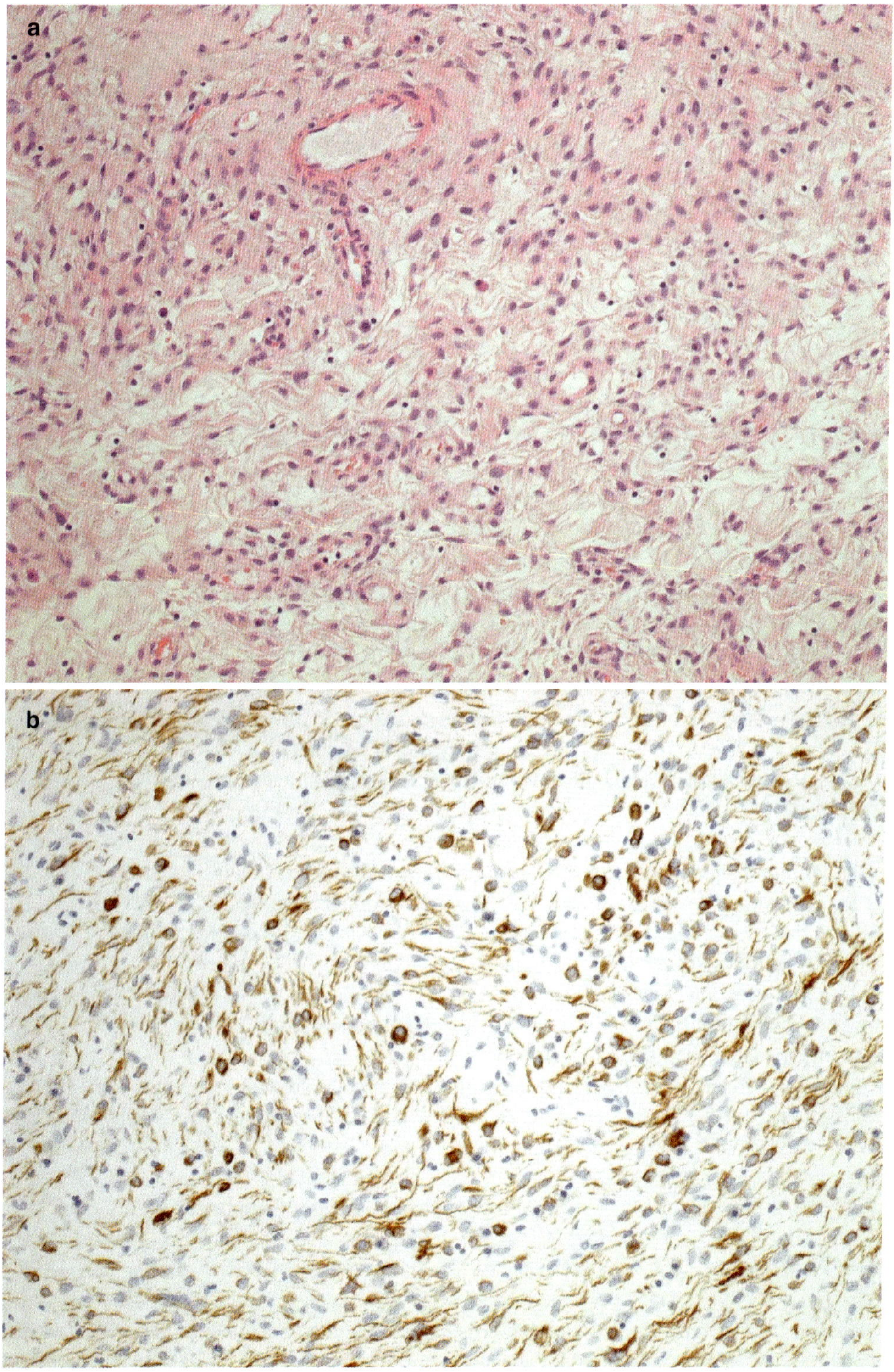

Fig. 8.16 Superficial myofibroblastoma of the lower female genital tract composed of bland spindle cells with cellular areas and hypocellular edematous areas (**a**). Desmin staining highlights the dendritic cell processes in some of the tumor cells (**b**)

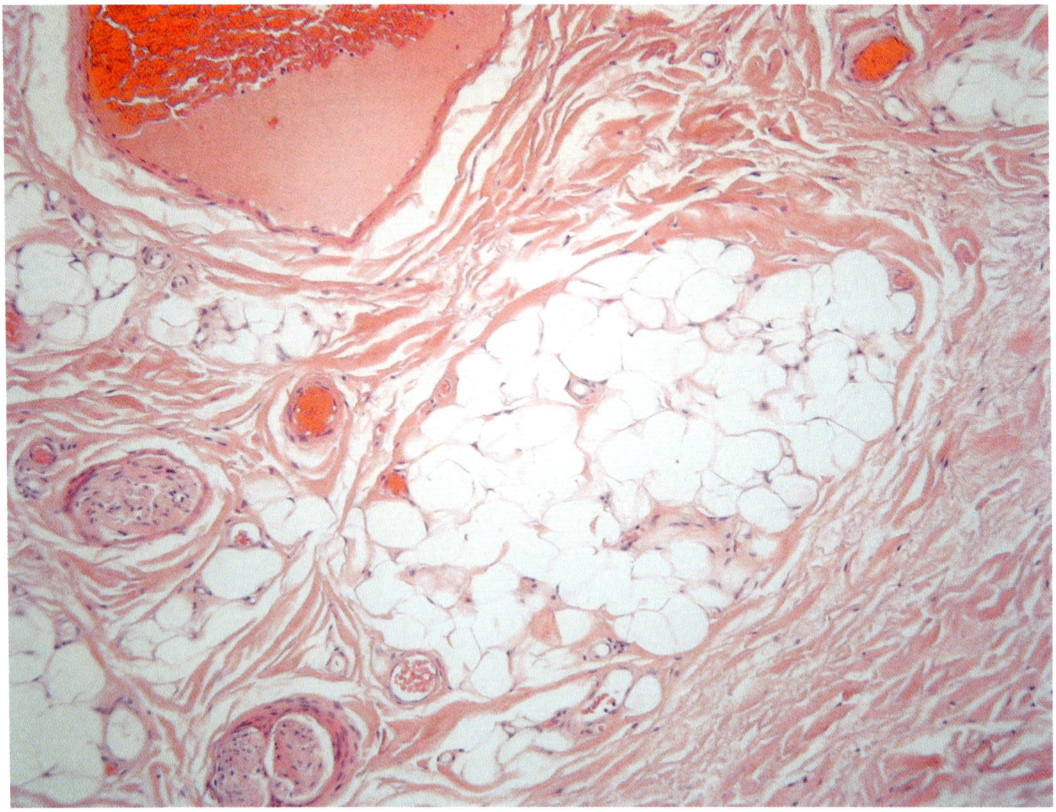

Fig. 8.17 Prepubertal vulval fibroma composed of haphazard admixture of hypocellular fibrous tissue, adipose tissue, vascular channels, and nerve fibers

[73]. The term prepubertal vulval fibroma is preferred and is now in widespread use. In one of the papers, it was suggested that this might represent the childhood equivalent of aggressive angiomyxoma, and in the other it was considered that this was a physiologic enlargement in response to the hormonal changes of pre- and early puberty with hormonal activation of otherwise normal native tissues [72, 73]. A hamartomatous lesion is also a possibility since there is an admixture of tissues normally found at this site.

Clinical Features

This lesion occurs largely in prepubertal girls aged 3–13 years. Almost all cases involve the labium majus, and these are usually unilateral lesions located in the submucosa or subcutaneous tissue. Occasional cases are bilateral. There may be recurrence following local excision [72, 73]. A seemingly identical case has been described in a 65-year-old female [74].

Gross Features

Macroscopically, these are poorly circumscribed and ill-defined lesions, usually with a fibrous cut surface.

Microscopic Features

These lesions are poorly circumscribed and composed of an admixture of adipose tissue and cells with bland spindle-shaped nuclei and indiscernible cytoplasm in a collagenous, edematous or focally myxoid stroma (Fig. 8.17). Vascular channels and nerve fibers are present. Mitotic activity is minimal.

Ancillary Techniques

CD34 is positive in most cases and ER may be positive. SMA, desmin, and S100 are negative. Cytogenetic analysis in a small number of cases has revealed a normal karyotype [73].

Differential Diagnosis and Pitfalls

Diagnosis is usually straightforward, given the characteristic age range and admixture of tissues normally found at this site.

Superficial Angiomyxoma

A benign myxoid mesenchymal neoplasm which has a wide distribution but which may occur on the vulva. A synonym is cutaneous myxoma.

Clinical Features

Although more commonly occurring at extragenital sites [75, 76], especially the head and neck, superficial angiomyxoma may involve the vulvovaginal region, almost always the vulva [77]. Occasionally, multiple cutaneous myxomas or angiomyxomas are a manifestation of the autosomal dominant Carney's complex, although this has not been a feature of those reported cases in the vulvovaginal region. However, especially if there are multiple superficial angiomyxomas, the possibility of Carney's complex should be raised since these patients are at risk for the development of cardiac myxomas. Superficial angiomyxoma is a benign lesion with no metastatic potential. However, since these are multinodular, local recurrence is not uncommon and the lesions should be excised with a rim of normal tissue where possible.

Gross Features

On gross examination, these are ill-defined nodular or multinodular lesions involving the dermis and/or subcutaneous tissue. The cut surface is myxoid or gelatinous.

Microscopic Features

Histologically, this is usually located within the dermis and subcutaneous tissue. Many, but not all, have a multinodular pattern, and the lesion is composed of morphologically bland cells with spindle- and stellate-shaped nuclei in an abundant myxoid stroma (Fig. 8.18a). Occasional multinucleate cells may be present. There may be acellular collections of myxoid material. There are few or no mitotic figures. Thin-walled capillary-like blood vessels are present, often with a curvilinear pattern, and a characteristic histological feature is the common presence of inflammatory cells, including neutrophils, which are a useful diagnostic aid (Fig. 8.18b). There may be entrapped epithelial elements derived from the overlying skin or skin appendages, especially towards the surface of the lesion (Fig. 8.19).

Ancillary Techniques

The lesional cells are typically positive with vimentin, CD34, and SMA but are generally negative with desmin, ER, and PR. S100 positivity has been reported in some, but not all, studies [77]. The immunophenotype is not specific, but negative staining with hormone receptors may be a useful clue to diagnosis since other myxoid lesions at this site are generally positive.

Differential Diagnosis and Pitfalls

The differential diagnosis includes many of the other site-specific vulvovaginal mesenchymal lesions, especially those with a myxoid stroma, and a variety of non-site-specific myxoid lesions. One of the main lesions in the differential diagnosis is aggressive (deep) angiomyxoma. In general, this is a larger deeper-seated lesion than superficial angiomyxoma and has an infiltrative margin that contrasts with the multinodular growth pattern of superficial angiomyxoma. The

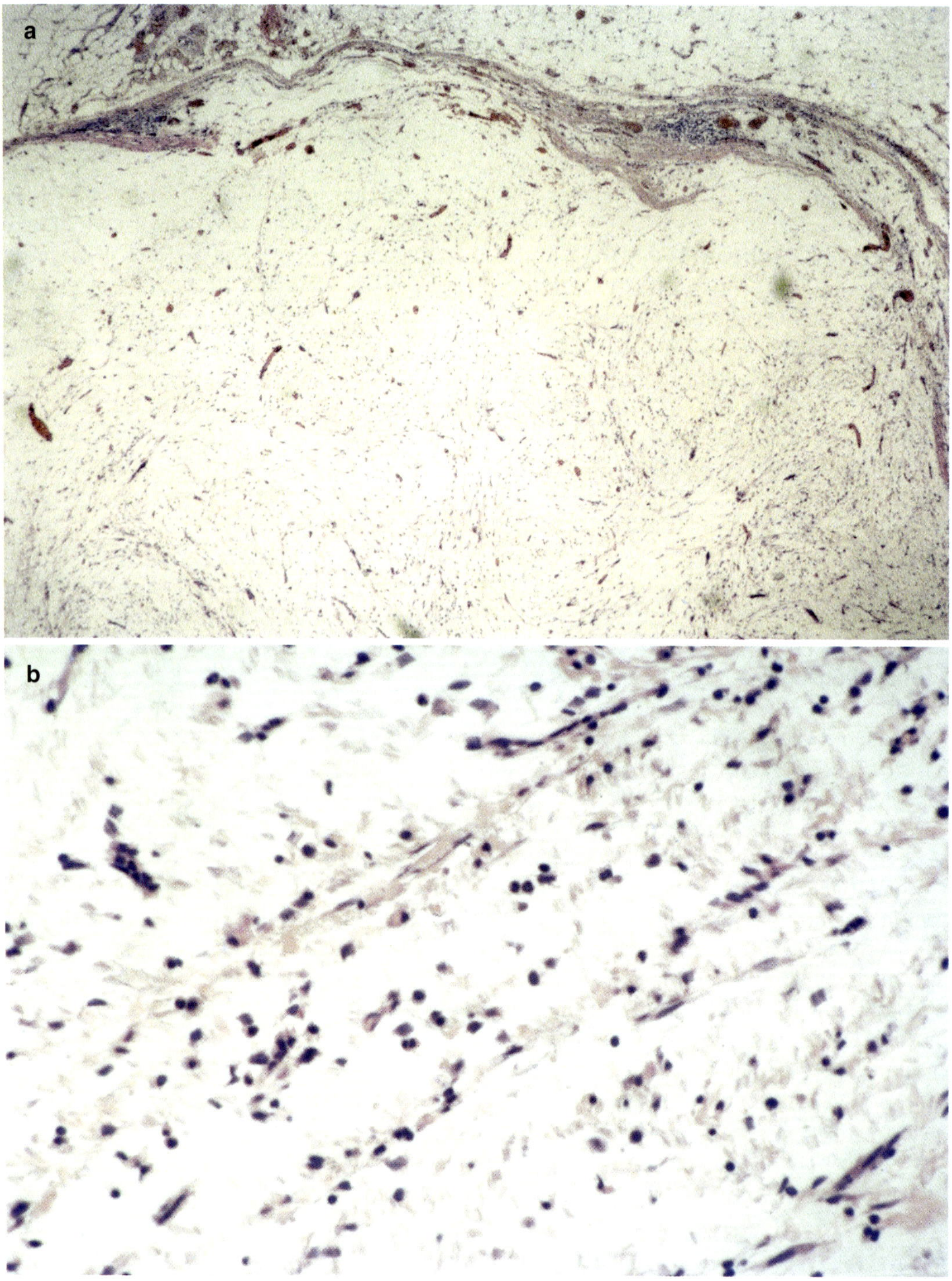

Fig. 8.18 Superficial angiomyxoma with nodular appearance and myxoid stroma (**a**). Collections of inflammatory cells are present (**b**)

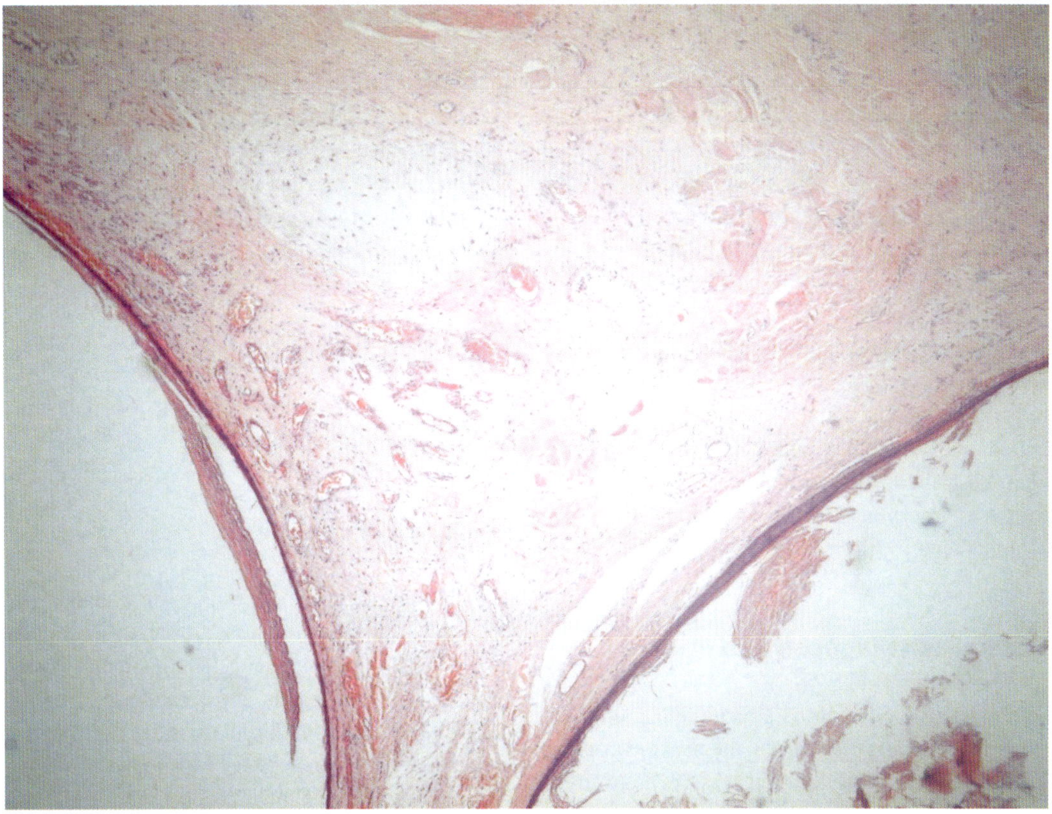

Fig. 8.19 Superficial angiomyxoma: Entrapped squamous elements are present in some cases

blood vessels are more variable in appearance in aggressive angiomyxoma, usually with a component of thick-walled vessels, while the presence of stromal neutrophils favors superficial angiomyxoma. An absence of ER and PR staining favors superficial angiomyxoma since most aggressive angiomyxomas are positive. Positive desmin staining is more in keeping with aggressive angiomyxoma. HMGA2 has been negative in all cases of superficial angiomyxoma studied [24].

Massive Vulval Edema

This is a rare cause of vulval swelling [78–80]. The pathogenesis is likely to be lymphedema secondary to chronic lymphatic obstruction. The term localized lymphedema of the vulva has also been proposed [80]. Similar cases have been described involving the upper and lower extremites of obese patients [81].

Clinical Features

The vulval swelling is usually bilateral [78–80]. Predisposing factors include obesity, immobilization, and prior surgery [78–80]. The swelling may be massive and present as a large polypoid lesion or as generalized vulval enlargement. Edema may also result in more modest vulval swelling, sometimes with multiple skin polyps or pedunculated plaques, which is clinically recognized as being due to edema and surgical removal not undertaken. Massive vulval edema is a benign condition but may recur following excision.

Gross Features

Most reported cases have comprised a large polypoid mass. The overlying skin may be erythematous or ulcerated. Sectioning reveals a thickened dermis and underlying edematous adipose tissue.

Micoscopic Features

Histology shows expanded edematous and fibrosed dermal tissue with widely spaced bland mesenchymal cells and numerous thin-walled vascular channels which are often dilated (Fig. 8.20a). Multinucleate stromal cells may be present as may collections of inflammatory cells. The underlying adipose tissue is also edematous (Fig. 8.20b). Perivascular cuffing by lymphocytes and plasma cells is a characteristic feature of massive edema. The overlying epidermis may exhibit hyperkeratosis and acanthosis. A single case associated with lymphangioma circumscriptum has been described; the lymphangioma circumscriptum was interpreted as being secondary to the lymphedema [80].

Differential Diagnosis and Pitfalls

The markedly edematous stroma and numerous vascular channels may mimic the myxoid appearance and vascularity of aggressive angiomyxoma. In contrast to aggressive angiomyxoma, which is a more deep seated lesion, massive edema usually presents as bilateral vulval swelling and the stroma is edematous (Alcian blue negative) rather than truly myxoid (Alcian blue positive). Perivascular cuffing by lymphocytes and plasma cells is often present in massive edema but not in aggressive angiomyxoma. HMGA2 is negative in massive edema [24]. Examples of vulval edema resulting in more modest swelling may mimic other mesenchymal lesions, including fibroepithelial polyp.

Reactive Fibroblastic and Myofibroblastic Proliferation of the Vulva ("Cyclist's Nodule")

This entity is characterized by the presence of a vulval nodule in female cyclists [82] and probably analogous to perineal nodules occurring in male cyclists, although the histologic features of the latter are not well documented.

Clinical Features

In the one reported series of four cases, the vulval nodules or swellings developed in competitive female cyclists aged 15–45 years. The lesions were unilateral and occurred on the right or left labium majus (two cases each). One case recurred following local excision.

Gross Features

Grossly these are poorly circumscribed lesions with a fibrous cut surface.

Microscopic Features

The histologic appearances are of a haphazard admixture of adipose tissue, variably cellular hyalinized tissue containing bland spindle-shaped fibroblasts, blood vessels, and nerve fibers. In some areas, thick cords of fibrous tissue may impart a keloid-like appearance. Other histologic features in some cases include plump mesenchymal cells with round or ovoid nuclei and abundant eosinophilic cytoplasm resulting in an epithelioid, plasmacytoid, or ganglion-like appearance (Fig. 8.21), a lymphocytic infiltrate around blood vessels, foci of fat necrosis, and collections of elastic fibers. The overall morphologic appearances, especially in the cases with plump mesenchymal cells, bear some resemblance to proliferative fasciitis.

Ancillary Techniques

Immunohistochemically, the cells are ER positive and the plump mesenchymal cells are SMA positive. Desmin, S100, CD34, and HMGA2 are negative [82].

Differential Diagnosis and Pitfalls

If the existence of the entity is known, diagnosis is usually straightforward given the characteristic clinical setting.

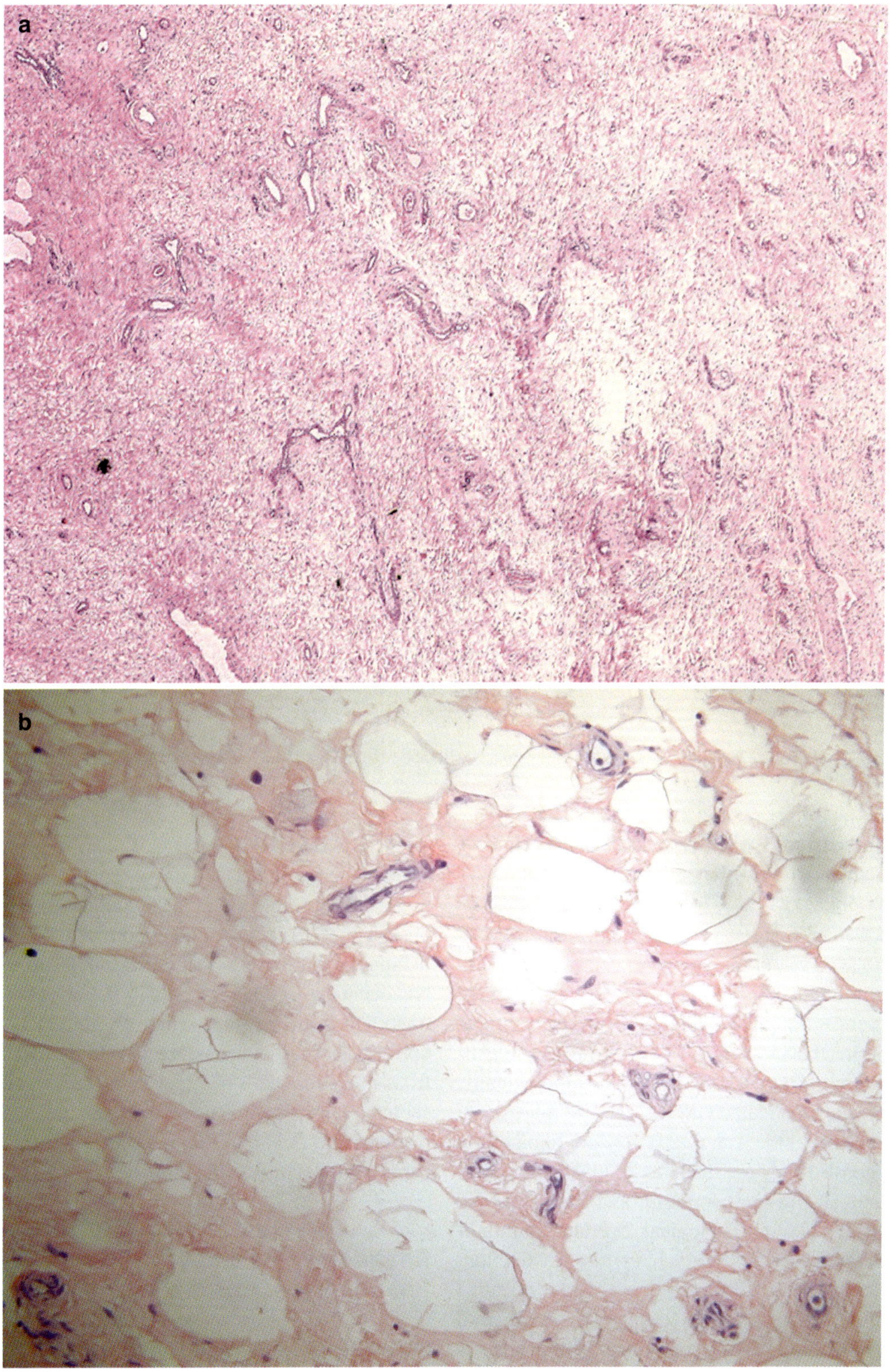

Fig. 8.20 Massive vulval edema exhibiting edematous dermal tissue (**a**) and adipose tissue (**b**)

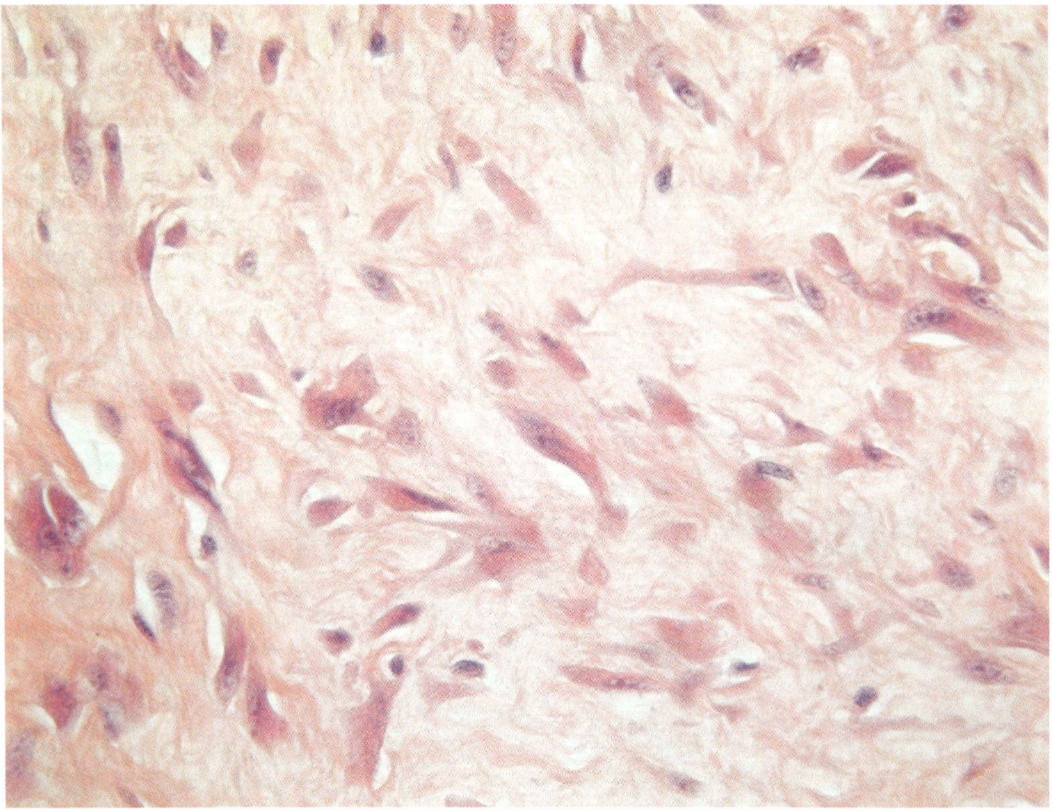

Fig. 8.21 "Cyclists" nodule containing myofibroblasts with abundant eosinophilic cytoplasm

Gastrointestinal Stromal Tumor of the Vagina and Rectovaginal Septum

Occasional gastrointestinal stromal tumors (GISTs) arise in the vagina or rectovaginal septum without connection to the rectal wall and present as a vaginal mass [83]. When occurring at this site, they are referred to as extragastrointestinal stromal tumors (eGISTs). Morphologically, these are identical to GISTs arising at more usual locations but the pathologist may not think of the diagnosis. They are likely to be misdiagnosed as a smooth muscle neoplasm, and there may be considerable morphological overlap; immunohistochemistry is crucial in the distinction. Desmin, ER, and PR are almost always negative in eGISTs but are positive in most vulvovaginal smooth muscle neoplasms. Once the diagnosis is considered, confirmation is usually straightforward since the majority of GISTs are positive with c-KIT and DOG-1. CD34 is positive in most cases. H-caldesmon, which is considered the most specific smooth muscle marker, may be positive in GISTs [84]. The importance of establishing the diagnosis is that these neoplasms usually contain activating c-KIT mutations and treatment with tyrosine kinase inhibitors is an option. These neoplasms are presumed to arise from interstitial cells of Cajal in the rectovaginal septum. It is recommended that because of the rarity of GISTs at this site, molecular studies are carried out to confirm the diagnosis.

Rhabdomyoma and Rhabdomyosarcoma

Occasional rhabdomyomas have been reported in the vulvovaginal region, usually in the vagina [85, 86]. These are usually polypoid lesions in women in the reproductive age group and are typically less than 3 cm. They are covered by unremarkable squamous epithelium, and within the stroma there are cells exhibiting skeletal muscle differentiation with eosinophilic cytoplasm and cross striations (Fig. 8.22). Cells with cross striations may be numerous or few in number and are set within a loose somewhat vascular stroma. There is no mitotic activity and the skeletal muscle cells exhibit nuclear positivity with skeletal muscle markers such as myogenin and myo-D1. The differential diagnosis may include a fibroepithelial polyp in those examples where cells exhibiting skeletal muscle differentiation are sparse. Embryonal rhabdomyosarcoma may also be in the differential and occasional tumors exhibit features of both rhabdomyoma and rhabdomyosarcoma [87].

Embryonal rhabdomyosarcoma (sarcoma botryoides) is the most common vaginal malignancy in infants and young children, about 90% of cases arising in females less than 5 years of age. Rare examples occur in young adults and postmenopausal women. Presentation is usually with vaginal bleeding and a vaginal mass which is typically in the form of multiple soft edematous polyps, sometimes grossly resembling a bunch of grapes. Histology shows a polypoid lesion lined by unremarkable squamous epithelium. There is usually an increased cellularity just deep to the surface epithelium resulting in a cambium layer (Fig. 8.23). Here, the cells are small and primitive with hyperchromatic nuclei and exhibit mitotic activity. Beneath the cambium layer, the lesion is usually less cellular with an edematous or myxoid stroma containing similar cells. The cells may be round, ovoid, or spindle shaped with strap cells. A proportion of the cells contain eosinophilic cytoplasm with cross striations, although the latter may be difficult to find. Islands of hyaline cartilage may be present. The tumor cells are usually positive with desmin, but this is of limited value since the normal vaginal stromal tissue is desmin positive. There is typically focal nuclear positivity with the specific skeletal muscle markers myogenin and myo-D1. The differential diagnosis may include a fibroepithelial polyp with atypical stromal cells and a rhabdomyoma; these lack the cambium layer and primitive cells of rhabdomyosarcoma. Although embryonal rhabdomyosarcomas are aggressive neoplasms with potential for local invasion and metastasis, they respond well to modern combination chemotherapeutic regimes and radiation and the overall prognosis is excellent with a cure rate of 90–95% [88, 89].

Mesenchymal Proliferations Associated with Prolapsed Fallopian Tube

Occasionally following vaginal or more uncommonly abdominal hysterectomy, the Fallopian tube prolapses (see Chap. 4) and presents as a nodule at the vaginal vault. Histology shows ciliated tubal type epithelium and often an associated inflammatory reaction. Occasional examples of prolapsed fallopian tube associated with a florid mesenchymal proliferation have been reported. In one case, the mesenchymal proliferation mimicked angiomyofibroblastoma and in the other aggressive angiomyxoma [90, 91]. Obviously, the clue to the correct diagnosis is the presence of ciliated tubal type epithelium.

Postoperative Spindle Cell Nodule

Postoperative spindle cell nodule (PSCN), similar to those described elsewhere within the genitourinary tract, may occur in the vulvovaginal region, especially the vagina [92–94]. This is a reactive but proliferative pseudosarcomatous lesion that develops following an operative procedure, usually after a period of 1–12 weeks but sometimes later. PSCN is a benign lesion that rarely recurs following surgical removal. The history of a recent operative procedure is crucial in establishing the diagnosis. PSCN is cellular and composed of a fascicular arrangement of spindle-shaped cells, often with prominent vascularity. There is no significant nuclear atypia, but mitotic figures may be numerous and the lesion can have a somewhat infiltrative appearance. The discrepancy between the degree of nuclear atypia and

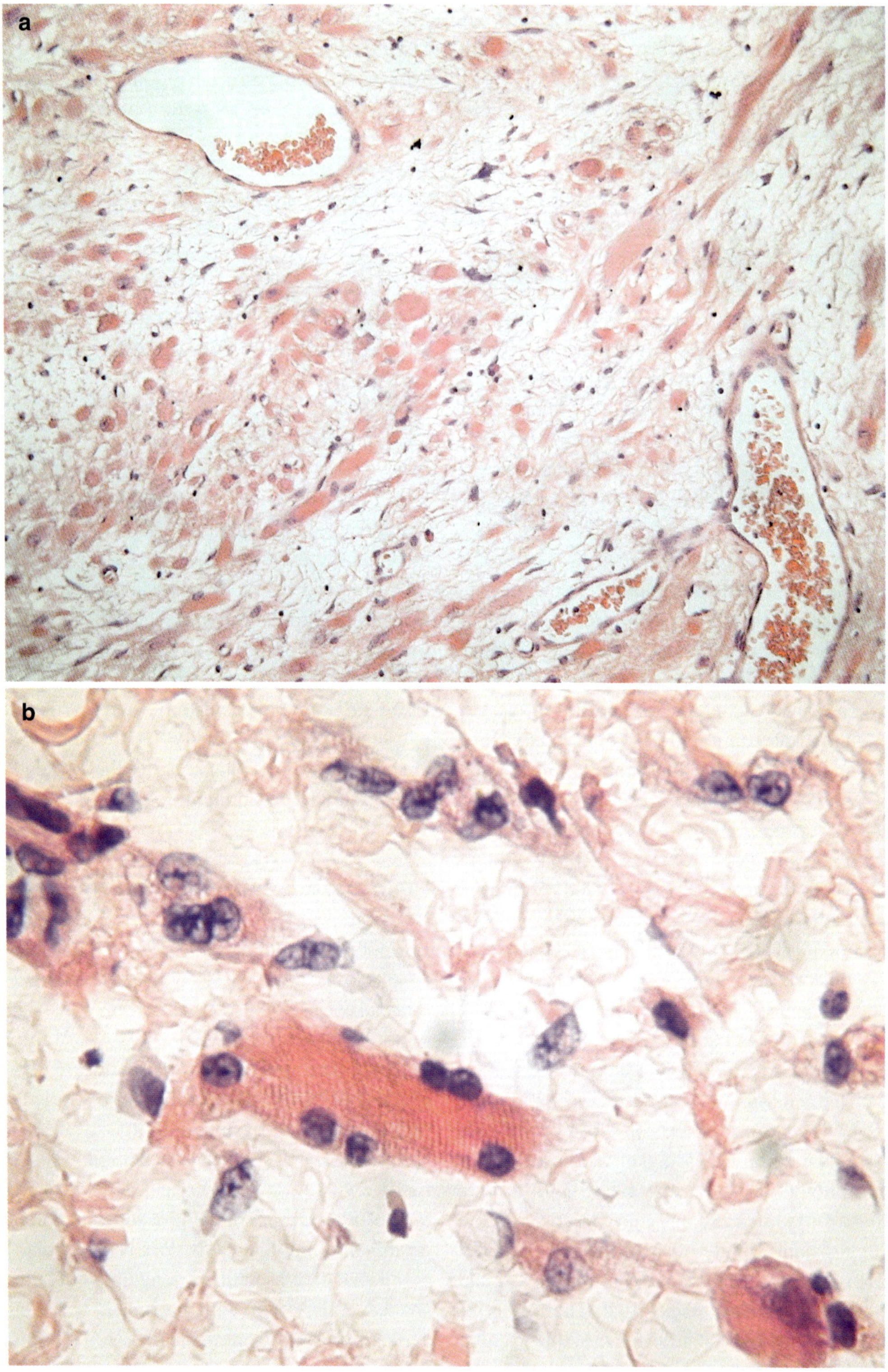

Fig. 8.22 Vulval rhabdomyoma containing cells with eosinophilic cytoplasm (**a**); on high-power examination, cross striations can be seen (**b**)

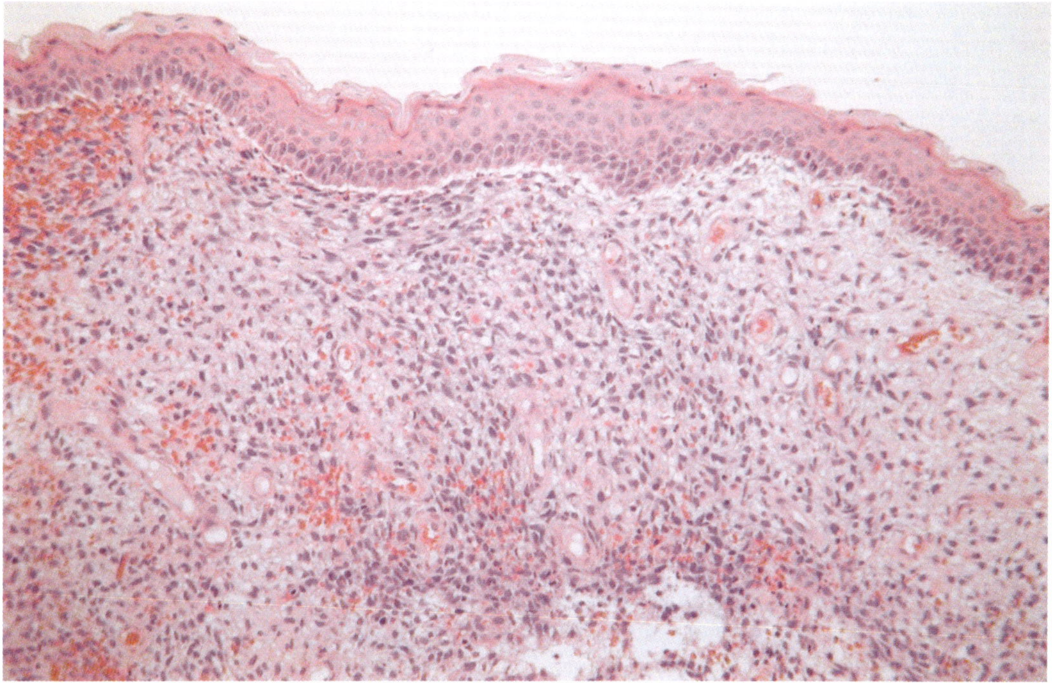

Fig. 8.23 Vulval embryonal rhabdomyosarcoma with cellular cambium layer beneath surface squamous epithelium

the mitotic rate may be a clue to diagnosis. Sometimes, there is ulceration of the overlying surface epithelium. There is immunoreactivity with vimentin and variably with SMA, desmin, and even cytokeratins [95].

Miscellaneous Lesions

A wide variety of other mesenchymal lesions may occasionally involve the vulvovaginal region, and it is stressed that when dealing with a mesenchymal lesion at this site, the pathologist should think widely and consider other lesions rather than just the site-specific ones discussed. Mesenchymal lesions that have been reported in the vulvovaginal region include nodular fasciitis, fibromatosis, spindle cell lipoma, liposarcoma, neural tumors (benign and malignant, including myxoid variants), hemangiopericytoma, solitary fibrous tumor, mammary-type myofibroblastoma, dermatofibrosarcoma protuberans (including myxoid variants), myoepithelial neoplasms (benign and malignant), epithelioid sarcoma, synovial sarcoma, angiosarcoma, alveolar soft part sarcoma, and neoplasms in the Ewing family of tumors [96–116].

It should also be remembered that some epithelial neoplasms may contain a population of spindle cells and, especially in a small biopsy, be mistaken for a mesenchymal lesion. Occasional vulval squamous carcinomas, especially in elderly women, are associated with a florid fibromyxoid stromal reaction [117]. These tumors often involve the clitoris. This represents a nonneoplastic stromal reaction to the tumor and, if this is florid, the epithelial component may be potentially overlooked. Spindle cell squamous carcinoma or carcinosarcoma in this region may also be misdiagnosed as a mesenchymal neoplasm. Cytokeratin or p63 positivity of the tumor cells may help in diagnosing a spindle cell squamous carcinoma. However, neither of these markers is specific; for example, cytokeratins may be positive in a variety of mesenchymal lesions and p63 is often positive in myoepithelial neoplasms. An origin from the overlying squamous epithelium and further sampling to identify areas of more typical squamous carcinoma may also assist in diagnosis. Malignant melanoma may occur in the vulva and vagina and be composed predominantly or exclusively of spindle cells [118].

Conclusions

An extremely large array of mesenchymal lesions may involve the vulvovaginal region, some relatively specific to this site and others with a more widespread distribution. When faced with such a lesion, the pathologist may need to think widely and consider a wide range of diagnoses and not just those lesions specific to the vulvovaginal region. It is important to establish a correct diagnosis since the behavior and management of the various lesions may differ markedly. Distinguishing the various site-specific lesions may be difficult because of overlapping morphological features. Histological examination is the mainstay in diagnosis and immunohistochemistry is of relatively limited value because of considerable immunophenotypic overlap. However, the distinction between certain lesions may be facilitated by a judiciously chosen immunohistochemical panel and HMGA2 is a useful marker of vulvovaginal aggressive angiomyxoma. It could be argued that the site-specific mesenchymal lesions, other than aggressive angiomyxoma, are largely well circumscribed and benign with limited tendency to local recurrence, and because of this and morphological overlap, there is little point in attempting to separate them. However, there is accumulating evidence that behavior may differ between lesions, and it is recommended that accurate diagnosis is important so that the outcome of these uncommon neoplasms can be more fully ascertained.

The full range of vulvovaginal mesenchymal lesions has probably not yet been described, and in recent years, there has been refinement and expansion of the morphological features of some lesions with the description of new entities. It is likely in the future that molecular techniques will contribute to more precise classification of some of these lesions, as in soft tissue tumors in general, by revealing characteristic chromosomal translocations and other molecular abnormalities.

References

1. Nucci MR, Fletcher CD. Vulvovaginal soft tissue tumours: update and review. Histopathology. 2000;36: 97–108.
2. McCluggage WG. A review and update of morphologically bland vulvovaginal mesenchymal lesions. Int J Gynecol Pathol. 2005;24:26–38.
3. Nielsen GP, Young RH. Mesenchymal tumors and tumor-like lesions of the female genital tract: a selective review with emphasis on recently described entities. Int J Gynecol Pathol. 2001;20:105–27.
4. McCluggage WG. Recent developments in vulvovaginal pathology. Histopathology. 2009;54:156–73.
5. Tavassoli FA, Devilee P. World Health Organisation Classification of Tumours. Pathology and genetics. Tumours of the breast and female genital organs. Lyon: IARC Press; 2003.
6. Steeper TA, Rosai J. Aggressive angiomyxoma of the female pelvis and perineum. Report of nine cases of a distinctive type of gynecologic soft-tissue neoplasm. Am J Surg Pathol. 1983;7:463–75.
7. Begin LR, Clement PB, Kirk ME, et al. Aggressive angiomyxoma of pelvic soft parts: a clinicopathologic study of nine cases. Hum Pathol. 1985;16:621–8.
8. Fetsch JF, Laskin WB, Lefkowitz M, et al. Aggressive angiomyxoma: a clinicopathologic study of 29 female patients. Cancer. 1996;78:79–90.
9. Skalova A, Michal M, Husek K, et al. Aggressive angiomyxoma of the pelvioperineal region. Immunohistological and ultrastructural study of seven cases. Am J Dermatopathol. 1993;15:446–51.
10. Iezzoni JC, Fechner RE, Wong LE. Aggressive angiomyxoma in males. A report of four cases. Am J Clin Pathol. 1995;104:391–6.
11. Siassi RM, Padapopoulos T, Matzel KE. Metastasizing aggressive angiomyxoma. N Engl J Med. 1999;341:1772.
12. Blandamura S, Cruz J, Faure Vergara L. Aggressive angiomyxoma: a second case of metastasis with patient's death. Hum Pathol. 2003;34:1072–4.
13. McCluggage WG, Jamieson TJ, Dobbs SP, et al. Aggressive angiomyxoma of the vulva: dramatic response to gonadotropin releasing hormone agonist therapy. Gynecol Oncol. 2006;100:623–5.
14. Fine BA, Munoz AK, Litx LE, et al. Primary medical management of recurrent aggressive angiomyxoma of the vulva with a gonadotropin-releasing hormone agonist. Gynecol Oncol. 2001;81:120–2.
15. McClean G, McCluggage WG. Unusual morphologic features of uterine leiomyomas treated with gonadotropin-releasing hormone agonists: massive lymphoid infiltration and vasculitis. Int J Surg Pathol. 2003;11:339–44.
16. McCluggage WG, Patterson A, Maxwell P. Aggressive angiomyxoma of pelvic parts exhibits oestrogen and progesterone receptor positivity. J Clin Pathol. 2000;53:603–5.
17. Htwe M, Deppisch LM, Saint-Julien JS. Hormone-dependent, aggressive angiomyxoma of the vulva. Obstet Gynecol. 1995;86:697–9.

18. Horman DE, Berean KW, Salski CB, et al. Aggressive angiomyxoma of the pelvis: cytogenetic findings in a single case. Cancer Genet Cytogenet. 1991;56:130–1.
19. Betz JL, Meloni AM, U'Ren LA, et al. Cytogenetic findings in a case of angiomyxoma of the vaginal wall. Cancer Genet Cytogenet. 1995;84:157.
20. Nucci MR, Weremowicz S, Neskey DM, et al. Chromosomal translocation t(8;12) induced aberrant HMGIC expression in aggressive angiomyxoma of the vulva. Genes Chromosomes Cancer. 2001;32: 172–6.
21. Medeiros F, Oliveira AM, Lloyd RV. HMGA2 expression as a biomarker for aggressive angiomyxoma. Mod Pathol. 2008;21:214A (abstract).
22. Rabban JT, Dal Cin P, Oliva E. HMGA2 rearrangement in a case of vulvar aggressive angiomyxoma. Int J Gynecol Pathol. 2006;25:403–7.
23. Tallini G, Vanni R, Manfioletti G, et al. HMGI-C and HMGI(Y) immunoreactivity correlates with cytogenetic abnormalities in lipomas, chondroid hamartomas, endometrial polyps, and uterine leiomyomas and is compatible with rearrangement of the HMGI-C and HMGI(Y) genes. Lab Invest. 2000;80:359–69.
24. McCluggage WG, Connolly L, McBride HA. HMGA2 is a sensitive but not specific immunohistochemical marker of vulvovaginal aggressive angiomyxoma. Am J Surg Pathol. 2010;34:1037–42.
25. Dal Cin P, Quade BJ, Neskey DM. Intravenous leiomyomatosis is characterized by a der(14)t(12;14) (q15;q24). Genes Chromosomes Cancer. 2003;36: 205–6.
26. Fletcher CDM, Tsang WY, Fisher C. Angiomyofibroblastoma of the vulva. A benign neoplasm distinct from aggressive angiomyxoma. Am J Surg Pathol. 1992;16:373–82.
27. Fukunaga M, Nomura K, Matsumoto K, et al. Vulval angiomyofibroblastoma. Clinicopathologic analysis of six cases. Am J Clin Pathol. 1997;107:45–51.
28. Hisaoka M, Kouho H, Aoki T, et al. Angiomyofibroblastoma of the vulva: a clinicopathologic study of seven cases. Pathol Int. 1995;45:487–92.
29. Sasano H, Date F, Yamamoto H, et al. Angiomyofibroblastoma of the vulva: case report with immunohistochemical, ultrastructural and DNA ploidy studies and a review of the literature. Pathol Int. 1997;47:647–50.
30. Vazquez MD, Ro JY, Park YW. Angiomyofibroblastoma. A clinicopathologic study of eight cases and review of the literature. Int J Surg Pathol. 1999;7:161–9.
31. Nielsen GP, Rosenberg AE, Young RH, et al. Angiomyofibroblastoma of the vulva and vagina. Mod Pathol. 1996;9:284–91.
32. McCluggage WG, White RG. Angiomyofibroblastoma of the vagina. J Clin Pathol. 2000;53:803.
33. Kobayashi T, Suzuki K, Arai T, et al. Angiomyofibroblastoma arising from the fallopian tube. Obstet Gynecol. 1999;94:833–4.
34. Laskin WB, Fetsch JF, Tavassoli FA. Angiomyofibroblastoma of the female genital tract: analysis of 17 cases including a lipomatous variant. Hum Pathol. 1997;28:1046–55.
35. Cao D, Srodon M, Montgomery EA, Kurman RJ. Lipomatous variant of angiomyofibroblastoma: report of two cases and review of the literature. Int J Gynecol Pathol. 2005;24:196–200.
36. Granter SR, Nucci MR, Fletcher CDM. Aggressive angiomyxoma: reappraisal of its relationship to angiomyofibroblastoma in a series of 16 cases. Histopathology. 1997;30:3–10.
37. Nielsen GP, Young RH, Dickersin GR, et al. Angiomyofibroblastoma of the vulva with sarcomatous transformation ("angiomyofibrosarcoma"). Am J Surg Pathol. 1997;21:1104–8.
38. Folpe AL, Tworek JA, Weiss SW. Sarcomatous transformation in angiomyofibroblastomas: a clinicopathological, histological and immunohistochemical study of eleven cases. Mod Pathol. 2001;14:12A (abstract).
39. Horiguchi H, Matsui-Horiguchi M, Fujiwara M, et al. Angiomyofibroblastoma of the vulva: report of a case with immunohistochemical and molecular analysis. Int J Gynecol Pathol. 2003;22:277–84.
40. Mucitelli DR, Charles EZ, Kraus FT. Vulvovaginal polyps. Histologic appearance, ultrastructure, immunocytochemical characteristics, and clinicopathologic correlations. Int J Gynecol Pathol. 1990;9:20–40.
41. Hartmann CA, Sperling M, Stein H. So-called fibroepithelial polyps of the vagina exhibiting an unusual but uniform antigen profile characterized by expression of desmin and steroid hormone receptors but no muscle-specific actin or macrophage markers. Am J Clin Pathol. 1990;93:604–8.
42. Rollason TP, Byrne P, Williams A. Immunohistochemical and electron microscopic findings in benign fibroepithelial vaginal polyps. J Clin Pathol. 1990;43:604–8.
43. Chirayil SJ, Tobon H. Polyps of the vagina: a clinicopathologic study of 18 cases. Cancer. 1981;47:2904–7.
44. Norris HJ, Taylor HB. Polyps of the vagina: a benign lesion resembling sarcoma botryoides. Cancer. 1966;19:227–32.
45. Miettinen M, Wahlstrom T, Vesterinen E, et al. Vaginal polyps with pseudosarcomatous features. A clinicopathologic study of seven cases. Cancer. 1983;51:1148–51.
46. Ostor AG, Fortune DW, Riley CB. Fibroepithelial polyps with atypical stromal cells (pseudosarcoma botryoides) of vulva and vagina. A report of 13 cases. Int J Gynecol Pathol. 1988;7:351–60.
47. Maenpaa J, Soderstrom KO, Salmi T, et al. Large atypical polyps of the vagina during pregnancy with concomitant human papilloma virus infection. Eur J Obstet Gynecol Reprod Biol. 1988;27:65–9.
48. O'Quinn AG, Edwards CL, Gallagher HS. Pseudosarcoma botryoides of the vagina in pregnancy. Gynecol Oncol. 1982;13:237–41.
49. Mitchell M, Talerman S, Sholl JS, et al. Pseudosarcoma botryoides in pregnancy: report of a case with ultrastructural observations. Obstet Gynecol. 1987;70:522–6.
50. Nucci MR, Young RH, Fletcher CDM. Cellular pseudosarcomatous fibroepithelial stromal polyps of the lower female genital tract: an underrecognized lesion often misdiagnosed as sarcoma. Am J Surg Pathol. 2000;24:231–40.

51. Nielsen GP, Rosenberg AE, Koerner FC. Smooth-muscle tumors of the vulva. A clinicopathologic study of 25 cases and review of the literature. Am J Surg Pathol. 1996;20:779–93.
52. Newman PL, Fletcher CDM. Smooth muscle tumours of the external genitalia: clinicopathological analysis of a series. Histopathology. 1991;18:523–9.
53. Tavassoli FA, Norris HJ. Smooth muscle tumors of the vulva. Obstet Gynecol. 1979;53:213–7.
54. Barricks RL. Multiple leiomyomata with associated clitoral hypertrophy. J Iowa Med Soc. 1973;63:535–8.
55. Faber K, Jones MA, Spratt D, et al. Vulvar leiomyomatosis in a patient with esophagogastric leiomyomatosis. Review of the syndrome. Gynecol Oncol. 1991;41:92–4.
56. Whalen T, Astedt B. Familial occurrence of coexisting leiomyoma of vulva and esophagus. Acta Obstet Gynecol Scand. 1965;44:197–203.
57. Shapiro RL, Sandrock AR. Esophagogastric and vulvar leiomyomatosis: a new radiologic syndrome. J Can Assoc Radiol. 1973;24:184–7.
58. Patil DT, Laskin WB, Fetsch JF, Miettinen M. Inguinal smooth muscle tumors in women – a dichotomous group consisting of Mullerian-type leiomyomas and soft tissue leiomyosarcomas: an analysis of 55 cases. Am J Surg Pathol. 2011;35:315–24.
59. Nucci MR, Granter SR, Fletcher CD. Cellular angiofibroma: a benign neoplasm distinct from angiomyofibroblastoma and spindle cell lipoma. Am J Surg Pathol. 1997;21:636–44.
60. McCluggage WG, Perenyei M, Irwin ST. Recurrent cellular angiofibroma of the vulva. J Clin Pathol. 2002;55:477–9.
61. Curry JL, Olejnik JL, Wojcik EM. Cellular angiofibroma of the vulva with DNA ploidy analysis. Int J Gynecol Pathol. 2001;20:200–3.
62. Dickmen Y, Yucebilgin MS, Kazandi M, et al. Cellular angiofibroma of the vulva: report of a case. Eur J Gynaecol Oncol. 2004;25:242–4.
63. Dargent JL, de Saint Aubain N, Galdon MG. Cellular angiofibroma of the vulva: a clinicopathological study of two cases with documentation of some unusual features and review of the literature. J Cutan Pathol. 2003;30:405–11.
64. Lane JE, Walker AN, Mullis Jr EN, et al. Cellular angiofibroma of the vulva. Gynecol Oncol. 2001;81:326–9.
65. McCluggage WG, Ganesan R, Hirschowitz L, Rollason TP. Cellular angiofibroma and related fibromatous lesions of the vulva: report of a series with a morphological spectrum wider than previously described. Histopathology. 2004;45:360–8.
66. Iwasa Y, Fletcher CD. Cellular angiofibroma: clinicopathologic and immunohistochemical analysis of 51 cases. Am J Surg Pathol. 2004;28:1426–35.
67. Chen E, Fletcher CD. Cellular angiofibroma with atypia or sarcomatous transformation: clinicopathologic analysis of 13 cases. Am J Surg Pathol. 2010;34:707–14.
68. Maggani F, Debiec-Rychter M, Vanbockrijk M, Sciot R. Cellular angiofibroma: another mesenchymal tumour with 13q14 involvement, suggesting a link with spindle cell lipoma and (extra)mammary myofibroblastoma. Histopathology. 2007;51:410–2.
69. Laskin WB, Fetsch JF, Tavassoli FA. Superficial cervicovaginal myofibroblastoma: fourteen cases of a distinctive mesenchymal tumor arising from the specialized subepithelial stroma of the lower female genital tract. Hum Pathol. 2001;32:715–25.
70. Ganesan R, McCluggage WG, Hirschowitz L, Rollason TP. Superficial myofibroblastoma of the lower female genital tract: report of a series including tumours with a vulval location. Histopathology. 2005;46:137–43.
71. Stewart CJ, Amanuel B, Brennan BA, et al. Superficial cervicovaginal myofibroblastoma: a report of five cases. Pathology. 2005;37:144–8.
72. Iwasa Y, Fletcher CDM. Distinctive prepubertal vulval fibroma. A hitherto unrecognized mesenchymal tumor of prepubertal girls: analysis of 11 cases. Am J Surg Pathol. 2004;28:1601–8.
73. Vargas SA, Kozakewich HP, Boyd TK, et al. Childhood asymmetric labium majus enlargement mimicking a neoplasm. Am J Surg Pathol. 2005;29:1007–16.
74. Ajibona OO, Richards CJ, Davies Q. A distinctive vulval fibroma of so-called prepubertal type in a postmenopausal patient. J Clin Pathol. 2007;60:437–8.
75. Allen PW, Dymock RB, MacCormac LB. Superficial angiomyxomas with and without epithelial components. Report of 30 tumors in 28 patients. Am J Surg Pathol. 1988;12:519–30.
76. Calonje E, Guerin D, McCormick D, et al. Superficial angiomyxoma: clinicopathologic analysis of a series of distinctive but poorly recognized cutaneous tumors with tendency for recurrence. Am J Surg Pathol. 1999;23:910–7.
77. Fetsch JF, Laskin WB, Tavassoli FA. Superficial angiomyxoma (cutaneous myxoma): a clinicopathologic study of 17 cases arising in the genital region. Int J Gynecol Pathol. 1997;16:325–34.
78. Vang R, Connelly JH, Hammill HA. Vulvar hypertrophy with lymphedema. A mimicker of aggressive angiomyxoma. Arch Pathol Lab Med. 2000;124:1697–9.
79. McCluggage WG, Young RH. Massive vulval edema secondary to obesity and immobilization: a potential mimic of aggressive angiomyxoma. Int J Gynecol Pathol. 2008;27:447–52.
80. Fadare O, Brannan SM, Arin-Salasi D, Parkash V. Localized lymphedema of the vulva: a clinicopathologic study of 2 cases and a review of the literature. Int J Gynecol Pathol. 2011;30:306–13.
81. Farshid G, Weiss S. Massive localized lymphedema in the morbidly obese: a histologically distinct reactive lesion simulating liposarcoma. Am J Surg Pathol. 1998;22:1277–83.
82. McCluggage WG, Smith JH. Reactive fibroblastic and myofibroblastic proliferation of the vulva (Cyclist's nodule); a hitherto poorly described lesion occurring in cyclists. Am J Surg Pathol. 2011;35:110–4.

83. Lam MM, Corless CL, Goldblum JR, et al. Extragastrointestinal stromal tumors presenting as vulvovaginal/rectovaginal septal masses: a diagnostic pitfall. Int J Gynecol Pathol. 2006;25:288–92.
84. Irving JA, Merwill MF, Young RH. Gastrointestinal stromal tumors metastatic to the ovary: a report of five cases. Am J Surg Pathol. 2005;29:920–6.
85. Chabrel CM, Beilby JOW. Vaginal rhabdomyoma. Histopathology. 1980;4:645–51.
86. Iversen UM. Two cases of benign vaginal rhabdomyoma. APMIS. 1996;104:575–8.
87. Jacques SM, Lawrence WD, Malviya VK. Uterine mixed embryonal rhabdomyosarcoma and fetal rhabdomyoma. Gynecol Oncol. 1993;48:272–6.
88. Andrassy RJ, Hays DM, Raney RB, et al. Conservative surgical management of vaginal and vulvar pediatric rhabdomyosarcoma: a report from the intergroup rhabdomyosarcoma study III. J Pediatr Surg. 1995;30:1034–7.
89. Hays DM, Shimada H, Raney Jr B, et al. Clinical staging and treatment results in rhabdomyosarcoma of the female genital tract among children and adolescents. Cancer. 1988;61:1893–903.
90. Varnholt H, Otis CN, Nucci MR. Fallopian tube prolapse mimicking aggressive angiomyxoma. Int J Gynecol Pathol. 2005;24:292–4.
91. Michal M, Rokyta Z, Mejchar B, et al. Prolapse of the fallopian tube after hysterectomy associated with exuberant angiomyofibroblastic stroma response: a diagnostic pitfall. Virchows Arch. 2000;437:436–9.
92. Proppe KH, Scully RE, Rosai J. Postoperative spindle cell nodules of genitourinary tract resembling sarcomas. A report of eight cases. Am J Surg Pathol. 1984;8:101–8.
93. Manson CM, Hirsch PJ, Coyne JD. Post-operative spindle cell nodule of the vulva. Histopathology. 1995;26:571–4.
94. Guillou L, Gloor E, De Grandi P, et al. Post-operative pseudosarcoma of the vagina. A case report. Pathol Res Pract. 1989;185:245–8.
95. Hughes DF, Biggart JD, Hayes D. Pseudosarcomatous lesions of the urinary bladder. Histopathology. 1991;18:67–71.
96. O'Connell JX, Young RH, Nielsen GP, et al. Nodular fasciitis of the vulva: a study of six cases and literature review. Int J Gynecol Pathol. 1997;16:117–23.
97. Moodley M, Moodley J. Dermatofibrosarcoma protuberans of the vulva: a case report and review of the literature. Gynecol Oncol. 2000;78:74–5.
98. Edelweiss M, Malpica A. Dermatofibrosarcoma protuberans of the vulva: a clinicopathologic and immunohistochemical study of 13 cases. Am J Surg Pathol. 2010;34:393–400.
99. Vanni R, Faa G, Dettori T, et al. A case of dermatofibrosarcoma protuberans of the vulva with a COL1A1/PDGFB fusion identical to a case of giant cell fibroblastoma. Virchows Arch. 2000;437:95–100.
100. Huang HJ, Yamabe T, Tagawa H. A solitary neurilemmoma of the clitoris. Gynecol Oncol. 1983;15:103–10.
101. Venter PF, Rohm GF, Slabber CF. Giant neurofibromas of the labia. Obstet Gynecol. 1981;57:128–30.
102. Sonnedecker EW, Cohen RJ, Dreyer L, et al. Neuroma of the vulva. A case report. J Reprod Med. 1993;38:33–6.
103. Nielsen GP, Young RH. Fibromatosis of soft tissue type involving the female genital tract: a report of two cases. Int J Gynecol Pathol. 1997;16:383–6.
104. Allen MV, Novotny DB. Desmoid tumor of the vulva associated with pregnancy. Arch Pathol Lab Med. 1997;121:512–4.
105. Kfuri A, Rosenshein N, Dorfman H, et al. Desmoid tumor of the vulva. J Reprod Med. 1981;26:272–3.
106. Ergeneli MH, Demirhan B, Duran EH. Desmoid tumor of the vulva. A case report. J Reprod Med. 1999;44:748–50.
107. Fukunaga M. Atypical solitary fibrous tumor of the vulva. Int J Gynecol Pathol. 2000;19:164–8.
108. Biedrzycki OJ, Singh N, Habeeb H, Wathen N, Faruqi A. Solitary fibrous tumor of the female genital tract: a case report and review of the literature. Int J Gynecol Pathol. 2007;26:259–64.
109. Biedrycki OJ, Singh N, Faruqi A. Nodular fasciitis of the vulva with an unusually long clinical history; the importance of making this unexpected diagnosis in such an unusual site. Histopathology. 2007;51:547–50.
110. Azzopardi JG, Eusebi V, Tison V, et al. Neurofibroma with rhabdomyomatous differentiation: benign 'Triton' tumour of the vagina. Histopathology. 1983;7:561–72.
111. Hiura M, Nogawa T, Nagai N, et al. Vaginal hemangiopericytoma: a light microscopic and ultrastructural study. Gynecol Oncol. 1985;3:376–84.
112. McMenamin ME, Fletcher CD. Mammary-type myofibroblastoma of soft tissue: a tumor closely related to spindle cell lipoma. Am J Surg Pathol. 2001;25:1022–9.
113. McCluggage WG, Sumathi VP, Nucci MR, et al. Ewing family of tumours involving the vulva and vagina: report of a series of four cases. J Clin Pathol. 2007;60:674–80.
114. Pelosi G, Luzzatto F, Landoni F, et al. Poorly differentiated synovial sarcoma of the vagina: first reported case with immunohistochemical, molecular and ultrastructural data. Histopathology. 2007;50:808–10.
115. Sumathi VP, Fisher C, Williams A, Meiss JM, Ganesan R, Kindblom LG, McCluggage WG. Synovial sarcoma of the vulva and vagina: a clinicopathologic and molecular genetic study of 4 cases. Int J Gynecol Pathol. 2011;30:84–91.
116. Meenakshi M, McCluggage WG. Myoepithelial neoplasms involving the vulva and vagina: report of 4 cases. Hum Pathol. 2009;40:1747–53.
117. Amros RA, Malfetano JH, Mihm Jr MC. Clinicopathologic features of vulvar squamous carcinomas exhibiting prominent fibromyxoid stromal response. Int J Gynecol Pathol. 1996;15:137–45.
118. Gupta D, Malpica A, Deavers MT, Silva EG. Vaginal melanoma: a clinicopathologic and immunohistochemical study of 26 cases. Am J Surg Pathol. 2002;26:1450–7.

Skin Adnexal Tumors

9

Dmitry V. Kazakov, Michal Michal,
and Denisa Kacerovska

Abstract

Adnexal tumors on the vulva do occur but less frequently compared to other anatomic sites. Histopathologically, they are identical to neoplasms occurring elsewhere on the integument and presumably have the same histogenesis. However, some lesions that are traditionally classified under the rubric of cutaneous adnexal neoplasms appear to be specific for the vulva and are histogenetically associated with specific anatomic structures named anogenital mammary-like glands (AGMLG). The latter resemble breast tissue and have long been considered as such, namely, to represent ectopic breast tissue. Recent research however demonstrated that AGMLG represent a normal constituent of the anogenital area, and the vulva in particular. Lesions originating in AGMLG, benign or malignant, epithelial or stromal, manifest a striking similarity to their mammary homologues. Discussed in this chapter, the most common lesions thought to be associated with AGMLG, including hidradenoma papilliferum, fibroadenoma, phyllodes tumor, extramammary Paget disease, and some other less common entities.

Anogenital Mammary-Like Glands

Anogenital mammary-like glands (AGMLG) mainly located in the sulcus between the labia minor and majora are nowadays considered by many to represent a normal constituent of the anogenital area [1]. The traditional viewpoint that these glands are ectopic breast tissue representing the caudal remnants of the milk ridges has been seriously questioned, mainly based on the fact that the milk line in humans does not exist in the form comparable to that in cetaceous animals [1, 2]. Lesions of AGMLG, benign or malignant, typically show a striking homology to their mammary counterparts; therefore, an approach through the eyes of a breast pathologist is advised in challenging cases [3–7].

The normal histology of AGMLG varies from simple glandular structures with round lumina surrounded by loosely or densely fibrotic stroma to complex lobular units closely imitating breast tissue (Fig. 9.1). Decapitation apocrine secretion is often evident [1]. The excretory duct opens

D.V. Kazakov, M.D., Ph.D. (✉) • M. Michal, M.D.
D. Kacerovska, M.D., Ph.D.
Sikl's Department of Pathology,
Medical Faculty Hospital, Charles University,
Alej Svobody 80, Pilsen 304 60, Czech Republic
e-mail: kazakov@medima.cz

L. Brown (ed.), *Pathology of the Vulva and Vagina*, Essentials of Diagnostic Gynecological Pathology,
DOI 10.1007/978-0-85729-757-0_9, © Springer-Verlag London 2013

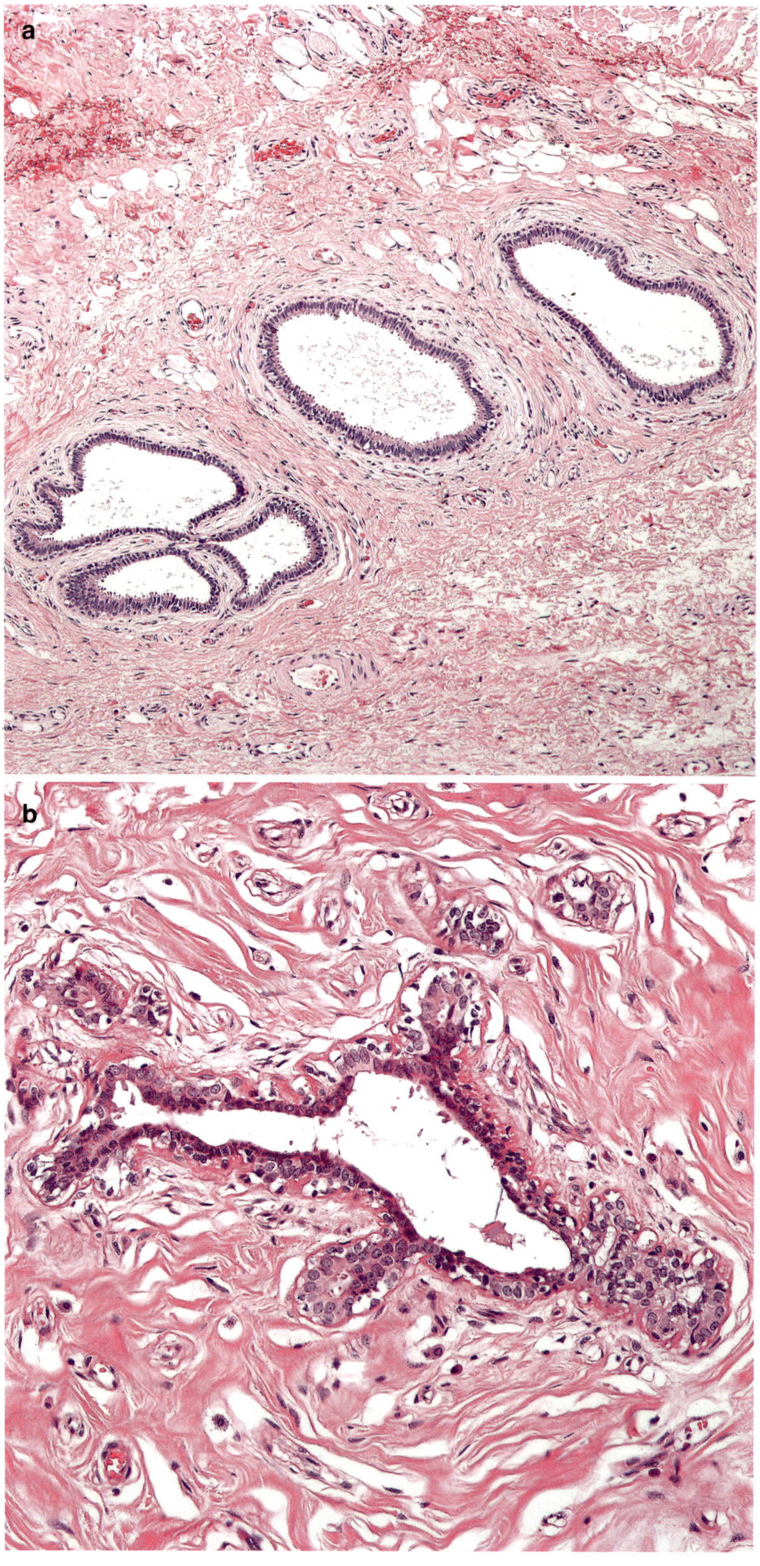

Fig. 9.1 Anogenital mammary-like glands. Note simple glandular structures with round lumens surrounded by loosely or densely fibrotic stroma (**a**) and more complex tubules with outpouchings (**b**)

onto the epidermal surface and has a peripheral myoepithelial cell layer and luminal columnar epithelium often showing apocrine secretion, but a short distance before it enters the epidermis, the duct becomes lined by squamous epithelium.

Hidradenoma Papilliferum

Hidradenoma papilliferum, probably the commonest benign neoplasm involving AGMLG, affects almost exclusively women at a mean age of 50–52 years and appears clinically as a solitary asymptomatic nodule or cyst-like lesion ranging in size from 0.5 to 2 cm with a marked predilection for the labia where about 90% of the lesions occur [8, 9]. Other reported locations included the fourchette, clitoris, perianal area, and perineum. The term "ectopic" hidradenoma papilliferum has been applied to extragenital lesions mostly involving the eyelid and external auditory canal, but these are probably better regarded as papillary adenomas arising in Moll's glands and ceruminous glands, respectively [10–12].

Hidradenoma papilliferum can conceptually be compared to intraductal papilloma of the breast. Microscopically, the neoplasm appears as an intradermal solid-cystic lesion with a complex pattern of branching and anastomosing tubules interconnected in a labyrinthine manner, with bands of fibrous tissue between them, focally forming papillae. The tubules and papillae are lined by a luminal layer of monomorphic, cuboidal to columnar cells with clear or eosinophilic cytoplasm displaying decapitation secretion and surrounded by a layer of myoepithelial cells (Fig. 9.2) [13]. The cells are bland and the mitotic index is usually low [14]. The epithelial cells are immunoreactive for various cytokeratins, gross cystic disease fluid protein (GCDFP-15), and estrogen receptors [15–17], whereas the myoepithelial cells express S-100 protein, calponin, and alpha-smooth muscle actin.

Various histopathological changes described in hidradenoma include metaplastic epithelial alterations (oxyphilic metaplasia, clear cell change, or rarely, mucinous metaplasia); connection to the overlying epidermis of the follicular infundibulum with an accompanying plasma cell-rich stromal infiltrate; changes reminiscent usual, florid, and atypical ductal hyperplasia as defined in the breast; sclerosing adenosis-like changes; marked cystic change; prominent necrosis conceptually similar to intraductal papilloma with necrosis of the breast; focal hyperplasia of stromal myofibroblast-like cells; and myoepithelial hyperplasia (Figs. 9.3, 9.4, and 9.5). Remnants of AGMLG may occasionally be seen adjacent to the neoplasm, and the glands may appear normal or manifest alterations compatible with columnar cell change or columnar hyperplasia (Fig. 9.6). The co-occurrence of hidradenoma papilliferum with extramammary Paget disease and melanoma has rarely been reported [18, 19].

Malignant transformation of hidradenoma papilliferum is extremely rare, and the term "hidradenocarcinoma papilliferum" has been used for the malignant counterpart of the lesion. Most of the convincing examples of hidradenocarcinoma papilliferum corresponded to ductal carcinoma in situ (DCIS) arising within a preexisting hidradenoma papilliferum. DCIS is characterized by the presence of one or more foci of crowded epithelial cells with pleomorphic hyperchromatic nuclei or vesicular nuclei with macronucleoli and exhibiting abnormal mitotic figures with retention of myoepithelial cells around such areas [20–22].

Fibroepithelial Neoplasms (Fibroadenoma and Phyllodes Tumor)

Clinically, the lesions have been reported as solitary asymptomatic nodules averaging 3 cm and occurring at a mean age of 38–39 years [23–25]. An extremely rare presentation is with multiple lesions [26–28]. Rare patients have also presented with analogous tumors in the breast, often metachronous [25, 29, 30].

Fibroadenoma and phyllodes tumor arising in AGMLG are microscopically identical to their mammary homologues. Fibroadenoma

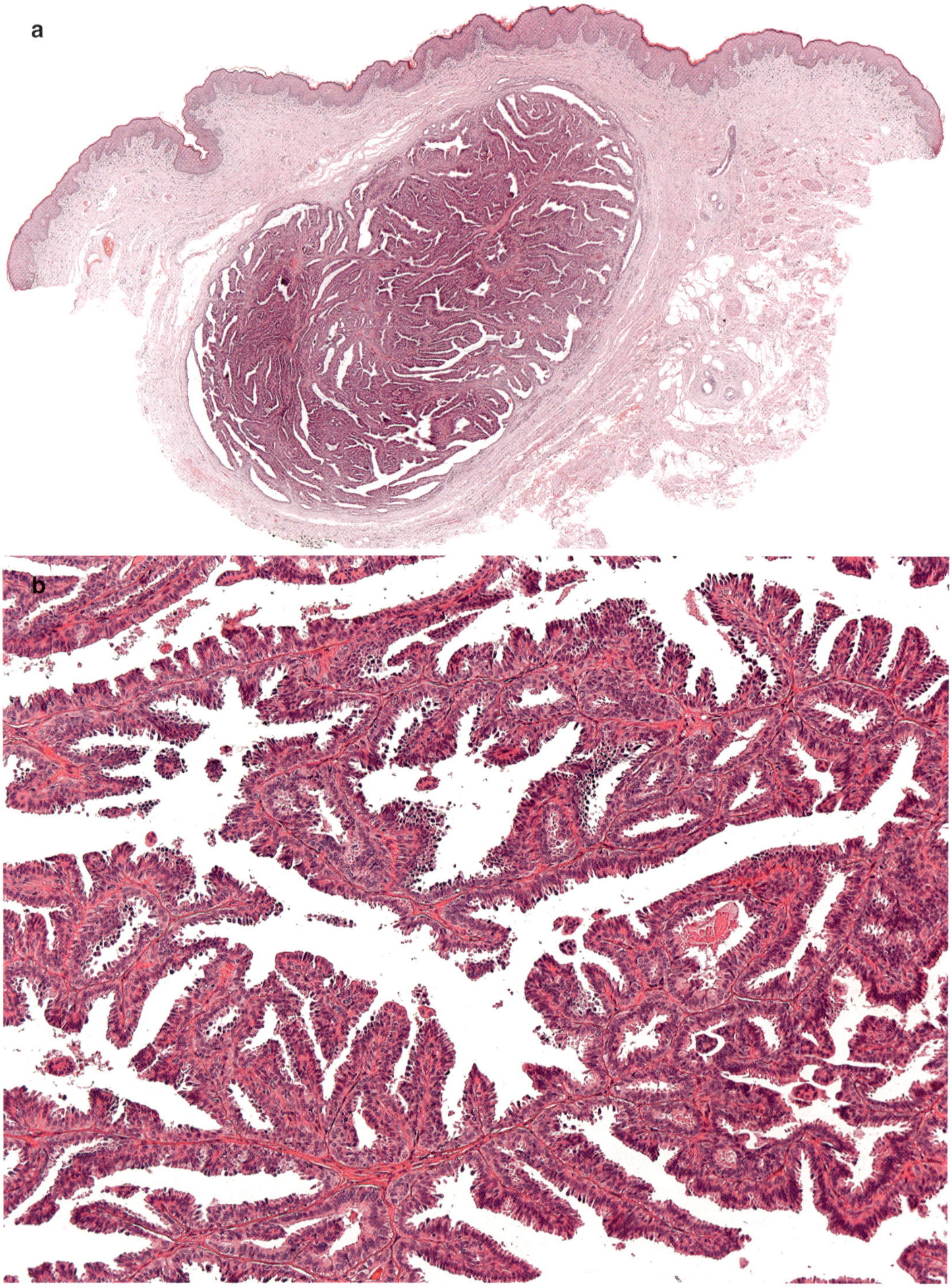

Fig. 9.2 Hidradenoma papilliferum. Intradermal solid-cystic lesion with a complex pattern of branching and anastomosing tubules interconnected in a labyrinthine manner, with bands of fibrous tissue between them, focally forming papillae. The tubules and papillae are lined by a luminal layer of monomorphic, cuboidal to columnar cells with clear or eosinophilic cytoplasm displaying decapitation secretion and surrounded by a layer of myoepithelial cells (**a**, **b**)

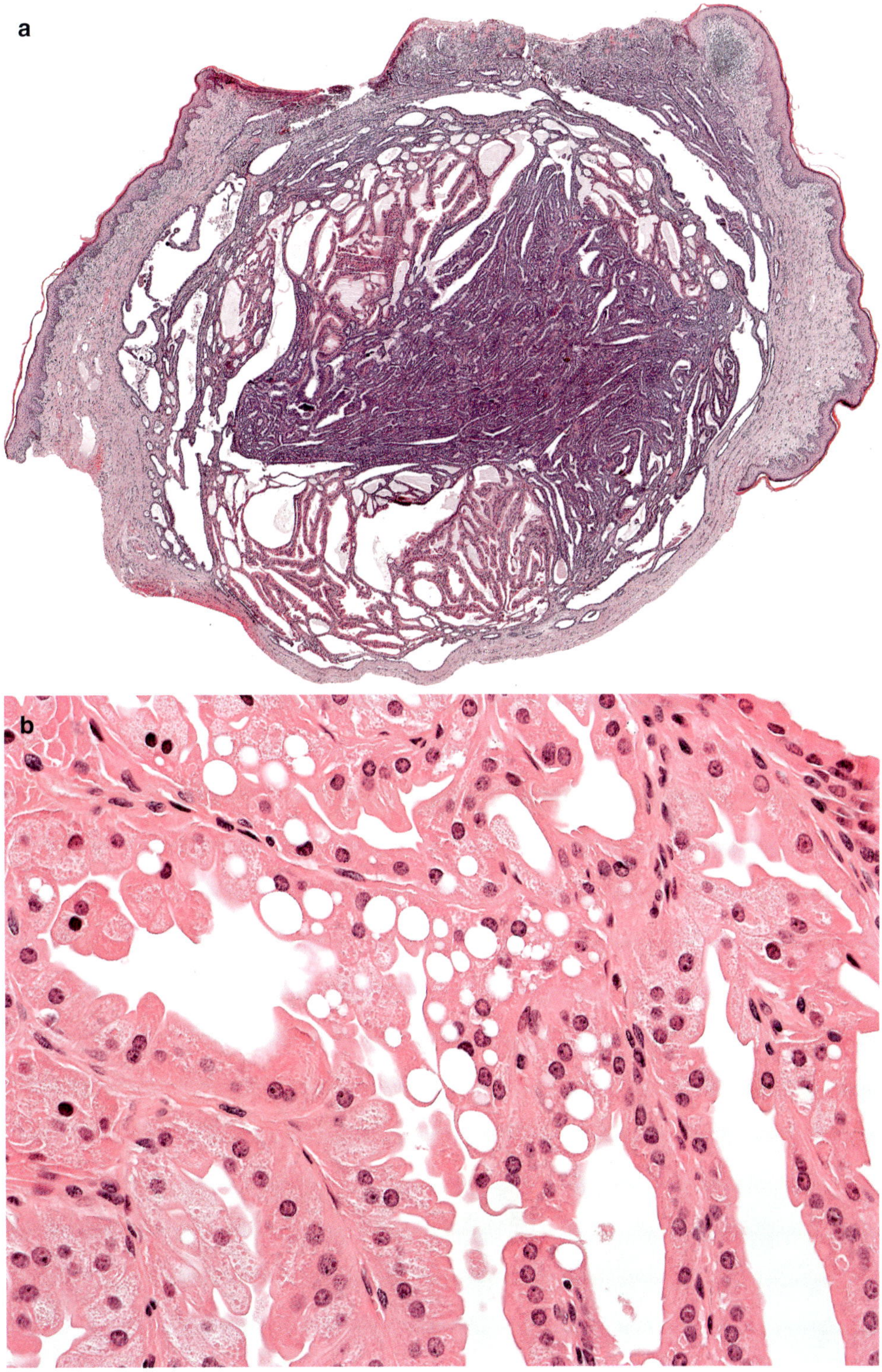

Fig. 9.3 Hidradenoma papilliferum with multiple areas of oxyphilic metaplasia (**a**). The cells possess abundant eosinophilic cytoplasm with zymogen granules. Note also numerous vacuoles. Mild nuclear pleomorphism is a common feature in areas with oxyphilic metaplasia (**b**)

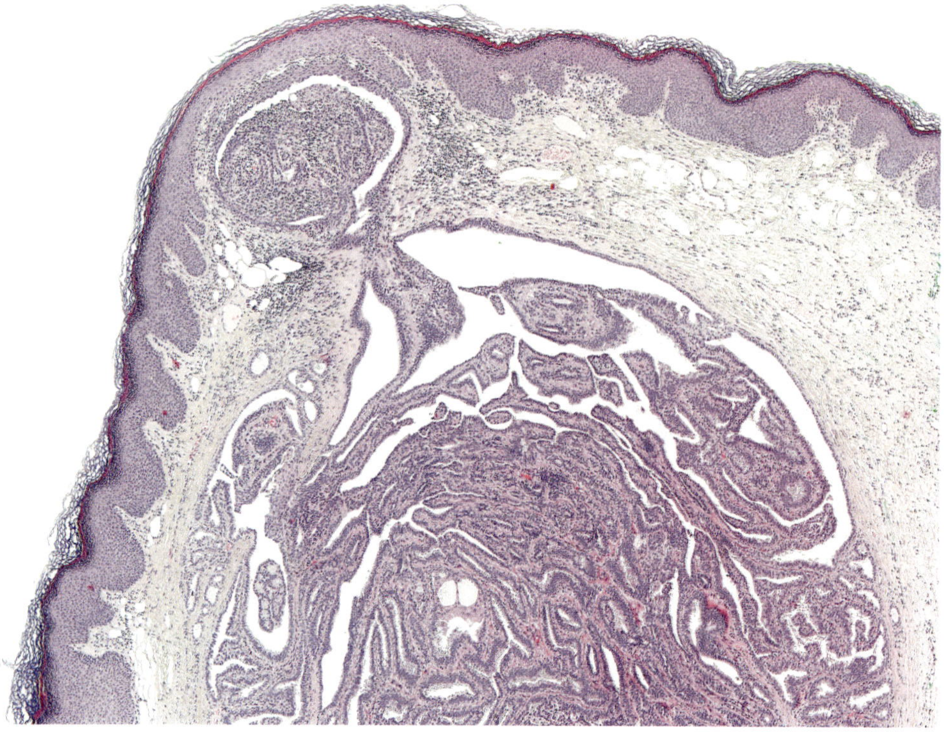

Fig. 9.4 Hidradenoma papilliferum with a focal connection to the overlying epidermis. In such areas, there is usually a dense plasma cell-rich stromal infiltrate occasioning a resemblance to syringocystadenoma papilliferum

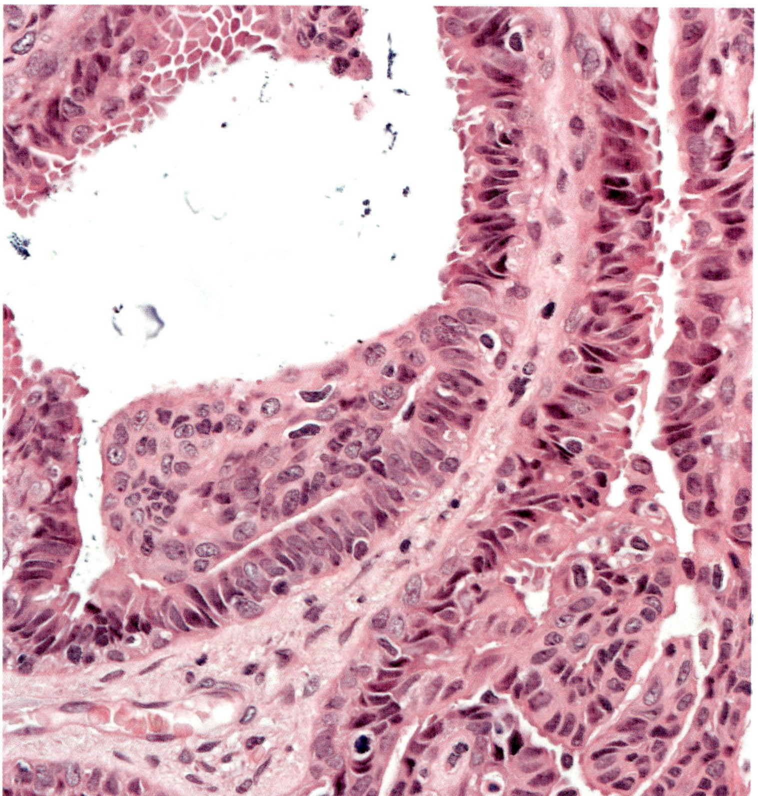

Fig. 9.5 Hidradenoma papilliferum. A focus compatible with atypical ductal hyperplasia as defined in mammary pathology

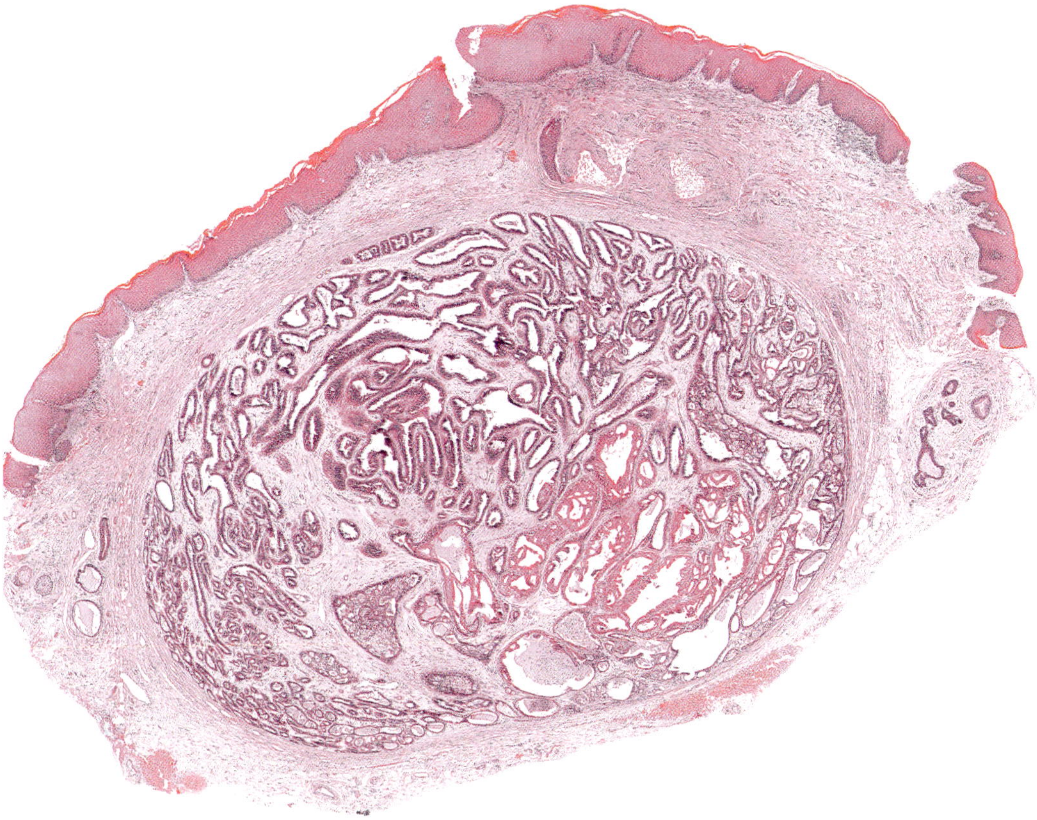

Fig. 9.6 Hidradenoma papilliferum. Note remnants of anogenital mammary-like glands in the vicinity of the tumor

appears as a well-circumscribed neoplasm composed of round or elongated, often branching and anastomosing, glandular structures surrounded by typically paucicellular stroma composed of bland spindled or stellate cells, showing low or absent mitotic activity. The stroma may be sufficiently abundant to compress the glandular elements into slit-like structures, or the lumina maintain their round or oval configuration (Fig. 9.7). A case of vulvar fibroadenoma identical to juvenile fibroadenoma of the breast has been reported [25]. Other changes documented include metaplastic epithelial alterations, ductal ectasia, and stromal sclerosis [5, 6, 24, 25, 30, 31]. Lactation-like change has also been described [25].

Phyllodes tumor grows as leaf-like projections into glandular lumina, and the stroma is usually hypercellular, with variable cellularity within a given neoplasm, typically with periglandular condensation (Figs. 9.8 and 9.9). Depending on stromal atypia, both benign and low-grade malignant variants have been reported in the vulva [25, 28, 30, 32, 33]. A single lesion classified as high-grade malignant phyllodes tumor has recently been described [34].

A distinct stromal alteration, pseudoangiomatous stromal hyperplasia (PASH), has been documented both in fibroadenomas and phyllodes tumors [30]. PASH appears as open, slit-like, often anastomosing channels devoid of erythrocytes and lined by discontinuous, often attenuated, inconspicuous stromal cells lacking atypia or mitotic activity (Fig. 9.10). The intervening collagen bundles are sometimes hyalinized. PASH with multinucleated stromal giant cells has been described in a patient having neurofibromatosis type 1 [25]. Apart from the two fibroepithelial neoplasms, PASH has rarely been documented in other lesions [6, 35].

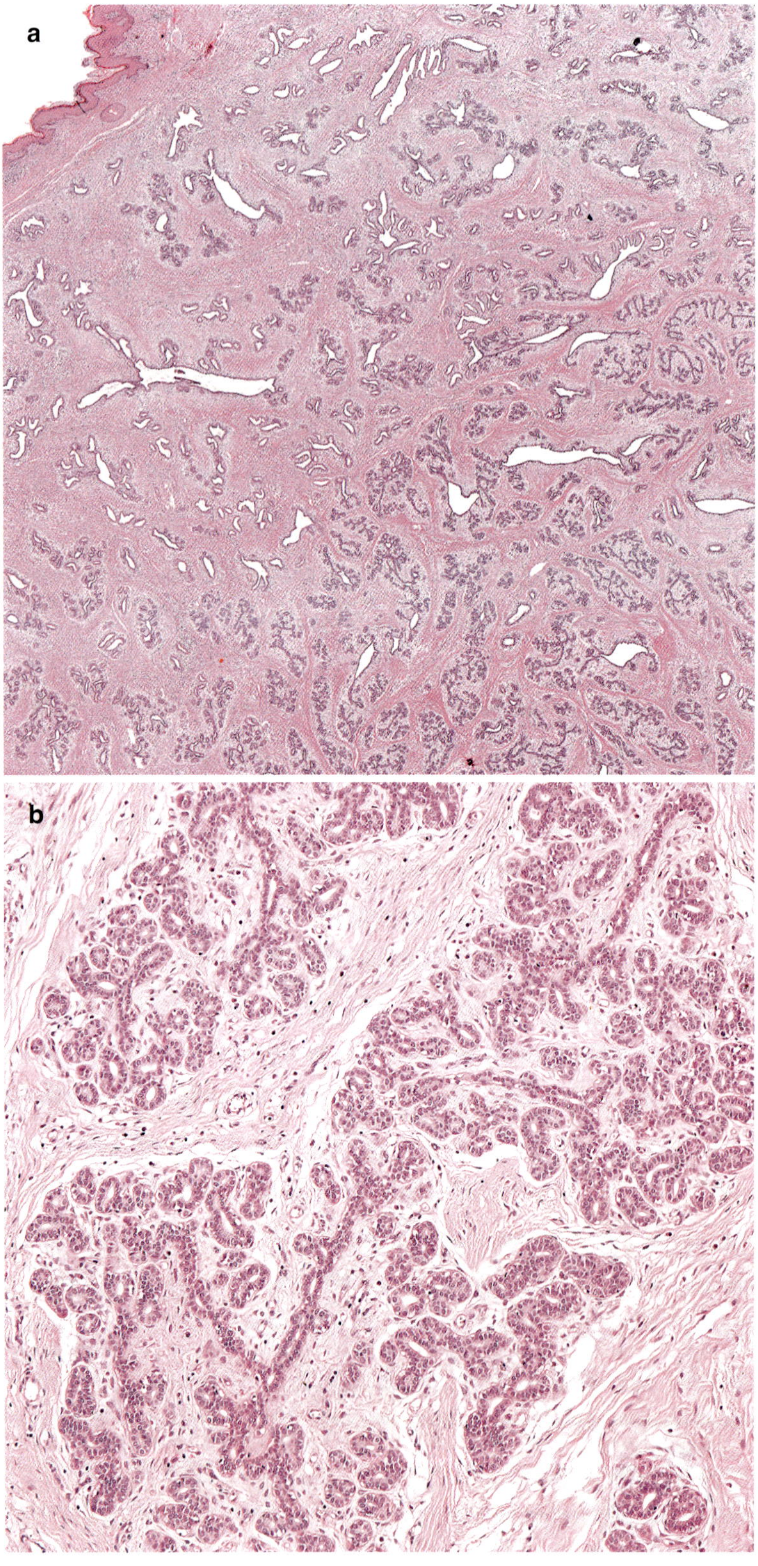

Fig. 9.7 Fibroadenoma originating from anogenital mammary-like glands is identical to its mammary counterpart and appears as a well-circumscribed neoplasm composed of round or elongated, often branching and anastomosing, glandular structures surrounded by typically paucicellular stroma composed of bland spindled or stellate cells (**a**, **b**)

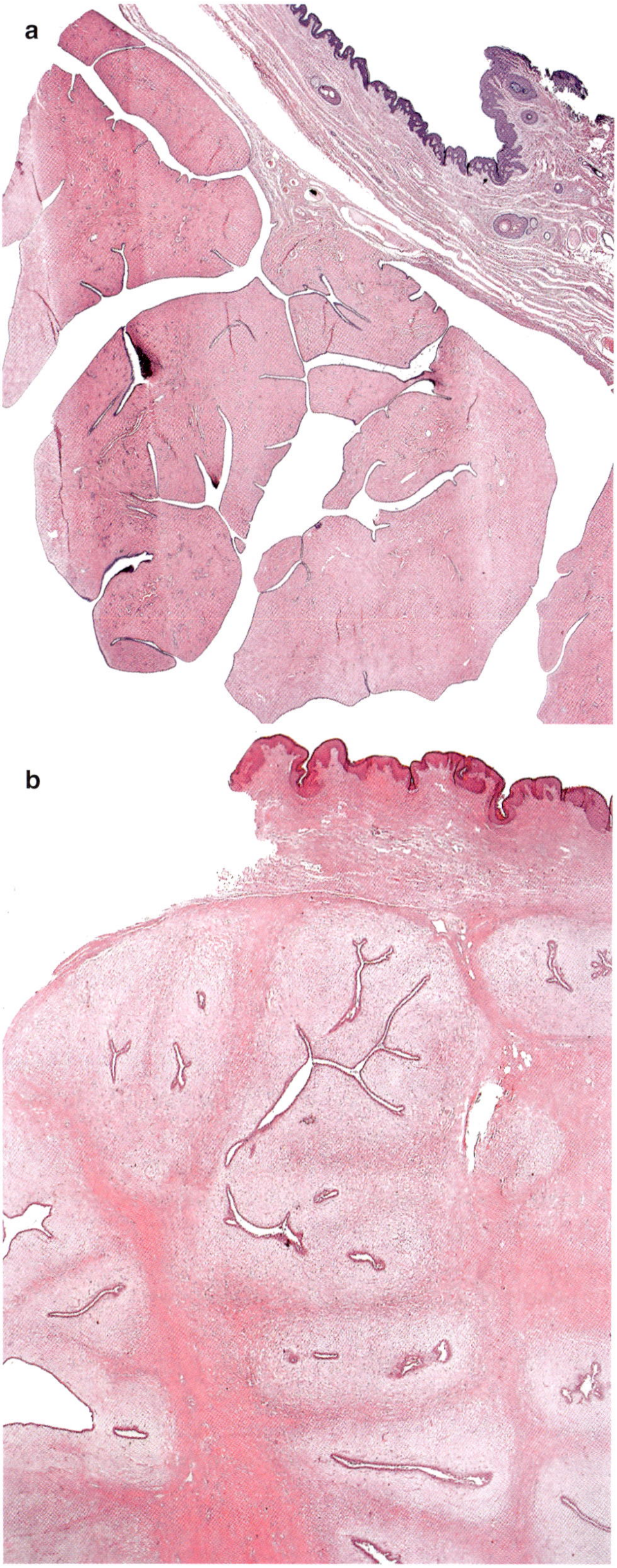

Fig. 9.8 (**a**, **b**) Phyllodes tumor. Both vulvar tumors depicted here display biphasic growth pattern with leaf-like projections into glandular lumina and cellular stroma, with variable cellularity throughout the tumors

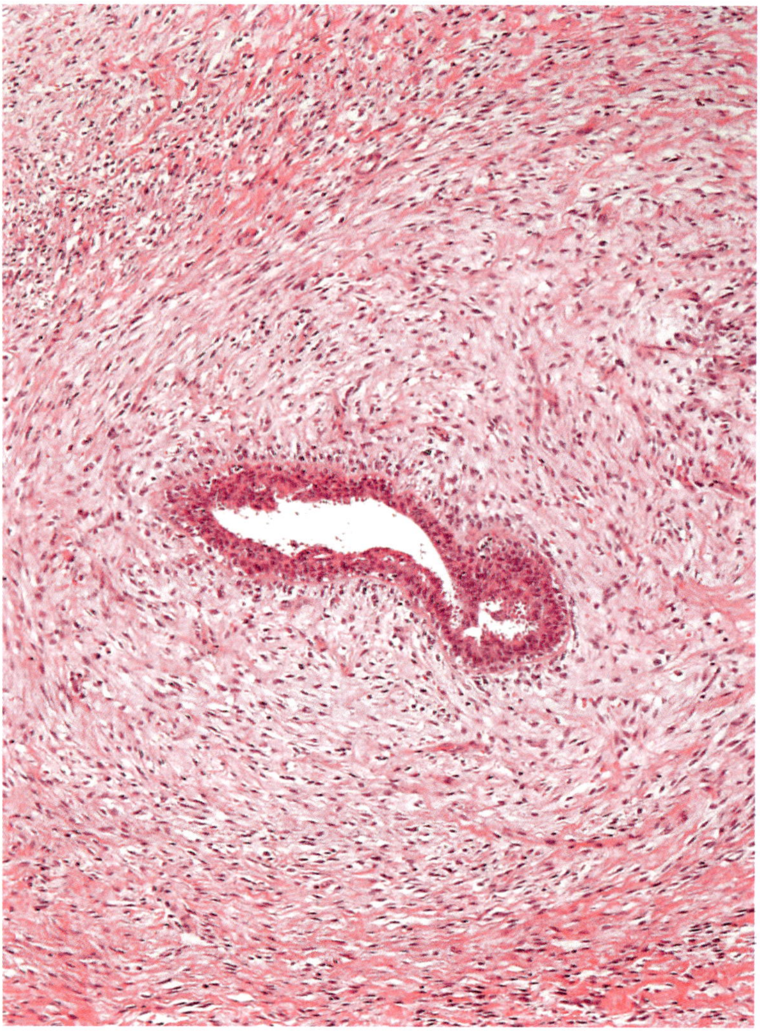

Fig. 9.9 Phyllodes tumor. Note periglandular condensation of the stroma

Immunohistochemically, both fibroepithelial neoplasms in questions appear to manifest an immunoprofile identical to that seen in their mammary homologues. The epithelial component reacts with epithelial markers, estrogen, and progesterone receptors. Staining for *c-erb*B-2 is negative. Myoepithelial markers may be used to visualize a myoepithelial cell layer around the glandular epithelial cells. Stromal cells are positive for vimentin, CD34, and, variably, positive for actins [6, 30, 31, 33]. In practice of course, one rarely needs to perform immunostaining in these lesions.

Extramammary Paget Disease

Extramammary Paget disease (EMPD) represents approximately 1% of neoplasms in the anogenital area. It can be classified into primary and secondary variants, the latter arising from an underlying carcinoma usually originating in the lower gastrointestinal or urinary tracts. The histogenesis of primary EMPD is still a subject of debate and controversy. Evidence indicates that at least a subset of cases may be associated with AGMLG. Other suggested origins include skin adnexa (eccrine or

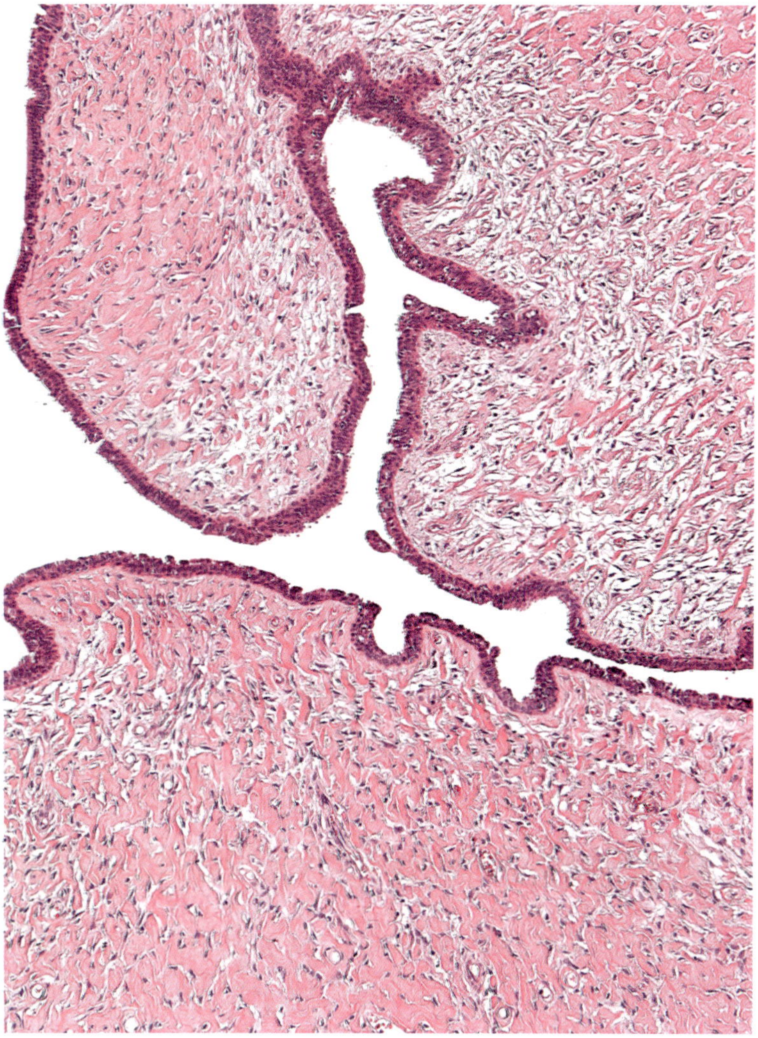

Fig. 9.10 Pseudoangiomatous stromal hyperplasia (*PASH*) in a vulvar phyllodes tumor. Note open, slit-like, often anastomosing channels devoid of erythrocytes and lined by discontinuous, often attenuated, inconspicuous stromal cells lacking atypia or mitotic activity

apocrine glands), vulvar Toker cells [36] (analogous to Toker cells of the nipple [37]), or pluripotential germinative cells [38].

Clinically, EMPD predominantly affects elderly women (median: 70–75 years), mainly involves the labia majora, and appears as relatively well-demarcated flat or slightly elevated erythematous or white-gray lesions, with or without scaling, excoriations, and/or crust. The lesions often mimic an inflammatory process, including contact dermatitis, eczema, or fungal infection (Fig. 9.11). The affected areas range in size considerable (1–20 cm) [39, 40]. Rarely, hyper-, hypo-, or depigmented lesions are seen, as are nodular lesions [41, 42]. Multicentric EMPD is a rare form in which the genital lesions are associated with synchronous or metachronous, uni- or bilateral axillary involvement (so-called triple EMPD) [43–46].

Histopathologically, the epidermis is infiltrated by carcinoma cells with vesicular nuclei, prominent nucleoli, and abundant pale, clear, basophilic, or amphophilic cytoplasm that grow as solitary units, small solid nests, or form gland-like structures (Figs. 9.12 and 9.13). Apocrine secretion is rarely seen within the gland-like

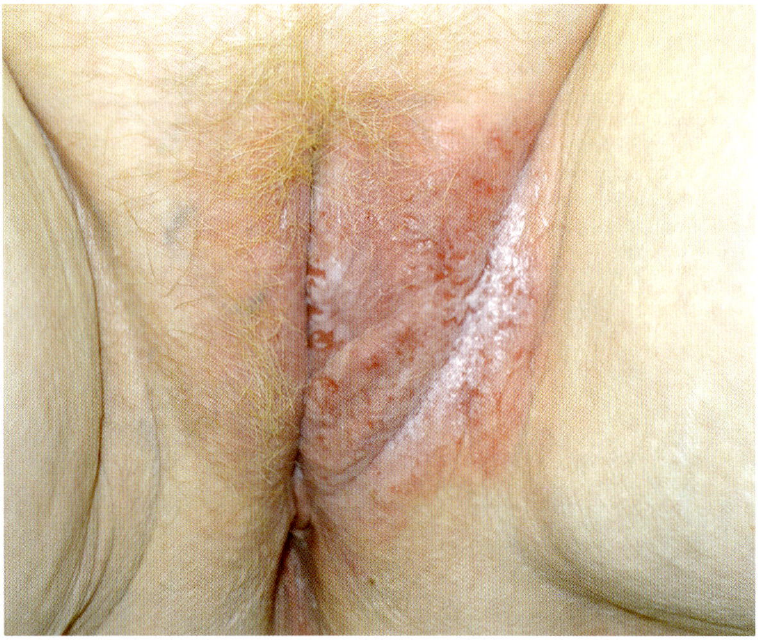

Fig. 9.11 Extrammamary Paget disease. A typical clinical presentation with a flat, erythematous, erosive lesion (Courtesy of Dr. Jiri Bouda, Jr, Pilsen, Czech Republic)

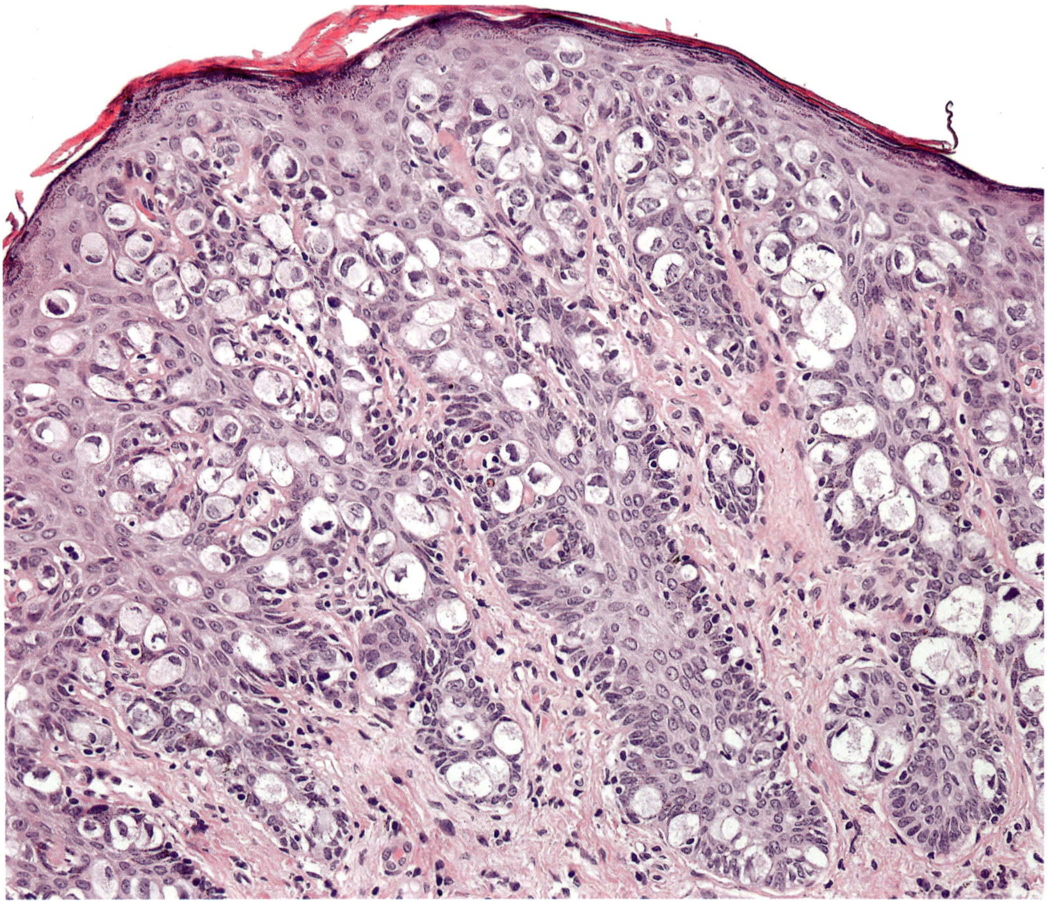

Fig. 9.12 Extrammamary Paget disease. The epidermis is infiltrated by singular carcinoma cells with vesicular nuclei, prominent nucleoli, and abundant pale cytoplasm

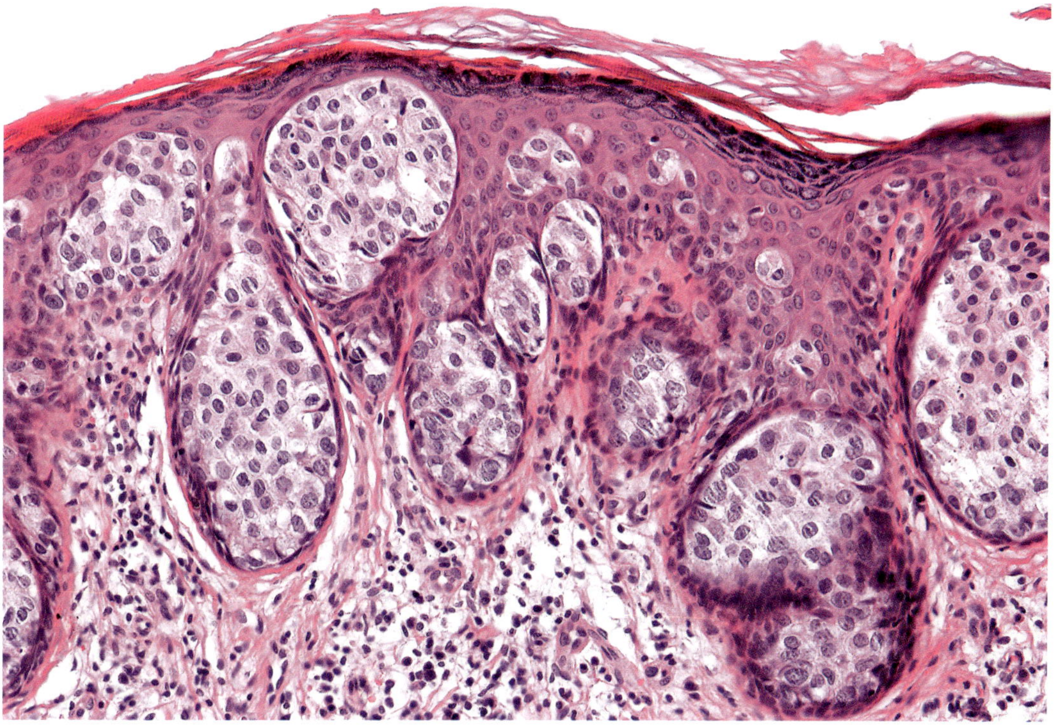

Fig. 9.13 Extrammamary Paget disease. In this example, the neoplastic cells form solid nests

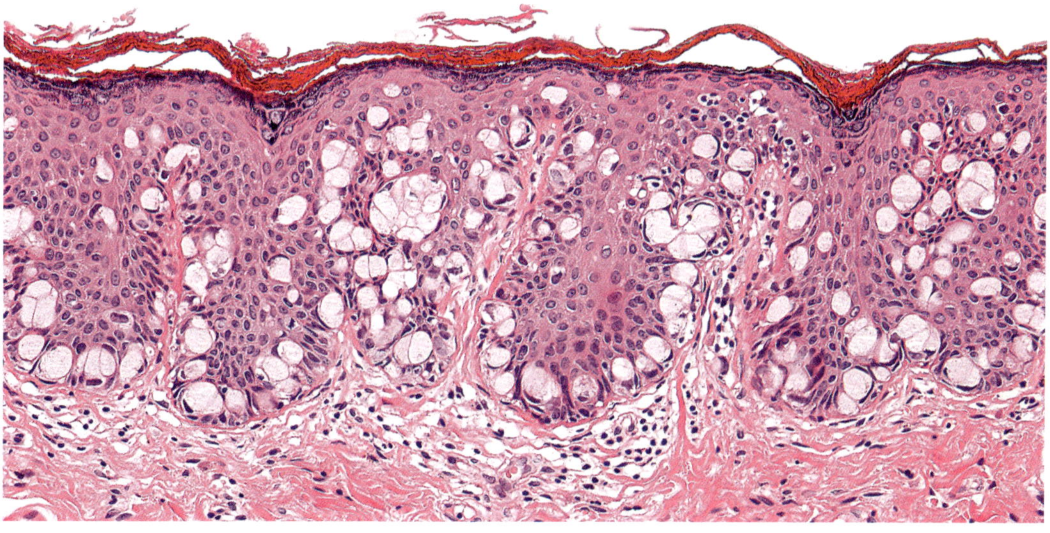

Fig. 9.14 Extrammamary Paget disease. In this example, the neoplastic cells have a signet-ring appearance due to large intracytoplasmic mucin droplets dislodging the nucleus eccentrically

elements. Cytological variations include cells with a signet-ring appearance (due to large intracytoplasmic mucin droplets displacing the nucleus eccentrically), cells with hyperchromatic nuclei, and multinucleated cells (Fig. 9.14).

The common approach nowadays is to classify EMPD into in situ and invasive. In the former, malignant cells are confined to the epidermis. When invasion into the dermis occurs, cases are designated as *invasive* or *microinvasive* carcinomas, the

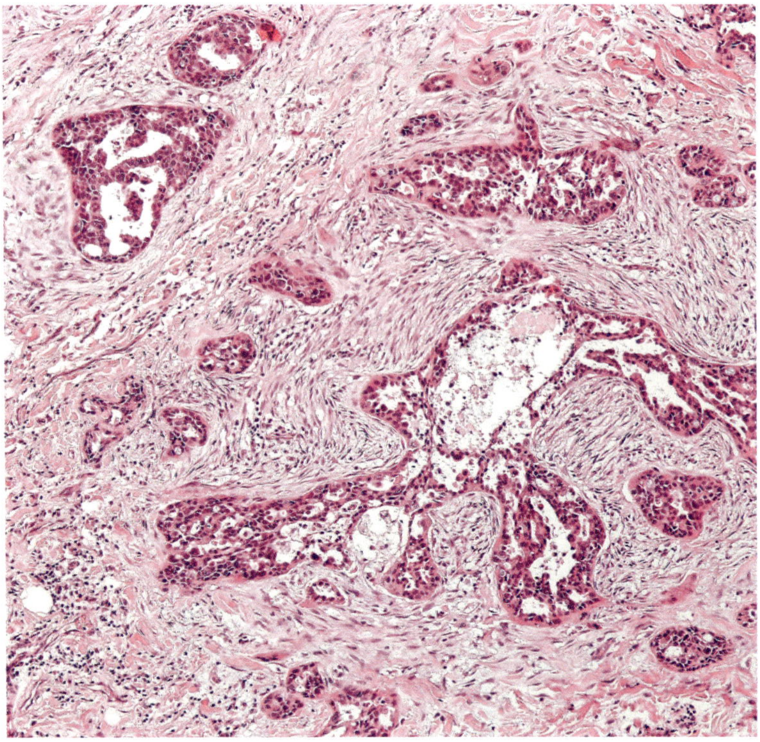

Fig. 9.15 Extrammamary Paget disease with invasive carcinoma corresponding to invasive ductal carcinoma as defined in mammary pathology

latter defined as stromal invasion to a depth of no more than 1.0 mm below the basement membrane [47]. However, limitations of this approach are demonstrated by rare cases of EMPD in which there is *both* intraepidermal pagetoid spread and an underlying carcinoma of mammary type for which the term *carcinoma* in situ (DCIS) equates to *ductal carcinoma* in situ of mammary type, whereas *invasive carcinoma* corresponds to invasive ductal carcinoma of mammary type (Fig. 9.15). DCIS is suggested to originate in AGMLG. Apart from DCIS, other ductal changes (atypical ductal hyperplasia, infiltration by carcinoma cells) in AGMLG in EMPD have rarely been reported (Fig. 9.16).

A common feature in EMPD is involvement of adnexal, especially eccrine, glands and hair follicles (Fig. 9.17). Some cases of EMPD are associated with various proliferative epidermal lesions [48–50]. Rare proliferative lesions may have abundant stromal plasma cells and papillary architecture occasioning a resemblance to syringocystadenocarcinoma papilliferum and should not be misinterpreted as such (Fig. 9.18). Epidermal acantholysis may occasionally be encountered [39]. Rarely, abundant melanin can be recognized within the cytoplasm of Paget cells [51]. The pigmentation may be clinically evident (pigmented form). In addition to phagocytosis of melanin by carcinoma cells, proliferation of heavily pigmented dendritic melanocytes between carcinoma cells can also contribute to the occurrence of pigmented lesions (Fig. 9.19).

Rarely, EMPD has been described to coexist with other lesions including melanoma [52], vulvar intraepithelial neoplasia [53, 54], invasive squamous cell carcinoma [48], basal cell carcinoma [55], condyloma acuminatum [56], and hidradenoma papilliferum [18, 19]. An association with an underlying mammary-type carcinoma is a rare event (<5%). The carcinomas are identical to those seen in the breast, and the presumption is that at least some may originate in AGMLG. The majority of the carcinomas have features of ductal carcinoma, mostly invasive [57–61].

Histochemically, Paget cells usually stain positively with mucicarmine, alcian blue, and PAS after diastase digestion (Fig. 9.20). Immunohistochemically, the neoplastic cells in primary EMPD consistently react with CK7 and

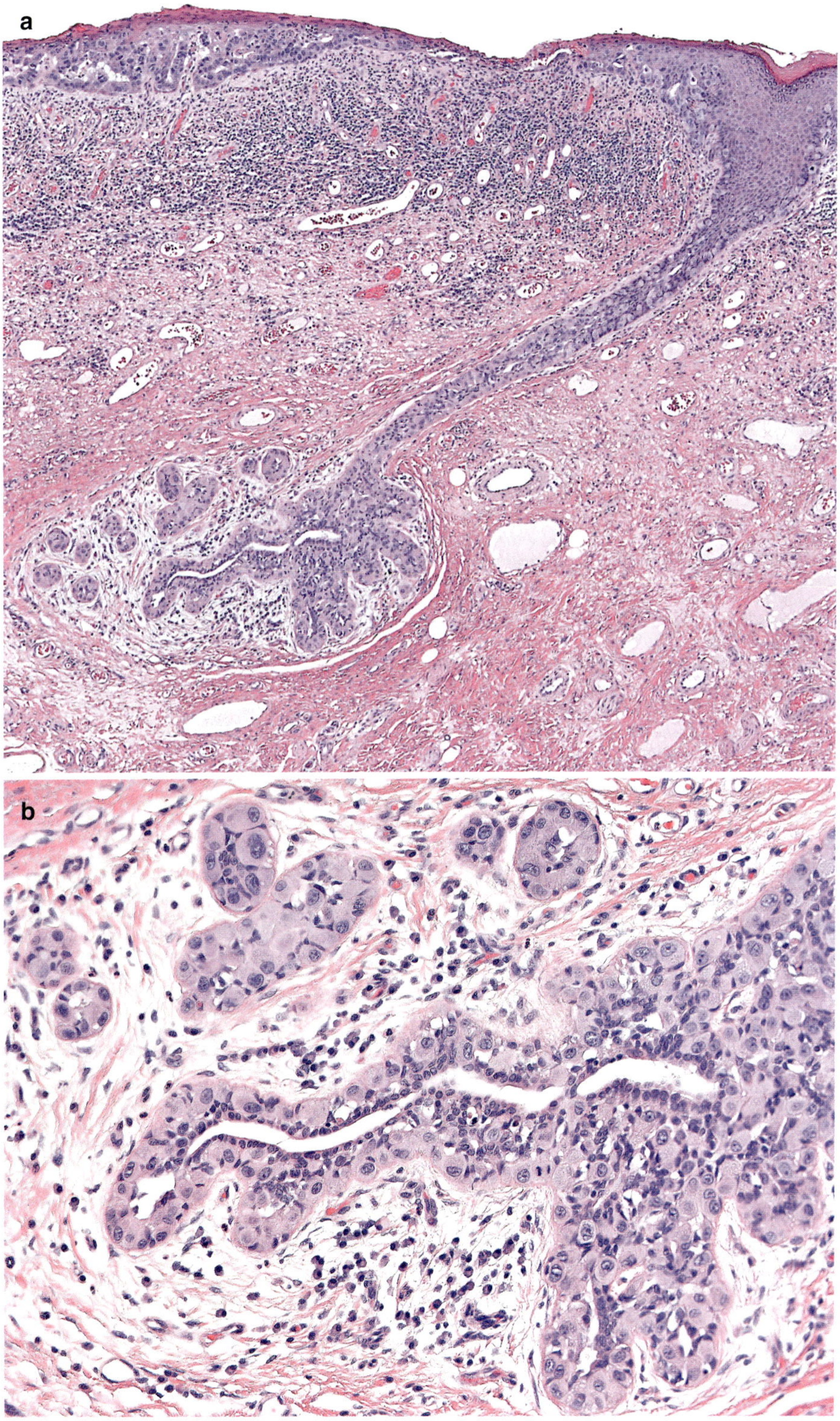

Fig. 9.16 Extrammamary Paget disease. Neoplastic cells infiltrate both the secretory portion (**a**) and the excretory duct (**b**) of anogenital mammary-like gland

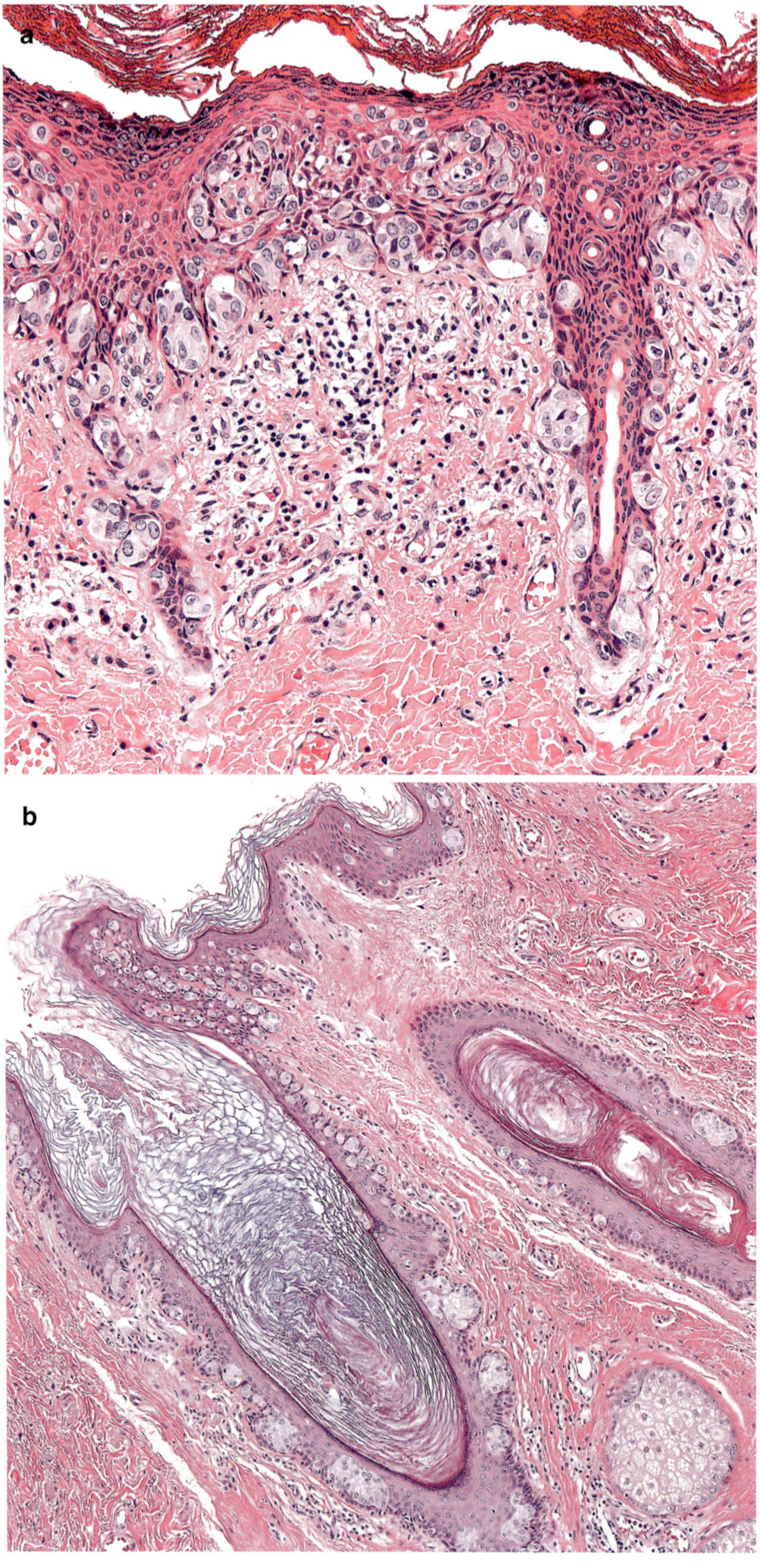

Fig. 9.17 Extrammamary Paget disease. Cutaneous adnexa are involved in majority of cases, especially eccrine ducts (**a**) and pilosebaceous units (**b**)

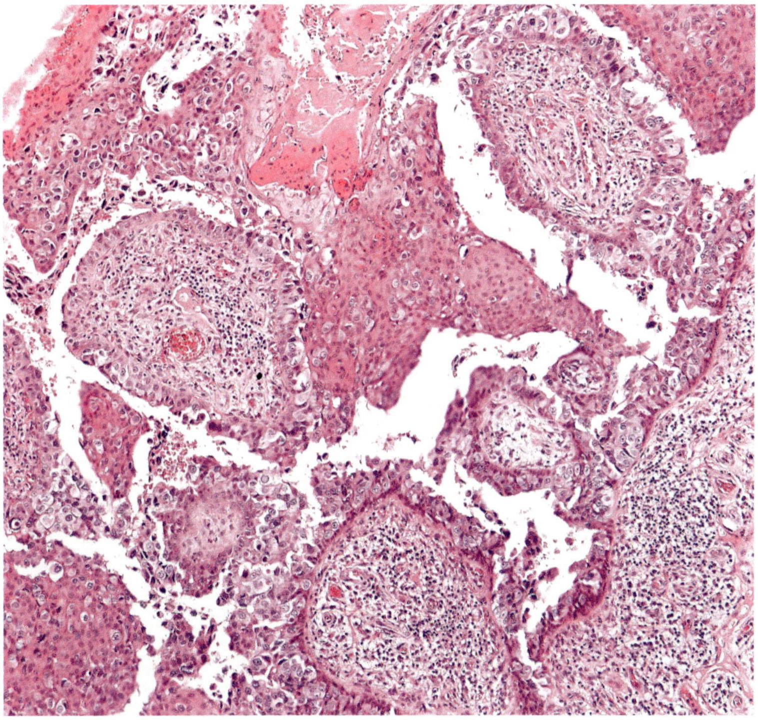

Fig. 9.18 Extrammamary Paget disease with a resemblance to syringocystadenocarcinoma papilliferum

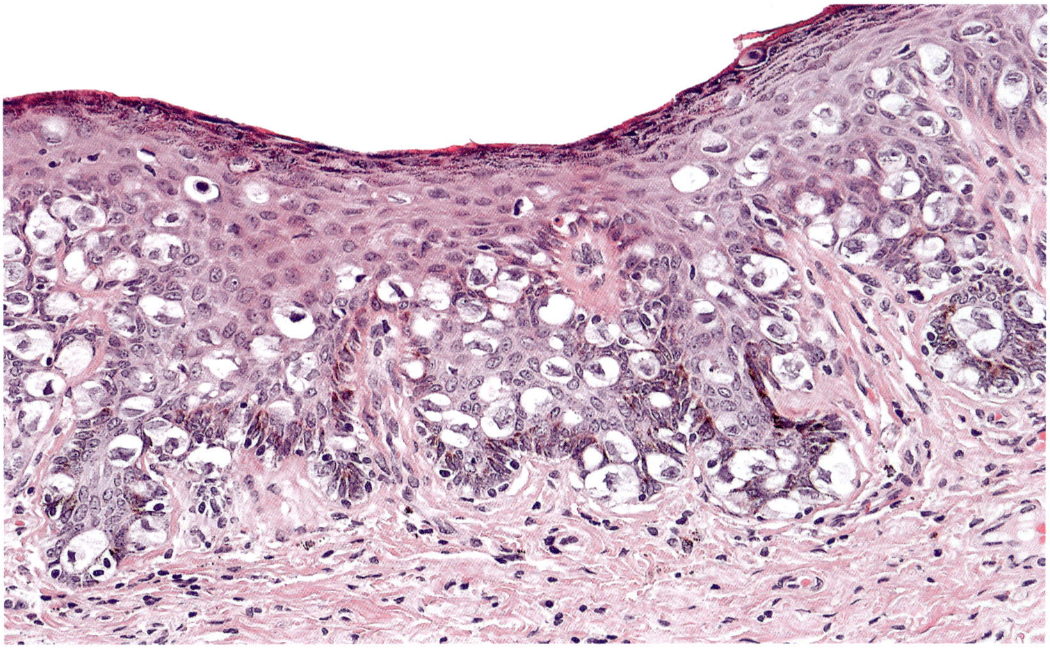

Fig. 9.19 Pigmented extrammamary Paget disease due to abundant melanin

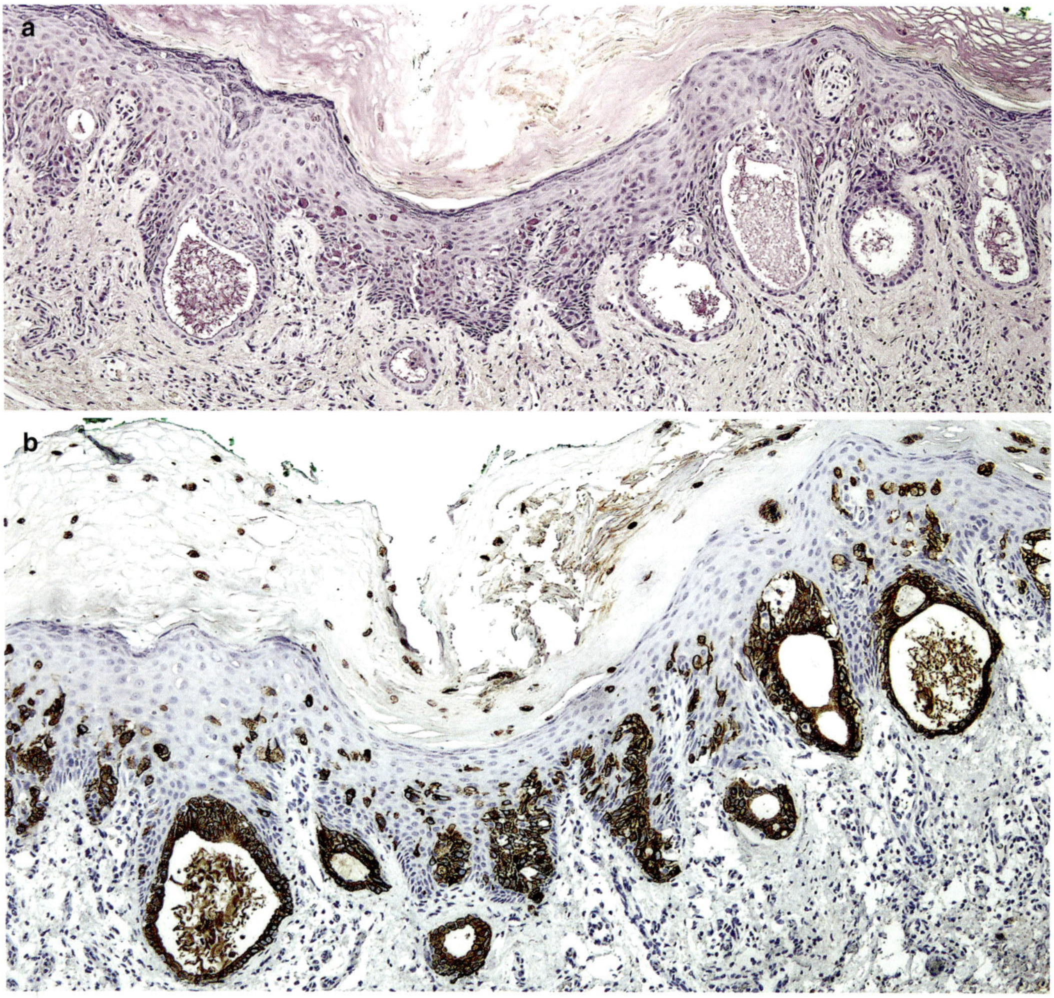

Fig. 9.20 Extrammamary Paget disease. Staining for mucicarmine (**a**) and CK7 (**b**)

often express CEA and GCDFP-15 (Fig. 9.20). Co-expression of CK20 and CDX2 by the Paget cells is indicative of secondary EMPD of colorectal origin [62, 63]. CDX2 is especially useful in the rare cases of CK20-negative and CK7-positive colorectal carcinomas causing secondary EMPD [64]. Uroplakin-III expression helps establish urothelial carcinoma as the cause of EMPD [65]. The combination of prostate-specific antigen (PSA) and prostate-specific acid phosphatase (PSAP) positivity is strongly indicative of an underlying prostatic carcinoma; however, expression of PSA has been documented in primary EMPD in males without any evidence of an underlying prostate carcinoma [66].

Apart from differentiation between primary and secondary EMPD and establishing its origin, the differential diagnostic considerations include vulvar Toker cells [36, 67], mucinous metaplasia of the vulval squamous epithelium [68–70], and VIN (especially if exhibiting a pagetoid pattern of involvement, CK7 positivity, and mucinous differentiation) [71–75]. Other major differential diagnoses include melanoma, lymphoma, pagetoid dyskeratosis [76–78], and cytopathic HPV changes. A further condition to be considered in the differential is clear cell

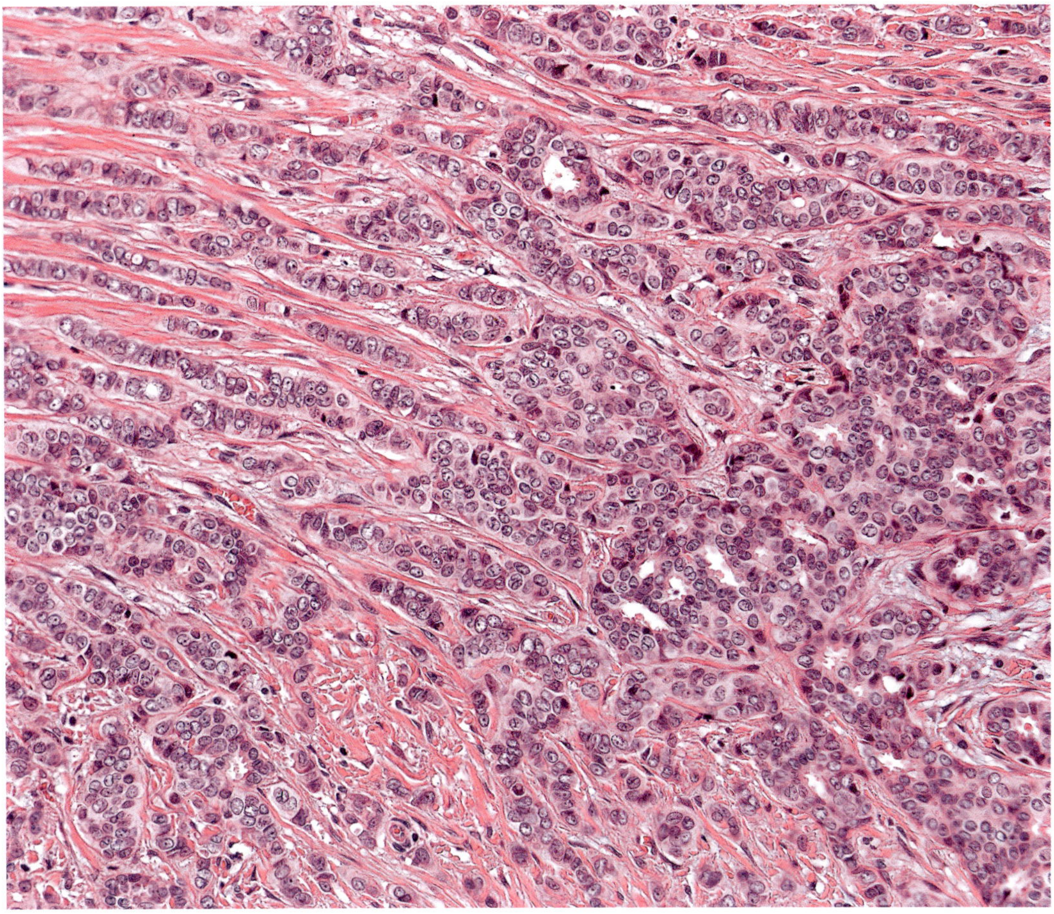

Fig. 9.21 Mammary-type tubulolobular carcinoma of the anogenital area. The neoplasm is composed of single-cell cords of neoplastic cells resembling an invasive lobular carcinoma but also tubular structures, with both components staining positive for E-cadherin

papulosis which is a rare condition, so far reported predominantly in Asians. This affects the pubic area, lower abdomen, and anterior trunk, manifesting clinically as multiple hypopigmented macules and histopathologically as round cells having ample clear cytoplasm and pale, sometimes grooved, nuclei, distributed among the basal keratinocytes [79–86].

Other Carcinomas of Anogenital Mammary-Like Glands

AGMLG have been suggested as a likely origin for some of carcinomas (other than EMPD) in the anogenital area based on their marked similarity to homologous carcinomas of the breast and the finding of AGMLG adjacent to the carcinomas, sometimes with transition between the benign residuum and the carcinoma [87, 88]. As a group, primary mammary-type carcinomas arising from AGMLG seem to be locally aggressive neoplasms associated with frequent lymph node metastases in approximately 60% of cases [87]. The most common variant is mammary-type ductal carcinoma [57, 58, 60, 87, 89–91]. Convincing examples of mammary-type lobular carcinoma are yet to be reported [92–94]. Extremely rare are carcinomas with mixed ductal and lobular features and tubulolobular carcinoma (Fig. 9.21) [95, 96]. Origin in AGMLG has been suggested for few mucinous carcinomas reported in the vulva

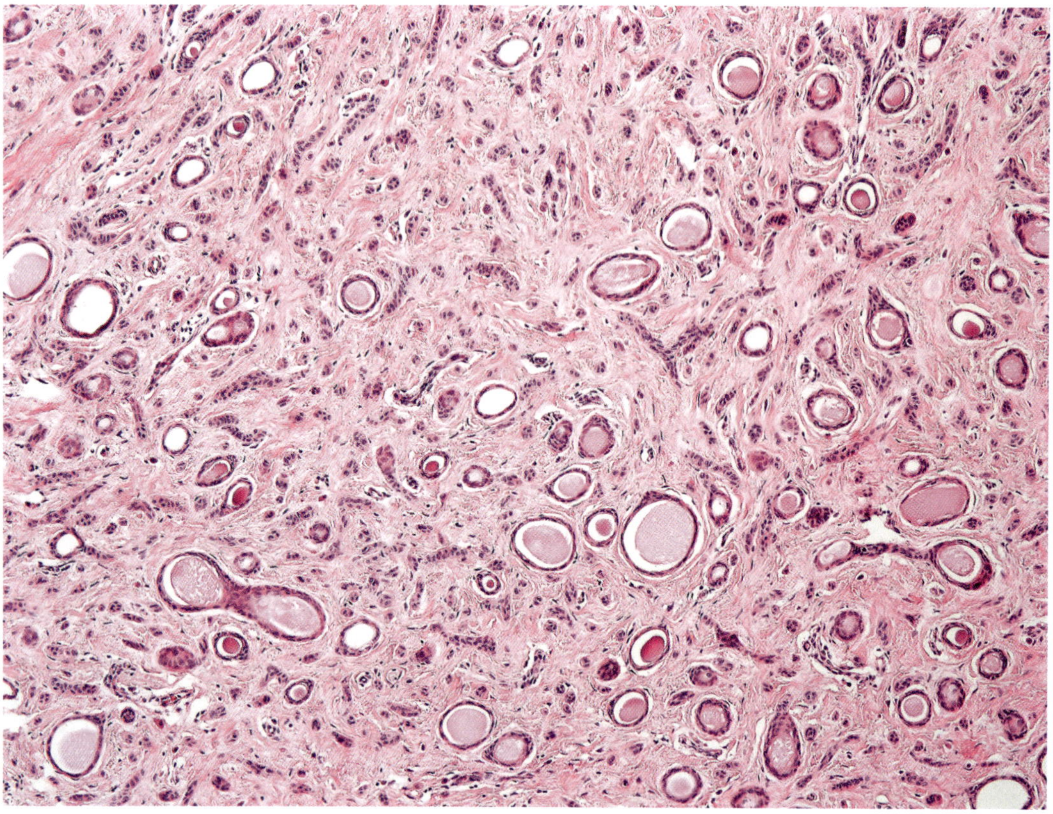

Fig. 9.22 Syringoma. The tumor is composed of small solid and ductal structures often having peculiar geometric shapes including "comma-like" or "tadpole-like" elements relatively evenly distributed in a sclerotic collagenous stroma

[97, 98] and for a rare distinctive carcinoma resembling adenoid cystic carcinoma [99].

Other Benign Lesions of Anogenital Mammary-Like Glands

Rare benign lesions of AGMLG include lactating adenoma [100, 101], so-called adenosis tumor (sclerosing adenosis associated with other patterns identical to those seen in benign breast disease) [7], and some poorly classified proliferations [3, 102].

Other Adnexal Neoplasms Occurring in the Vulva

Practically, any cutaneous adnexal neoplasm can occur in the vulva, but in general occurrence of adnexal tumors in this anatomic site is rare. Perhaps, the only exception is vulvar syringoma for which the vulva is not an uncommon site. The neoplasm occurs as numerous, small (1–4 mm), smooth-surfaced, skin-colored, or pink papules. The lesions are often associated with pruritus [103]. Increase in size in summer or during menstruation has been observed. Histopathologically, syringoma is usually a small, well-circumscribed neoplasm confined to the upper part of the dermis, composed of small solid and ductal structures often having peculiar geometric shapes ("comma-like" or "tadpole-like") relatively evenly distributed in a sclerotic collagenous stroma (Fig. 9.22). A distinct variant is clear cell syringoma, which results from glycogen accumulation is occasionally seen in the vulva. Extension into the deeper dermis or subcutis requires distinction from microcystic adnexal carcinoma [104].

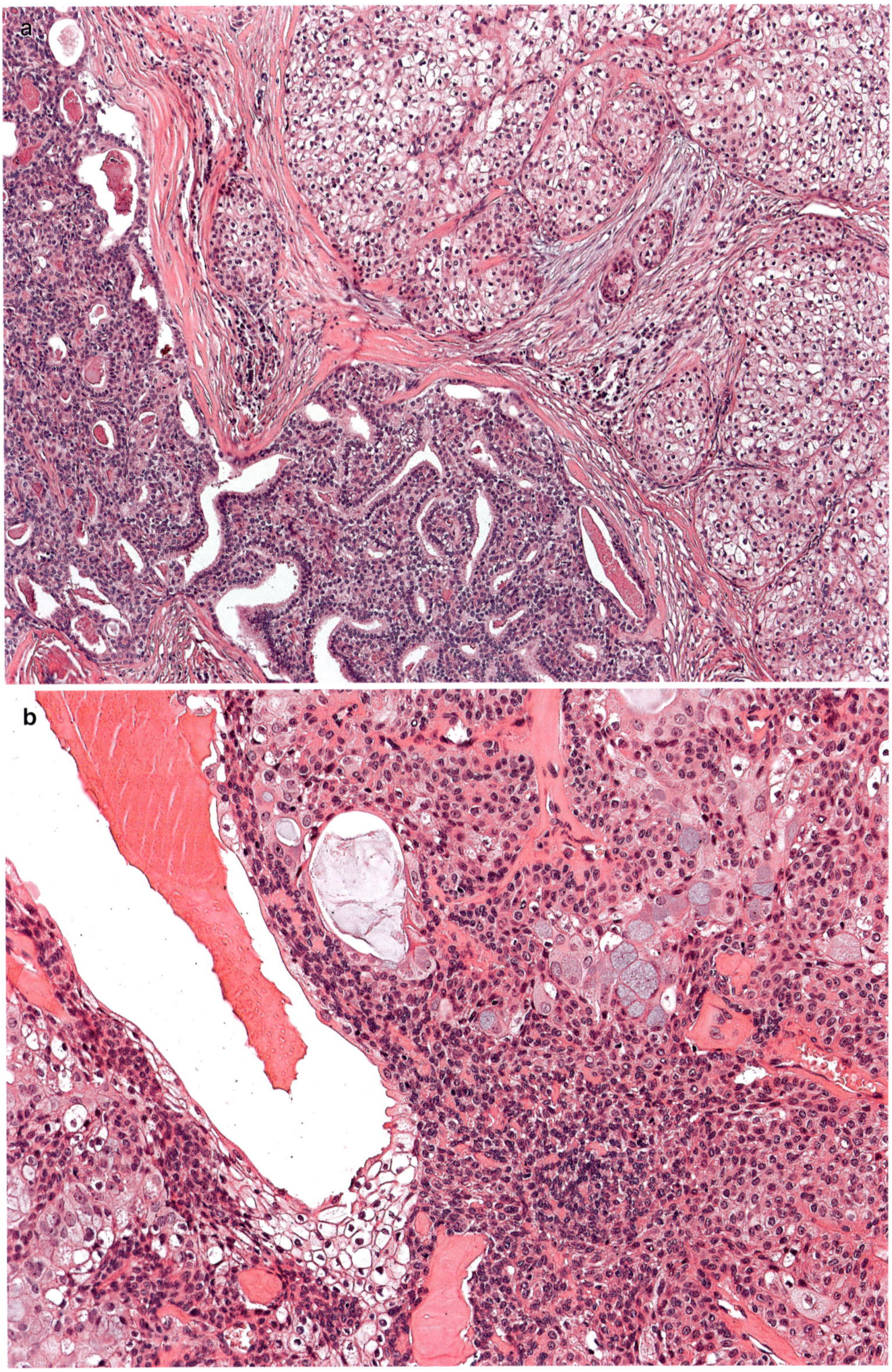

Fig. 9.23 Hidradenoma. This neoplasm is rare in the vulva. There are glandular structures and solid areas composed of clear cells (**a**), polyhedral eosinophilic cells, mucinous cells, and transitional elements (**b**)

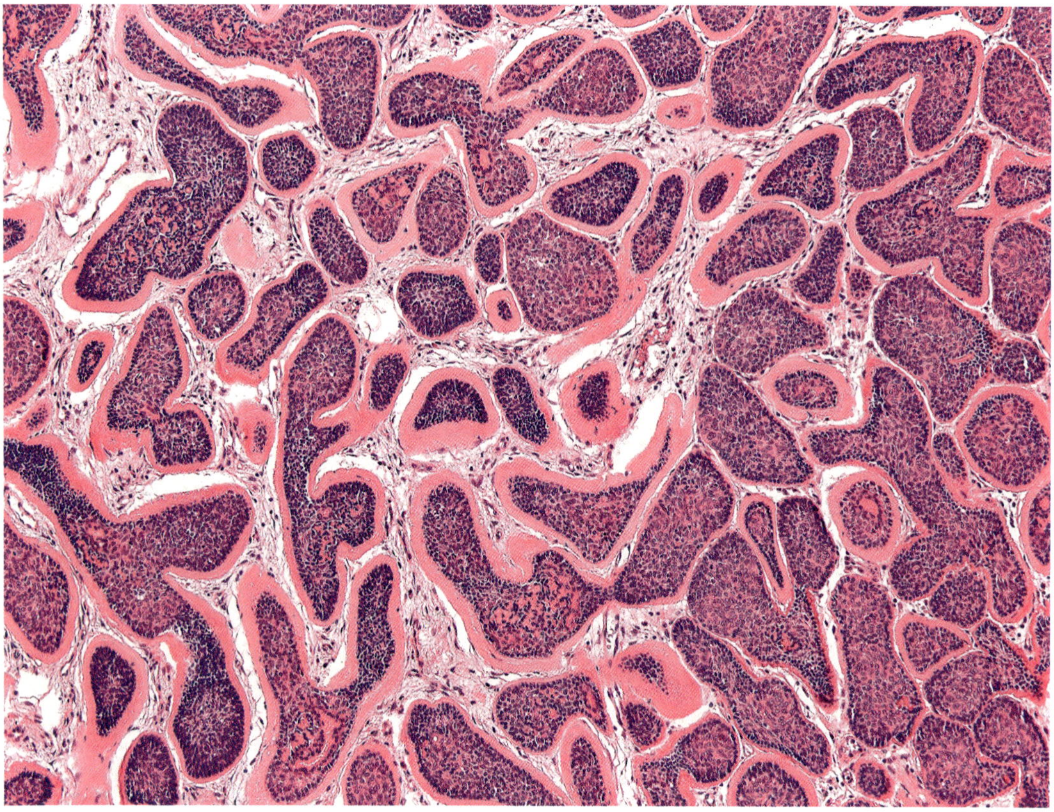

Fig. 9.24 Cylindroma. This neoplasm is also rare in the vulva compared to other anatomic sites, but the vulva may be involved by multiple tumors in Brooke-Spiegler syndrome. The neoplasm is composed of nodules of basaloid cells surrounded by eosinophilic basement membrane material. A typical feature is the so-called jigsaw puzzle arrangement of the neoplastic cell nodules and absence of intratumoral lymphocytes

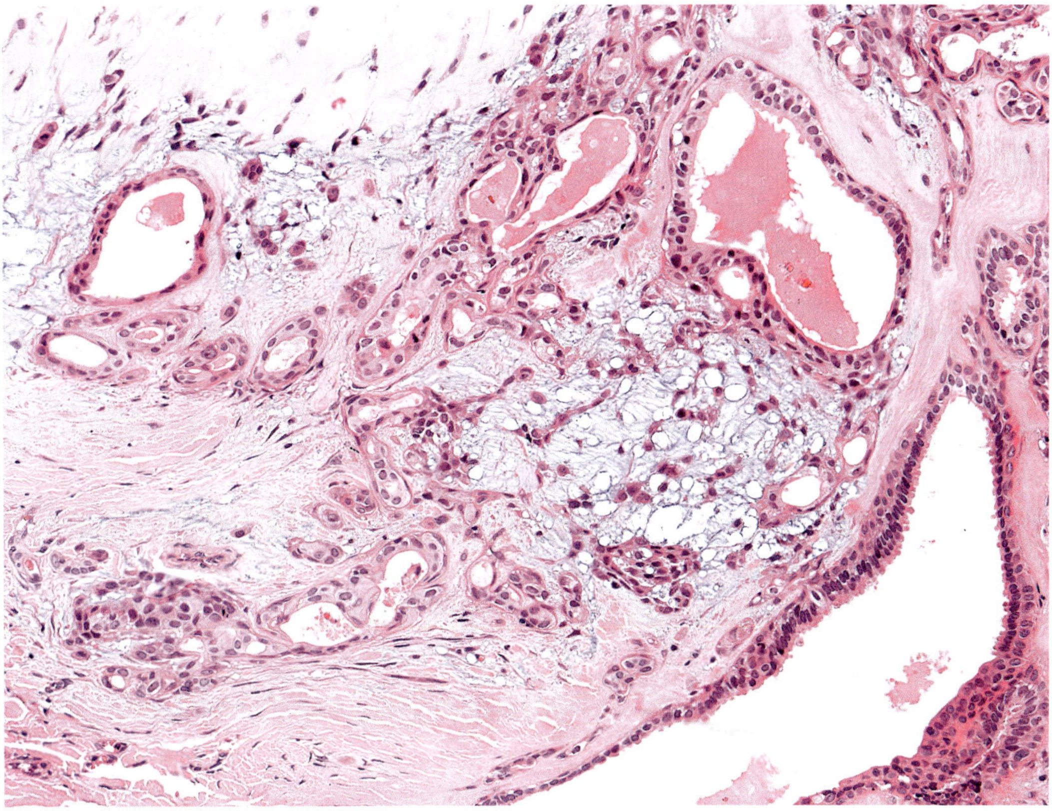

Fig. 9.25 Apocrine mixed tumor (chondroid syringoma). Note glandular elements with apocrine secretion and myxohyaline stroma

The histopathological features of all adnexal neoplasms are identical to those seen elsewhere in the skin (Figs. 9.23, 9.24, and 9.25); therefore the reader is referred to other sources. [105–120].

References

1. van der Putte SC. Anogenital "sweat" glands. Histology and pathology of a gland that may mimic mammary glands. Am J Dermatopathol. 1991;13:557–67.
2. van der Putte SC. Mammary-like glands of the vulva and their disorders. Int J Gynecol Pathol. 1994;13:150–60.
3. Kinkor Z, Michal M. Anogenital mammary type sclerosing adenosis – two case reports and the review of literature. Ceska Gynekol. 2004;69:292–7.
4. Kazakov DV, Mikyskova I, Kutzner H, et al. Hidradenoma papilliferum with oxyphilic metaplasia: a clinicopathological study of 18 cases, including detection of human papillomavirus. Am J Dermatopathol. 2005;27:102–10.
5. Higgins CM, Strutton GM. Papillary apocrine fibroadenoma of the vulva. J Cutan Pathol. 1997;24:256–60.
6. Vella JE, Taibjee SM, Sanders DS, et al. Fibroadenoma of the anogenital region. J Clin Pathol. 2008;61: 871–2.
7. Kazakov DV, Bisceglia M, Sima R, et al. Adenosis tumor of anogenital mammary-like glands: a case report and demonstration of clonality by HUMARA assay. J Cutan Pathol. 2006;33:43–6.
8. Meeker JH, Neubecker RD, Helwig EB. Hidradenoma papilliferum. Am J Clin Pathol. 1962;37:182–95.
9. Scurry J, van der Putte SC, Pyman J, et al. Mammary-like gland adenoma of the vulva: review of 46 cases. Pathology. 2009;41:372–8.
10. Netland PA, Townsend DJ, Albert DM, et al. Hidradenoma papilliferum of the upper eyelid arising from the apocrine gland of Moll. Ophthalmology. 1990;97:1593–8.

11. Nissim F, Czernobilsky B, Ostfeld E. Hidradenoma papilliferum of the external auditory canal. J Laryngol Otol. 1981;95:843–8.
12. Santa Cruz DJ, Prioleau PG, Smith ME. Hidradenoma papilliferum of the eyelid. Arch Dermatol. 1981;117: 55–6.
13. Cooper PH. Mitotic figures in sweat gland adenomas. J Cutan Pathol. 1987;14:10–4.
14. Sington J, Chandrapala R, Manek S, et al. Mitotic count is not predictive of clinical behavior in hidradenoma papilliferum of the vulva: a clinicopathologic study of 19 cases. Am J Dermatopathol. 2006;28:322–6.
15. Mazoujian G, Margolis R. Immunohistochemistry of gross cystic disease fluid protein (GCDFP-15) in 65 benign sweat gland tumors of the skin. Am J Dermatopathol. 1988;10:28–35.
16. Plumb SJ, Argenyi ZB, Stone MS, et al. Cytokeratin 5/6 immunostaining in cutaneous adnexal neoplasms and metastatic adenocarcinoma. Am J Dermatopathol. 2004;26:447–51.
17. Swanson PE, Mazoujian G, Mills SE, et al. Immunoreactivity for estrogen receptor protein in sweat gland tumors. Am J Surg Pathol. 1991;15:835–41.
18. Stefanato CM, Finn R, Bhawan J. Extramammary Paget disease with underlying hidradenoma papilliferum: guilt by association? Am J Dermatopathol. 2000;22:439–42.
19. Simpson WA, Burke M, Frappell J, et al. Paget's disease, melanocytic neoplasia and hidradenoma papilliferum of the vulva. Histopathology. 1988;12:675–9.
20. Castro CY, Deavers M. Ductal carcinoma in-situ arising in mammary-like glands of the vulva. Int J Gynecol Pathol. 2001;20:277–83.
21. Shah SS, Adelson M, Mazur MT. Adenocarcinoma in situ arising in vulvar papillary hidradenoma: report of 2 cases. Int J Gynecol Pathol. 2008;27:453–6.
22. Vazmitel M, Spagnolo DV, Nemcova J, et al. Hidradenoma papilliferum with a ductal carcinoma in situ component: case report and review of the literature. Am J Dermatopathol. 2008;30:392–4.
23. Donati P, Amantea A. Adenoma of anogenital mammary-like glands. Am J Dermatopathol. 1996;18: 73–6.
24. Carter JE, Mizell KN, Tucker JA. Mammary-type fibroepithelial neoplasms of the vulva: a case report and review of the literature. J Cutan Pathol. 2008;35: 246–9.
25. Kazakov DV, Spagnolo DV, Stewart CJ, et al. Fibroadenoma and phyllodes tumors of anogenital mammary-like glands: a series of 13 neoplasms in 12 cases, including mammary-type juvenile fibroadenoma, fibroadenoma with lactation changes, and neurofibromatosis-associated pseudoangiomatous stromal hyperplasia with multinucleated giant cells. Am J Surg Pathol. 2010;34:95–103.
26. Assor D, Davis JB. Multiple apocrine fibroadenomas of the anal skin. Am J Clin Pathol. 1977;68:397–9.
27. Hassim AM. Bilateral fibroadenoma in supernumerary breasts of the vulva. J Obstet Gynaecol Br Commonw. 1969;76:275–7.
28. Tbakhi A, Cowan DF, Kumar D, et al. Recurring phyllodes tumor in aberrant breast tissue of the vulva. Am J Surg Pathol. 1993;17:946–50.
29. Burger RA, Marcuse PM. Fibroadenoma of vulva. Am J Clin Pathol. 1954;24:965–80.
30. Kazakov DV, Bisceglia M, Mukensnabl P, et al. Pseudoangiomatous stromal hyperplasia in lesions involving anogenital mammary-like glands. Am J Surg Pathol. 2005;29:1243–6.
31. Sington JD, Manek S, Hollowood K. Fibroadenoma of the mammary-like glands of the vulva. Histopathology. 2002;41:563–5.
32. Chulia MT, Paya A, Niveiro M, et al. Phyllodes tumor in ectopic breast tissue of the vulva. Int J Surg Pathol. 2001;9:81–3.
33. Giger OT, Lacoste E, Honegger C, et al. Expression of the breast differentiation antigen NY-BR-1 in a phyllodes tumor of the vulva. Virchows Arch. 2007;450: 471–4.
34. Fu L, Lau S, Roy I, et al. Phyllodes tumor with malignant stromal morphology of the vulva: a case report and review of the literature. Int J Gynecol Pathol. 2011;30:198–202.
35. Vazmitel M, Pavlovsky M, Kacerovska D, et al. Pseudoangiomatous stromal hyperplasia in a complex neoplastic lesion involving anogenital mammary-like glands. J Cutan Pathol. 2009;36: 1117–20.
36. Willman JH, Golitz LE, Fitzpatrick JE. Vulvar clear cells of Toker: precursors of extramammary Paget's disease. Am J Dermatopathol. 2005;27:185–8.
37. Toker C. Clear cells of the nipple epidermis. Cancer. 1970;25:601–10.
38. Belousova IE, Kazakov DV, Michal M, et al. Vulvar Toker cells: the long-awaited missing link: a proposal for an origin-based histogenetic classification of extramammary Paget disease. Am J Dermatopathol. 2006;28:84–6.
39. Shaco-Levy R, Bean SM, Vollmer RT, et al. Paget disease of the vulva: a histologic study of 56 cases correlating pathologic features and disease course. Int J Gynecol Pathol. 2010;29:69–78.
40. Siesling S, Elferink MA, van Dijck JA, et al. Epidemiology and treatment of extramammary Paget disease in the Netherlands. Eur J Surg Oncol. 2007;33:951–5.
41. Chen YH, Wong TW, Lee JY. Depigmented genital extramammary Paget's disease: a possible histogenetic link to Toker's clear cells and clear cell papulosis. J Cutan Pathol. 2001;28:105–8.
42. Kakinuma H, Iwasawa U, Kurakata N, et al. A case of extramammary Paget's disease with depigmented macules as the sole manifestation. Br J Dermatol. 1994;130:102–5.
43. Duperrat B, Mascaro JM. Extra-mammary Paget's disease. Presse Med. 1965;73:1019–24.
44. Kawatsu T, Miki Y. Triple extramammary Paget's disease. Arch Dermatol. 1971;104:316–9.
45. Miyakawa T, Togawa Y, Matushima H, et al. Squamous metaplasia of Paget's disease. Clin Exp Dermatol. 2004;29:71–3.

46. Hilliard NJ, Huang C, Andea A. Pigmented extramammary Paget's disease of the axilla mimicking melanoma: case report and review of the literature. J Cutan Pathol. 2009;36:995–1000.
47. Feuer GA, Shevchuk M, Calanog A. Vulvar Paget's disease: the need to exclude an invasive lesion. Gynecol Oncol. 1990;38:81–9.
48. Brainard JA, Hart WR. Proliferative epidermal lesions associated with anogenital Paget's disease. Am J Surg Pathol. 2000;24:543–52.
49. Hurt MA, Hardarson S, Stadecker MJ, et al. Fibroepithelioma-like changes associated with anogenital epidermotropic mucinous carcinoma. Fibroepitheliomatous Paget phenomenon. J Cutan Pathol. 1992;19:134–41.
50. Ishida-Yamamoto A, Sato K, Wada T, et al. Fibroepithelioma-like changes occurring in perianal Paget's disease with rectal mucinous carcinoma: case report and review of 49 cases of extramammary Paget's disease. J Cutan Pathol. 2002;29:185–9.
51. Helwig EB, Graham JH. Anogenital (extramammary) Paget's disease. A clinicopathological study. Cancer. 1963;16:387–403.
52. Manabe T, Moriya T, Inagaki Y, et al. Malignant melanoma and extramammary Paget's disease in the same patient. Am J Dermatopathol. 1985;7(Suppl):29–34.
53. Hawley IC, Husain F, Pryse-Davies J. Extramammary Paget's disease of the vulva with dermal invasion and vulval intra-epithelial neoplasia. Histopathology. 1991;18:374–6.
54. Orlandi A, Piccione E, Sesti F, et al. Extramammary Paget's disease associated with intraepithelial neoplasia of the vulva. J Eur Acad Dermatol Venereol. 1999; 12:183–5.
55. Ishizawa T, Mitsuhashi Y, Sugiki H, et al. Basal cell carcinoma within vulvar Paget's disease. Dermatology. 1998;197:388–90.
56. Egawa K, Honda Y. Simultaneous human papillomavirus 6 (HPV 6) -positive condyloma acuminatum, HPV 31-positive Bowen's disease, and non HPV-associated extramammary Paget's disease coexisting within an area presenting clinically as condyloma acuminatum. Am J Dermatopathol. 2005;27:439–42.
57. Di Bonito L, Patriarca S, Falconieri G. Aggressive "breast-like" adenocarcinoma of vulva. Pathol Res Pract. 1992;188:211–4; discussion 214–6.
58. Kennedy DA, Hermina MS, Xanos ET, et al. Infiltrating ductal carcinoma of the vulva. Pathol Res Pract. 1997;193:723–6.
59. Piura B, Gemer O, Rabinovich A, et al. Primary breast carcinoma of the vulva: case report and review of literature. Eur J Gynaecol Oncol. 2002;23:21–4.
60. van der Putte SC, van Gorp LH. Adenocarcinoma of the mammary-like glands of the vulva: a concept unifying sweat gland carcinoma of the vulva, carcinoma of supernumerary mammary glands and extramammary Paget's disease. J Cutan Pathol. 1994;21:157–63.
61. Irvin WP, Cathro HP, Grosh WW, et al. Primary breast carcinoma of the vulva: a case report and literature review. Gynecol Oncol. 1999;73:155–9.
62. De Nisi MC, D'Amuri A, Toscano M, et al. Usefulness of CDX2 in the diagnosis of extramammary Paget disease associated with malignancies of intestinal type. Br J Dermatol. 2005;153:677–9.
63. Ohnishi T, Watanabe S. The use of cytokeratins 7 and 20 in the diagnosis of primary and secondary extramammary Paget's disease. Br J Dermatol. 2000;142: 243–7.
64. Zhang PJ, Shah M, Spiegel GW, et al. Cytokeratin 7 immunoreactivity in rectal adenocarcinomas. Appl Immunohistochem Mol Morphol. 2003;11:306–10.
65. Brown HM, Wilkinson EJ. Uroplakin-III to distinguish primary vulvar Paget disease from Paget disease secondary to urothelial carcinoma. Hum Pathol. 2002;33:545–8.
66. Inoguchi N, Matsumura Y, Kanazawa N, et al. Expression of prostate-specific antigen and androgen receptor in extramammary Paget's disease and carcinoma. Clin Exp Dermatol. 2007;32:91–4.
67. van der Putte SC. Clear cells of Toker in the developing anogenital region of male and female fetuses. Am J Dermatopathol. 2011;33:811–8.
68. Coghill SB, Tyler X, Shaxted EJ. Benign mucinous metaplasia of the vulva. Histopathology. 1990;17: 373–5.
69. Thomson MA, Carr RA, Ganesan R, et al. Extensive mucinous metaplasia of the vulva arising within Zoon's vulvitis. Br J Dermatol. 2007;156:750–2.
70. Val-Bernal JF, Hernandez-Nieto E. Benign mucinous metaplasia of the penis. A lesion resembling extramammary Paget's disease. J Cutan Pathol. 2000;27:76–9.
71. Armes JE, Lourie R, Bowlay G, et al. Pagetoid squamous cell carcinoma in situ of the vulva: comparison with extramammary Paget disease and nonpagetoid squamous cell neoplasia. Int J Gynecol Pathol. 2008;27:118–24.
72. Raju RR, Goldblum JR, Hart WR. Pagetoid squamous cell carcinoma in situ (pagetoid Bowen's disease) of the external genitalia. Int J Gynecol Pathol. 2003;22: 127–35.
73. Williamson JD, Colome MI, Sahin A, et al. Pagetoid Bowen disease: a report of 2 cases that express cytokeratin 7. Arch Pathol Lab Med. 2000;124: 427–30.
74. Fulling KH, Strayer DS, Santa Cruz DJ. Adnexal metaplasia in carcinoma in situ of the skin. J Cutan Pathol. 1981;8:79–88.
75. McCluggage WG. Recent developments in vulvovaginal pathology. Histopathology. 2009;54:156–73.
76. Val-Bernal JF, Pinto J. Pagetoid dyskeratosis is a frequent incidental finding in hemorrhoidal disease. Arch Pathol Lab Med. 2001;125:1058–62.
77. Pique-Duran E, Palacios-Llopis S, Moreno-Ramis P, et al. Comparative study of pagetoid dyskeratosis between acrochordons and soft fibromas. Am J Dermatopathol. 2006;28:478–81.
78. Tschen JA, McGavran MH, Kettler AH. Pagetoid dyskeratosis: a selective keratinocytic response. J Am Acad Dermatol. 1988;19:891–4.

79. Benouni S, Kos L, Ruggeri SY, et al. Clear cell papulosis in Hispanic siblings. Arch Dermatol. 2007;143:358–60.
80. Gianotti R, Cambiaghi S, Locatelli A, et al. Clear cell papulosis (pagetoid papulosis) in a non-Asian patient. Dermatology. 2001;203:260–1.
81. Kim YC, Mehregan DA, Bang D. Clear cell papulosis: an immunohistochemical study to determine histogenesis. J Cutan Pathol. 2002;29:11–4.
82. Kumarasinghe SP, Chin GY, Kumarasinghe MP. Clear cell papulosis of the skin: a case report from Singapore. Arch Pathol Lab Med. 2004;128:e149–52.
83. Kuo TT, Chan HL, Hsueh S. Clear cell papulosis of the skin. A new entity with histogenetic implications for cutaneous Paget's disease. Am J Surg Pathol. 1987;11:827–34.
84. Kuo TT, Huang CL, Chan HL, et al. Clear cell papulosis: report of three cases of a newly recognized disease. J Am Acad Dermatol. 1995;33:230–3.
85. Lee JY, Chao SC. Clear cell papulosis of the skin. Br J Dermatol. 1998;138:678–83.
86. Mohanty SK, Arora R, Kakkar N, et al. Clear cell papulosis of the skin. Ann Diagn Pathol. 2002;6:385–8.
87. Abbott JJ, Ahmed I. Adenocarcinoma of mammary-like glands of the vulva: report of a case and review of the literature. Am J Dermatopathol. 2006;28:127–33.
88. Guerry RL, Pratt-Thomas HR. Carcinoma of supernumerary breast of vulva with bilateral mammary cancer. Cancer. 1976;38:2570–4.
89. Bailey CL, Sankey HZ, Donovan JT, et al. Primary breast cancer of the vulva. Gynecol Oncol. 1993;50:379–83.
90. Fracchioli S, Puopolo M, De La Longrais IA, et al. Primary "breast-like" cancer of the vulva: a case report and critical review of the literature. Int J Gynecol Cancer. 2006;16 Suppl 1:423–8.
91. Levin M, Pakarakas RM, Chang HA, et al. Primary breast carcinoma of the vulva: a case report and review of the literature. Gynecol Oncol. 1995;56:448–51.
92. Guercio E, Cesone P, Saracino A, et al. Adenocarcinoma occurring in an aberrant mammary gland located in the vulva. Minerva Ginecol. 1984;36:315–9.
93. Neumann I, Strauss HG, Buchmann J, et al. Ectopic lobular breast cancer of the vulva. Anticancer Res. 2000;20:4805–8.
94. Gull SE, Al-Rufaie HK. Paget's disease of the vulva with underlying in situ and invasive classical lobular breast carcinoma. J Obstet Gynaecol. 1999;19:320–1.
95. Kazakov DV, Belousova IE, Sima R, et al. Mammary type tubulolobular carcinoma of the anogenital area: report of a case of a unique tumor presumably originating in anogenital mammarylike glands. Am J Surg Pathol. 2006;30:1193–6.
96. Fernandez-Figueras MT, Michal M, Kazakov DV. Mammary-type tubulolobular carcinoma of anogenital mammary-like glands with prominent stromal elastosis. Am J Surg Pathol. 2010;34:1224–6.
97. Kazakov DV, Suster S, LeBoit PE, et al. Mucinous carcinoma of the skin, primary, and secondary: a clinicopathologic study of 63 cases with emphasis on the morphologic spectrum of primary cutaneous forms: homologies with mucinous lesions in the breast. Am J Surg Pathol. 2005;29:764–82.
98. Yin C, Chapman J, Tawfik O. Invasive mucinous (colloid) adenocarcinoma of ectopic breast tissue in the vulva: a case report. Breast J. 2003;9:113–5.
99. Kazakov DV, Spagnolo DV, Kacerovska D, et al. Lesions of anogenital mammary-like glands: an update. Adv Anat Pathol. 2011;18:1–28.
100. Gugliotta P, Fibbi ML, Fessia L, et al. Lactating supernumerary mammary gland tissue in the vulva. Appl Pathol. 1983;1:61–5.
101. O'Hara MF, Page DL. Adenomas of the breast and ectopic breast under lactational influences. Hum Pathol. 1985;16:707–12.
102. Kazakov DV, Hugel H, Vanecek T, et al. Unusual hyperplasia of anogenital mammary-like glands. Am J Dermatopathol. 2006;28:134–7.
103. Young Jr AW, Herman EW, Tovell HM. Syringoma of the vulva: incidence, diagnosis, and cause of pruritus. Obstet Gynecol. 1980;55:515–8.
104. Kazakov DV, Bouda Jr J, Kacerovska D, et al. Vulvar syringomas with deep extension: a potential histopathologic mimic of microcystic adnexal carcinoma. Int J Gynecol Pathol. 2011;30:92–4.
105. Carlson JW, McGlennen RC, Gomez R, et al. Sebaceous carcinoma of the vulva: a case report and review of the literature. Gynecol Oncol. 1996;60:489–91.
106. Kazakov DV, Zelger B, Rutten A, et al. Morphologic diversity of malignant neoplasms arising in preexisting spiradenoma, cylindroma, and spiradenocylindroma based on the study of 24 cases, sporadic or occurring in the setting of Brooke-Spiegler syndrome. Am J Surg Pathol. 2009;33:705–19.
107. Cruz-Jimenez PR, Abell MR. Cutaneous basal cell carcinoma of vulva. Cancer. 1975;36:1860–8.
108. Gibson GE, Ahmed I. Perianal and genital basal cell carcinoma: a clinicopathologic review of 51 cases. J Am Acad Dermatol. 2001;45:68–71.
109. Kazakov DV, Belousova IE, Bisceglia M, et al. Apocrine mixed tumor of the skin ("mixed tumor of the folliculosebaceous-apocrine complex"). Spectrum of differentiations and metaplastic changes in the epithelial, myoepithelial, and stromal components based on a histopathologic study of 244 cases. J Am Acad Dermatol. 2007;57:467–83.
110. Kazakov DV, Kacerovska D, Hantschke M, et al. Cutaneous mixed tumor, eccrine variant: a clinicopathologic and immunohistochemical study of 50 cases, with emphasis on unusual histopathologic features. Am J Dermatopathol. 2011;33:557–68.

111. Requena L, Kiryu H, Ackerman AB. Neoplasms with apocrine differentiation. Philadelphia: Lippincott-Raven; 1998.
112. Ackerman AB, Böer A. Histopathologic diagnosis of adnexal epithelial neoplasms. New York: Ardor Scribendi; 2008.
113. Ackerman AB, Nussen-Lee S, Aldrene Tan ML. Histopathologic diagnosis of neoplasms with sebaceous differentiation. New York: Ardor Scribendi; 2009.
114. Gilks CB, Clement PB, Wood WS. Trichoblastic fibroma. A clinicopathologic study of three cases. Am J Dermatopathol. 1989;11:397–402.
115. Malliah R, Gilhooly P, Lambert WC, et al. Sebaceous hyperplasia of the vulva: case report and review of the literature. J Low Genit Tract Dis. 2006; 10:55–7.
116. Calonje E, Brenn T, Lazar AJ, et al. McKee's pathology of the skin. Philadelphia: Elsevier; 2011.
117. Weedon D. Weedon's skin pathology. 3rd ed. London: Churchill Livingstone Elsevier; 2010.
118. LeBoit PE, Burg G, Weedon D, et al. World Health Organization classification of tumours. Pathology and genetics of skin tumours. Lyon: IARC Press; 2006.
119. Kazakov DV, Michal M, Kacerovska D, et al. Cutaneous adnexal tumors. Lippincott Williams and Wilkins; Philadelphia 2012.
120. Michal M, Miettinen M. Myoepitheliomas of the skin and soft tissues. Report of 12 cases. Virchows Arch. 1999;434:393–400.

Appendices

Laurence Brown and Asma Zaman Faruqi

Appendix A

Surgical Cut-up of Specimens

Laurence Brown

Essential Information on the Request Form

- Identifying patient details, history, and the results of past biopsies.
- Clear details of the surgical procedure. The site of biopsy is often not clear on the vulvectomy specimen and can be marked with a suture.
- An accompanying diagram of the site of operation/biopsy with orientation markings/sutures (Fig. A.1).
- Full identifying details of specimens from multiple sites.
- Specimen containers labeled to correspond to the specimen details on the request form.

Desirable Information on the Request Form

- The results of ultrasound, fine needle aspiration cytology, computerized tomography (CT), and magnetic resonance imaging (MRI) to identify nodal involvement
- Lymphangiography, including dye injections and scintillography for sentinel node assessment

L. Brown B.Sc., MBBS, FRCPath
Department of Histopathology, Leicester Royal Infirmary, Leicester, UK

A.Z. Faruqi MBBS, LMCK FRCPath
Department of Cellular Pathology, The Royal London and St. Bartholomew's Hospitals, London, UK

Usual Types of Specimens

- Radical vulvectomy and lymph node dissection (with or without sentinel node dissection)
- Partial vulvectomy and lymph node dissection (with or without sentinel node dissection)
- Radical vulvectomy
- Partial vulvectomy
- Wide local excision
- Diagnostic biopsy

It might be necessary to paint the excision margins with ink or dye prior to block taking in larger specimens. A photographic record and/or schematic graphic of the orientated vulval specimen (Fig. A.1) may be useful. It is easier to take

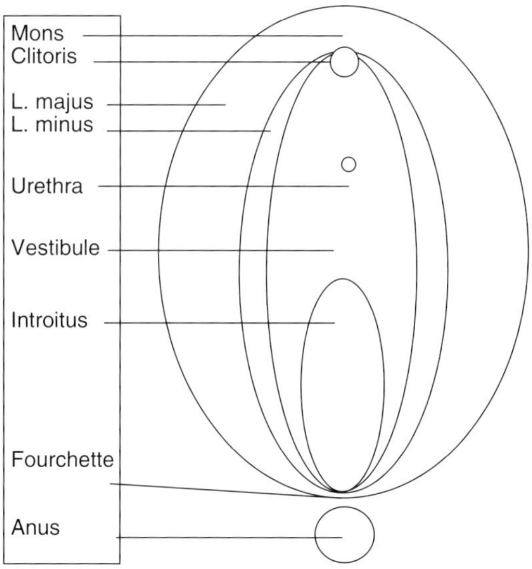

Fig. A.1 Diagram to assist the orientation of specimens and selected blocks (Modified from Brown and McCluggage [1]. With permission from the Royal College of Pathologists)

L. Brown (ed.), *Pathology of the Vulva and Vagina*, Essentials of Diagnostic Gynecological Pathology, DOI 10.1007/978-0-85729-757-0, © Springer-Verlag London 2013 blocks from pinned out, fixed specimens, but this is not essential. Identification of the lesion is made easier if the surgeons mark the site of previous biopsy with a suture or ink.

Block Taking

Take blocks to record the:

- Type and grade of the lesion.
- Measurement of tumor depth (or thickness, if ulcerated) and width.
- Distance to epithelial resection margin.
- Distance to urethral resection margin (if appropriate).
- Distance to vaginal resection margin (if appropriate).
- Distance to anal resection margin (if appropriate).
- Distance to soft tissue (deep) resection margin.
- Any grossly normal or abnormal epithelium to identify VIN, Paget's disease, and nonneoplastic epithelial diseases (NNED).
- Any incidental cysts or other abnormalities.
- The status of all lymph nodes from each side. Include macroscopic involvement of lymph nodes with the dimensions of involved nodes.
- Oversize blocks can give good overview of the tumor and resection margins but are not necessary if adequate measurements are given.
- For sentinel nodes:
  - Each lymph node must be examined histologically.
  - Only one block is necessary from any grossly involved node.
  - Resected lymph nodes not obviously involved by tumor must be examined in their entirety.
  - Larger nodes may require more than one block.
  - Nodes larger than 5 mm should be blocked out at 2–3-mm intervals cut perpendicular to the long axis.
  - Nodes smaller than 5 mm can be bisected or embedded whole.
  - Levels are only required for clarification of suspicious groups of cells.
  - The sentinel node is highly predictive for inguinofemoral node involvement with a negative predictive value of 95–100% [1]. Although step sectioning and immunohistochemistry have been performed in some studies, there is no evidence that ultrastaging is prognostically significant.
- Record the origin/designation of all tissue blocks on the pathology report. This facilitates review.

Excisional or Small Biopsies

- Sample-wide local excisions in a similar manner to vulvectomy specimens.
- The initial diagnosis of malignancy can be made by a small punch biopsy: bisect in vertical section if larger than 3 mm and the epithelium is clearly visible for orientation.
- A larger ellipse or oval specimen can be orientated by the surgeon with a stitch to allow identification of the margins: embed as received if narrower than 3 mm and cut longitudinally if wider.
- The biopsy site on the vulva must be identified to allow sampling of residual disease in any subsequent vulvectomy specimen.
- Take care not to damage the surface epithelium.
- Count fragments and embed as received.
- Measure larger pieces individually.

Cut wider or larger biopsies with an identifiable lesion in transverse section to include the nearest resection margins. Identify the margins with ink or nicks.

Frozen Sections

Frozen sections are rarely used for confirmation of malignancy or assessment of margins, particularly with Paget's disease, but this is not routine.

Reference

1. Brown L, McCluggage G, on behalf of the Royal College of Pathologists Working Group on Cancer Services. Standards and datasets for reporting cancers – Datasets for the histopathological reporting of vulval neoplasms. 3rd edn. 2010. At: http://www.rcpath.org/publications-media/publications/datasets/dataset-for-histological-reporting-of-vulval-neoplasms-3rd-edition.htm. January 30th 2012

Appendix B

Reporting proforma for vulval cancer resection specimens

Surname		Forenames	Date of birth...................	
Hospital		Hospital no	NHS/CHI no	
Date of receipt		Date of report	Report no	
Pathologist		Surgeon...................		
Nature of Vulvectomy Specimen				
Radical □		Simple □	Anterior □	Posterior □
Left hemi □		Left nodes □	Right hemi □	Right nodes □
3 parts with nodes □		Y excision with nodes □	Local excision □	
Other................				
Gross Description				
Size of specimen:		Length .... mm	Width .... mm	Thickness .... mm
Size of tumor:		Length .... mm	Width .... mm	Thickness .... mm
Site(s) of tumor (please state):				
No macroscopic residual tumor: □				
Histology				
Histological type:		Squamous (usual) □	Verrucous □	
		Adenocarcinoma □	Basal cell □	
		(For melanoma, use appropriate skin dataset)		
Other (please specify) □...				
Histological differentiation:		Well □	Moderate □	Poor □
Tumor size (for staging):		Maximum horizontal dimension .... mm		
		Thickness/depth of invasion....................... mm		
		(NB requires correlation of macro-/micromeasurements)		
Lymphovascular invasion:		Present □	Absent □	
Minimum Tumor-Free Margin				
Skin/epithelial.........mm		N/A □	Involved □ (position).........o'clock	
Urethral.................mm		N/A □	Involved □	
Vaginal ....mm		N/A □	Involved □	
Anal ....mm		N/A □	Involved □	
Soft tissue ....mm		N/A □	Involved □	
VIN 1 □	VIN 2 □	VIN 3 □	Differentiated VIN □	Paget's □
VIN or Paget's excised		Yes □	No □	

(continued)

Appendix B (continued)

Minimum Margin			
Skin/epithelial.........mm	N/A □	Involved □ (position).........o'clock	
Urethral.................mm	N/A □	Involved □	
Vaginal ....mm	N/A □	Involved □	
Anal ....mm	N/A □	Involved □	
Presence of nonneoplastic epithelial disease (NNED):		Yes □	No □
Lichen sclerosus □		Lichen planus □	
Squamous hyperplasia □		HPV-associated features □	
NNED excised:	Yes □	No □	
Groin Nodes			
Sentinel node, if sent – (right) positive □		Sentinel node, if sent – (left) positive □	
Total number of nodes (right)		Total number of nodes (left)	
Total number of positive nodes (right)		Total number of positive nodes (left)	
Extranodal extension:	Yes □	No □	
>5-mm metastasis	Yes □	No □	
Comments/Additional Information			
Provisional FIGO Stage.................. (May Change Following MDTM Discussion)			
SNOMED Codes: T...... M...........			
Signature.......................................		**Date....../......./......**	

Modified with permission from [1]

Reference

1. Royal College of Pathologists Standards and datasets for reporting cancers Datasets for the histopathological reporting of vulval neoplasms. 3rd edn. 2010 – partial revision. http://www.rcpath.org/publications-media/publications/datasets/dataset-for-histological-reporting-of-vulval-neoplasms-3rd-edition.htm. January 30th 2012

Appendix C

Staging of Vulval Carcinoma

Asma Zaman Faruqi

The two main staging systems for vulval carcinoma are the FIGO (International Federation of Gynecology and Obstetrics) system and the UICC/TNM (International Union Against Cancer) classification. The system used by the AJCC (American Joint Committee on Cancer) is based on the TNM classification.

Changes to the FIGO System

In 2008, the FIGO staging system for vulval carcinoma was revised after nearly a decade [1, 2]. The changes were made because it was felt that the previous FIGO system lacked predictive value. In the old system stage III was a heterogeneous group in which the survival rates ranged from 34% to 100% [3]. Furthermore, the number and morphology of positive lymph nodes were not taken into account. The collected data show that the size of nodal metastasis is of prognostic significance [4, 5]. In one study, the survival rate was 90% if the size of the nodal metastatic deposit was less than 5 mm and fell to 20.6% when nodal deposits exceeded 15 mm [6]. The presence of extracapsular spread further decreases the survival rate.

The GOG report [3] showed that when lymph node metastases were absent, even primary lesions up to 8 cm were of low risk. This is reflected in the new staging system; once the lesional size exceeds 2 cm and/or stromal invasion exceeds 1 mm in depth (i.e., stage II and above), size is no longer considered to be of prognostic significance if lymph nodes are negative.

Stage IA remains unchanged because there is a negligible risk of lymph node metastases. Stages IB and II are now combined, and the number and morphology of lymph node metastases have been incorporated in stage III. Tumor bilaterality is now discounted [7, 8].

TNM Classification

The latest TNM classification (TNM seventh edition) of vulval cancer has also been amended and is largely similar to FIGO staging apart from the T0 and Tis categories which are not included in the FIGO system. There is no T4 category, and a FIGO IVA or IVB is classified using the N and M categories [9].

FIGO Stage 1/T1 Tumors

The term "microinvasive" is not recommended; instead, the depth of the tumor should be measured in millimeters. The depth of invasion is measured from the point of deepest invasion to the adjacent most superficial epithelial–stromal junction. The tumor thickness is the distance between surface of the tumor or the base of the granular layer to the point of deepest invasion. It is useful to measure both depth of invasion and thickness especially when there is surface ulceration of the tumor; as in such a case, tumor thickness may underestimate the depth of invasion [7, 9, 10].

Vascular Invasion

Lymphovascular invasion is not included in either staging system. Nevertheless, it is important to mention the presence or absence of this feature in the pathology report as it may affect surgical procedure and the decision to perform lymphadenectomy.

FIGO 2008

STAGE I: *Confined to vulva, negative nodes*

IA: Tumor confined to the vulva or perineum, ≤2 cm in size with stromal invasion ≤1 mm, negative nodes.

IB: Tumor confined to the vulva or perineum, >2 cm in size or with stromal invasion >1 mm, negative nodes.

STAGE II: *Tumor of any size extending to adjacent structures*

II: Tumor of any size with adjacent spread (1/3 lower urethra, 1/3 lower vagina, anus), negative nodes.

Stage III: *Tumor of any size with or without extension to adjacent perineal structures but with positive nodes*

IIIA: Tumor of any size with positive inguinofemoral lymph nodes

(i) One lymph node metastasis greater than or equal to 5 mm

(ii) One to two lymph node metastasis (es) of less than 5 mm

IIIB:

(i) Two or more lymph node metastases greater than or equal to 5 mm

(ii) Three or more lymph node metastases less than 5 mm

IIIC: Positive node(s) with extracapsular spread.

Stage IV: *Invasion of other regional structures (upper 2/3 urethra or vagina or distant metastases)*

IVA:

(i) Tumor invades other regional structures (2/3 upper urethra, 2/3 upper vagina), bladder mucosa, rectal mucosa, or fixed to pelvic bone.

(ii) Fixed or ulcerated inguinofemoral lymph nodes.

IVB: Any distant metastasis including pelvic lymph nodes.

The depth of invasion is defined as the measurement of the tumor from the epithelial–stromal junction of the adjacent most superficial dermal papilla to the deepest point of invasion.

TNM/FIGO Categories

Primary Tumor (*T*)

- *TX*: Primary tumor cannot be assessed
- *T0*: No evidence of primary tumor
- *Tis*/0: Carcinoma in situ (preinvasive carcinoma, VIN III)
- *T1*/*I*: Tumor confined to the vulva or vulva and perineum, 2 cm or less in greatest dimension
  - *T1a*/*IA*: Tumor confined to the vulva or vulva and perineum, 2 cm or less in greatest dimension and with stromal invasion no greater than 1 mm
  - *T1b*/*IB*: Tumor confined to the vulva or vulva and perineum, 2 cm or less in greatest dimension and with stromal invasion greater than 1 mm
- *T2*/*II*: Tumor confined to the vulva or vulva and perineum, more than 2 cm in greatest dimension extending to adjacent perineal structures: lower third of urethra, lower third vagina, anus
- *T3*/*IVA*: Tumor of any size with extension to the upper 2/3 urethra, upper 2/3 vagina, or anus
- [*Note*: The depth of invasion is defined as the measurement of the tumor from the epithelial–stromal junction of the adjacent most superficial dermal papilla to the deepest point of invasion.]

Regional Lymph Nodes (*N*)

- *NX*: Regional lymph nodes cannot be assessed
- *N0*: No regional lymph node metastasis
- *N1a*/*IIIA*: One or two lymph nodes, less than 5 mm
- *N1b*/*IIIA*: One node equal to or more than 5 mm
- *N2a*/*IIIB*: Three or more nodes, less than 5 mm
- *N2b*/*IIIB*: Two or more nodes equal to more than 5 mm
- *N2c*/*IIIC*: Extracapsular spread
- *N3*/*IVA*: Fixed
- *M1*/*IVB*: Distant

Every effort should be made to determine the site and laterality of lymph node metastases. However, if "regional lymph node metastases, NOS" is the final diagnosis, then the patient should be staged as N1.

Distant Metastasis (*M*)

- *MX*: Distant metastasis cannot be assessed
- *M0*: No distant metastasis
- *M1*/*IVB*: Distant metastasis (including pelvic lymph node metastasis)

UICC Stage Groupings [9]

Stage 0: Tis, N0, M0
Stage I: T1, N0, M0
Stage IA: T1a, N0, M0
Stage IB: T1b, N0, M0
Stage II: T2, N0, M0
Stage IIIA: T1/T2, N1a/N1b, M0
Stage IIIB: T1/T2, N2a/N2b, M0
Stage IIIC: T1/T2, N2c, M0
Stage IVA: T1/T2, N3, M0 or T3, Any N, M0
Stage IVB: Any T, Any N, M1

References

1. Pecorelli S. Revised FIGO staging for carcinoma of the vulva, cervix, and endometrium. Int J Gynaecol Obstet. 2009;105(2):103–4. Erratum in: Int J Gynaecol Obstet. 2010;108(2):176.

2. Mutch D. The new FIGO staging system for cancers of the vulva, cervix endometrium and sarcomas. Gynecol Oncol. 2009;115 (3):325–8.
3. Homesley HD, Bundy BN, Sedlis A, Yordan E, Berek JS, Jahshan A, Mortel R. Assessment of current International Federation of Gynecology and Obstetrics staging of vulvar carcinoma relative to prognostic factors for survival (a Gynecologic Oncology Group study). Am J Obstet Gynecol. 1991;164(4):997–1003; discussion 1003–4.
4. Hacker NF, Berek JS, Lagasse LD, Leuchter RS, Moore JG. Management of regional lymph nodes and their prognostic influence in vulvar cancer. Obstet Gynecol. 1983;61(4):408–12.
5. Hoffman JS, Kumar NB, Morley GW. Prognostic significance of groin lymph node metastases in squamous carcinoma of the vulva. Obstet Gynecol. 1985;66(3):402–5.
6. Origoni M, Sideri M, Garsia S, Carinelli SG, Ferrari AG. Prognostic value of pathological patterns of lymph node positivity in squamous cell carcinoma of the vulva stage III and IVA FIGO. Gynecol Oncol. 1992;45(3):313–6.
7. Hacker NF. Revised FIGO staging for carcinoma of the vulva. Int J Gynaecol Obstet. 2009;105(2):105–6.
8. van der Steen S, de Nieuwenh of HP, Massuger L, Bulten J, de Hullu JA. New FIGO staging system of vulvar cancer indeed provides a better reflection of prognosis. Gynecol Oncol. 2010;119(3):520–5.
9. Sobin L, Gospodarwicz MK, Wittekind Ch. TNM classification of malignant tumors. New York: Wiley-Blackwell; 2009.
10. Wilkenson EJ. Premalignant and malignant tumours of the vulva. [book auth.] Ellenson LH, Ronnett BM Kurman RJ. Blaustein's pathology of the female genital tract. 6th edn. New York: Springer; 2011.

Index

L. Brown (ed.), *Pathology of the Vulva and Vagina*, Essentials of Diagnostic Gynecological Pathology,
DOI 10.1007/978-0-85729-757-0, © Springer-Verlag London 2013